P9-CJD-174

Handbook of Experimental Pharmacology

Volume 112

Conjugation–Deconjugation Reactions in Drug Metabolism and Toxicity

Contributors

K.W. Bock, B. Burchell, M. Chiba, D.J. Clarke, C.R. Creveling
C. Fenselau, F.C. Kauffman, G.Y. Kwei, S.S. Lau, W. Lilienblum
A.Y.H. Lu, J.A. Miller, T.J. Monks, E.K. Novak, D. Otterness
K.S. Pang, C.B. Pickett, L.A. Reinke, T.H. Rushmore, Y.-J. Surh
R.T. Swank, D.R. Thakker, R.G. Thurman, K.P. Vatsis, M. Vore
C.Y. Wang, W.W. Weber, R. Weinshilboum, J. Zaleski, L. Zhen

Editor

Frederick C. Kauffman

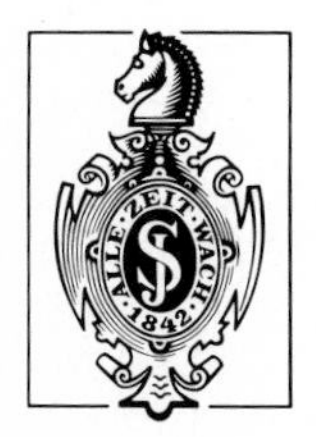

Springer-Verlag
Berlin Heidelberg New York London Paris
Tokyo Hong Kong Barcelona Budapest

Professor FREDERICK C. KAUFFMAN, Ph.D.
Director
Laboratory for Cellular and Biochemical Toxicology
College of Pharmacy
Rutgers University
Kilmer Campus
41 Gordon Road
Piscataway, NJ 08854
USA

With 109 Figures and 34 Tables

ISBN 3-540-57122-1 Springer-Verlag Berlin Heidelberg New York
ISBN 0-387-57122-1 Springer-Verlag New York Berlin Heidelberg

Library of Congress Cataloging-in-Publication Data. Conjugation–deconjugation reactions in drug metabolism and toxicity / contributors, K.W. Bock . . . [et al.]; editor, Frederick C. Kauffman. p. cm. — (Handbook of experimental pharmacology; v. 112) Includes bibliographical references and index. ISBN 3-540-57122-1 (acid-free paper: Berlin). — ISBN 0-387-57122-1 (acid-free paper: New York) 1. Drugs—Metabolism. 2. Drugs—Metabolic detoxication. 3. Metabolic conjugation. 4. Xenobiotics—Metabolism. 5. Xenobiotics—Metabolic detoxication. I. Kauffman, Frederick, C. II. Bock, K. W. (Karl Walter), 1935- . III. Series. QP905.H3 vol. 112 [RM301.55] 615′.1 s—dc20 [615′.7] 93-43134

Printed in Germany

Typesetting: Best-set Typesetter Ltd., Hong Kong
SPIN: 10077708 27/3130/SPS – 5 4 3 2 1 0 – Printed on acid-free paper

List of Contributors

BOCK, K.W., Institut für Toxikologie, Universität Tübingen, Wilhelmstr. 56, D-72074 Tübingen, Germany

BURCHELL, B., Department of Biochemical Medicine, University of Dundee, Ninewells Hospital and Medical School, Dundee DD1 9SY, Scotland, U.K.

CHIBA, M., Department of Pharmacology, Faculty of Pharmacy, University of Toronto, 19 Russel Street, Toronto, Ontario M5S 1A1, Canada. Present Address: Merck Sharp and Dohme Research Laboratories, West Point, PA19486, U.S.A.

CLARKE, D.J., Department of Biochemical Medicine, University of Dundee, Ninewells Hospital and Medical School, Dundee DD1 9SY, Scotland, U.K.

CREVELING, C.R., Laboratory of Bioorganic Chemistry, NIDDK, NIH, Bldg. 8A, Room 1A27, Bethesda, MD 20892, USA

FENSELAU, C., Chemistry and Biochemistry Department, University of Maryland Baltimore County, Structural Biochemistry Center, 5401 Wilkins Avenue, Baltimore, MD 21228, USA

KAUFFMAN, F.C., Laboratory for Cellular and Biochemical Toxicology, College of Pharmacy, Rutgers University, 41 Gordon Road, Piscataway, NJ 08854, USA

KWEI, G.Y., Pharmaceutical Research, 44I 130, Merck Sharp & Dohme Research Laboratories, West Point, PA 19486, USA

LAU, S.S., Division of Pharmacology and Toxicology, College of Pharmacy, University of Texas at Austin, Austin, TX 78712-1074, USA

LILIENBLUM, W., Niedersächsisches Landesamt für Immissionsschutz, Göttinger Straße 14, D-30449 Hannover, Germany

LU, A.Y.H., Drug Metabolism, Merck Sharp & Dohme Research Laboratories, P.O. Box 2000, Rahway, NJ 07065-0900, USA

MILLER, J.A., McArdle Laboratory for Cancer Research, University of Wisconsin Medical School, Department of Oncology, 1400 University Avenue, Madison, WI 53706, USA

MONKS, T.J., Division of Pharmacology and Toxicology, College of Pharmacy, University of Texas at Austin, Austin, TX 78712-1074, USA

NOVAK, E.K., Department of Molecular and Cellular Biology, Roswell Park Cancer Institute, Elm and Carlton Streets, Buffalo, NY 14263, USA

OTTERNESS, D., Department of Pharmacology, Mayo Medical School, Mayo Clinic, Mayo Foundation, Rochester, MN 55905, USA

PANG, K.S., Faculty of Pharmacy, and Department of Pharmacology, Faculty of Medicine, University of Toronto, 19 Russel Street, Toronto, Ontario M5S 1A1, Canada

PICKETT, C.B., Merck Frosst Center for Therapeutic Research, Merck Frosst Canada Inc., P.O. Box 1005, Point-Claire-Dorval, Quebec H9R 4P8, Canada

REINKE, L.A., Department of Pharmacology, University of Oklahoma Health Sciences Center, Biomedical Sciences Building, Rm. 753, P.O. Box 26901, Oklahoma City, OK 73190, USA

RUSHMORE, T.H., Merck Frosst Center for Therapeutic Research, Merck Frosst Canada, Inc., P.O. Box 1005, Point-Claire-Dorval, Quebec H9R 4P8, Canada

SURH, Y.-J., Department of Epidemiology and Public Health, Yale University School of Medicine, New Haven, CT 06510, USA

SWANK, R.T., Department of Molecular and Cellular Biology, Roswell Park Cancer Institute, Elm and Carlton Streets, Buffalo, NY 14263, USA

THAKKER, D.R., Department of Drug Metabolism, Glaxo Inc., Research Institute, Research Triangle Park, NC 27709, USA

THURMAN, R.G., Laboratory of Hepatobiology and Toxicology, Department of Pharmacology, University of North Carolina at Chapel Hill, 1124 FLOB, CB#7365, Chapel Hill, NC 27599-7365, USA

VATSIS, K.P., Department of Pharmacology, M6322/0626 Medical Science Building I, Medical School, The University of Michigan, Ann Arbor, MI 48109-0626, USA

VORE, M., Department of Pharmacology, MS-305 Chandler Medical Center, University of Kentucky College of Medicine, Lexington, KY 40536, USA

WANG, C.Y., Department of Chemical Carcinogenesis, Michigan Cancer Foundation, 110 East Warren Avenue, Detroit, MI 48201, USA

WEBER, W.W., Department of Pharmacology, M6322/0626 Medical Science Building I, Medical School, The University of Michigan, Ann Arbor, MI 48109-0626, USA

WEINSHILBOUM, R., Department of Pharmacology, Mayo Medical School, Mayo Clinic, Mayo Foundation, Rochester, MN 55905, USA

ZALESKI, J., Laboratory for Cellular and Biochemical Toxicology, College of Pharmacy, Rutgers University, 41 Gordon Road, Piscataway, NJ 08854, USA

ZHEN, L., Department of Molecular and Cellular Biology, Roswell Park Cancer Institute, Elm and Carlton Streets, Buffao, NY 14263, USA

Preface

This volume is entitled *Conjugation–Deconjugation Reactions in Drug Metabolism and Toxicity* to emphasize the important functions of both synthetic and hydrolytic enzymes in determining the net production and utilization of xenobiotic and biotic conjugates. The role of hydrolytic enzymes in determining the formation and fate of phase II metabolites, to date, has been often overlooked. The present volume was stimulated by the enormous progress made over the last five years in applying molecular biological approaches to defining the expression and regulation of transferases and hydrolases involved in the conjugation and deconjugation of biologically important drugs and toxic chemicals. Based on the work of many investigators, it is now apparent that multiple gene families have evolved for most, if not all, enzymes involved in conjugation–deconjugation reactions in mammalian tissues.

There are three main parts in this book. Chapters 1–7 deal largely with advances made in describing the expression and regulation of enzymes involved in conjugation–deconjugation reactions. Chapters 8–11 review work concerning the regulation of these reactions in intact cells. The last part, Chaps. 12–16, is focused primarily on recent research indicating that a broad range of biologically active, as well as the more commonly known inactive, products are generated by this important group of drug metabolizing enzymes. The final chapter reflects the editor's view of challenges and important directions for future research.

Research on conjugating–deconjugating reactions has progressed rapidly over the last decade through efforts of many laboratories worldwide. Selection of authors and work reviewed was the choice of the editor, who by necessity could not include all who have made important contributions. Editing was limited to avoiding overlap and providing continuity to the views of authors who generously contributed to this book. The editor enjoyed working with colleagues who submitted chapters and is deeply grateful for their thoughtful and timely contributions.

Ms. Marybeth Sarsfield is thanked for her excellent help with typing and maintaining bibliographic data bases. The editor is especially thankful to Ms. Doris M. Walker of Springer-Verlag for her insights and cheerful assistance, and to the editors of the series and publisher for encouraging a volume on conjugation–deconjugation reactions at this time.

Piscataway
April 1994

FREDERICK C. KAUFFMAN

Contents

Section I: Transferases and Hydrolases Involved in Phase II Conjugation–Deconjugation Reactions, Genetic Polymorphism and Regulation of Expression

CHAPTER 4

Human *N*-Acetyltransferases

CHAPTER 5

Genetic Regulation of the Subcellular Localization and Expression of Glucuronidase

CHAPTER 6

Microsomal Amidases and Carboxylesterases

Section II: Regulation of Phase II Conjugation: Deconjugation Reactions in Intact Cells and Tissues

CHAPTER 8

Cofactor Supply as a Rate-Limiting Determinant of Hepatic Conjugation Reactions
L.A. REINKE, F.C. KAUFFMAN, and R.G. THURMAN.

Section III: Pharmacology and Toxicology of Drug Conjugates

CHAPTER 13

Acyl Glucuronides as Chemically Reactive Intermediates

CHAPTER 14

Roles of Uridine Diphosphate Glucuronosyltransferases in Chemical Carcinogenesis

CHAPTER 17

Challenges and Directions for Future Research

Section I
Transferases and Hydrolases Involved in Phase II Conjugation–Deconjugation Reactions, Genetic Polymorphism and Regulation of Expression

CHAPTER 1

The Uridine Diphosphate Glucuronosyltransferase Multigene Family: Function and Regulation

D.J. CLARKE and B. BURCHELL

A. Introduction

Glucuronidation is a major detoxication pathway in all vertebrates examined, from the most primitive (fish; CLARKE et al. 1991) to the most evolved (man; DUTTON 1980) and accounts for most of the detoxified material in bile and urine (DUTTON 1980).

The uridine diphosphate (UDP) glucuronosyltransferases (UDPGTs; EC 24.1.17) are a family of closely related membrane-bound enzymes that are responsible for the transfer of the glucuronyl group from uridine 5′-diphosphoglucuronate (UDPGA) to millions of biological, and pharmacologically active endogenous and exogenous molecules having nucleophilic functional groups of oxygen, nitrogen, sulphur and carbon (TEPHLY and BURCHELL 1990). The mechanism of the reaction catalysed by UDPGTs is a SN_2 reaction, the acceptor group of the substrate attacking the C_1 of the pyranose acid ring of UDPGA, which results in the formation of a glucuronide (a β-D-glucopyranosiduronic acid conjugate; Fig. 1). The resulting glucuronide is generally water soluble, less toxic and more easily excreted than the parent compound.

B. The Physiological Roles of Uridine Diphosphate Glucuronosyltransferases

I. Endogenous Compound Metabolism

Of the endogenous compounds glucuronidated bilirubin, the end product of haem catabolism, has been the most extensively studied substrate of UDPGTs. The requirement for the body to remove bilirubin is paramount, as at high concentrations it has been shown to elicit cellular damage. In severe prolonged hyperbilirubinaemic disease states (see Sect. E.11), plasma albumin, which transports circulating bilirubin, becomes saturated and unbound bilirubin is capable of crossing membranes, including the blood–brain barrier. This results in kernicterus, which may elicit neurological damage and eventual death. Conjugation of bilirubin with glucuronic acid prevents such consequences occurring, as under normal physiological condi-

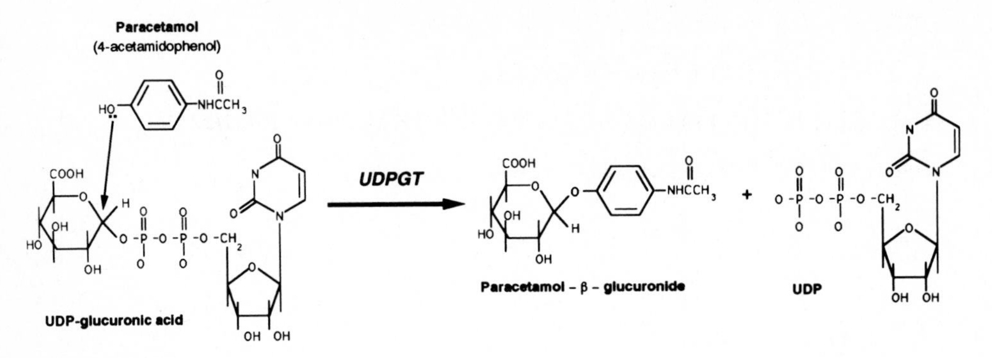

Fig. 1. Glucuronidation of a phenolic compound catalysed by uridine diphosphate (*UDP*) glucuronosyltransferase (*UDPGT*)

tions, bilirubin is excreted from the body as biliary bilirubin mono- and diglucuronides (see ROY CHOWDHURY et al. 1989 for an extensive review).

The biological purpose of glucuronidation for other endogenous compounds (i.e., steroid hormones, bile acids, thyroid hormones, 5-hydroxytryptamine; for a comprehensive list see DUTTON 1980) is grossly under-investigated; however, it seems reasonable to postulate that it plays mainly a catabolic role, as their glucuronides are found in bile.

Interestingly, glucuronidation at the D-ring of estriol, testosterone and dihydroxytestosterone have been shown to possess pharmacological activity in that they mediate cholestasis (MEYERS et al. 1981; VORE et al. 1983; VORE and SLIKKER 1985). In contrast, A-ring conjugates of these steroids are inactive (SLIKKER et al. 1983). Other examples of biologically active conjugates are reviewed in Chap. 12 of this volume.

Recently, glucuronidation of retinoic acid has been demonstrated to prevent binding of the parent compound to retinoic acid receptor proteins (SANI et al. 1992). Similarly, thyroxine glucuronide has been shown to have a markedly reduced plasma-binding capacity compared to the free hormone (HAYS and HSU 1988). These studies indicate that as well as enhancing the excretion of endogenous compounds, glucuronidation also terminates the biological activity of some compounds.

II. Drug and Xenobiotic Conjugation

Drugs from almost all therapeutic classes are glucuronidated (for a list of those glucuronidated in humans, see Table 1). Many of these drugs have narrow therapeutic indices (e.g., morphine, chloramphenicol), and glucuronidation is likely to have important consequences in their clinical use.

Glucuronidation of drug molecules containing a wide range of acceptor groups have been reported, including phenols (e.g., propofol, paracetamol, naloxone), alcohols (e.g., chloramphenicol, codeine, oxazepam), aliphatic

Table 1. Drug glucuronidation in humans[a]

Drug	Therapeutic class	References
Acetaminophen	Analgesic	CUMMINGS et al. (1967)
Alclonfenac	Anti-inflammatory	BROGDEN et al. (1977)
Alprazolam	Anxiolytic	FRASER et al. (1991)
Alprenolol	Antihypertensive	BODIN (1974)
Amitriptyline	Antidepressant	VANDEL et al. (1982)
Benazepril	Antihypertensive	WALDMEIER et al. (1991)
Benoxaprofen	Anti-inflammatory	SMITH et al. (1977)
Bromperidol	Antipsychotic	BENFIELD et al. (1988)
Carprofen	Anti-inflammatory	SPAHN et al. (1989)
Carvediolol	Antihypertensive	NEUGEBAUER and NEUBERT (1991)
Chloramphenicol	Antibiotic	AMBROSE (1984)
Ciclopiroxalamine	Antifungal	KELLNER et al. (1981)
Ciprofibrate	Antihyperlipoproteinemic	OELSCHLAGER et al. (1991)
Ciramadol	Analgesic	SISENWINE et al. (1986)
Clofibric acid	Antihyperlipoproteinaemic	HOUIN et al. (1975)
Codeine	Analgesic	ADLER et al. (1955)
Cyclobenzaprine	Muscle relaxant	HUCKER et al. (1978)
Cyproheptadine	Antihistaminic	PORTER et al. (1975)
Diflunisal	Analgesic	LOEWEN et al. (1988)
Enciprazine	Anxiolytic	SCATINA et al. (1991)
Epirubicin	Antineoplastic	MORRIS et al. (1991)
Etodolac	Anti-inflammatory	FERDINANDI et al. (1983)
Fenofibric acid	Antihyperlipoproteinaemic	WEIL et al. (1990)
Fenoprazone	Anti-inflammatory	YAMAGUCHI et al. (1979)
Fenoprofen	Anti-inflammatory	RUBIN et al. (1972)
Haloperidol	Antipsychotic	SOMEYA et al. (1992)
Imiloxan	Adrenoceptor antagonist	RUSH et al. (1992)
Isoxepac	Anti-inflammatory	PAUL et al. (1981)
Ketoprofen	Anti-inflammatory	UPTON et al. (1980)
Ketorolac	Anti-inflammatory	MROSZCZAK et al. (1987)
Ketotifen	Antihistaminic	LE BIGOT et al. (1987)
Labetalol	Antihypertensive	MARTIN et al. (1976)
Lamotrigine	Anticonvulsant	COHEN et al. (1987)
Lorazepam	Anxiolytic	GREENBLATT et al. (1979)
Lormetazepam	Sedative	DOENICKE et al. (1991)
Meptazinol	Analgesic	MURRAY et al. (1989)
Mexiletine	Antiarrhythmic	GRECH-BELANGER et al. (1985)
Morphine	Analgesic	OSBORNE et al. (1990)
Nalidixic acid	Antiseptic	PORTMANN et al. (1966)
Naloxone	Narcotic antagonist	BERKOWITZ (1976)
S-Naproxen	Anti-inflammatory	UPTON et al. (1980)
Nitecapone	Narcotic antagonist	TASKINEN et al. (1991)
Nortriptyline	Antidepressant	DAHL et al. (1991)
Oxaprozin	Anti-inflammatory	JANSSEN et al. (1980)
Oxazepam	Anxiolytic	ALVAN et al. (1977)
Oxprenolol	Antihypertensive	RIESS et al. (1974)
Perindopril	Antihypertensive	VERPOOTEN et al. (1991)
Phenprocoumon	Anti-inflammatory	TOON et al. (1985)
Phenylbutazone	Anti-inflammatory	DIETERLE et al. (1976)
Pirprofen	Anti-inflammatory	EGGER et al. (1982)
Probencid	Uricosuric	UPTON et al. (1980)
Propofol	Analgesic	SIMONS et al. (1988)

Table 1. (*Continued*)

Drug	Therapeutic class	References
Ritrodrine	Antihypertensive	BRASHEAR et al. (1988)
Salicylamide	Analgesic	LEVY and MATSUZAWA (1967)
Salicylic acid	Anti-inflammatory	LEVY et al. (1972)
Sulfamethomidine	Antibacterial	VREE et al. (1991)
Sulfadimethoxine	Antibacterial	ADAMSON et al. (1970)
Sulfinpyrazone	Uricosuric	DIETERLE et al. (1975)
Suprofen	Anti-inflammatory	MORI et al. (1985)
Temazepam	Sedative	SCHWARTZ (1979)
Tiaprofenic acid	Anti-inflammatory	POTTIER et al. (1977)
Tocainide	Antiarrhythmic	ELVIN et al. (1980)
Tripelennamine	Antihistamine	CHAUDHURI et al. (1976)
Valproic acid	Anticonvulsant	DICKINSON et al. (1989)
Zidovudine	Antiviral	BLUM et al. (1988)
Zomepirac	Analgesic	O'NEILL et al. (1982)

[a] All drugs listed in this table are excreted as at least 20% glucuronic acid conjugates. Drugs which are excreted at less than this value are not included.

amines (e.g., ciclopiroxalamine, lamotrigine, amitriptyline), acidic carbon atoms (e.g., feprazone, phenylbutazone, sulphinpyrazone) and carboxylic acids (e.g., naproxen, zomepirac, ketoprofen). This indicates the variability of acceptor groups that can be glucuronic acid-conjugated in humans.

Table 1 shows that humans have the ability to form N-linked glucuronides of several tertiary amine drugs (e.g., cyclobenzaprine, cyproheptadine, tripelannamine). This is not, however, the case with laboratory animals such as rats and monkeys which have an inability to form such quaternary ammonium glucuronides (FISCHER et al. 1980), indicating that it is important not to rely exclusively on laboratory animals for drug metabolism studies.

The enantioselective and stereoselective glucuronidation of many drugs has been demonstrated in humans for oxazepam (SEIDEMAN et al. 1981), focainide (HOFFMAN et al. 1984), ibuprofen (EL MOUELHI et al. 1987), mexiletine (GRECH-BELANGER et al. 1986), naproxen (EL MOUELHI et al. 1987), benoxaprofen (EL MOUELHI et al. 1987), picenadol (FRANZ et al. 1990), prenylamine (GIETL et al. 1990), morphine (COUGHTRIE et al. 1989), 4′-hydroxypropanolol (WALLE et al. 1988) and *E*-10-hydroxynortriptyline (DAHL-PUUSTINEN et al. 1989); however, the enzymes responsible for this selectivity have yet to be identified.

The primary physiological role of drug glucuronidation is the metabolically initiated clearance of drugs from the body in bile and urine. Such a mechanism, therefore, terminates the otherwise prolonged and possibly deleterious pharmacological action of many drugs. The pharmacokinetics of drug action is thus dependent on, amongst other variables, the rate of glucuronidation, which in turn varies for different drug substrates due to the catalytic activity of individual UDPGTs (see Sect. D.11) and factors affecting UDPGT expression (see Sect. E). Until the characterisation of all UDPGT enzymes and factors that control their differential expression in humans is achieved, it will be impossible to forecast accurately UDPGTs' role in the pharmacokinetics of drug metabolism and disposition.

Most investigators have ignored the possibility that glucuronic acid-conjugated metabolites of drugs have any pharmacological properties, assuming that such glucuronides are inactive. There are, however, two notable exceptions reported, where such metabolites have been found to be pharmacologically active. (−)-Morphine is glucuronidated in a stereoselective manner to (−)-morphine-3-glucuronide and (−)-morphine-6-glucuronide in the liver (WAHLSTROM et al. 1988; COUGHTRIE et al. 1989). Detailed pharmacological characterisation of the glucuronides has established that (−)-morphine-6-glucuronide is 650 times more potent than the parent drug as an analgesic, whereas morphine-3-glucuronide is a potent antagonist of morphine and has no analgesic activity (PASTERNAK et al. 1987; FRANCES et al. 1990; PAUL et al. 1989; SMITH et al. 1990). This discovery has led to (−)-morphine-6-glucuronide being commercially marketed as a drug recently. In addition to (−)-morphine-6-glucuronide, a number of carboxylic acid drug glucuronides have been demonstrated to have biological activity. Acylglucuronides of a number of carboxylic acid drugs (e.g., zomepirac, clofibrate, valproate) have been implicated in adverse drug reactions (e.g., anaphylaxis) by virtue of the observation that they are able to undergo acyl migration and bind to cellular proteins (reviewed in SPAHN-LANGGUTH and BENET 1992 and Chap. 8 of this volume). Similar events may take place in cholestasis or conjugated hyperbilirubinaemia, thereby causing liver damage (BLANCKAERT et al. 1978). Acyl migration is discussed in more detail in Chap. 13.

Apart from glucuronides of morphine and carboxylic acid drugs, there have been few reports of pharmacologically active drug glucuronides; however, it is likely that many others will be found with interesting properties.

The role of glucuronidation in the metabolism of carcinogens and other environmental pollutants, whether ingested, inhaled or absorbed, are discussed elsewhere. The reader is referred to Chap. 14 of this textbook and DUTTON (1980) for comprehensive reviews on these areas, respectively.

III. Role of Glucuronidation in Olfaction and Glycolipid Biosynthesis

Recently several hydroxyl-containing odorants (e.g., borneal, 2-ethyl-1-hexanol, guaiacol, eugenol) have been shown to be glucuronidated by an olfactory-specific UDPGT in rodent and bovine species (LAZARD et al. 1990, 1991; BURCHELL 1991). Evidence suggests that glucuronidation of such odorants prevents them stimulating an increase in adenylate cyclase activity (LAZARD et al. 1991; BURCHELL 1991), thus ceasing an olfactory response. In contrast, steroid glucuronides such as 3α, 17α-dihydroxy-5β-pregnan-20-one-3-glucuronide, which is a male pheromone in fish, are extremely potent odorants which are capable of initiating olfactory neural impulses in piscine species (CLARKE et al. 1991; LAMBERT and RESINK 1991). Thus, glucuronides appear to be involved in both the termination and initiation of olfactory stimuli.

As well as the glucuronidation of the aforementioned compounds, a novel UDPGT is involved in the biosynthesis of sulphated glucuronic acid-containing glycolipids which are localised in peripheral nerves and in caudal equina (CHOU et al. 1991; DAS et al. 1991; OKA et al. 1992). It has been suggested that the carbohydrate moieties of these lipids are involved in cell–cell interactions and cellular adhesion in the cerebellum and in the regulation of myelinogenesis (CHOU et al. 1991). At present, however, the exact physiological purpose of such glycolipids still requires further investigation.

C. Localisation of Uridine Diphosphate Glucuronosyltransferases

I. Tissue Distribution

Of all the organs in the body, the liver has been established to be, quantitatively and qualitatively, the most important site for glucuronidation (DUTTON 1980; the study of the numerous hepatic UDPGTs is discussed in Sects. D.I and D.III). The localisation of glucuronidation within the liver is predominantly periportal (BRANCH et al. 1983; MITCHELL et al. 1989). Immunohistochemical analysis has also revealed that phenol UDPGT is also located in the epithelial cells of the bile duct and the endothelial cells of the hepatic artery and portal vein (KNAPP et al. 1988). Bile duct epithelial cells have also recently been shown to have steroid UDPGTs (FRANSON et al. 1990).

As well as the liver, it should be emphasised that other extra-hepatic tissues have the capacity to glucuronidate compounds, albeit with a more restricted substrate specificity and capacity than hepatic tissue. In rat kidney, UDPGT activity twards (−)-morphine (RUSH et al. 1983) and testosterone (LUCIER and MCDANIEL 1977) is absent in contrast to the liver; however, transferase activities towards phenols and bilirubin are present (LILIENBLUM et al. 1982). In contrast to rats, human kidney does not conjugate bilirubin (FEVERY et al. 1977), but is capable of conjugating both the (−) and (+) enantiomers of morphine at the 3-hydroxy position (COUGHTRIE et al. 1989). In addition, 3- and 6-hydroxylated bile acids are also glucuronidated by human renal tissue (MATERN et al. 1984; MARSCHALL et al. 1987; PARQUET et al. 1988). Microdissection of rabbit kidney has revealed that the highest glucuronidation activities were found in the proximal tubule area (HJELLE et al. 1986).

In rats, the gastro-intestinal tract exhibits glucuronidation capacity for phenols, (−)-morphine, certain steroids and bilirubin (KOSTER et al. 1986; ROY CHOWDHURY et al. 1985). The activity towards phenols increases from the stomach to the duodenum and then decreases towards the colon (SCHWENK 1989). In humans, the intestine can metabolise planar phenols (PETERS and JANSEN 1988; PACIFICI et al. 1989) and bilirubin (PETERS and JANSEN 1988).

Other organs proximate to the external environment – i.e., lungs (AITIO 1976; COUGHTRIE et al. 1985), bronchus (GIBBY and COHEN 1984), skin (COOMES et al. 1983; PHAM et al. 1989), nasal tissue (GERVASI et al. 1991; LAZARD et al. 1990b; LONGO et al. 1992) – also have appreciable activity to simple phenolic xenobiotics. Phenol UDPGT activity also appears ubiquitous to many other tissues including spleen, thymus, brain and heart, albeit at low levels (AITIO 1974). The variations in the tissue-specific expression of individual UDPGT isoforms has recently been demonstrated by immunochemical analysis in rats (KOSTER et al. 1986; BURCHELL and COUGHTRIE 1989) and humans (PETERS and JANSEN 1988).

II. Topology of Uridine Diphosphate Glucuronosyltransferases in the Endoplasmic Reticulum

The location of UDPGTs has wide-ranging implications on the biochemical and pharmacological role of these enzymes. UDPGTs are primarily located in the endoplasmic reticulum (ER) of both hepatic and extra-hepatic tissues (DUTTON 1980; ROY CHOWDHURY et al. 1985). Early studies reviewed by DUTTON (1980) revealed that UDPGT activity was latent, the total enzyme activity not being expressed until membrane disrupting agents (e.g., detergents) were added to microsomal preparations. Following such membrane disruption, the activity increased up to 20-fold. Thus, the active site of the enzyme was thought to lie in the lumen of the ER. This theory has recently been substantiated by experiments using proteases (VANSTAPEL and BLANCKAERT 1988), proteases and antibodies (SHEPHERD et al. 1989; YOKOTA et al. 1992) and computer-aided prediction based on UDPGT sequences (JACKSON and BURCHELL 1986; MACKENZIE 1986a; IYANAGI et al. 1986), which demonstrated that the bulk of the enzyme is located in the lumen of the ER and that there is only one transmembrane spanning region near the carboxy terminal end. Additional support for the luminal orientation is provided by the fact that most UDPGTs are N-glycosylated (ROY CHOWDHURY et al. 1985; HARDING et al. 1988; GREEN and TEPHLY 1989; MACKENZIE 1990a,b; JACKSON et al. 1990; CLARKE et al. 1992; YOKOTA et al. 1992); hence, a proportion of the enzyme must be facing the lumen. Very recently, a motif that contains a retention signal for proteins in the ER membrane has been found in UDPGTs (NILSSON et al. 1989; JACKSON et al. 1990).

The luminal orientation of the UDPGT active site has led several groups to postulate that at least two membrane transporters must exist to transport

(a) the highly charged co-substrate UDPGA from the cytoplasm, where it is synthesised to the lumen of the ER and (b) the product of the glucuronidation from the lumen to the cytoplasm (JANSEN et al. 1992). Figure 2 shows a model of the topology of UDPGT and the proposed transporters based on current knowledge.

D. The Uridine Diphosphate Glucuronosyltransferase Multigene Family

I. Elucidation of Uridine Diphosphate Glucuronosyltransferase Heterogeneity

A plethora of indirect evidence for the multiplicity of UDPGTs has been demonstrated. Indications of UDPGT heterogeneity are: (a) tissue differences in UDPGT expression (see Sect. C.II), (b) the differential induction of UDPGTs by xenobiotics (see Sect. E.III), (c) the ontogenic development of UDPGTs (see Sect. E.I) and (d) the genetic deficiency of UDPGTs in animals and man (see Sect. E.11). The most direct approach towards determining the heterogeneity of UDPGTs has been the physical separation of UDPGTs by protein purification and cloning and expression of individual enzyme forms.

Purification of UDPGTs proved to be inherently difficult due to their relative instability in the high concentrations of detergent required for

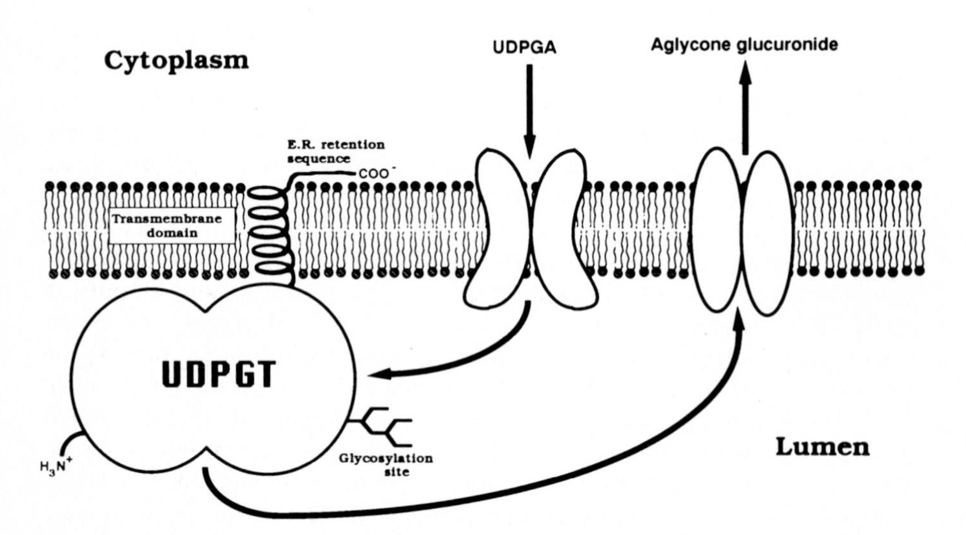

Fig. 2. Topology of uridine diphosphate glucuronosyltransferase (*UDPGT*) and proposed transporters in the endoplasmic reticulum (*E.R.*) membrane. *UDPGA*, uridine 5′-diphosphoglucuronate

solubilisation (see BURCHELL 1981 for a review of earlier studies), their phospholipid dependence (GRAHAM and WOOD 1969; GRAHAM et al. 1977; TUKEY et al. 1979; SINGH et al. 1981; BURCHELL 1982; HOCHMAN et al. 1981) and the great similarity between different isoforms of the enzyme (BURCHELL et al. 1991). Chromatofocusing (column isoelectric focusing) together with affinity chromatography on UDP-hexanolamine sepharose has been found to be the most useful technique for the resolution of UDPGT isoenzymes. This was first applied by FALANY and TEPHLY (1983) to purify a phenol UDPGT, a 17β-hydroxysteroid UDPGT and 3α-hydroxysteroid UDPGT to homogeneity from rat liver. Since then, this technique has allowed the resolution of several other rat UDPGT isoforms, including those that catalyse the glucuronidation of morphine (PUIG and TEPHLY 1986), 4-hydroxybiphenyl (STYCZYNSKI et al. 1991) and bilirubin (CLARKE et al. 1992). Anion exchange and affinity chromatography have also been successful in purifying an isoform that glucuronidates the neurotransmitter 5-hydroxytryptamine (ABE and YUASA 1988) and a novel phenol UDPGT from rat liver (YOKOTA et al. 1988).

The isolation of human UDPGTs has proved to be even more difficult than rat UDPGTs, due to the scarcity of quality human tissue and the lability of the enzymes. TEPHLY's group purified two human isoforms to apparent homogeneity which displayed overlapping specificity towards phenols, but could also be distinguished by glucuronidation of oestriol by one form, while the other conjugated 4-aminobiphenyl (IRSHAID and TEPHLY 1987; COFFMAN et al. 1990). More recently, a UDPGT isoform that conjugates 6α-bile acids has been purified from human liver (MATERN et al. 1991).

Due to the apparent overlapping substrate specificities (Tables 2, 3) and the similarity of molecular masses (50–57 kDa) of the enzymes in this multigene family, purity of most of the aforementioned transferases were assessed by N-terminal sequence analysis to ensure only one polypeptide was present. The requirement of this purity check further accentuates the problems associated with studying this group of enzymes by protein purification techniques.

The tedium and difficulties involved in purifying homogenous preparations of a single UDPGT isoform have now largely been superceeded by the powerful techniques of recombinant DNA technology. Cloning of UDPGTs was initially made possible by the generation of anti-UDPGT antibodies utilising purified UDPGTs as immunogens (MACKENZIE et al. 1984; JACKSON et al. 1985, 1987) and the use of degenerate oligonucleotides based on peptide sequences derived from partial amino acid sequence analysis of purified UDPGTs (IYANAGI et al. 1986). The cloning of UDPGT cDNAs and their subsequent expression in tissue culture by transfection has proved an invaluable tool for determining the function and structure of a large number of UDPGTs, especially the elusive human UDPGTs.

Table 2. The heterogeneity and substrate specificity of rat liver uridine diphosphate glucuronosyltransferases

Isoform	Subunit Mass (kDa)	Substrates	References
Phenol UDPGT[a,c,d] (UGT1*06)	56	4-Nitrophenol 1-Naphthol BP-3,6-quinol BP-3,6-quinol MG	FALANY and TEPHLY (1983) BOCK et al. (1988) JACKSON et al. (1988)
Morphine UDPGT[c] (–)	56	(−)-Morphine	PUIG and TEPHLY (1986)
5-Hydroxytryptamine[c] (–)	55	5-Hydroxytryptamine 4-Hydroxybiphenyl	ABE and YUASA (1988)
Phenol UDPGT[b,c] (–)	54	4-Nitrophenol 1-Naphthol Eugenol 5-Hydroxytryptamine	YOKOTA et al. (1988)
Bilirubin UDPGT[a,c] (UGT1*01)	54	Bilirubin Bilirubin monoglucuronide 1-Naphthol 7,7,7-Triphenylheptanoic acid	BURCHELL (1980) BURCHELL and BLANCKAERT (1984) CLARKE et al. (1992)
Chloramphenicol UDPGT[d] (UGT2B1)	53	Chloramphenicol 4-Hydroxybiphenyl Testosterone	MACKENZIE (1987) MACKENZIE (1990)
4-Hydroxybiphenyl[c,d] UDPGT (UGT2B15)	52	4-Hydroxybiphenyl 4-Nitrophenol	STYCZYNSKI et al. (1992)

3α-Hydroxysteroid[c,d] UDPGT (UGT2B2)	52	Androsterone Etiocholanolone Lithocholic acid 3,5Bc$_{20-23}$ bile acids	Falany and Tephly (1983) Falany et al. (1986) Mackenzie (1986) Radominska et al. (1988)
17β-Hydroxysteroid[a,c,d] UDPGT (UGT2B3)	50	Testosterone Dihydroxytestosterone	Falany and Tephyly (1983) Falany et al. (1986) Mackenzie (1986) Harding et al. (1987)
17β-Hydroxysteroid[b,d] UDPGT (UGT2B6)	50	Testosterone Dihydroxytestosterone	Mackenzie (1990a)
Bilirubin UDPGTB[d] (UGT1*04)	?	Bilirubin	Sato et al. (1990)
Digitoxigenin monodigitoxide UDPGT[c] (–)	?	Digitoxigenin monodigitoxoside Digitoxigenin bisdigitoxoside	von Meyerinck et al. (1985)
Estrone UDPGT[c] (–)	?	Estrone	Weatherill and Burchell (1980) Roy Chowdhury et al. (1986)

The nomenclature for the gene encoding these enzymes is given in parenthesis based on Burchell et al. 1991. (–) indicates gene not cloned.
BP, Benzo(a)pyrene; MG, monoglucuronide; UDPGT, uridine diphosphate glucuronosyltransferase.
[a,b] Arbitrary symbols used to designate two different isoenzymes differentiated by amino acid sequence that have similar substrate preferences.
[c] Protein purification used to resolve isoenzyme.
[d] cDNA cloning used to resolve isoenzyme.

Table 3. Characteristics of human liver uridine diphosphate glucuronosyltransferase isoenzymes

Isoform	Subunit Mass (kDa)	Substrates	References
Bulky phenol UDPGT[a] (UGT1*02)	56	4-Tertiary butylphenol Propafol Carvacrol Galangin Other bulky phenols	Wooster et al. (1991) Ebner and Burchell (1993)
Bilirubin UDPGT[a,c] (UGT1*1)	55	Bilirubin Bilirubin monoglucuronide Ethinylestradiol 1-Naphthol Octylgallate	Ritter et al. (1991) Sutherland et al. (1992) Ebner et al. (1993) bin Senafi et al. (1994)
Planar phenol UDPGT[a] (UGT1*6)	55	1-Naphthol BP-3,6-quinol Paracetamol Vanillin	Harding et al. (1988) Wooster et al. (1991) Bock et al. (1992) Bock et al. (1993)
4-Aminobiphenyl UDPGT[b] (–)	54	4-Aminobiphenyl 4-Nitrophenol 1-Naphthylamine	Irshaid and Tephly (1987)
Estriol UDPGT[a] (UGT2B8)	53	Estriol 4-Nitrophenol 1-Naphthylamine	Irshaid and Tephly (1987) Coffman et al. (1990)

Estrogen UDPGT[a,c] (UGT2B4)	52	Hyodeoxycholic acid 4-Hydroxyestrone 17-Epiestriol Estriol	Jackson et al. (1987) Fournel-Gigleux et al. (1989) Ritter et al. (1992)
Estrogen UDPGT[a,d] (UGT2B7)	52	Hyodeoxycholic acid 4-Hydroxyestrone 17-Epiestriol Estriol	Ritter et al. (1990) Ritter et al. (1992)
Bilirubin UDPGT[a,d] (UGT1*4)	?	Bilirubin Bilirubin monoglucuronide	Ritter et al. (1991)

The nomenclature for the gene encoding these enzymes is given in parenthesis based on Burchell et al. 1991. (–) indicates gene not cloned.
UDPGT, uridine diphosphate glucuronosyltransferase.
[a] Protein purification used to resolve isoenzyme.
[b] cDNA cloning used to resolve isoenzyme.
[c,d] Arbitrary symbols used to designate two different isoenzymes differentiated by amino acid sequence that have similar substrate preferences.

Eight different rat UDPGTs and ten human UDPGTs have been identified to date (BURCHELL et al. 1991) by cDNA cloning. Tables 2 and 3 show the extent of our current knowledge of the heterogeneity of UDPGTs in rat and human liver, respectively, derived from purification and cloning studies.

II. Primary Structure and Post-Translational Processing of Uridine Diphosphate Glucuronosyltransferases

Studies on the primary sequence of UDPGTs has revealed a number of important features regarding UDPGTs. Comparison of the deduced amino acid sequences of 26 UDPGTs cloned from mammalian species has indicated that UDPGTs may be split into two families based on amino acid identities (BURCHELL et al. 1991). Within a single family, the UDPGT protein sequences exhibit greater than 55% resemblance. Figure 3 illustrates the current status of the human UDPGT family tree. Although these gene families have been based on amino acid sequence identities, the primary structure of the proteins from each of the two families also differ greatly. The members of the *UGT1* gene family, which comprises phenol- and bilirubin-metabolising isoforms, all share an identical 246 amino acid carboxy terminus, whereas their N-terminal halves show a striking lack of identity (34%–49%). In contrast, comparison of members of the *UGT2* gene family, which comprises steroid-metabolising isoforms, indicates that amino acid differences between different isoforms of this family occur throughout the length of the protein.

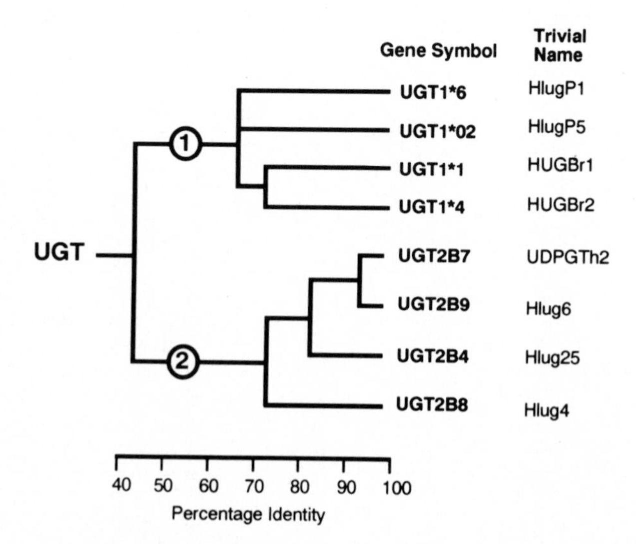

Fig. 3. The human uridine diphosphate glucuronosyltransferase (UDPGT) family tree based on *percentage amino acid identity*

As well as enabling the UDPGTs to be split into two families of proteins, analysis of the primary sequences of UDPGTs has revealed that several important structural motifs and domains exist in UDPGTs. Comparison of the amino acid sequence of all UDPGTs indicates that the N-terminal half of the proteins are more variable, especially between residues 60 and 120, suggesting that this half of UDPGT proteins may be involved in binding the aglycone substrate. Experimental evidence supporting this hypothesis is that *UGT1* family members have different substrate specificities, but share a common C-terminal domain. Furthermore, studies by MACKENZIE (1990a) in which he assayed a series of chimeric proteins prepared by recombinant techniques from two rat UGTB cDNAs for catalytic activity indicate that the N-terminal half of these cDNAs encode the critical determinants for substrate specificity. This analysis also suggested that the UDP sugar-binding domain was situated at the C-terminal half of UDPGT proteins. Indeed, comparison of the *UGT1* and *UGT2* family members from different species with other UDP sugar-binding proteins indicates a highly homologous region between residues 352 and 403 which may be involved in UDP binding (Fig. 4).

Putative N-terminal signal sequences have been demonstrated in all UDPGTs. However, such leader sequences are not always removed during membrane insertion of proteins into the ER (GONZALEZ 1980). Conclusive proof that UDPGTs are cleaved by microsomal signal peptidase has been demonstrated with five UDPGTs. Comparison of the N-terminal sequences from purified UDPGTs and those derived from cDNAs has revealed that 23–27 amino acids are cleaved off during membrane insertion, resulting in a mature protein (HARDING et al. 1987; IYANAGI et al. 1986; MACKENZIE 1986b; TEPHLY et al. 1988; COFFMAN et al. 1990; CLARKE et al. 1992). Recently,

```
Human UGT1*6    W L P Q N D L L G H P K A R A F I T H S G S H G I Y E G I C N G V P M V M M P L F G D Q M D N A K R M
Human UGT2B4    W I P Q N D L L G H P K T R A F I T H G G A N G I Y K A I S P R I P M V G M P L F A D Q P D N I A H M
Rat UGT1*06     W L P Q N D L L G H P K A R A F I T H S G S H G I Y E G I C N G V P M V M M P L F G D Q M D N A K R M
Rat UGT2B2      W L P Q N D I L G H P K T K A F V T H G G A N G L Y E A I Y H G I P M I G I P L F G D Q P D N I A H M
Murine UGT1*6   W L P Q N D L L G H P K A R A F I T H S G S H G I Y E G I C N G V P M V M M P L F G D Q M D N A K R M
Murine UGT2B5   W L P Q N D L I G H P K T K A F V T H G G A N G V Y E A I Y H G I P M I G I P L F G E Q H D N I A H M
Bovine UGT2A1   W I P Q N D L L G H P K T K A F I T H G G A N G V F E A I Y H G I P M V G L P L F G D Q L D N I V Y M
Plant ugt       W A P Q V A V L R H P S V G A F V T H A G W A S V L E G L S S G V P M A C R P F F G D Q R M N A R S V
Virus ugt       W F N Q R A V L R H K K M A A F I T G G G L Q S S D E A L E A G I P M V C L P M M G D Q F Y H A H K L
Bacteria ugt    F V D Q P R Y V A E A N     L V I T H G G L N T V L D A L A A A T P V L A V P L S F D Q P A V A A R L
```

Fig. 4. The proposed uridine diphosphate (UDP)-binding site in UDP-glucuronosyltransferases (UDPGTs) based on a region of high amino acid identity with UDP-glucosyltransferases (ugt). The predicted amino acid sequence corresponding to residues 352–403 of human phenol UDPGT (UGT1*6) was compared to that of other UDPGTs and ugts. The *boxed areas* indicate regions of conservative amino acid replacements between the ten proteins. The reader is referred to the following references describing each of the DNA sequences encoding these proteins: human UGT1*6 (HARDING et al. 1988); human UGT2B4 (JACKSON et al. 1987); rat UGT1*06 (IYANAGI et al. 1986); rat UGT2B2 (JACKSON and BURCHELL 1986; MACKENZIE 1986b); murine UGT1*6 (BURCHELL et al. 1991); murine UGT2B5 (KIMURA and OWENS 1987); bovine UGT2A1 (LAZARD et al. 1991); Plant ugt (RALSTON et al. 1988); virus ugt (O'REILLY and MILLER 1989); bacteria ugt (HUNDLE et al. 1992) using recombinant DNA techniques, TOGHROL et al. (1990) have shown that the signal sequence of UDPGTs is required for the correct insertion of the transferase into the ER, as a truncated UDPGT without this sequence was expressed as a unstable cytosolic form.

There is only one stretch of amino acids in UDPGTs that have the potential to cross the lipid bilayer. This hydrophobic domain of 17 amino acids is located near the C terminus and is flanked by two highly charged areas, which is characteristic of the half-transfer signals of other transmembrane proteins (SABATINI et al. 1982). Also at the carboxy terminal end of UDPGTs, elegant molecular biological studies have revealed that positively charged lysines at −3, −4 and −5 from the carboxy terminus are responsible for the retention of UDPGTs in the ER (NILSSON et al. 1989; JACKSON et al. 1990). Most UDPGTs are also post-translationally modified by glycosylation. All UDPGTs so far isolated, with the exception of two rat 17β-hydroxysteroid UDPGT (MACKENZIE 1987, 1990b), possess a putative asparagine-linked glycosylation consensus sequence (Asn-X-Ser/Thr) in the translated protein (for references, see Tables 2 and 3). The glycosylation of the asparagine in this consensus sequence has been illustrated by a mobility shift of UDPGTs on sodium dodecyl sulphate polyacrylamide gels following endoglycosidase treatment of purified UDPGTs (BURCHELL et al. 1987; GREEN and TEPHLY 1989; CLARKE et al. 1992; YOKOTA et al. 1992) or tunicamycin (an inhibitor of N-linked glycosylation; ELBEIN 1984) treatment of cell cultures expressing UDPGT cDNAs (HARDING et al. 1988; JACKSON et al. 1988; MACKENZIE 1990c). Figure 5 summarises what is known about UDPGT domain structure to date. Future work using photoaffinity labelling probes such as flunitrazepam (THOMASSIN and TEPHLY 1990), chlorpromazine (STYCZYNSKI et al. 1992) and 5-azido-UDP-glucuronic acid (DRAKE et al. 1992) and site-directed mutagenesis studies should provide evidence of residues required for UDPGTs catalytic activities.

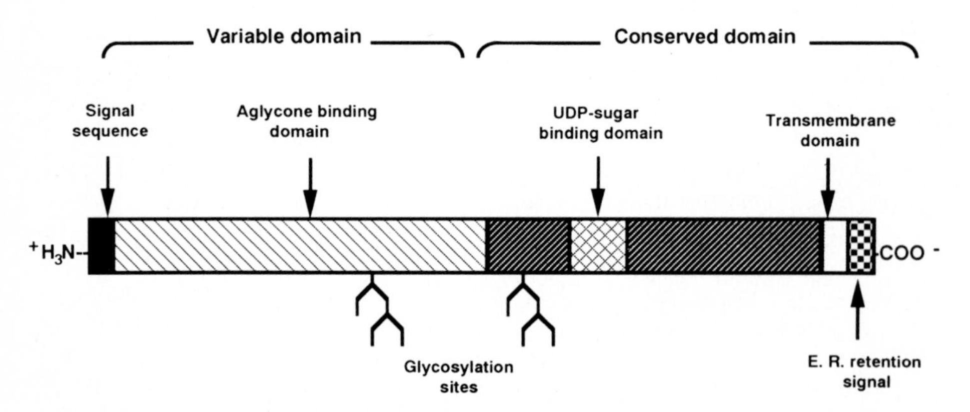

Fig. 5. Functional domains on a linearised uridine diphosphate (*UDP*) glucuronosyltransferase protein map. *E.R.*, endoplasmic reticulum

III. Substrate Specificity of Uridine Diphosphate Glucuronosyltransferase Isoforms

Studies on the substrate specificity of individual UDPGT isoforms has been achieved by either assaying purified UDPGT proteins or whole cell extracts derived from tissue culture cells expressing single UDPGT cDNA clones. For the reasons outlined in the previous section, the latter source is the most attractive, as a comprehensive study of the substrate specificity of a UDPGT isoform isolated by protein purification requires the protein to be isolated in large yields several times by time-consuming and tedious methodologies. The development of eukaryotic vectors that allow the transient or stable expression of individual cDNAs and thus single gene products in tissue culture cells has revolutionised the study of the substrate specificity of UDPGTs. These cell lines can relatively rapidly and easily be prepared, providing a "constant" source of catalytic material in a membrane environment for substrate specificity studies. The current methodology used to prepare stable cell lines in our laboratory is as follows: cDNAs encoding the complete coding sequence of UDPGTs are cloned into the expression vector pCDNAneo and are used to transfect hamster lung fibroblast V79 cells, which are almost devoid of intrinsic UDPGT activity. Next, the cells are selected for geneticin resistance due to the expression of the aminoglycoside phosphotransferase encoded by the vector. Following selection, stable cell lines are grown to approximately 70% confluency, and after harvesting and sonication they are assayed for UDPGT activity either by conventional methods or by the universal thin-layer chromatographic assay described by BANSAL and GESSNER (1980).

1. Rat Uridine Diphosphate Glucuronosyltransferase Isoforms

Examination of the substrate specificity of each of the rat UDPGT isoforms has revealed that they have overlapping substrate specificities. Three different cloned and expressed rat isoforms of 84%–93% similarity in amino acid sequence glucuronidate the 17β-hydroxysteroids, testosterone and dihydroxytestosterone (MACKENZIE 1986a, 1987, 1990b). They may be distinguished by the fact that only one of them can conjugate chloramphenicol and 4-hydroxybiphenyl. The other two may be differentiated by the fact that only one of them has the ability to conjugate β-estradiol (Table 2).

As with the glucuronidation of 17β-hydroxysteroids, bilirubin is also metabolised by more than one UDPGT isoform. Two isoforms have been demonstrated in rat liver (SATO et al. 1990; CLARKE et al. 1992). Of these, only one has been characterised to any extent. CLARKE et al. (1992) found that in addition to bilirubin, this isoform conjugated bilirubin monoglucuronide and a xenobiotic arylalkanoic acid, indicating that this isoform has the potential of forming toxic acylglucuronides. The neurotransmitter 5-hydroxytryptamine appears to be glucuronidated by two isoforms which have a preferential substrate specificity towards phenols (ABE and YUASA 1988; YOKOTA et al. 1988). Only one isoform has been demonstrated to conjugate 3α-hydroxysteroids and 3α,5β-short chain bile acids (FALANY and TEPHLY 1983; MACKENZIE 1986b; RADOMINSKA et al. 1988).

Although all the other UDPGT isoforms glucuronidate at least one endogenous acceptor substrate, no endogenous compound has been found for the planar phenol UDPGT despite extensive studies. This isoform has a strict substrate specificity for xenobiotic planar phenols such as 4-nitrophenol and cannot glucuronidate phenols with bulkier substituents such as 4-propyl phenol (JACKSON et al. 1988).

To date, three rat isoforms have been demonstrated to be involved in carcinogen metabolism. The planar phenol UDPGT glucuronidates oxidation products of the proximate carcinogen benzo(a)pyrene (BP) such as BP-3,6-quinol, 3-hydroxy BP and 7-hydroxy BP (LILIENBLUM et al. 1987; BOCK et al. 1988, 1992). N-Glucuronidation of the carcinogenic aromatic amines α-naphthylamine and β-naphthylamine is catalysed by 3α-hydroxysteroid, 17β-hydroxysteroid and the planar phenal UDPGT (GREEN and TEPHLY 1987). In addition, the 3-hydroxysteroid UDPGT isoform glucuronic acid conjugates the tumour promoter 4-aminobiphenyl (GREEN and TEPHLY 1987).

2. Human Uridine Diphosphate Glucuronosyltransferase Isoforms

Eight human UDPGTs have been characterised to date and as with their rodent counterparts, they also have overlapping substrate specificities. Three human isoforms of 75%–86% amino acid sequence identity that catalyse the glucuronidation of estriol (IRSHAID and TEPHLY 1987; COFFMAN et al. 1990; RITTER et al. 1992a) may be distinguished by the fact that only one of the forms also glucuronidates 4-nitrophenol and 1-naphthylamine. The other two of 86% identity have parallel aglycone specificities for dihydroxy- and trihydroxy-substituted steroid ring structures, including 3,4-catechol oestrogen and hyodeoxycholic acid. They may be distinguished by one of them being a better catalyst than the other (RITTER et al. 1992a).

Recently, three human UGTs which were stably expressed in hamster fibroblasts have been extensively characterised for their substrate specificity towards more than 100 compounds in this laboratory. One of these, UGT1*02 (trivial name UGT-HP4), is extremely promiscuous in that it accepts a diverse range of compounds (WOOSTER et al. 1991; EBNER and BURCHELL 1993). These include non-planar phenols, anthraquinones, flavones, aliphatic alcohols, aromatic carboxylic acids, steroids (4-hydroxyestrone, estrone) and many drugs (see Table 3) of varied structure (EBNER and BURCHELL 1993). This human transferase is apparently a key enzyme in the detoxication of many xenobiotic compounds and drugs. Another isoform, UGT1*1 (trivial name UGT-HP3), which has the primary purpose of conjugating bilirubin (RITTER et al. 1991; SUTHERLAND et al. 1992), is the major human UDPGT responsible for the glucuronidation of the oral contraceptive ethinylestradiol

(EBNER et al. 1993). We have also demonstrated that this isoform has the capacity to glucuronidate phenols, flavones and certain steroids, but in a much restricted spectrum compared with UGT1*02 (trivial name UGT-HP4) (BIN-SENAFI et al., submitted). Another human UDPGT, UGT1*6 (trivial name UGT-HP1), the analogue of the rat planar phenol UDPGT, exhibited a limited substrate specificity for planar phenolic compounds (see Table 3) in contrast to the other human UDPGTs. The coumarin 4-methylumbelliferone, which is a compound that was previously believed to be specific for phenol UDPGTs, is a substrate for most UDPGTs (for references see Tables 2 and 3), indicating its redundancy as a specific substrate for any particular isoform. The effective specificity of individual isoforms towards overlapping substrates in vivo has yet to be determined, but measurement of K_m and V_{max} in vitro may indicate the catalytic potential in vivo.

Table 4 summarises the drug specificity of human UDPGTs. It is noteworthy that isoforms that are able to glucuronidate many of the drugs in Table 1, such as morphine and tertiary amine drugs, have not been discovered yet. It is, therefore, obvious that many more UDPGTs still have to be identified either by purification or cDNA cloning. Thus, it is possible that the UDPGT gene family may be of a similar size to the cytochrome P-

Table 4. Drug glucuronidation by human uridine diphosphate glucuronosyltransferase

Isoform			
Planar phenol UDPGT (UGT1*6)[a]	Complex phenol UDPGT (UGT1*02)[b]	Bilirubin UDPGT (UGT1*1)[c]	Estrogen UDPGT (UGT2B9)[d]
Paracetamol	Propofol[e]	Ethinylestradiol[e]	Clofibrate
	Bumetanide		Valproate
	Ibuprofen		Naproxen
	Ketoprofen		Fenoprofen
	Labetalol		Zomepirac
	Naproxen		
	Propranolol		
	Ethinylestradiol		
	Dapsone		

Gene symbols corresponding to each of the enzymes are given in parenthesis.
Amitryptiline, 3-azido-3-deoxythymidine, carbamazepine, cyproheptadine, chloramphenicol, chlorpheniramine, daunomycin, fenoterol, imipramine, ketotifen, lorazepam, mitoxantrone, (−)-morphine, (+)-morphine, oxazepam, probenecid, rifampicin, temazepam, tetracycline and tripelennamine are not substrates for any of the four enzymes above.

[a] BOCK et al. (1993).
[b] EBNER and BURCHELL (1993).
[c] EBNER et al. (1993).
[d] BURCHELL et al. (unpublished).
[e] The major drug substrate which is glucuronidated at a ten fold greater rate than the other compounds in each column.

450 monooxygenase gene family, which has over 30 members (GONZALEZ 1992).

IV. Structure and Mapping of Uridine Diphosphate Glucuronosyltransferase Gene Loci

The four human UDPGT isoforms that belong to the *UGT1* family share identical C-terminal ends (Table 2 and Sect. D.III). There has been much speculation regarding how such proteins might be biosynthesised (SATO et al. 1990; RITTER et al. 1991; WOOSTER et al. 1991) due to their unusual structure. Recently, RITTER et al. (1992b) have isolated a large gene complex of approximately 95 kb that encodes several *UGT1* family isoforms. Examination of the structure of this complex indicated that it was composed of at least six alternative isoform specific exons, three of which have been identified as those that encode the variable regions of the bilirubin UDPGTs (UGT1*1 and UGT1*4) and the planar phenol (UDPGT1*6). Sequence analysis of the other three exons demonstrated that they have a high degree of homology (>90%) with the bilirubin UDPGT variable UGT1*4 exon. One of these, designated UGT1*2P, has a stop codon at position 65 and was thus a pseudogene. As yet, the function of the other two exons (UGT1*3 and UGT1*5) has not been elucidated. A schematic diagram of the *UGT1* gene complex is shown in Fig. 6. In addition to the variable exon 1 identified by RITTER and colleagues, another specific exon also exists in the *UGT1* gene complex that encodes the bulky phenol UDPGT (UGT1*02; CLARKE et al., in preparation).

Although alternative splicing of a common precursor RNA has been proposed as a mechanism for the generation of the different isoforms in this complex, this scenario is unlikely. Each of the variable exons has recently been found to have TATA boxes and transcriptional start sites (OWENS and RITTER 1992). Thus, a more likely explanation is that each UGT1 transcriptional unit is under the control of its own promoter, thus allowing independent regulation of each isoform at the level of transcription, as has been shown recently for the angiotensin-converting enzyme gene (KUMAR et al. 1991). Such co-ordinated control of gene expression would explain how the

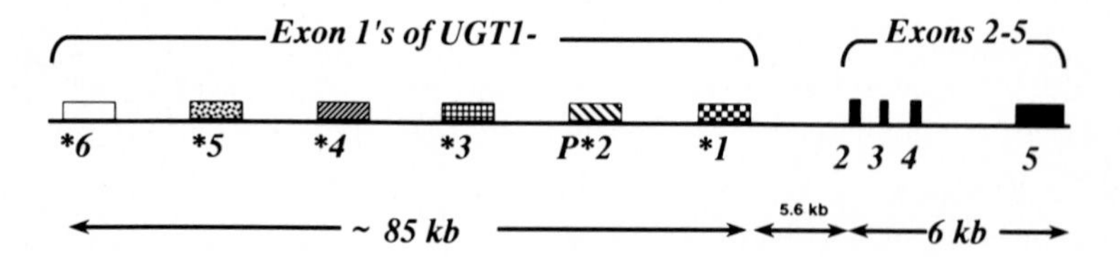

Fig. 6. The *UGT1* gene complex that encodes human bilirubin and phenol uridine diphosphate glucuronosyltransferases. *Black boxes* indicate C-terminal exons; the *patterned boxes*, N-terminal exons; and the *black bar*, introns

different gene products are differentially regulated in tissues (Sect. C.II), at ontogenic periods (Sect. E.I) and by xenobiotics (Sect. E.III).

As well as the *UGT1* gene complex, two rodent *UGT2B* genes that code for chloramphenicol UDPGT and 3α-hydroxysteroid UDPGTs have been cloned (MACKENZIE and RODBOURN 1991; HAQUE et al. 1991). The *UGT2B1* and *UGT2B2* genes both have six exons and are 12 kb and 15 kb in size, respectively (Fig. 7). Interestingly, the sizes of each of the exons of these two genes are remarkably conserved, indicating conservative evolution of genes in this subfamily. Comparison of these *UGT2B* genes and the *UGT1* gene complex indicates that the distribution and size of exons encoding the approximately 240 amino acids at the C terminus of the encoded proteins are very similar. Exons 3–6 of the *UGT2B* genes code for 44, 29, 74 and 91 amino acids, respectively, whereas exons 2–5 of the *UGT1* locus code for 44, 29, 74 and 99 amino acids. In contrast, the approximately 290 amino acids of the variable exon 1 of the *UGT1* complex are encoded by two exons in the *UGT2B* genes. Studies in this laboratory have indicated that a human gene, *UGT2B4*, has a similar structure to the two rat *UGT2B* genes (MONAGHAN et al., in preparation).

Transcriptional start sites of all the *UGT* genes so far characterised have been within 120 bp of their respective ATG translation start codons. In addition, both *UGT2B* genes contain consensus binding sites for the ubiquitous *trans*-acting regulatory protein hepatocyte specific factor 1 within 70 bp of their transcriptional start sites. The *UGT2B1* gene has also several other DNA promoter elements, including the binding site for the transcriptional factor AP-1 and DNA motifs characteristic of liver-specific genes (MACKENZIE and RODBOURN 1991). The ability of the 5′-flanking region of this gene to function as a promoter in cultured cells is both species and tissue specific.

As well as the structural organisation of *UGT* genes, studies have also revealed the chromosomal localisation of these genes. The human *UGT1* gene complex has been assigned to chromosome 2 (HARDING et al. 1990; MOGHRABI et al. 1992), and recent studies in this laboratory have revealed that it is localised to the long arm of this chromosome at 2q37 (CLARKE et

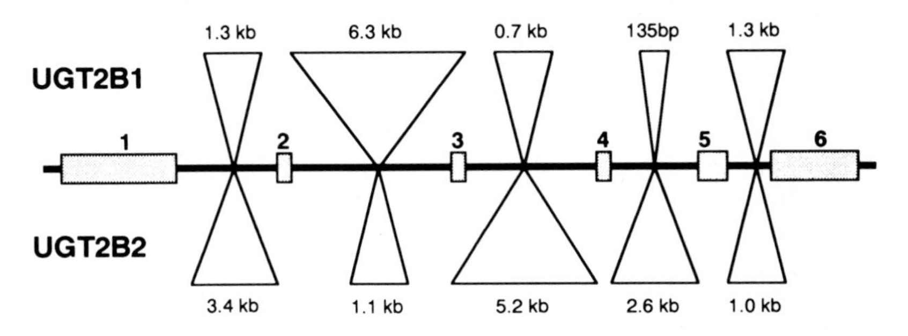

Fig. 7. Rat *UGT2B* family genes. *Shaded boxes* represent exons; the *black bar*, introns

al., in preparation). The human *UGT2B4* gene has recently been assigned to chromosome 4 (MONAGHAN et al. 1992). It is of interest to note that the murine genes encoding the *UGT1* complex and a *UGT2B* gene are present on chromosome 1 (MILES et al. 1991) and chromosome 5 (KRASNEWICH et al. 1987), respectively, which are known to have syntenic regions with the aforementioned human chromosomes (NADEAU and REINER 1989).

E. Factors Affecting Uridine Diphosphate Glucuronosyltransferase Expression

I. Ontogeny

One of the major factors that affects UDPGT expression and hence glucuronidation reactions is ontogeny. Extensive studies on rats have demonstrated that there are three distinct developmental "clusters". The late fetal cluster of UDPGT activities towards simple planar phenols (4-nitrophenol, 2-aminophenol, 1-naphthol) develop immediately prior to birth and surge to maximum levels at about 2 days post partum. After a temporary postnatal decline (SCRAGG et al. 1985), these activities surge again to a second peak at about 1 month, then gradually decrease into adult values by >70 days. In contrast, glucuronidation activity towards a second group of substrates develops immediately after birth and does not exhibit a postnatal decline. This group, termed the neonatal cluster, includes the endogenous compounds bilirubin and testosterone and the drug chloramphenicol. These activities reach a maximum at about 1 month. Finally, a third distinct developmental cluster, the postweaning cluster, develops after weaning (approximately 25 days), when activities towards androsterone (MATSUI and WATANABE 1982) and digitoxigenin monodigitoxoside (WATKINS and KLAASSEN 1985) appear and rise quickly to adult levels.

Immunoblot analysis has recently been used to demonstrate the level of individual enzyme proteins at these different developmental stages in rats. This indicated that phenol UDPGT protein was the only detectable UDPGT in fetal rat liver, whereas bilirubin UDPGT and testosterone UDPGT isoforms appeared postnatally (COUGHTRIE et al. 1988). Recently, the development of two rat steroid UDPGTs has been demonstrated to be regulated at the transcriptional level (HAQUE et al. 1991; MARIE and CRESTEIL 1989).

Development of human UDPGT enzyme activities and proteins have also been investigated. Only one isoform that catalyses the glucuronidation of 5-hydroxytryptamine appears to be present in the fetus at levels comparable to the adult (LEAKEY et al. 1987; COUGHTRIE et al. 1988). The remaining UDPGTs that glucuronidate bilirubin, simple phenols, androsterone and testosterone are present at less than 20% of adult levels in fetal liver (LEAKEY et al. 1987). These activities gradually develop postnatally (LEAKEY et al. 1987; COUGHTRIE et al. 1988).

As well as the in vitro assays of UDPGT activity in human biopsy samples, in vivo studies have revealed that neonates have an inadequacy to glucuronidate bilirubin and several drugs when compared to adult subjects. Unconjugated hyperbilirubinaemia in newborn infants is due to an inadequacy to glucuronidate bilirubin (DONE 1964).

Glucuronidation of chloramphenicol is markedly decreased in neonates (WEISS et al. 1960) and leads to "grey baby" syndrome. The clearance of paracetamol from the body has also been shown to be impaired in neonates, due to a deficiency in paracetamol glucuronidation (LEDERMAN et al. 1983; LEVY et al. 1975; MILLER et al. 1976; ROBERTS et al. 1984). At present the factors that regulate the ontogenic expression of UDPGTs are poorly understood, although corticosteroids (DUTTON 1980) and thyroid hormones (LABRUNE et al. 1992) have been implicated in the developmental surge of phenol and bilirubin UDPGTs after birth.

II. Induction by Xenobiotics

It is well documented that exposure to xenobiotic agents such as drugs and environmental pollutants can result in an increase of certain UDPGT activities. Generally, in the rat, polycyclic aromatic hydrocarbons (e.g., 3-methylcholanthrene, β-naphthoflavone) induce UDPGT activity towards simple phenolic compounds such as 1-naphthol and 4-nitrophenol (BOCK et al. 1973; LILIENBLUM et al. 1982; WATKINS and KLAASSEN 1982), the process being dependent on the Ah receptor as the analogous induction process for the cytochrome P450 1A subfamily (OWENS 1977; NEBERT and GONZALEZ 1985). Phenobarbitol-type compounds increase UDPGT activity towards a number of structurally dieverse compounds, including morphine, chloramphenicol, bilirubin, testosterone and androsterone, to varying degrees (BOCK et al. 1973; LILIENBLUM et al. 1982; WATKINS and KLAASSEN 1982; WATANABE and MATSUI 1984). The steroid-like compound pregnenolone-16α-carbonitrile induces UDPGT activity towards digitoxigenin monodigitoxoside (WATKINS and KLAASSEN 1982). Several arylcarboxylic acids (i.e., clofibrate, fenofibrate) and perfluorodecanoic acid specifically induce the glucuronidation of bilirubin (FOLIOT et al. 1977; LILIENBLUM et al. 1982; FOURNEL et al. 1987; ARAND et al. 1991).

Recently, the development of immunological and nucleic acid probes has allowed the examination of the differential induction of UDPGT isoforms at the molecular level. Several laboratories have shown that the induction of rat phenol UDPGT activity by polycyclic aromatic hydrocarbons was due to an increased de novo synthesis of the enzyme protein (COUGHTRIE et al. 1987; BOCK et al. 1988) resulting from transcriptional activation of the rat phenol *UGT1*06* gene (IYANAGI et al. 1987; HARDING et al. 1989). Similarly, phenobarbital induction of steroid UDPGTs has also been shown to be controlled at this level (MACKENZIE 1986a; JACKSON and BURCHELL 1986; MARIE and CRESTEIL 1989). Following administration of clofibrate bilirubin, UDPGT protein was induced approximately twofold (SCRAGG et al. 1985) due to transcriptional activation of the gene (ROY CHOWDHURY et al. 1991), whereas other UDPGT isoforms were repressed (SCRAGG et al. 1985).

In humans, induction of glucuronidation reactions has also been reported, although it is much less well defined. Polycyclic aromatic hydrocarbons in cigarette smoke induce the glucuronidation of mexiletine (GRECH-BELANGER et al. 1986), paracetamol (BOCK et al. 1987) and propranolol (WALLE et al. 1987), but do not appear to affect the glucuronidation of codeine (ROGERS et al. 1982), clofibric acid (DRAGACCI et al. 1987) or diflusinal (MACDONALD et al. 1990). Indoles present in cruciferous vegetables (brussels sprouts and cabbage) appear to enhance oxazepam and paracetamol glucuronidation modestly (PANTUCK et al. 1984). The anticonvulsant agents phenobarbitone, phenytoin and carbamazepine either separately or in combination induce the glucuronidation of paracetamol (MINERS et al. 1984a; BOCK and BOCK-HENNIG 1987; PRESCOTT et al. 1981). Carbamazepine also induces valproic acid glucuronidation (PANESAR et al. 1989). Co-administration of phenobarbitone and phenytoin induces chloramphenicol glucuronidation (BLOXHAM et al. 1979; POWELL et al. 1981). Several oral contraceptive drugs have been demonstrated to increase the glucuronidation of paracetamol (ABERNETHY et al. 1982; MINERS et al. 1983; MITCHELL et al. 1983), clofibric acid (MINERS et al. 1984b), temazepam (STOEHR et al. 1984), salicylic acid (MINERS et al. 1986), diflusinal (MACDONALD et al. 1990) and phenoprocoumon (MONIG et al. 1990). Rifampicin and sulfinpyazone have also been reported to induce paracetamol glucuronidation (BOCK et al. 1987; MINERS et al. 1984a).

Very recently, the bilirubin UDPGT RNA transcript encoded by the *UGT1*1* gene has been reported to be selectively induced in human livers from patients treated with phenytoin and phenobarbital (SUTHERLAND et al. 1993), indicating a similar induction pattern to that found in rats.

III. Genetic Deficiencies

1. Deficiency of Androsterone Uridine Diphosphate Glucuronosyltransferase

The low androsterone UDPGT phenotype of Wistar rat (MATSUI et al. 1979), which has approximately 2% of the capacity of glucuronidate androsterone compared with normal rats, has been observed in Wistar rat colonies throughout the world (GREEN et al. 1985; CORSER et al. 1987). UDPGT activities towards bilirubin, testosterone, oestradiol, 4-nitrophenol and 2-aminophenol are unaffected by this deficiency (MATSUI et al. 1979; MATSUI and WATANABE 1982; GREEN et al. 1985). The molecular basis for this defect has recently been found to be due to a large deletion in the androsterone UDPGT gene (*UGT2B2*) including exon 1 (CORSER et al. 1987; HOMMA et al. 1992). This results in no androsterone UDPGT mRNA being transcribed (JACKSON and BURCHELL 1986; CORSER et al. 1987) and a corresponding lack of androsterone UDPGT protein (GREEN et al. 1985; MATSUI and NAGAI 1986; CORSER et al. 1987).

2. The Gunn Rat

The Gunn rat, a mutant strain of Wistar rat, is genetically deficient in the conjugation of a number of aglycones including bilirubin, planar and bulky phenols and 5-hydroxytryptamine (GUNN 1938; LATHE and WALKER 1957; BURCHELL 1981), whereas activity to steroid substrates and the drugs morphine, chloramphenicol and valproic acid are normal (WATKINS and KLAASSEN 1982). As a result of their inability to glucuronidate bilirubin, these animals suffer from non-haemolytic unconjugated hyperbilirubinaemia (GUNN 1938; LATHE and WALKER 1957). Molecular analysis of the defect with antibody probes indicated that bilirubin- and phenol-metabolising enzymes of 53–54 kDa were absent in Gunn rats (SCRAGG et al. 1985; COUGHTRIE et al. 1987; CLARKE et al. 1992) and that truncated non-functional versions of these enzymes of approximately 43 kDa were detectable (EL AWADY et al. 1990). This was found to be due to a −1 frameshift mutation which deletes a guanosine residue and introduces an in-frame stop codon in the shared 3′-terminals of RNAs encoding five UGT1 family proteins (IYANAGI et al. 1989; EL AWADY et al. 1990; SATO et al. 1991; ROY CHOWDHURY et al. 1991; IYANAGI 1991).

3. Crigler-Najjar Syndrome

Crigler-Najjar Syndrome is a familial form of severe unconjugated hyperbilirubinaemia caused by a dysfunction in bilirubin glucuronidation in man (CRIGLER and NAJJAR 1952; ROY CHOWDHURY et al. 1989). As a result of the high bilirubin concentrations, infants often develop severe neurological damage from bilirubin encephalopathy (kernicterus) unless treated with phototherapy, plasmapheresis or liver transplantation. Two forms of this syndrome have been identified. Crigler-Najjar syndrome type 1 patients have unconjugated serum bilirubin levels greater than 340 μM, whereas type 2 patients have levels ranging from 60–340 μM. The two subtypes of the disease may also be clinically differentiated by their response to barbiturate therapy (ROY CHOWDHURY et al. 1989). Only patients with type 2 disease respond to phenobarbital administration, their serum bilirubin levels being reduced by approximately 20%–30% as a result (ROY CHOWDHURY et al. 1989; SINAASAPPEL and JANSEN 1991). Recently, analysis of bile aspirates has proved to be a more definitive method of diagnosing the disease type (SINAASAPPEL and JANSEN et al. 1992; CLARKE and BURCHELL, in preparation). The molecular basis of these syndromes has recently been characterised by catalytic, immunochemical and molecular genetic analysis. In vitro analysis of Crigler-Najjar type 1 liver samples has revealed that as well as complete absence of bilirubin UGT activity, these patients also poorly glucuronidate phenols, 5-hydroxytryptamine and the drugs ethinylestradiol and propofol (VAN ES et al. 1990; ROBERTSON et al. 1991; BOSMA et al. 1992a,b; EBNER et al. 1993b; MOGHRABI et al., submitted). In some, but not all patients, this correlates with an absence of anti-UGT immunoreactive polypeptides upon immunoblot analysis (VAN ES et al. 1990; ROBERTSON et al. 1991; BOSMA et al. 1992a,b; MOGHRABI et al., submitted).

Very recently, as a result of the elucidation of the *UGT1* gene complex (Sect. D.IV), several groups have discovered the genetic lesions that cause Crigler-Najjar syndrome type 1. As with the animal model for this syndrome, the Gunn rat, the mutations that result in Crigler-Najjar syndrome type 1 have been found in the exons 2, 3 and 4 encoding the constant region of all UGT1 proteins, thus explaining the decreased activity towards other aglycones as well as bilirubin (BOSMA et al. 1992a,b; RITTER et al. 1992c; MOGHRABI et al., 1993a).

Crigler-Najjar syndrome type 2 is caused by a reduced capacity to glucuronidate bilirubin (ROY CHOWDHURY et al. 1989; ROBERTSON et al. 1991; SINAASAPPEL and JANSEN 1992). The genetic cause of the disease has been identified in three patients which have point mutations causing amino acid substitutions encoded by exon UGT1*1 (BOSMA et al. 1993; MOGHRABI, in preparation) and exon 2 of the gene complex (MOGHRABI et al., 1993b).

4. Gilbert Syndrome

Gilbert syndrome is a benign, mild, unconjugated hyperbilirubinaemia that is found in approximately 5% of the population (GILBERT and LEREBOULLET 1901; ODELL and CHILDS 1980; ROY CHOWDHURY et al. 1989). The disease is characterised by decreased bilirubin diglucuronide and increased levels of bilirubin monoglucuronide in bile as a result of a reduced hepatic bilirubin UGT activity (FEVERY et al. 1977; MACKLON et al. 1979; FEVERY 1981). Also associated with Gilbert syndrome is an apparent decrease in menthol (BECK and KIANI 1960; ARIAS et al. 1969) and acetaminophen (DE MORIAS et al. 1992) glucuronidation. Despite its prevalence in the population and pharmacogenetic consequences, there have been no reports on the molecular basis of Gilbert syndrome to date.

F. Concluding Remarks

The application of molecular biology to the study of glucuronidation has considerably advanced our understanding of the biological mechanisms underlying this important function. Stably expressed cloned UDPGTs have proved to be invaluable tools for studying the substrate specificity of individual isoforms. Such cell cultures should prove to be of great benefit to the pharmaceutical industry as drugs which have cytotoxic glucuronides or are metabolised too rapidly to be of therapeutic value can be identified, chemically modified and improved.

The elucidation of the structure of UDPGT genes has recently led to the elucidation of the genetic lesions that cause hyperbilirubinaemias. In future the identification of *cis* and *trans* elements that regulate UDPGT gene expression will enable us to understand the molecular mechanisms involved in the differential induction, tissue distribution and ontogeny of the different UDPGT isoforms.

Acknowledgements. The studies from our laboratory reported here were supported by the Medical Research Council (UK) and the Wellcome Trust. The authors wish to thank Rosemary Cooper for her expert secretarial assistance in typing this manuscript.

References

Abe N, Yuasa A (1988) Purification and properties of 5-hydroxytryptamine UDP-glucuronyltransferase from rat liver microsomes. J Biochem 104:421–426

Abernethy DR, Divoll M, Ochs HR, Ameer B, Greenblatt DJ (1982) Increased metabolic clearance of acetaminophen with oral contraceptive use. Obstet Gynecol 60:338–341

Adamson RH, Bridges JW, Kibby MR, Walker SR, Williams RT (1970) The fate of sulphadimethoxine in primates compared with other species. Biochem J 118:41–45

Adler TK, Fujimoto JM, Way EL, Baker EM (1955) The metabolic fate of codeine in man. J Pharmacol Exp Ther 114:251–262

Aitio A (1974) UDP-glucuronyltransferase activity in various rat tissues. Int J Biochem 5:325–330

Aitio A (1976) Glucuronide conjugation in the lung. Agents Actions 6:531–533

Alvan G, Siwers B, Vessman J (1977) Pharmacokinetics of oxazepam in healthy volunteers. Acta Pharmacol Toxicol (Copenh) 40 Suppl 1:40–51

Ambrose PJ (1984) Clinical pharmacokinetics of chloramphenicol and chloramphenicol succinate. Clin Pharmacokinet 9:222–238

Arand M, Coughtrie MW, Burchell B, Oesch F, Roberston LW (1991) Selective induction of bilirubin UDP-glucuronosyltransferase by perfluorodecanoic acid. Chem Biol Interact 77:97–105

Arias IM, Gartner LM, Cohen M, Ben Esser J, Levi AJ (1969) Chronic non-haemolytic unconjugated hyperbilirubinaemia with glucuronosyltransferase deficiency. Am J Med 47:395–409

Bansal SK, Gessner T (1980) A unified method for the assay of uridine diphosphoglucuronosyltransferase activities towards various aglycones using uridine diphospho [U-^{14}C] glucuronic acid. Anal Biochem 109:321–329

Beck K, Kiani B (1960) Zur Frage der Glucuronobildung bei der funktionellen Hyperbilirubinamie. Berücksichtigung der fenalen Glucuronid-Clearance. Klin Wochenschr 38:428–433

Benfield P, Ward A, Clark BG, Jue SG (1988) Bromperidol: a preliminary review of its pharmacodynamic and pharmacokinetic properties and therapeutic efficacy in psychoses. Drugs 35:670–684

Berkowitz BA (1976) The relationship of pharmacokinetics to pharmacological activity: morphine, methadone and naloxone. Clin Pharmacokinet 1:219–230

Blanckaert N, Compernolle F, Leroy P, Van Houte R, Fevery J, Heirwegh KPM (1978) The fate of bilirubin-IXa glucuronide in cholestasis and during storage in vitro. Biochem J 171:203–214

Bloxham RA, Durbin GM, Johnson T, Winterborn MH (1979) Chloramphenicol and phenobarbitone – a drug interaction. Arch Dis Child 54:76–77

Blum MR, Liao SHT, Good SS, De Miranda P (1988) Pharmacokinetics and bioavailability of zidovudine in humans. Am J Med 85 Suppl 2A:189–194
Bock KW, Frohling W, Remmer H, Rexer IS (1973) Effects of phenobarbital and 3-methylcholanthrene on substrate specificity of rat liver microsomal UDP-glucuronosyltransferase. Biochim Biophys Acta 327:46–56
Bock KW, Bock-Hennig BS (1987) Differential induction of human liver UDP-glucuronosyltransferase activities by phenobarbital-type inducers. Biochem Pharmacol 36:4137–4144
Bock KW, Schrimer G, Green MD, Tephly TR (1988) Properties of a 3-methylcholanthrene-inducible phenol UDP-glucuronosyltransferase from rat liver. Biochem Pharmacol 37:1439–1443
Bock KW, Wiltfang J, Blume R, Ullrich D, Bircher J (1987) Paracetamol as a test drug to determine glucuronide formation in man. Effects of inducers and of smoking. Eur J Clin Pharmac 31:677–683
Bock KW, Gschaidmeier H, Seidel A, Baird S, Burchell B (1992) Mono- and di-glucuronide formation of chrysene and benzo(a)pyrene phenols by 3-methylcholanthrene-inducible phenol UDP-glucuronosyltransferase (UGT1A1) Mol Pharmacol 42:613–618
Bock KW, Forster A, Gschaidmeier H, Bruck M, Munzel P, Schareck W, Fournel-Gigleux S, Burchell B (1993) Paracetamol glucuronidation by recombinant rat and human phenol UDP-glucuronosyltransferases. Biochem Pharmacol 45: 1809–1814
Bodin N-O (1974) Identification of the major urinary metabolite of alprenolol in man, dog and rat. Life Sci 14:685–692
Bosma PJ, Roy Chowdhury N, Goldhoorn BG, Hofker MH, Oude-Elferink RPJ, Jansen PLM, Roy Chowdhury J (1992a) Sequence of exons and the flanking regions of human bilirubin UDP-glucuronosyl-transferase gene complex and identification of a genetic mutation in a patient with Crigler-Najjar syndrome type I. Hepatology 15:941–947
Bosma PJ, Roy Chowdhury J, Huang TJ, Lahiri P, Oude-Elferink RPJ, Van Es HHG, Lederstein M, Whitington PF, Jansen PLM, Roychowdhury N (1992b) Mechanisms of inherited deficiencies of multiple UDP-glucuronosyltransferase isoforms in two patients with Crigler-Najjar syndrome type I. FASEB J 6:2859–2863
Branch RA, Cothman R, Johnson R, Porter J, Desmond PV, Schenker S (1983) Periportal localisation of lorazepam glucuronidation in the isolated perfused rat liver. J Lab Clin Med 102:805–812
Brashear WT, Kuhnert BR, Wei R (1988) Maternal and neonatal urinary excretion of sulfate and glucuronide ritodrine conjugates. Clin Pharmacol Ther 44:634–641
Brogden RN, Heel RC, Speight TM, Avery S (1977) Alclofenac: a review of its pharmacological properties and therapeutic efficacy in rheutmatoid arthritis and allied rheumatoid disorders. Drugs 14:241–259
Burchell B (1980) Isolation and purification of bilirubin UDP-glucuronyltransferase from rat liver. FEBS Lett 111:131–135
Burchell B (1981) Identification and purification of multiple forms of UDP-glucuronosyltransferase. Rev Biochem Toxicol 3:1–39
Burchell B (1982) Reconstitution of purified Wistar rat liver bilirubin UDP-glucuronyltransferase into Gunn rat liver microsomes. Biochem J 201:567–573
Burchell B (1991) Turning on and turning off the sense of smell. Nature 350:16–17
Burchell B, Blanckaert N (1984) Bilirubin mono- and diglucuronide formation by purified rat liver microsomal bilirubin UDP-glucuronyltransferase. Biochem J 223:461–465
Burchell B, Coughtrie MWH (1989) UDP-glucuronosyltransferases. Pharmacol Ther 43:261–289
Burchell B, Coughtrie MWH, Jackson MR, Shepherd SRP, Harding D, Hume R (1987) Genetic deficiency of bilirubin glucuronidation in rats and humans. Mol Aspects Med 9:429–455

Burchell B, Nebert DW, Nelson DR, Bock KW, Iyanagi T, Jansen PLM, Lancet D, Mulder GJ, Roychowdhury J, Siest G, Tephly TR, Mackenzie PI (1991) The UDP-glucuronosyltransferase gene superfamily: suggested nomenclature based on evolutionary divergence. DNA Cell Biol 10:487–494

Chaudhuri NK, Servando OA, Manniello MJ, Luders RC, Chao DK, Bartlett MF (1976) Metabolism of tripelennamine in man. Drug Metab Dispos 4:372–378

Cheymol G, Cheymol A, Jozefczak C, Lecoq V, Jaillon P (1990) Pharmacokinetic characteristics of bornaprolol in healthy volunteers. Xenobiotica 20:855–860

Chou DKH, Flores S, Jungalwala FB (1991) Expression and regulation of UDP-glucuronate: neolactotetraosylceramide glucuronyltransferase in the nervous system. J Biol Chem 266:17941–17949

√Clarke DJ, George SG, Burchell B (1991) Glucuronidation in fish. Aquat Toxicol 20:35–56

Clarke DJ, Keen JN, Burchell B (1992) Isolation and characterisation of a new hepatic bilirubin UDP-glucuronosyltransferase – absence from Gunn rat liver. FEBS Lett 299:183–186

Coffman BL, Tephly TR, Irshaid YM, Green MD, Smith C, Jackson MR, Wooster R, Burchell B (1990) Characterisation and primary sequence of human hepatic microsomal estriol UDP-glucuronosyltransferase. Arch Biochem Biophys 281:170–175

Cohen AF, Land GS, Breimer DD, Yuen WC, Winton C, Peck AW (1987) Lamotrigine, a new anticonvulsant: pharmacokinetics in normal humans. Clin Pharmacol Ther 42:535–541

Coomes MW, Norsling A, Pohl RJ, Miller D, Fouts JR (1983) Foreign compounds metabolism by isolated skin cells from the hairless mouse. J Pharmacol Exp Ther 225:770–777

Corser RB, Coughtrie MWH, Jackson MR, Burchell B (1987) The molecular basis of the inherited deficiency of androsterone UDP-glucuronyltransferase in Wistar rats. FEBS Lett 213:448–452

Coughrite MWH, Burchell B, Bend JR (1985) Characterisation of rat pulmonary UDP-glucuronyltransferase. Pharmacologist 27:262

Coughtrie MWH, Burchell B, Shepherd IM, Bend JR (1987) Defective induction of phenol glucuronidation by 3-methylcholanthrene in Gunn rats is due to the absence of a specific UDP-glucuronsyltransferase isoenzyme. Mol Pharmacol 31:585–591

Coughtrie MWH, Burchell B, Leakey JEA, Hume R (1988) The inadequacy of perinatal glucuronidation. Mol Pharmacol 34:729–735

Coughtrie MWH, Ask B, Rane A, Burchell B, Hume R (1989) The enantioselective glucuronidation of morphine in rats and humans. Evidence for the involvement of more than one UDP-glucuronosyltransferase isozyme. Biochem Pharmacol 38:3273–3280

Crigler JF, Najjar VA (1952) Congenital familial non-haemolytic jaundice with kernicterus. Paediatrics 10:169–180

Cummings AJ, King ML, Martin BK (1967) A kinetic study of drug elimination: the elimination of paracetamol and its metabolites in man. Br J Pharmacol Chemother 29:150–157

Dahl ML, Nordin C, Bertilsson L (1991) Enantioselective hydroxylation of nortriptyline in human liver microsomes, intestinal homogenate, and patients treated with nortriptyline. Ther Drug Monit 13:189–194

Dahl-Puustinen MJ, Perry TL, Dumont E, von Bahr C, Nordin C, Bertilsson L (1989) Stereoselective disposition of racemic E-10-hydroxynortriptyline in human beings. Clin Pharmacol Ther 45:650–656

Das KK, Basu M, Basu S, Chou DKH, Jungalwala FB (1991) Biosynthesis in vitro of GlcAB1 – 3nLcOse4Cer by a novel glucuronosyltransferase (GlcAT-1) from embryonic chicken brain. J Biol Chem 266:5238–5243

De Morias SMF, Uetrecht JP, Wells PG (1992) Decreased glucuronidation and increased bioactivation of acetaminophen in Gilbert's Syndrome. Gastroenterology 102:577–586
Dickinson RG, Hooper WD, Dunstan PR, Eadie MJ (1989) Urinary excretion of valproate and some metabolites is chronically treated patients. Ther Drug Monit 11:127–133
Dieterle W, Faigle JW, Richter WJ, Theobald W (1975) Biotransformation and pharmacokinetics of sulfinpyrazone (Anturan) in man. Eur J Clin Pharmacol 9:135–145
Dieterle W, Faigle JW, Fruh F, Mory H, Theobald W, Alt KO, Richter WJ (1976) Metabolism of phenylbutazone in man. Arzneimittelforschlung 26:572–577
Doenicke A, Dorowe R, Tauber U (1991) The pharmokinetics of lormetaxepam following cimetidine. Anaesthesis 40:675–679
Done AK (1964) Developmental pharmacology. Clin Pharmacol Ther 5:432–479
Dragacci S, Hamar-Hansen C, Fournel-Gigleux S, Lafaurie C, Magdalou J, Siest G (1987) Comparative study of clofibric acid and bilirubin glucuronidation in human liver microsomes. Biochem Pharmacol 36:3923–3927
Drake RR, Igari Y, Lester R, Elbein AD, Radominska A (1992) Application of 5-azido-UDP-glucose and 5-azido-UDP-glucuronic acid photoaffinity probes for the determination of the active site orientation of microsomal UDP-glucosyltransferases and UDP-glucuronosyltransferases. J Biol Chem 267:11360–11365
Dutton GJ (1980) Glucuronidation of drugs and other compounds. CRC, Boca Raton
Ebner T, Burchell B (1993) Substrate specificities of two stably expressed human liver UDP-glucuronosyltransferases of the UGT1 family. Drug Metab Dispos 21:50–55
Ebner T, Remmel RP, Burchell B (1993) Human bilirubin UDP-glucuronosyltransferase catalyses the glucuronidation of ethinylestradiol. Mol Pharmacol 43: 649–654
Egger H, Bartlett F, Yuan H-P, Karliner J (1982) Metabolism of pirprofen in man, monkey, rat and mouse. Drug Metab Dispos 10:529–536
El Awady M, Roy Chowdhury J, Kesarl K, van Es H, Jansen PLM, Lederstein M, Arias IM, Roy Chowdhury N (1990) Mechanism of the lack of induction of UDP-glucuronsyltransferase activity in Gunn rats by 3-methylcholanthrene. Identification of a truncated enzyme. J Biol Chem 265:10752–10758
Elbein AD (1984) Inhibitors of the biosynthesis and processing of N-linked oligosaccharides. CRC Crit Rev Biochem 16:21–49
El-Mouelhi M, Ruelius HW, Feneslau C, Dulik DM (1987) Species dependent enantioselective glucuronidation of three 2-arylpropionic acids, naproxen, ibuprofen and benoxaprofen. Drug Metab Dispos 15:767–772
Elvin AT, Lalka D, Stoeckel K, Du Souich P, Axelson JE, Golden LH, McLean AJ (1980) Tocainide kinetics and metabolism: effects of phenobarbital and substrates for glucuronyl-transferase. Clin Pharmacol Ther 28:652–658
Falany CN, Tephly TR (1983) Separation, purification and characterisation of three isoenzymes of UDP-glucuronyltransferase from rat liver microsomes. Arch Biochem Biophys 227:248–258
Falany CN, Green MD, Swain E, Tephly TR (1986) Substrate specificity and characterization of rat liver p-nitrophenol, 3α-hydroxysteroid and 17β-hydroxysteroid UDP-glucuronyltransferases. Biochem J 238:65–73
Ferdinandi ES, Cayen MN, Kraml M, Dvornik D (1983) Disposition of etodolac. 2nd World Congress on Clinical Pharmacology and Therapy, Washington, Abstr 81
Fevery J (1981) Pathogenesis of Gilbert's syndrome. Eur J Clin Invest 11:417–418
Fevery J, Blanckaert N, Heirwegh KPM, Preaux AM, Berthelot P (1977) Unconjugated bilirubin and an increased proportion of bilirubin monoconjugates in the

bile of patients with Gilbert's syndrome and Crigler-Najjar disease. J Clin Invest 60:970–979
Fischer LJ, Thien RL, Charkowski D, Darham KJ (1980) Formation and urinary excretion of cyproheptidine in monkeys, chimpanzees and humans. Drug Metab Dispos 8:422–424
Foliot A, Drocourt J-L, Etienne J-P, Housset E, Fiessinger J-N, Christoforov B (1977) Increase in hepatic glucuronidation and clearance of bilirubin in clofibrate-treated rats. Biochem Pharmacol 26:547–549
Fournel S, Magdalou J, Pinon P, Siest G (1987) Differential induction profile of drug metabolising enzymes after treatment with hypolipidaemic agents. Xenobiotica 17:445–457
Fournel-Gigleux S, Jackson MR, Wooster R, Burchell B (1989) Expression of a human liver UDP-glucuronosyltransferase catalysing the glucuronidation of hyodeoxycholic acid in cell culture. FEBS Lett 243:119–122
Fournel-Gigleux S, Sutherland L, Sabolovic N, Burchell B, Siest G (1990) Stable expression of two human UDP-glucuronosyltransferase cDNAs in V79 cell cultures. Mol Pharmacol 39:177–183
Frances B, Gout R, Campistron G, Panconi E, Cros J (1990) Morphine-6-glucuronide is more mu-selective and potent in analgesis tests than morphine. Prog Clin Biol Res 328:477–480
Franson KL, Burchell B, Mathis GA (1990) 17β-Hydroxysteroid UDP-glucuronosyltransferase is expressed in bile ductular epithelial cells under physiological conditions. Biochem Biophys Rec Commun 173:1001–1007
Franz PM, Anliker SL, Callahan JT, DeSante KA, Dhahir PH, Nelson RL, Rubin A (1990) Disposition in humans of racemic picenadol, an opioid analgesic. Drug Metab Dispos 18:968–973
Fraser AD, Bryan W, Isner AF (1991) Urinary screening for alprazolam and its major metabolites by the Abbot ADx and TDx analysers with confirmation by GC/MS. J Anal Toxicol 15:25–29
Gervasi PG, Longo V, Naldi F, Panattoni G, Ursino F (1991) Xenobiotic-metabolising enzymes in human respiratory nasal mucosa. Biochem Pharmacol 41:177–184
Gibby EM, Cohen GM (1984) Conjugation of l-naphthol by human bronchus and bronchoscopy samples. Biochem Pharmacol 33:739–743
Gietl Y, Spahn H, Knauf H, Mutschler E (1990) Single- and multiple-dose pharmacokinetics of R-(−)- and S-(+)-prenylamine in man. Eur J Clin Pharmacol 38:587–593
Gilbert A, Lereboullet P (1901) La cholamie simple familiale. Sem Med 21:241–245
Gonzalez FJ (1992) Molecular genetics of the P-450 superfamily. In: Kalow W (ed) Pharmacogenetics of drug metabolism. Pergamon, New York, pp 413–452
Graham AB, Wood GC (1969) The phospholipid-dependence of UDP-glucuronyltransferase. Biochem Biophys Res Commun 37:567–575
Graham AB, Wood GC (1973) Factors affecting the response of microsomal UDP-glucuronyltransferase to membrane perturbants. Biochim Biophys Acta 311: 45–50
Graham AB, Pechey DT, Toogood KC, Thomas SB, Wood GC (1977) The phospholipid-dependence of uridine diphosphate glucuronosyltransferase: phospholipid depletion and re-activation of guinea pig liver microsomal enzyme. Biochem J 163:117–124
Grech-Belanger O, Gilbert M, Turgeon J, LeBlanc P-L (1985) Effect of cigarette smoking on mexiletine kinetics. Clin Pharmacol Ther 37:638–643
Grech-Belanger O, Turgeon J, Gilbert M (1986) Stereoselective disposition of mexiletine in man. Br J Clin Pharmacol 21:481–487
Green MD, Falany CN, Kirkpatrick RB, Tephly TR (1985) Strain differences in purified rat hepatic 3α-hydroxysteroid UDP-glucuronosyltransferase. Biochem J 230:496–534

Green MD, Tephly TR (1987) N-Glucuronidation of carcinogenic aromatic amines catalysed by rat hepatic microsomal preparations and purified rat liver uridine 5′-diphosphate-glucuronosyltransferases. Cancer Res 47:2028–2031
Green MD, Tephly TR (1989) N-Glycosylation of purified rat and rabbit hepatic UDP-glucuronosyltransferase. Arch Biochem Biophys 273:72–78
Greenblatt DJ, Allen MD, Locniskar A, Harmatz JS, Shader RI (1979) Lorazepam kinetics in the elderly. Clin Pharmacol Ther 26:103–113
Gunn CH (1938) Hereditary alcoholuric jaundice. J Hered 29:137–139
Haque SJ, Petersen DD, Nebert DW, MacKenzie PI (1991) Isolation, sequence and developmental expression of rat UGT2B2: the gene encoding a constitutive UDP-glucuronosyltransferase that metabolises etiocholanolone and androsterone. DNA Cell Biol 10:515–524
Harding D, Wilson SM, Jackson MR, Burchell B, Green MD, Tephly TR (1987) Nucleotide and deduced amino acid sequence of rat liver 17β-hydroxy steroid UDP-glucuronosyltransferase. Nucleic Acids Res 15:3936
Harding D, Fournel-Gigleux S, Jackson MR, Burchell B (1988) Cloning and substrate specificity of a human phenol UDP-glucuronosyltransferase expressed in COS-7 cells. Proc Natl Acad Sci USA 85:8381–8385
Harding D, Jackson MR, Corser R, Burchell B (1989) Phenol UDP-glucuronosyltransferase deficiency in Gunn rats: mRNA levels are considerably reduced. Biochem Pharmacol 38:1013–1017
Harding D, Jeremiah SJ, Povey S, Burchell B (1990) Chromosomal mapping of a human phenol UDP-glucuronosyltransferase GNT1. Ann Hum Genet 54:17–21
Hayball PJ, Nation RL, Bochner F (1992) Stereoselective interactions of ketoprofen glucuronides with human plasma protein and serum albumin. Biochem Pharmacol 44:291–299
Hays MT, Hsu L (1988) Equilibrium dialysis of plasma binding of thyroxine, triiodothyronine and other glucuronide and sulphate conjugates in human and cat plasma. Endocr Res 14:51–58
Hazelton A, Klaassen CD (1988) UDP-glucuronosyltransferase activity towards digitoxigenin-monodigitoxoside. Differences in activation and induction properties in rat and mouse liver. Drug Metab Dispos 16:30–36
Hjelle JT, Hazelton GA, Klaasen CD, Hjelle JJ (1986) Glucuronidation and sulphation in rabbit kidney. J Pharmacol Ther 236:150–156
Hochman Y, Zakim D, Vessey DA (1981) A kinetic mechanism for modulation of the activity of microsomal UDP-glucuronosyltransferase by phospholipids. J Biol Chem 256:4783–4788
Hoffman K-J, Renberg J, Baarnhielm C (1984) Stereoselective disposition of RS-tocainide in man. Eur J Drug Metab Pharmacokinet 9:215–222
Homma H, Kawai H, Kubota M, Matsui M (1992) Large deletion of androsterone UDP-glucuronosyltransferase gene in the inherited deficient strain of Wistar rats. Biochim Biophys Acta 1138:34–40
Houin G, Thebault JJ, D'Athis P, Tillement J-P, Beaumont J-L (1975) A glc method for the estimation of chlorophenoxyisobutyric acid in plasma. Pharmacokinetics of a single oral dose of clofibrate in man. Eur J Clin Pharmacol 8:433–437
Hucker HB, Stauffer SC, Balletto AJ, White SD, Zacchei AG, Arison BH (1978) Physiological disposition and metabolism of cyclobenzaprine in the rat, dog, rhesus monkey and man. Drug Metab Dispos 6:659–672
Hundle BS, O'Brien DA, Alberti M, Beyer P, Hearst JE (1992) Functional expression of zeaxanthin glucosyltransferase from Erwinal herbicola and a proposed uridine diphosphate binding site. Proc Natl Acad Sci USA 89:9321–9325
Illing PHA, Wilson ID (1981) pH dependent formation of beta-glucuronidase resistant conjugates from the biosynthetic ester glucuronide of isoxepac. Biochem Pharmacol 30:3381–3384
Irshaid YM, Tephly TR (1987) Isolation and purification of two human liver UDP-glucuronosyltransferases. Mol Pharmacol 31:27–34

Irshaid YM, Radominska A, Ziminak P, Ziminak Z, Lester R, Tephly T (1991) Glucuronidation of monohydroxylated short chain bile acids by human liver microsomes and purified human liver UDP-glucuronosyltransferases. Drug Metab Dispos 19:173–176

Iyanagi T (1991) Molecular basis of multiple UDP-glucuronsyltransferase isoenzyme deficiencies in the hyperbilirubinemic rat (Gunn rat). J Biol Chem 266:24048–24052

Iyanagi T, Haniv M, Sagawa K, Fujii-Kuriyama Y, Watanabe S, Shively JE, Anan KF (1986) Cloning and characterisation of cDNA encoding 3-methylcholanthrene-inducible rat mRNA for UDP-glucuronosyltransferase. J Biol Chem 261:15607–15614

Iyanagi T, Watanage T, Uchiyama Y (1989) The 3-methylcholanthrene-inducible UDP-glucuronosyltransferase deficiency in the hyperbilirubinaemic rat (Gunn rat) is caused by a −1 frameshift mutation. J Biol Chem 264:21304–21307

Jackson MR, Burchell B (1986) The full length coding sequence of rat liver androsterone UDP-glucuronosyltransferase cDNA and comparison with other members of this gene family. Nucleic Acids Res 14:779–795

Jackson MR, Nilsson T, Peterson PA (1990) Identification of a consensus motif for retention of transmembrane proteins in the endoplasmic reticulum. EMBO J 9:3153–3162

Jackson MR, Fournel-Gigleux S, Harding D, Burchell B (1988) Examination of the substrate specificity of cloned rat kidney phenol UDP-glucuronosyltransferase expressed in COS-7 cells. Mol Pharmacol 34:638–642

Jackson MR, McCarthy LR, Corser RB, Barr GC, Burchell B (1985) Cloning of cDNAs coding for rat hepatic microsomal UDP-glucuronyltransferases. Gene 34:147–153

Jackson MR, McCarthy LR, Harding D, Wilson S, Coughtrie MWH, Burchell B (1987) Cloning of a human liver microsomal UDP-glucuronosyltransferase cDNA. Biochem J 242:581–588

Jansen PLM, Mulder GJ, Burchell B, Bock KW (1992) New developments in glucuronidation research: report of a workshop on glucuronidation – it's role in health and disease. Hepatology 15:532–544

Janssen FW, Jusko WJ, Chiang ST, Kirkman SK, Southgate PJ, Coleman AJ, Ruelius HW (1980) Metabolism and kinetics of oxaprozin in normal subjects. Clin Pharmacol Ther 27:352–362

Kimura T, Owens IS (1987) Mouse UDP-glucuronosyltransferase-cDNA and complete amino acid sequence and regulation. Eur J Biochem 168:515–521

Knapp SA, Green MD, Tephly TR, Baron J (1988) Immunohistochemical demonstration of isozyme- and strain-specific differences in the intralobular localizations and distributions of UDP-glucuronosyltransferases in livers of untreated rats. Mol Pharmacol 33:14–21

Kontoghiorghes GJ, Goddard JG, Bartlett AN, Sheppard L (1990) Pharmacokinetic studies in humans with the oral iron chelator 1,2-dimethyl-3-hydroxypyrid-4-one. Clin Pharmacol Ther 48:255–261

Koster A, Schirmer G, Bock KW (1986) Immunochemical and functional characterisation of UDP-glucuronosyltransferase from rat liver, intestine and kidney. Biochem Pharmacol 35:3971–3975

Krasnewich D, Kozak CA, Nebert DW, MacKenzie PI (1987) Localisation of UDP-glucuronosyltransferase gene(s) on mouse chromosome 5. Somatic Cell Mol Genet 13:179–182

Kumar RS, Thekkumkara TJ, Sen GC (1991) The mRNAs encoding the two angiotensin-converting isozymes are transcribed from the same gene by a tissue specific choice of alternative transcription initiation sites. J Biol Chem 266: 3854–3862

Labrune P, Myara A, Huguet P, Foliot A, Vial M, Trivin F, Odievre M (1992) Bilirubin UDP-glucuronosyltransferase hepatic activity in jaundice associated with congenital hypothyroidism. J Pediatr Gastroenterol Nutr 14:79–82

Lambert JGD, Resink JW (1991) Steroid glucuronides as male pheromones in the reproduction of the African catfish Clarias Gariepinus – a brief review. J Steriod Biochem Mol Biol 40:549–556

Lathe GH, Walker M (1957) An enzymatic defect in human neonatal jaundice and in Gunn's strain of jaundiced rats. Biochem J 67:9P

Lazard D, Tal N, Rubinstein M, Khen M, Lancet D, Zupko K (1990) Identification and biochemical analysis of novel olfactory-specific cytochrome P-450IIA and UDP-glucuronosyltransferase. Biochemistry 29:7433–7440

Lazard D, Zupko K, Poira Y, Nef P, Lazarovits J, Horn S, Khen M, Lancet D (1991) Odorant signal termination by olfactory UDP-glucuronosyltransferase. Nature 349:790–793

Leakey JEA, Hume R, Burchell B (1987) Development of multiple activities of UDP-glucuronosyltransferase in human liver. Biochem J 245:859–861

Le Bigot JF, Begue JM, Kiechel JR, Guillouzo A (1987) Species differences in the metabolism of ketotifen in rat, rabbit and man: demonstration of similar pathways in vivo and in cultured hepatocytes. Life Sci 40:883–890

Lederman S, Fysh WJ, Tredger M, Gamsu HR (1983) Neonatal paracetamol poisoning. Treatment by exchange transfusion. Arch Dis Child 58:631–633

Levy G, Matsuzawza T (1967) Pharmacokinetics of salicylamide formation in man. J Pharmacol Exp Ther 156:285–293

Levy G, Tsuchiya T, Amsel LP (1972) Limited capacity for salicyl glucuronide and its effect on the kinetics of salicylate elimination in man. Clin Pharmacol Ther 13:258–268

Levy G, Khanna NN, Soda DM, Tsuzuki O, Stern L (1975) Pharmacokinetics of acetominophen in the human neonate: formation of acetaminophen glucuronide and sulphate in relation to plasma bilirubin concentration and D-glucaric acid excretion. Pediatrics 55:818–825

Lilienblum W, Walli AK, Bock KW (1982) Differential induction of rat liver microsomal UDP-glucuronosyltransferase activities by various inducing agents. Biochem Pharmacol 31:907–913

Lilienblum W, Platt KL, Schrimer G, Oesch F, Bock KW (1987) Regioselectivity of rat liver microsomal UDP-glucuronosyltransferase activities towards phenols of benzo(*a*)pyrene and dibenz(*a,h*)anthracene. Mol Pharmacol 32:173–177

Loewen GR, Herman RJ, Ross SG, Verbeeck RK (1988) Effect of dose on the glucuronidation and sulphation kinetics of diflunisal in man: single dose studies. Br J Clin Pharmacol 26:31–39

Longo V, Mazzaccaro A, Naldi F, Gervasi PG (1991) Drug-metabolising enzymes in liver, olfactory, and respiratory epithelium of cattle. J Biochem Toxicol 6: 123–128

Longo V, Mazzaccaro A, Ventura P, Gervasi PG (1992) Drug-metabolizing enzymes is respiratory nasal mucosa and liver of Cynomolgus monkey. Xenobiotica 22:427–431

Lucier GW, McDaniel OS (1977) Steroid and non-steroid UDP-glucuronosyltransferase: glucuronidation of synthetic estrogens as steroids. J Steroid Biochem 8:867–872

MacDonald JI, Herman RJ, Verbeeck RK (1990) Sex-difference and the effects of smoking and oral contraceptive steroids on the kinetics of diflunisal. Eur J Clin Pharmacol 38:175–179

Mackenzie PI (1986a) Rat liver UDP-glucuronosyltransferase. Sequence and expression of a cDNA encoding a phenobarbital-inducible form. J Biol Chem 261: 6119–6125

Mackenzie PI (1986b) Rat liver UDP-glucuronosyltransferase. cDNA sequence and expression of a form glucuronidating 3-hydroxyandrogens. J Biol Chem 261: 14112–14117

Mackenzie PI (1987) Rat liver UDP-glucuronyltransferase. Identification of cDNA encoding two enzymes which glucuronidate testosterone, dihydrotestosterone and β-estradiol. J Biol Chem. 262:9744–9749

Mackenzie PI (1990a) Expression of chimeric cDNAs in cell culture defines a region of UDP-glucuronosyltransferase involved in substrate selection. J Biol Chem 265:3432–3435

Mackenzie PI (1990b) The cDNA sequence and expression of a variant 17B hydroxysteroid UDP glucuronosyltransferase. J Biol Chem 265:8699–8703

Mackenzie PI (1990c) The effect of N-linked glycosylation on the substrate preferences of UDP-glucuronosyltransferases. Biochem Biophys Res Commun 166: 1293–1299

Mackenzie PI, Rodbourn L (1990) Organisation of the rat UDP-glucuronosyltransferase UDPGTr-2 gene and organisation of its promoter. J Biol Chem 265: 11328–11332

Mackenzie PI, Gonzalez FJ, Owens IS (1984) Cloning and characterisation of DNA complementary to rat liver UDP-glucuronosyltransferase. J Biol Chem 259: 12153–12160

Macklon AF, Savage RL, Rawlins MD (1979) Gilbert's syndrome and drug metabolism. Clin Pharmacokinet 4:223–232

Magdalou J, Herber R, Bidault R, Siest G (1992) In vitro N-glucuronidation of a novel antiepileptic drug, lamotrigine by human liver microsomes. J Pharmacol Exp Ther 260:1166–1173

Marie S, Cresteil T (1989) Phenobarbital-inducible gene expression in developing rat liver: relationship to hepatocyte function. Biochem Biophys Acta 1009:221–228

Marschall HU, Matern H, Egestad B, Matern S, Sjovall S (1987) 6-alpha-glucuronidation of hyodeoxycholic acid by human liver, kidney and small bowel microsomes. Biochim Biophys Acta 921:392–397

Martin LE, Hopkins R, Bland R (1976) Metabolism of labetalol by animals and man. Br J Clin Pharmacol 3:695–710

Matern S, Matern H, Farthmann EH, Gerok W (1984) Hepatic and extrahepatic glucuronidation of bile acids in man. Characterisation of bile acid uridine 5′-diphosphate-glucuronosyltransferase in hepatic, renal and intestinal microsomes. J Clin Investig 74:402–410

Matern H, Lappas N, Matern S (1991) Isolation and characterisation of hyodeoxycholic acid: UDP-glucuronosyltransferase from human liver. Eur J Biochem 200:393–400

Matsui M, Nagai F (1986) Genetic deficiency of androsterone UDP-glucuronosyltransferase activity in Wistar rats is due to the loss of enzyme protein. Biochem J 234:139–144

Matsui M, Watanabe HK (1982) Developmental alteration of hepatic UDP-glucuronosyltransferase and sulphotransferase towards androsterone and 4-nitrophenol in Wistar rats. Biochem J 204:441–447

Matsui M, Nagai F, Aoyagi S (1979) Strain differences in rat liver UDP-glucuronyltransferase activity towards androsterone. Biochem J 179:483–457

Meyers M, Slikker W, Vore M (1981) Steroid D-ring glucuronides: characterisation of a new class of cholestatic agents in the rat. J Pharmacol Exp Ther 218:63–73

Miles JS, Moss JE, Taylor BA, Burchell B, Wolf CR (1991) Mapping genes encoding drug metabolising enzymes in recombinant inbred mice. Genomics 11: 309–316

Miller RP, Roberts RJ, Fischer LJ (1976) Acetaminophen elimination kinetics in neonates, children and adults. Clin Pharmacol Ther 19:284–294

Miners JO, Attwood J, Birkett DJ (1983) Influence of sex and oral contraceptive steroids on paracetamol metabolism. Br J Clin Pharmacol 16:503–509

Miners JO, Attwood J, Birkett DJ (1984a) Determinants of acetaminophen metabolism: effect of inducers and inhibitors of drug metabolism on acetaminophen's metabolic pathways. Clin Pharmacol Ther 35:480–486

Miners JO, Robson RA, Birkett D (1984b) Gender and oral contraceptive steroids as determinants of drug glucuronidation: effects on clofibric acid elimination. Br J Clin Pharmacol 18:240–243

Miners JO, Grgurinovich N, Whitehead AG, Robson RA, Birkett DJ (1986) Influence of gender and oral contraceptive steroids on the metabolism of salicylic acid and acetylsalicylic acid. Br J Clin Pharmacol 22:359–362
Mitchell MC, Hanew T, Meredith CG, Schenker S (1983) Effects of oral contraceptive steroids on acetaminophen metabolism and elimination. Clin Pharmacol Ther 34:48–53
Mitchell MC, Hamilton R, Wacker L, Branch RA (1989) Zonal distribution of paracetamol glucuronidation in the isolated perfused rat liver. Xenobiotica 19:389–400
Moghrabi N, Sutherland L, Wooster R, Povey S, Boxer M, Burchell B (1992) Chromosome assignment of human phenol and bilirubin UDP-glucuronosyltransferase genes (UGT1A subfamily). Ann Hum Genet 56:83–93
Moghrabi N, Clarke DJ, Burchell B, Boxer M (1993a) Cosegregation of intragenic markers with a novel mutation that causes Crigler-Najjar syndrome type 1: Implication in carrier detection and prenatal diagnosis. Am J Hum Genet 53:722–729
Moghrabi N, Clarke DJ, Boxer M, Burchell B (1993b) Identification of an A-to-G missense mutation in exon 2 of the *UGT1* gene complex that causes Crigler-Najjar Syndrome type 2. Genomics 18:171–173
Monaghan G, Povey S, Burchell B, Boxer M (1992) Localization of a bile acid UDP-glucuronosyltransferase gene (UGT2B) to chromosome 4 using the polymerase chain reaction. Genomics 13:908–909
Monig H, Baese C, Heidemann HT, Ohnhaus EE, Schulte HM (1990) Effect of oral contraceptive steroids on the pharmacokinetics of phenprocoumon. Br J Clin Pharmacol 30:115–118
Mori Y, Kuroda M, Sakai Y, Yokyoa F, Toyoshi K, Baba S (1985) Species differences in the metabolism of suprofen in laboratory animals and man. Drug Metab Dispos 13:239–245
Morris RG, Kotasek D, Paltridge G (1991) Disposition of epirubicin and metabolites with repeated courses to cancer patients. Eur J Clin Pharmacol 40:481–487
Mroszczak EJ, Lee JW, Combs D, Sarnquist FH, Huang BL, Wu AT, Tokes LG, Maddox ML, Cho DK (1987) Ketorolac trimethamine absorption, distribution, metabolism, excretion and pharmacokinetics in animals and humans. Drug Metab Dispos 15:618–626
Murray GR, Whiffen GM, Franklin RA, Henry JA (1989) Quantitative aspects of the urinary excretion of meptazinol and its metabolites in human volunteers. Xenobiotica 19:669–675
Nadeau JH, Reiner AH (1989) Linkage and synteny homologies in mouse and man. In: Lyon MF, Searle AG (eds) Genetic variants and strains of the laboratory mouse, vol 2. Oxford University Press, London, pp 506–536
Nebert DW, Gonzalez F (1985) Autoregulation plus upstream positive and negative control regions associated with transcriptional activation of the mouse P1-450 gene. Nucleic Acids Res 13:7269–7288
Neugebauer G, Neubert P (1991) Metabolism of carvedilol in man. Eur J Drug Metab Pharmacokinet 16:257–260
Nilsson T, Jackson M, Peterson PA (1989) Short cytoplasmic sequences serve as retention signals for transmembrane proteins in the endoplasmic reticulum. Cell 58:707–718
Odell GB, Childs B (1980) Hereditary hyperbilirubinaemias. Prog Med Genet 4:103–134
Oelschlager H, Kohl C, Armstrong DW, Rothley D (1991) The pharmokinetics of antilipemic agents 8. Unequivocal characterisation of ciprofibrate-O-beta-d-glucuronide. Arch Pharm (Weinheim) 324:505–508
Oka S, Terayama K, Kawashima C, Kawaski T (1992) A novel glucuronosyltransferase in nervous system presumably associated with the biosynthesis of HNK-1 carbohydrate epitope on glycoproteins. J Biol Chem 267:22711–22714

O'Neill PJ, Yorgey KA, Renzi NL, Williams RL, Benet LZ (1982) Disposition of zomepirac sodium in man. J Clin Pharmacol 22:470–476
O'Reilly DR, Miller LK (1989) A baculovirus blocks insect molting by producing ecdysteroid UDP-glucosyl transferase. Science 245:1110–1112
Osborne R, Joel S, Trew D, Slevin M (1990) Morphine and metabolite behaviour after different routes of morphine administration: demonstration of the importance of the active metabolite morphine-6-glucuronide. Clin Pharmacol Ther 47:12–19
Owens IS (1977) Genetic regulation of UDP-glucuronosyltransferase induction by polycyclic aromatic compounds in mice. J Biol Chem 252:2827–2833
Owens IS, Ritter JK (1992) The novel bilirubin/phenol UDP-glucuronosyltransferase UGT1 gene locus: implications for multiple non-hemolytic familial hyperbilirubinaemia phenotypes. Pharmacogenetics 2:93–108
Pacifici GM, Franchi M, Bencini C, Repetti F, Di Lascio N, Muraro GB (1988) Tissue distribution of drug-metabolising enzymes in humans. Xenobiotica 18: 849–856
Panesar SK, Orr JM, Farrell K, Burton RW, Kassahun K, Abbott FS (1989) The effect of carbamazepine on valproic acid disposition in adult volunteers. Br J Clin Pharmacol 27:322–328
Pantuck EJ, Pantuck CB, Anderson KE, Wattenburg LW, Conney AH, Kappas A (1984) Effect of brussels sprouts on drug conjugation. Clin Pharmacol Ther 35:161–169
Parquet M, Pessah M, Sacquet E, Salvat C, Raizman A (1988) Effective glucuronidation of 6α-hydroxylated bile acids by human hepatic and renal microsomes. Eur J Biochem 171:329–334
Pasternak GW, Bodnar RJ, Clark JA, Inturrisi CE (1987) Morphine-6-glucuronide, a potent MU agonist. Life Sci 41:2845–2849
Paul D, Standifer KM, Inturrisi CE, Pasternak GW (1989) Pharmacological characterisation of morphine-6-β-glucuronide, a very potent morphine metabolite. J Pharmacol Exp Ther 251:477–483
Paul H, Illing A, Wilson ID (1981) pH dependent formation of beta-glucuronidase resistant conjugates from the biosynthetic ester glucuronide of isoxepac. Biochem Pharmac 30:3381–3384
Peters WHM, Jansen PLM (1988) Immuno-characterisation of UDP-glucuronosyltransferase isoenzymes in human liver, intestine and kidney. Biochem Pharmacol 37:564–567
Pham MA, Magdalou J, Totis D, Fournel-Gigleux S, Siest G, Hammock BD (1989) Characterization of distinct forms of cytochrome P-450, epoxide metabolising enzymes and UDP-glucuronosyltransferases in rat skin. Biochem Pharmacol 38:2187–2194
Porter CC, Arison BH, Gruber VF, Titus DC, Vandenheuvel WJA (1975) Human metabolism of cyproheptadine. Drug Metab Dispos 3:189–197
Portmann GA, McChesney EW, Stander H, Moore WE (1966) Pharmacokinetic model for nalidixic acid in man. II. Parameters for absorption, metabolism and elimination. J Pharm Sci 55:72–78
Pottier J, Berlin D, Raynaud JP (1977) Pharmacokinetics of the anti-inflammatory tiaprofenic acid in humans, mice, rats, rabbits and dogs. J Pharm Sci 66:1030–1036
Powell DA, Nahata MC, Durrell DC, Glazer JP, Hilty MD (1981) Interactions among chloramphenicol, phenytoin and phenobarbitol in a pediatric patient. J Pediatr 98:1001–1003
Prescott LF, Critchley JAJH, Balali-Mood M, Pentland B (1981) Effects of microsomal enzyme induction on paracetamol metabolism in man. Br J Clin Pharmacol 12:149–153
Puig JF, Tephly TR (1986) Isolation and purification of rat liver morphine UDP-glucuronosyltransferase. Mol Pharmacol 33:97–101

Radominska A, Green MD, Zimniak P, Lester R, Tephly TR (1988) Biosynthesis of hydroxy-linked glucuronides of short-chain bile acids by rat liver 3-hydroxysteroid UDP-glucuronosyltransferase. Lipid Res 29:501–508
Ralston EJ, English JJ, Dooner HK (1988) Sequence of three bronze alleles of maize and correlation with the genetic fine structure. Genetics 119:185–197
Riess W, Huerzeler H, Raschdorf F (1974) The metabolites of oxprenolol (Trasicor) in man. Xenobiotica 4:365–373
Ritter JK, Sheen YY, Owens IS (1990) Cloning and expression of human liver UDP glucuronosyltransferase in COS-1 cells. 3,4-Catechol estrogens and estriol as primary substrates. J Biol Chem 265:7900–7906
Ritter JK, Crawford JM, Owens IS (1991) Cloning of two human liver bilirubin UDP-glucuronosyltransferase cDNA's with expression in COS-1 cells. J Biol Chem 266:1043–1047
Ritter JK, Fan C, Yhun YS, Lubet RA, Owens IS (1992a) Two human liver cDNAs encode UDP-glucuronosyltransferase with 2 log differences in activity toward parallel substrates including hyodeoxycholic acid and certain estrogen derivatives. Biochemistry 31:3409–3414
Ritter JK, Chen F, Sheen YY, Tran HM, Kimura S, Yeatman MT, Owens IS (1992b) A novel complex locus UGT1 encodes human bilirubin, phenol and other UDP-glucuronosyltransferase isoenzymes with identical carboxyl termini. J Biol Chem 267:3257–3261
Ritter JK, Yeatman MT, Ferreira P, Owens IS (1992c) Identification of a genetic alteration in the code for bilirubin UDP-glucuronosyltransferase in the UGT1 gene complex of a Crigler-Najjar type I patient. J Clin Invest 90:150–155
Roberts I, Robinson MJ, Mughal MZ, Ratcliffe JG, Prescott LF (1984) Paracetamol metabolites in the neonate following maternal overdose. Br J Clin Pharmacol 18:201–206
Robertson KJ, Clarke D, Sutherland L, Wooster R, Coughtrie MWH, Burchell B (1991) Investigation of the molecular basis of the genetic deficiency of UDP-glucuronosyltransferase in Crigler-Najjar syndrome. J Inherited Metab Dis 14:563–579
Rogers JF, Findlay JWA, Hull JH, Butz RF, Jones EC, Bustrack JA, Welch RM (1982) Codeine disposition in smokers and nonsmokers. Clin Pharmacol Ther 32:218–227
Roy Chowdhury J, Novikoff P, Roy Chowdhury N, Novikoff AB (1985) Distribution of UDP-glucuronosyltransferase in rat tissue. Proc Natl Acad Sci USA 82: 2990–2994
Roy Chowdhury J, Roy Chowdhury N, Falany CN, Tephly TR, Arias IM (1986) Isolation and characterisation of multiple forms of rat liver UDP-glucuronate glucuronosyltransferase. Biochem J 233:827–837
Roy Chowdhury J, Wolkoff AW, Arias IM (1989) Hereditary jaundice and disorders of bilirubin metabolism. In: Scriver CR, Beaudet AL, Sly WS, Valle D (eds) The metabolic basis of inherited disease, 6th edn. McGraw-Hill, New York, pp 1085–1094
Roy Chowdhury J, Huang T, Kesari K, Lederstein M, Arias IM, Roy Chowdhury N (1991) Molecular basis for the lack of bilirubin–specific and 3-methylcholanthrene – inducible UDP-glucuronosyltransferase activities in Gunn rats. J Biol Chem 266:18294–18298
Rubin A, Warrick P, Wolen RL, Ridolfo AS, Gruber CM (1972) The metabolism of fenoprofen in man. Clin Pharmacol Ther 13:151
Rush GF, Newton JF, Hook JB (1983) Sex differences in the excretion of glucuronide conjugates: the role of intrarenal glucuronidation. J Pharmacol Exp Ther 227: 658–662
Rush WR, Hall DJ, Graham DJ, Selby IA (1992) The metabolism of imiloxan hydrochloride in healthy male volunteers. Xenobiotica 22:237–246
Sabatini DD, Kreibich G, Morimoto T, Adesnik M (1982) Mechanisms for the incorporation of proteins into membranes and organelles. J Cell Biol 92:1–22

Samuel SA (1981) Apparent anaphylactic reaction to zomepirac (Zomax). N Engl J Med 304:978
Sani BP, Barua AB, Hill DL, Shih TW, Olson JA (1992) Retinoyl β-glucuronide: lack of binding to receptor proteins of retinioc acid as related to biological activity. Biochem Pharmacol 43:919–922
Sato H, Koiwai O, Tanabe K, Kashiwamata S (1990) Isolation and sequencing of rat liver bilirubin UDP-glucuronosyltransferase cDNA: possible alternate splicing of a common primary transcript. Biochem Biophys Res Commun 169:260–264
Sato H, Aono S, Kashiwamata S, Koiwai O (1991) Genetic defect of bilirubin UDP-glucuronosyltransferase in the hyperbilirubinaemic Gunn rat. Biochem Biophys Res Commun 177:1161–1164
Scatina JA, Lockhead SR, Cayen MN, Sisenwine SF (1991) Metabolic disposition of enciprazine, a non-benzodiazepine anxiolytic drug, in rat, dog and man. Xenobiotica 21:1591–1604
Scragg IM, Celier C, Burchell B (1985) Congenital jaundice in rats due to the absence of hepatic bilirubin UDP-glucuronosyltransferase enzyme protein. FEBS Lett 183:37–42
Schwartz HJ (1979) Pharmacokinetics and metabolism of temazepam in man and several animal species. Br J Clin Pharmacol 8:23S–29S
Schwenk M (1989) Glucuronidation and sulfation in the gastrointestinal tract. Prog Pharmacol Clin Pharmacol 7:153–169
Seideman P, Ericsson N, Groningsson K, Von Bahr C (1981) Effect of pentobarbital on the formation of diastereomeric oxazepam glucuronides in man: analysis by high performance liquid chromatography. Acta Pharmacol Toxic (Copenh) 49:200–204
Shepherd SRP, Baird SJ, Hallinan T, Burchell B (1989) An investigation of the transverse topology of bilirubin UDP-glucuronosyltransferase in rat endoplasmic reticulum. Biochem J 259:617–620
Simons PJ, Cockshott ID, Douglas EJ, Gordon EA, Hopkins K, Rowland M (1988) Disposition in male volunteers of a subanaesthetic intravenous dose of an oil in water emulsion of 14C-propofol. Xenobiotica 18:429–440
Sinaasappel M, Jansen PLM (1991) The differential diagnosis of Crigler-Najjar disease, types 1 and 2, by bile pigment analysis. Gastroenterology 100:783–789
Singh OMP, Graham AB, Wood GC (1981) The phospholipid-dependence of UDP-glucuronosyltransferase. Purification, delipidation and reconstitution of microsomal enzyme from guinea pig liver. Eur J Biochem 116:311–316
Sisenwine SF, Liu AL, Tio C, Kimmell H, Freeland G (1986) The metabolic disposition of 14C-ciramadol in humans. Xenobiotica 16:335–340
Slikker W Jr, Vore M, Bailey JR, Meyers M, Montgomery C (1983) Hepatotoxic effects of estradiol-17-B-D-glucuronide in the rat and monkey. J Pharmacol Exp Ther 225:138–143
Smith GL, Goulbourn RA, Burt RAP, Chatfield DH (1990) Preliminary studies of absorption and excretion of benoxaprofen in man. Br J Clin Pharmacol 4:585–590
Someya T, Shibasaki M, Noguchi T, Takahashi S, Inaba T (1992) Haloperidol metabolism in psychiatric patients: importance of glucuronidation and carbonyl reduction. J Clin Psychopharmacol 12:169–174
Spahn H, Spahn I, Benet LZ (1989) Probenecid-induced changes in the clearance of carprofen enantiomers: a preliminary study. Clin Pharmacol Ther 45:500–505
Spahn-Langguth H, Benet LZ (1992) Acyl glucuronides revisited: is the glucuronidation process a toxification as well as a detoxification mechanism? Drug Metab Rev 24:5–48
Stoehr GP, Kroboth PD, Juhl RP, Wender DB, Phillips JP, Smith RB (1984) Effect of oral contraceptives on triazolam, temazepam, alprazolam and lorazepam kinetics. Clin Pharmacol Ther 36:683–690

Styczynski PB, Green M, Puig J, Coffman B, Tephly TR (1991) Purification and properties of a rat liver phenobarbital-inducible 4-hydroxybiphenyl UDP-glucuronosyltransferase. Mol Pharmacol 40:80–84
Styczynski PB, Green MD, Coffman B, Tephly TR (1992) Studies on tertiary amine UDP-glucuronosyltransferase from human and rabbit hepatic microsomes. Drug Metab Dispos 20:896–901
Sutherland L, bin-Senafi S, Ebner T, Clarke DJ, Burchell B (1992) Characterisation of a human bilirubin UDP-glucuronosyltransferase stably expressed in hamster lung fibroblast cell cultures. FEBS Lett 308:161–164
Sutherland L, Ebner T, Burchell B (1993) The expression of UDP-glucuronosyltransferases of the UGT1 family in human liver and kidney and in response to drugs. Biochem Pharmacol 45:295–301
Tanaka M, Ono K, Hakusui H, Takegoshi T, Watanabe Y, Kanao M (1990) Identification of DP-1904 and its ester glucuronide in urine and determination of their enantiomeric compositions. Drug Metab Dispos 18:698–703
Taskinen J, Wikberg T, Ottoila P, Kanner L, Lotta T, Pippuri A, Backstrom R (1991) Identification of major metabolites of the catechol-O-methyltransferase-inhibitor nitecapone in human urine. Drug Metab Dispos 19:178–183
Tephly TR, Burchell B (1990) UDP-Glucuronosyltransferases: a family of detoxifying enzymes. Trends Pharmacol Sci 11:276–279
Tephly TR, Townsend M, Coffman B, Puig J, Green M (1988) Characterisation of UDP-glucuronosyltransferases from animal and human liver. In: Siest G, Magdalou J, Burchell B (eds) Molecular and cellular aspects of glucuronidation, vol 173. Eds. Libbey, Montrouge, pp 37–42
Thomassin J, Tephly TR (1990) Photoaffinity labelling of rat liver microsomal morphine UDP-glucuronosyltransferase by [3H] flunitrazepam. Mol Pharmacol 38:294–298
Toghrol F, Kimura T, Owens IS (1990) Expression of UDP-glucuronosyltransferase cDNA in Saccharomyces cerevisiae as a membrane-bound and as a cytosolic form. Biochemistry 29:2349–2356
Toon S, Heimark LD, Trager WF, O'Reilly RA (1985) The metabolic fate of phenprocoumon in man. J Pharm Sci 74:1037–1040
Tukey RH, Billings RE, Autor AP, Tephly TR (1979) Phospholipid-dependence of oestrone UDP-glucuronosyltransferase and p-nitrophenol UDP-glucuronosyltransferase. Biochem J 179:59–65
Upton RA, Buskin JN, Williams RL, Holford NGH, Riegelman S (1980) Negligible excretion of unchanged ketoprofen, naproxen and probenecid in urine. J Pharm Sci 69:1254–1257
Vandel B, Sandoz M, Vandel S, Volmat R (1982) Biotransformation of amitriptyline in depressive patients: urinary excretion of seven metabolites. Eur J Clin Pharmac 22:239–245
Van Es HHG, Goldhoorn BG, Paul-Abrahamse M, Oude Elferink RPJ, Jansen PLM (1990) Immunochemical analysis of uridine diphosphate-glucuronosyltransferase in four patients with the Crigler-Najjar syndrome type I. J Clin Invest 85:1199–1205
Van Hecken A, Verbesselt R, Tjandra-Maga TB, De Schepper PJ (1989) Pharmacokinetic interaction between indomethacin and diflunisal. Eur J Clin Pharmacol 36:507–512
Vanstapel F, Blanckaert N (1988) Topology and regulation of bilirubin UDP-glucuronyltransferase in sealed native microsomes from rat liver. Arch Biochem Biophys 263:216–225
Verpooten GA, Genissel PM, Thomas JR, De Broe ME (1991) Single dose pharmacokinetics of perindopril and its metabolites in hypertensive patients with various degrees of renal insufficiency. Br J Clin Pharmacol 32:187–192
Von Meyernick L, Coffman BL, Green MD, Kirkpatrick RB, Schmoldt A, Tephly TR (1985) Separation, purification and characterisation of digitoxigenin mono-

digitoxoside UDP-glucuronosyltransferase activity. Drug Metab Dispos 13: 700–704
Vore M, Slikker W (1985) Steroid D-ring glucuronides: a new class of cholestatic agents. TIPS 6:256–259
Vore M, Hadd H, Slikker W Jr (1983) Ethinylestradiol-17β-D-ring glucuronide conjugates are potent cholestatic agents in the rat. Life Sci 32:2989–2993
Vree TB, Benenken Kolmer EW, Hekster YA (1991) Pharmacokinetics, N1-glucuronidation and N4-acetylation of sulfamethomidine in humans. Pharm Weekbl [Sci] 13:198–206
Wahlstrom A, Persson K, Rane A (1989) Metabolic interaction between morphine and naloxone in human liver – a common pathway of glucuronidation? Drug Metab Dispos 17:218–220
Waldmeier F, Kaiser G, Ackermann R, Faigle JW, Wagner J, Barner A, Lasseter KC (1991) The disposition of [14C]-labelled benadzepril HCl in normal adult volunteers after single and repeated oral dose. Xenobiotica 21:251–256
Walle T, Walle UK, Cowart TD, Conradi EC, Gaffney TE (1987) Selective induction of propranolol metabolism by smoking. Additional effects on renal clearance of metabolities. J Pharmacol Exp Ther 241:928–933
Walle T, Webb J, Bagwell EE, Walle UK, Daniell HB, Gaffney TE (1988) Stereoselective delivery and actions of beta receptor antagonists. Biochem Pharmacol 37:115–124
Walls CM, Gray A, Vose LW, Robinson Y, Lopez N, Brownshill RD, Steiner JA (1988) Disposition of bemitradine, a renal vasodilator and diuretic, in man. Xenobiotica 18:1413–1423
Watanabe HK, Matsui M (1984) Effects of steroid hormones and xenobiotics on the pubertal development of UDP-glucuronosyltransferase activities towards androsterone and 4-nitrophenol in Wistar rats. Biochem J 222:321–326
Watkins JB, Klaassen CD (1982) Induction of UDP-glucuronosyltransferase activities in Gunn, heterozygous and Wistar rat livers by pregnenolone-16α-carbonitrile. Drug Metab Dispos 10:590–594
Watkins JB, Klaassen CD (1985) Development of UDP-glucuronosyltransferase activity towards digitoxigenin monodigitoxoside in neonatal rats. Drug Metab Dispos 13:186–191
Weatherill PJ, Burchell B (1980) Purification and separation of testosterone and oestrone UDP-glucuronyltransferase activities. Biochem J 189:377–380
Weil A, Caldwell J, Strolin-Benedetti M (1990) The metabolism and disposition of 14C-fenofibrate in human volunteers. Drug Metab Dispos 18:115–120
Weiss CF, Glazko AJ, Weston JK (1960) Chloramphenicol in the newborn infant. A physiologic explanation of its toxicity when given in excessive doses. N Engl J Med 262:787–794
Wooster R, Sutherland L, Ebner T, Clarke D, Da Cruz e Silva O, Burchell B (1991) Cloning and stable expression of a new member of the human liver phenol/bilirubin: UDP-glucuronosyltransferase cDNA family. Biochem J 278: 456–469
Yamaguchi H, Kubo J, Sekine K, Naruchi T, Hashimoto Y, Kato R (1979) Metabolites of feprazone in man. Drug Metab Dispos 7:340–344
Yokota H, Yuasa A, Sato R (1988) Purification and properties of a form of UDP-glucuronosyltransferase from liver microsomes of 3-methylcholanthrene-treated rats. J Biochem 104:531–536
Yokota H, Yuasa A, Sato R (1992) Topological disposition of UDP-glucuronosyltransferase in rat liver microsomes. J Biochem 112:192–196

CHAPTER 2

Sulfotransferase Enzymes

R. WEINSHILBOUM and D. OTTERNESS

A. Introduction

Sulfate conjugation is an important pathway in the biotransformation of many drugs, xenobiotic compounds, neurotransmitters, and hormones. Sulfation increases the water solubility of most compounds and, therefore, their renal excretion. It also usually results in a decrease in biological activity, but, in some cases, sulfate conjugation is required to "activate" drugs such as the antihypertensive medication minoxidil (JOHNSON et al. 1982; MEISHERI et al. 1988). It can also play a role in the bioactivation of procarcinogens (WATABE et al. 1982). Even though sulfation was discovered by BAUMANN (1876) over a century ago, only within the past 30 years has the enzymology of this important reaction been studied in detail. One important step in that process was the development of accurate assays for the measurement of the activities of sulfotransferase (ST) enzymes, followed by characterization of the reactions catalyzed by those enzymes in tissue preparations. Simultaneously, attempts were made to separate and purify ST enzymes to make it possible to characterize the molecular species that catalyzed specific reactions. Unfortunately, overlap in substrate specificities of these enzymes has led to confusion with regard to their number and properties. That confusion has been compounded by the existence of at least two broad streams of ST research, one involving the biotransformation of drugs and xenobiotic compounds and the other involving the sulfation of hormones, especially steroid hormones. These two fields have developed in parallel, but they have also frequently developed in isolation. That fact has often made it difficult to determine whether pharmacologists and endocrinologists were describing the same or different enzymes. The problem was further exacerbated by the adoption of different systems of enzyme nomenclature by individual laboratories. The end result has been that as more and more has been learned about ST enzymes, the field has become increasingly difficult to follow, even for those directly involved. That sequence of events is not unique to sulfation research, but is merely a recapitulation of the history of studies performed with other families of drug metabolizing enzymes, e.g., the cytochromes P450 and the glucuronosyltransferases. Recently, application of the techniques of molecular biology has resulted in the molecular cloning, sequencing, and in vitro expression of cDNAs for several

ST enzymes. The cloning of ST cDNAs offers hope that a simple nomenclature can be developed that will help investigators to communicate and to organize information about these enzymes. As the subject of ST enzymes has been reviewed several times during the past two decades (DODGSON and ROSE 1970; DODGSON 1977; JAKOBY et al. 1980; ROY 1981; SINGER 1985; WEINSHILBOUM 1986a,b; MULDER and JAKOBY 1990; FALANY 1991), the present chapter will focus on newer information and on placing the results of older studies within the context of more recent observations.

Previous reviews have classified ST enzymes on the basis of their substrate specificities or the general nature of the reactions that they catalyzed, e.g., *O*-sulfation, *N*-sulfation, or *S*-sulfation (JAKOBY et al. 1980; SINGER 1985; MULDER and JAKOBY 1990). Included among the broad classes of compounds that can undergo *O*-sulfation catalyzed by cytoplasmic enzymes are "simple" phenols such as 4-nitrophenol, phenolic catecholamine neurotransmitters such as dopamine, phenolic steroids such as the estrogens, nonphenolic hydroxysteroids such as dehydroepiandrosterone (DHEA), and, in plants, flavonols such as quercetin. Examples of substrates for each of these reactions are shown in Fig. 1. The figure indicates the usual sites of sulfate conjugation for each compound as well as the fact that compounds such as quercetin can undergo sulfation at multiple points, in this case at the 3 and at the 3′ or 4′ positions (VARIN and IBRAHIM 1989). Figure 1 also indicates that the N-sulfation of arylamines such as 2-naphthylamine can occur (HERNÁNDEZ et al. 1991), but the nature of the enzyme(s) that catalyze this reaction remains a subject of controversy. The compounds shown in Fig. 1 were chosen both for illustrative purposes and, as described subsequently, because each of them has been used as a prototypic substrate for a class of ST enzymes. Finally, it should be emphasized that although the subsequent review will deal only with the cytoplasmic ST enzymes that play an important role in pharmacology, membrane-bound STs also exist. Included among this class of enzymes are the *trans* Golgi tyrosyl protein ST that catalyzes the post-translational modification of several biologically active peptides and proteins (HUTTNER 1982), the Golgi complex-associated *N*-heparan sulfate ST (HASHIMOTO et al. 1992), and a galactolipid ST that is also localized in the Golgi complex (SAKAI et al. 1992). The relationship among these enzymes as well as the relationship between the cytoplasmic and membrane-bound ST enzymes is unclear; the subsequent discussion will thus deal only with the cytoplasmic ST enzymes that catalyze the sulfation of drugs, xenobiotic compounds, hormones, bile acids, and neurotransmitters.

Before describing the ST enzymes themselves, it is necessary to discuss briefly the cosubstrate for the reaction, 3′-phosphoadenosine-5′-phosphosulfate (PAPS) (Fig. 2). PAPS is synthesized from inorganic sulfate and adenosine triphosphate (ATP) in a two-step enzymatic process (DODGSON and ROSE 1970; JAKOBY et al. 1980; SINGER 1985). The enzymes which catalyze the formation of PAPS are sulfate adenylyltransferase (EC 2.7.7.4), also referred to as ATP sulfurylase, and adenylylsulfate kinase (EC

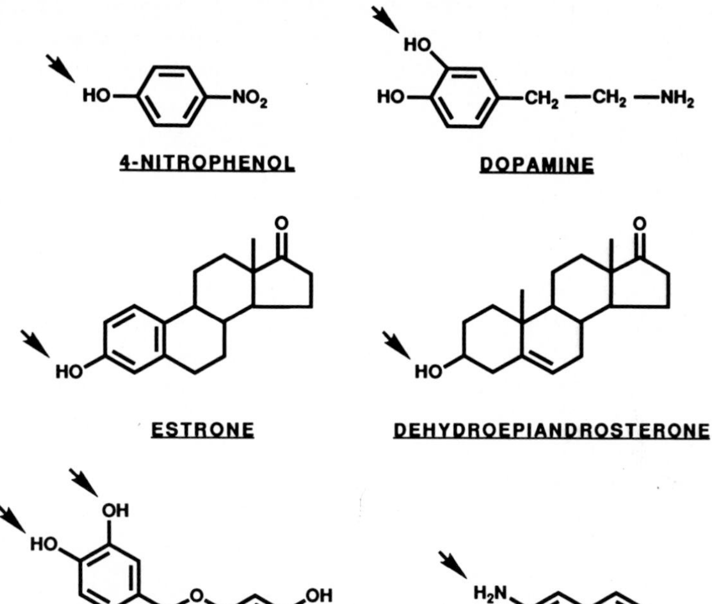

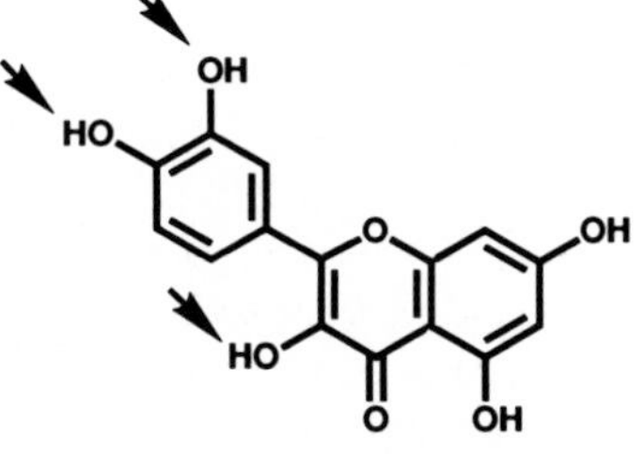

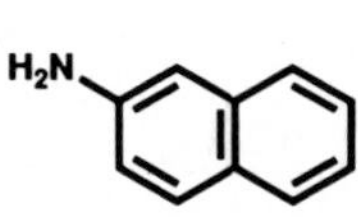

Fig. 1. Selected cytoplasmic sulfotransferase enzyme sulfate acceptor substrates. *Arrows* indicate sites of sulfate conjugation

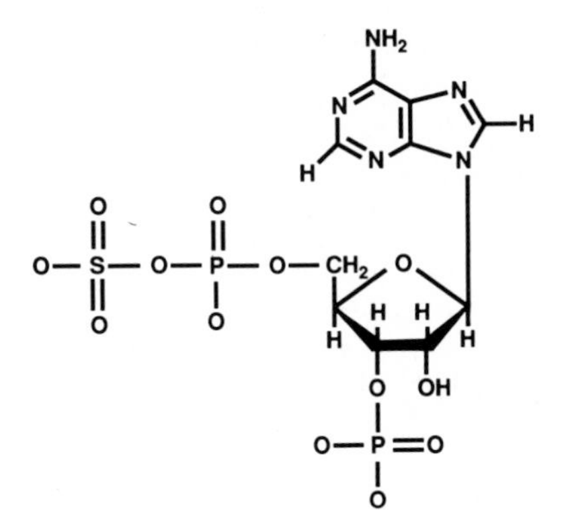

Fig. 2. Structure of 3′-phosphoadenosine-5′-phosphosulfate

2.7.1.25), or adenosine 5′-phosphosulfate (APS) kinase (Fig. 3). The reaction catalyzed by sulfate adenylyltransferase results in the formation of APS from ATP and inorganic sulfate. The subsequent reaction catalyzed by adenylylsulfate kinase results in the formation of PAPS from APS and a second molecule of ATP (Fig. 3). Although concentrations of ATP in tissues are usually adequate for these reactions, under certain circumstances the concentration of inorganic sulfate may be limiting. Therefore, sulfate conjugation may be regulated, at least in part, by limited availability of PAPS as a result of a relative lack of inorganic sulfate (MULDER and KRIJGSHELD 1981; LEVY 1986; MULDER and JAKOBY 1990). As will be discussed subsequently when assays for the measurement of ST enzyme activities are described, the availability of highly purified PAPS played a critical role in making it possible to assay accurately the activities of cytoplasmic ST enzymes.

B. Classification of Sulfotransferase Enzymes

I. Introduction

ST enzyme classification schemes have most often been based on substrate specificities. Therefore, some authors have classified these enzymes as phenol (aryl) STs (PSTs), hydroxysteroid (alcohol) STs (HSSTs), or arylamine STs (MULDER and JAKOBY 1990). Other classifications further subdivided STs so that enzymes which catalyzed the sulfate conjugation of phenolic hydroxyl groups on steroid hormones such as estrone were regarded as separate from other phenol STs (SINGER 1985). All of these enzymes are included within the International Union of Biochemistry nomenclature category of sulfotransferases, EC 2.8.2 (NOMENCLATURE COMMITTEE OF THE INTERNATIONAL UNION OF BIOCHEMISTRY 1984). Unfortunately, since the sulfation of many substrates can be catalyzed by more than one enzyme, it is often difficult to compare results reported by one laboratory with those from another group of investigators or to determine whether the two laboratories have studied the same enzyme. Ultimately, the only way in which to dispel

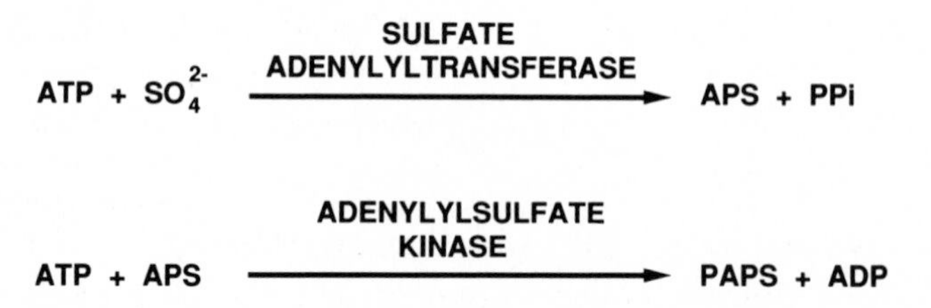

Fig. 3. Synthesis of 3′-phosphoadenosine-5′-phosphosulfate. *ATP*, adenosine 5′-triphosphate; *APS*, adenosine 5′-phosphosulfate; ADP, adenosine 5′-diphosphate

such uncertainty would be to determine the primary sequence of each ST enzyme. As a result of the cloning of cDNAs for cytoplasmic ST enzymes from both animals and plants, that information is becoming available. Sequence data obtained from cDNAs may make it possible to begin to develop an unambiguous scheme for the classification of these enzymes, just as similar studies of the molecular biology of the cytochromes P450 have made it possible to classify those enzymes (NEBERT et al. 1991). However, before a preliminary classification of cytoplasmic ST enzymes based on cDNA sequences is described, the current status of the classification of these enzymes for the two most intensively studied vertebrate species, humans and rats, will be described.

II. Human Sulfotransferase Enzyme Classification

Human tissues contain at least three separate, well-characterized cytoplasmic ST enzymes. These enzymes differ with regard to their substrate specificities, inhibitor sensitivities, thermal stabilities, and regulation, i.e., their levels of activity are regulated independently. Two of these enzymes are PSTs, whereas the other is an HSST. One form of PST is thermostable (TS), catalyzes the sulfate conjugation of micromolar concentrations of 4-nitrophenol and other "simple" phenols, and is sensitive to inhibition by 2,6-dichloro-4-nitrophenol (DCNP). The other form of PST in human tissue is thermolabile (TL), catalyzes the sulfate conjugation of micromolar concentrations of dopamine and other catechol or phenolic monoamines, and is relatively resistant to inhibition by DCNP (REIN et al. 1981, 1982; REITER and WEINSHILBOUM 1982a; REITER et al. 1983; YOUNG et al. 1984; CAMPBELL et al. 1987a; SUNDARAM et al. 1989a). The third cytosolic ST enzyme in human tissue that has been thoroughly characterized catalyzes the sulfation of DHEA as well as other steroid hormones and bile acids, has a thermal stability intermediate to those of TS and TL PST, and is resistant to inhibition by DCNP (FALANY et al. 1989; HERNÁNDEZ et al. 1992). The general characteristics of these three enzymes are listed in Table 1, and differences in their thermal stabilities and inhibition by DCNP in preparations of human liver, an organ in which all three enzymes are expressed, are depicted graphically in Fig. 4. These three enzymes can be separated physically and purified by the use of chromatographic techniques, and, as discussed below, cDNAs for two of them have been cloned and expressed. Unfortunately, there is overlap in the substrate specificities of these three enzymes, since millimolar concentrations of 4-nitrophenol and other phenols can serve as substrates for TL PST (REITER et al. 1983; SUNDARAM et al. 1989a), millimolar concentrations of dopamine can serve as a substrate for TS PST (CAMPBELL et al. 1987a), and both DHEA ST and TS PST can catalyze the sulfation of estrogen hormones (FALANY et al. 1989; HERNÁNDEZ et al. 1992). TS PST has also been referred to as the "phenolic" or "P" form of PST, while TL PST has also been referred to as the "monoamine" or

Table 1. General characteristics of the three well-characterized human tissue cytoplasmic sulfotransferase enzymes

	Enzyme		
	TS or P PST	TL or M PST	DHEA ST
Substrates	"Simple" phenols	Phenolic monoamines	Hydroxysteroids
Prototypic substrate	4-Nitrophenol	Dopamine	DHEA
Thermal stability	Stable	Labile	Intermediate
DCNP inhibition	Sensitive	Resistant	Resistant

DCNP, 2,6-dichloro-4-nitrophenol; TS, thermostable; P, phenolic; PST, phenol sulfotransferase; TL, thermolabile; M, monoamine; DHEA, dehydroepiandrosterone; ST, sulfotransferase.

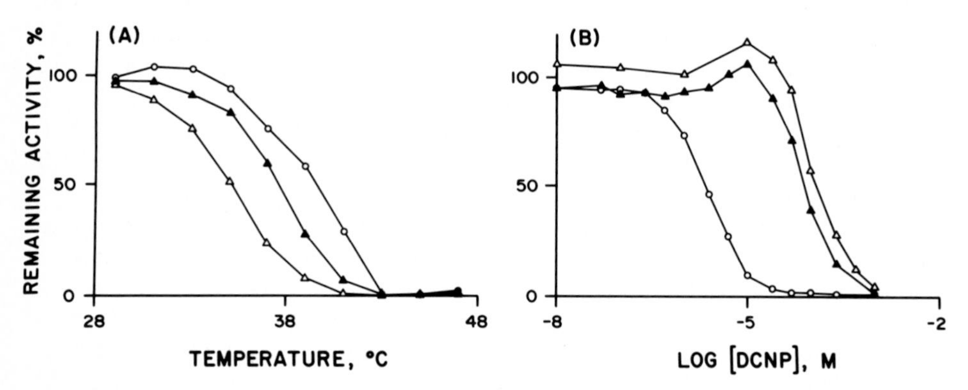

Fig. 4A,B. Human liver sulfotransferase (ST) enzymes. **A** Thermal inactivation by preincubation for 15 min at the temperatures indicated; **B** inhibition by 2,6-dichloro-4-nitrophenol. ○, Thermostable PST; △, thermolabile PST; ▲, DHEAST. Details of experimental procedures have been described by HERNÁNDEZ et al. (1992)

"M" form (REIN et al. 1982). However, because of the overlap in their substrate specificities, these two enzymes will be referred to subsequently as the TS and TL forms of PST on the basis of their unequivocal differences in thermal stability. The HSST present in human tissue has usually been referred to as DHEA ST (FALANY et al. 1989; HERNÁNDEZ et al. 1992; OTTERNESS et al. 1992).

III. Rat Sulfotransferase Enzyme Classification

Classification of cytosolic ST enzymes in rat tissue is less clear-cut than is that of ST enzymes in human tissue. One approach that has been used to study and to classify these enzymes is chromatographic separation of different activities, most often by anion exchange chromatography, followed by purification and bichemical characterization. However, different groups of investigators have tended to use only a single substrate or a single class of substrates during enzyme purification, making it difficult to compare results among laboratories. For example, rat liver appears to contain several cytoplasmic aryl or phenol STs. These enzymes were initially named on the basis of their sequential elution from an ion exchange column as aryl STs I, II, III, and IV (SEKURA and JAKOBY 1979, 1981). Form III is very labile, so it has never been fully characterized (JAKOBY et al. 1980; SEKURA and JAKOBY 1979). Subsequently, on the basis of substrate specificity, form IV has also been referred to as rat liver tyrosine methyl ester ST, while peaks I and II have been regarded as isoforms that can each catalyze the sulfation of simple phenols such as 4-nitrophenol (MULDER and JAKOBY 1990). Rat liver also contains at least three HSST activities which can catalyze the sulfation of DHEA and other primary or secondary alcohols (SINGER 1985). Although this situation is complex, it is probably manageable until the results of studies of rat liver glucocorticoid STs (three separate peaks of activity by ion exchange chromatography), mineralocorticoid ST (at least one additional peak separate from the glucocorticoid ST peaks), estrone ST, and estradiol-17β ST are considered (SINGER 1985). One review of this area of research included a table that listed the characteristics of sixteen different rat liver ST "activities" (SINGER 1985). However, the author of the review was unable to determine how many of these activities might represent the same enzyme studied with different substrates. This confusing situation emphasizes the need for a simple, specific, and unambiguous method for the classification of ST enzymes, and recent results obtained by cloning cDNAs for these enzymes offer hope that this goal might be achieved.

IV. Molecular Classification of Sulfotransferase Enzymes

At the time of this review, cDNAs for 11 eukaryotic ST enzymes have been cloned. These cDNAs appear to fall into four large groups on the basis of the amino acid sequences of their encoded proteins. Because of the diverse nomenclature for ST enzymes used by different laboratories, for purposes of this review the species from which each cDNA was cloned is indicated by a small letter or letters in which "h" represents human, "r" rat, "gp" guinea pig, "b" bovine, and "fc" *Flaveria chloraefolia*. The names of the enzymes are abbreviated PST, EST (for estrogen ST), HSST, FST (for flavonol ST), and SMP (for senescence marker protein). The reason for the inclusion of the SMP designation will be discussed below. Alignment of the amino acid sequences for these 11 enzymes (Fig. 5) shows many areas of sequence homology, including at least two long, very highly conserved regions, one located toward the amino terminus between the positions in the multiple alignment numbered 67 and 74, and the other located toward the carboxy terminus between the positions numbered 291 and 303. The conserved

```
          1                                                  50
hTSPST    .......... ........ME LIQDTSRPPL EYVKGVPL.. IKYFAEALGP
rPST      .......... ........ME F....SRPPL VHVKGIPL.. IKYFAETIGP
rEST      .......... ........ME TSMPEYYDVF GDFHGFLM.. DKRFTKYWED
bEST      .......... ........MS SSKPSFSDYF GKLGGIPM.. YKKFIEQFHN
gpEST     .......... .......MMD SSEHDYYEYF DEFRGILL.. YKQFIKYYDN
hDHEAST   .......... .......... .....MSDDF LWFEGIAFPT MGFRSETLRK
rHSST1    .......... .......... ......MPDY TWFEGIPFHA FGISKETLQN
rHSST2    .......... .......... ......MPDY TWFEGIPFPA FGIPKETLQN
rSMP2     .......... .......... .....MMSDY NWFEGIPFPA ISYQREILED
fcFST3    .......... MEDIIKTLPQ HTCSFLKHRF TLYKYKDAWN HQEFLEGRIL
fcFST4´   METTKTQFES MAEMIKKLPQ HTCSSLKGRI TLYKYQDFWG LQNNIEGAIL

          51                                                100
hTSPST    L.QSFQARPD DLLISTYPKS GTTWVSQILD MIYQGGDLEK CHRAPI....
rPST      L.QNFTAWPD DLLISTYPKS GTTWMSEILD MIYQGGKLEK CGRAPI....
rEST      V.ETFLARPD DLLIVTYPKS GSTWISEIVD MIYKEGDVEK CKEDAL....
bEST      V.EEFEARPD DLVIVTYPKS GTTWLSEIIC MIYNNGDVEK CKEDVI....
gpEST     V.EAFQARPD DLVIAAYPKS GTTWISEVVC MIYAEGDVKK CRQDAI....
hDHEAST   VRDEFVIRDE DVIILTYPKS GTNWLAEILC LMHSKGDAKW IQSVPI....
rHSST1    VCNKFVVKDE DLILLAYPKS GTNWLIEIVC LIQTKGDPKW IQSVTI....
rHSST2    VCNKFVVKEE DLILLTYPKS GTNWLIEIVC LIQTKGDPKW IQSVTI....
rSMP2     IRNKFVVKEE DLIILTYPKS GTNWLNEIVC LIQTKGDPKW IQSCPF....
fcFST3    SEQKFKAHPN DVFLASYPKS GTTWLKAWIC .IITREKFDD STSPLLTTMP
fcFST4´   AQQSFKARPD DVFLCSYPKS GTTWLKALAY AIVTREKFDE FTSPLLTNIP

          101                                               150
hTSPST    FMRVPFLEFK APGIPSGMET LKDTPAPRLL KTHLPLALLP QTLLDQKVKV
rPST      YARVPFLEFK CPGVPSGLET LEETPAPRLL KTHLPLSLLP QSLLDQKVKV
rEST      FNRIPDLECR NEDLINGIKQ LKEKESPRIV KTHLPAKLLP ASFWEKNCKI
bEST      FNRVPYLECS TEHVMKGVKQ LNEMASPRIV KSHLPVKLLP VSFWEKNCKI
gpEST     FNRVPFLECR NDKMMNGVKQ LEEMNSPRII KTHLPPRLLP ASFWEKRCKM
hDHEAST   WERSPWVESE I.....GYTA LSETESPRLF SSHLPIQLFP KSFFSSKAKV
rHSST1    WDRSPWIETD V.....GYDI LIKKKGPRLM TSHLPMHLFS KSLFSSKAKV
rHSST2    WDRSPWIETD L.....GYDM LIKKKGPRLI TSHLPMHLFS KSLFSSKAKV
rSMP2     ...GTVYPDE I.....EWIF RNNHGGPRLI TSHLPIHLFS KSFFSSKAKA
fcFST3    HDCIPLLEKD LEKIQEN... .QRNSLYTPI STHFHYKSLP ESARTSNCKI
fcFST4´   HNCIPYIEKD LKKIVEN... .QNNSCFTPM ATHMPYHVLP KSILALNCKM

          151                                               200
hTSPST    VYVARNAKDV AVSYYHF.YH MAKVHPEPGT WDSFLEKFMV GEVSYGSWYQ
rPST      IYIARNAKDV VVSYYNF.YN MAKLHPDPGT WDSFLENFMD GEVSYGSWYQ
rEST      IYLCRNAKDV VVSYYYF.FL IMKSYPNPKS FSEFVEKFME GQVPYGSWYD
bEST      IYLSRNAKDV VVSYYFL.IL MVTAIPDPDS FQDFVEKFMD GEVPYGSWFE
gpEST     ICICRNAKDV AVSYYYF.FL MVANHPDPGS FPEFVEKFMQ GQVPYGSWYD
hDHEAST   IYLMRNPRDV LVSGYFF.WK NMKFIKKPKS WEEYFEWFCQ GTVLYGSWFD
rHSST1    IYLVRNPRDV LVSGYYF.WG NSTLAKKPDS LGTYVEWFLK GNVLYGSWFE
rHSST2    IYLIRNPRDV LVSGYYF.WG KTTLAKKPDS LGTYVEWFLK GYVPYGSWFE
rSMP2     IYLMRNPRDI LVSGYFF.WG NTNLVKNPGS LGTYFEWFLQ GNVLFGSWFE
fcFST3    VYIYRNMKDV IVSYYHFLRQ IVKLSVEEAP FEEAFDEFCQ GISSCGPYWE
fcFST4´   VYIYRNIKDV IVSFYHFGRE ITKLPLEDAP FEEAFDEFYH GISQFGPYWD
```

Fig. 5. Amino acid sequence alignment of cytoplasmic sulfotransferase (ST) enzymes for which cDNAs have been cloned. The sequences were aligned with the PILEUP program (Feng and Doolittle 1987) from the Genetics Computer Group package (Madison, WI) (Devereux et al. 1984). White type on a black background indicates that at least seven of the amino acids at that position are identical. Abbreviations used for enzyme names are those listed in Table 2

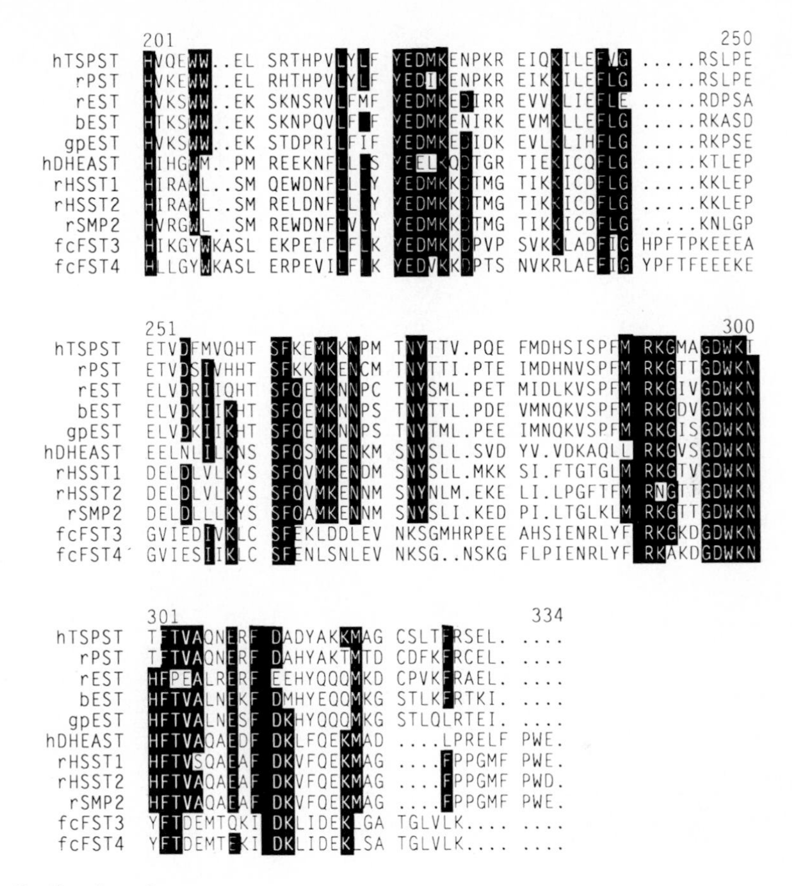

Fig. 5. *Continued*

sequence near the amino terminus is YPKSGTXW, while that near the carboxy terminus is RKGXXGDWKNXFT, in which X represents any amino acid. It is tempting to speculate that these two regions, conserved across phylogeny from eukaryotic plants to vertebrates, might be related to the binding site(s) for PAPS, the high-energy sulfate donor for the reactions catalyzed by all of these enzymes. Obviously, that hypothesis must eventually be tested experimentally. In addition to these two long sequences, shorter homologous regions, i.e., regions in which an identical amino acid is present in seven of the 11 proteins, are scattered throughout the enzymes (Fig. 5). The presence of such a high degree of similarity indicates that it might be helpful to compare the degree of homology of the complete sequences of these 11 proteins (Table 2). Table 2 shows that the sequences of the two PSTs included in the group are 79.7% identical; those of the three ESTs vary from 65.8% to 70.2% identity; the sequences of the four HSSTs vary from 61.3% to 89.8% identity; and the sequences of the two plant FSTs are

Table 2. Comparison of amino acid sequences of cloned cytosolic sulfotransferase enzymes

	hTSPST	rPST	rEST	bEST	gpEST	hDHEAST	rHSST1	rHSST2	rSMP2	fcFST3	fcFST4'
hTSPST	–	79.7 (89.0)	49.0 (68.6)	50.7 (69.7)	48.8 (68.8)	36.6 (59.8)	36.5 (56.6)	36.6 (57.6)	35.7 (59.2)	28.7 (52.4)	29.2 (55.2)
rPST		–	50.5 (67.4)	52.6 (70.1)	50.9 (68.4)	38.8 (59.4)	37.7 (56.5)	39.9 (58.3)	38.3 (60.2)	29.4 (55.9)	29.2 (56.3)
rEST			–	65.8 (81.7)	68.1 (84.7)	36.7 (59.8)	36.0 (58.3)	36.7 (59.0)	35.7 (62.5)	28.9 (54.0)	28.9 (54.0)
bEST				–	70.2 (85)	39.2 (62.2)	39.1 (59.5)	39.8 (60.6)	36.0 (60.1)	32.0 (55.3)	29.6 (54.3)
gpEST					–	36.9 (61.6)	36.2 (59.1)	36.8 (58.1)	37.0 (61.2)	32.5 (56.4)	31.2 (56.8)
hDHEAST						–	63.3 (78.8)	62.1 (79.8)	61.3 (79.8)	30.9 (56.4)	26.3 (53.0)
rHSST1							–	89.8 (93.7)	74.4 (85.8)	29.9 (55.5)	26.2 (54.1)
rHSST2								–	74.7 (86.5)	30.9 (54.5)	26.2 (54.1)
rSMP2									–	30.4 (57.0)	25.9 (55.8)
fcFST3										–	69.9 (82.8)
fcFST4'											–

The enzymes compared include human liver TS PST (hTSPST; Wilborn et al. 1993), rat liver PST (rPST; Ozawa et al. 1990), rat liver EST (rEST; Demyan et al. 1992), bovine placental EST (bEST; Nash et al. 1988), guinea pig adrenal EST (gpEST; Oeda et al. 1992), human liver DHEA ST (hDHEAST; Otterness et al. 1992), rat liver HSST (rHSST1 and rHSST2; Ogura et al. 1989, 1990), rat liver SMP-2 (rSMP2; Chatterjee et al. 1987), and *Flaveria chloraefolia* flavonol 3-ST and flavonol 4′-ST (fcFST3, fcFST4′; Varin et al. 1992). The top value in each cell represents the percentage identity, while the value in parentheses represents the percentage similarity of amino acid sequences as determined by use of the BESTFIT program (Smith and Waterman 1981) from the Genetics Computer Group package (Madison, WI; Devereux et al. 1984). The stippled cells represent enzymes with greater than 60% sequence identity, whereas the cross-hatched cells represent enzymes with greater than 40%, but less than 60% sequence identity.
TS, thermostable; ST, sulfotransferase; PST, phenol ST; EST, estrogen ST; DHEA, dehydroepiandrosterone; HSST, hydroxysteroid ST; SMP, senescence marker protein.

69.9% identical. In addition, the two PSTs show 48.8%–52.6% sequence identity with the three ESTs. However, the sequences of the HSSTs are less than 40% identical with those of the other ST enzymes, and the plant enzymes, the FSTs, show less than 32.5% identity with any of the other enzymes. These sequence relationships make it possible to begin to develop a classification for cytoplasmic ST enzymes analogous to classification schemes that have been developed for the cytochrome P450 and uridine diphosphate (UDP) glucuronosyltransferase gene superfamilies of drug-metabolizing enzymes (NEBERT et al. 1991; BURCHELL et al. 1991). In these cases, an arbitrary value of 40% sequence identity was chosen to classify enzyme families, and 60% sequence identity was chosen for subfamilies. If a similar and equally arbitrary approach were used to classify proteins encoded by the ST cDNAs reported thus far, these proteins could be separated into three families, the PSTs, HSSTs, and FSTs (Fig. 6). The PST family would consist, at present, of two subfamilies, the PSTs and ESTs. This provisional classification scheme (Fig. 6) is neither intended to be final nor all-inclusive, but it does begin to outline an approach that might eventually make it possible to decrease the confusion that has arisen during three decades of biochemical studies of these enzymes. Finally, it should be emphasized that although "functional" designations have been retained in the names assigned to the ST families and subfamilies depicted in Fig. 6, the classification is based entirely on amino acid sequence, not on function.

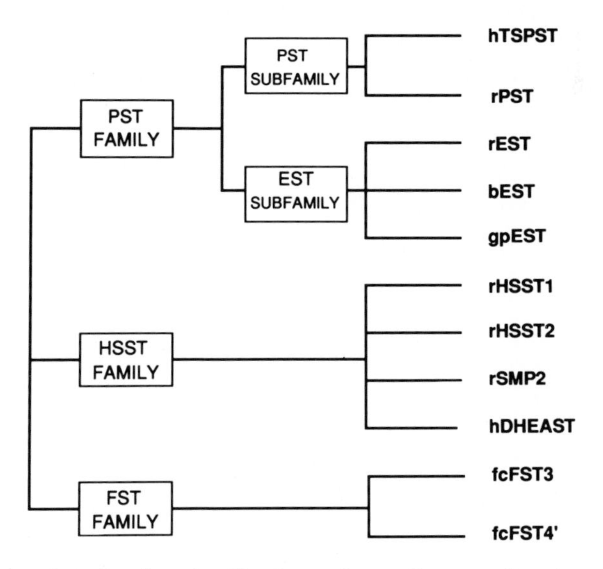

Fig. 6. Provisional molecular classification scheme for cytoplasmic sulfotransferase (ST) enzymes. Enzymes have been included in the same family if their amino acid sequences are more than 40% identical, and they have been included in the same subfamily if their amino acid sequences are more than 60% identical. Abbreviations used for enzyme names are those listed in Table 2. See text for details

Therefore, the scheme outlined in Fig. 6 represents only a "way station" on a path eventually leading to a nomenclature that will be entirely neutral as far as function is concerned, a nomenclature such as that presently used for the cytochromes P450 (NEBERT et al. 1991). However, in the subsequent discussion, the information will be organized under the names used in Fig. 6 for families and subfamilies, i.e., PSTs, ESTs, HSSTs, and FSTs.

C. Assays for Sulfotransferase Enzymes

The increase in understanding of the biochemistry of STs that has occurred during the past three decades was made possible by the development of accurate and sensitive assays for the measurement of these enzyme activities. Early assay procedures had to include a provision for the generation of PAPS. Therefore, they measured variation in at least three separate enzyme activities, the ST being studied and the two enzymes required for the generation of PAPS (see Fig. 3). The assays described subsequently removed that complication because they used exogenously added PAPS. These very sensitive assay procedures also made it possible to deal with another problem that complicated attempts to measure ST activities in tissue preparations, the presence of endogenous inhibitors and of competing enzyme systems capable of degrading PAPS (ANDERSON and WEINSHILBOURM 1979). One practical approach that has been used to negate the effects of endogenous ST inhibitors is to highly dilute tissue preparations. For example, human hepatic cytosolic preparations are diluted approximately 20000-fold for the assay of TS PST activity (CAMPBELL et al. 1987a). Obviously, extremely sensitive assays are required to measure enzyme activities at that degree of tissue dilution. The use of radioactively labeled ^{35}S-PAPS or of nonradioactive PAPS with a radioactive sulfate acceptor substrate has provided assays with the required degree of sensitivity.

The underlying principle of the most frequently used ST assay procedure was described by WENGLE (1964). This procedure is based on the precipitation of ^{35}S-PAPS and $^{35}SO_4^{2-}$ by barium. Barium salts of most sulfated reaction products are soluble in water, so they are not precipitated. Specifically, these assays involve incubation of a sulfate acceptor substrate with ^{35}S-PAPS, followed by termination of the reaction by the addition of $Ba(OH)_2$ and $ZnSO_4$. Centrifugation removes the precipitated ^{35}S-PAPS, while the radioactively labeled sulfated substrate remains in the aqueous phase. Radioactivity in the supernatant can then be measured in a liquid scintillation counter. This general procedure has undergone several modifications (FOLDES and MEEK 1973; ANDERSON and WEINSHILBOUM 1980), but it remains the most frequently used ST assay procedure performed with ^{35}S-PAPS. However, it does have limitations. The most important is that some sulfated reaction products, particularly carboxylic acid derivatives, are precipitated by barium (FOLDES and MEEK 1973). Furthermore, even reaction products that are soluble in the aqueous phase in the presence of barium may be precipitated to variable degrees (TOTH et al. 1987), resulting in difficulty in the estimation of absolute reaction velocities. As a result of these limitations, several alternative procedures for the separation of ^{35}S-PAPS from sulfated reaction products have been reported, including the use of thin layer chromatography (SEKURA et al. 1979), Ecteola cellulose chromatographic columns (BORCHARDT et al. 1983; WHITTEMORE and ROTH 1985), high-pressure liquid chromatography (HPLC) (HONKASALO and NISSINEN 1988), and organic solvent extraction performed in the presence of ion-pairing reagents (VARIN et al. 1987). Another issue that must be addressed when ^{35}S-PAPS is used as a cosubstrate for reactions catalyzed by ST enzymes is the presence of endogenous sulfate acceptor substrates in tissue preparations or even in partially purified enzyme preparations (BROOKS et al. 1987). Therefore, the choice of a "blank" for these assays is critical, and the use of heated enzyme or zero incubation time blanks is inappropriate. In most circumstances, a sample that does not contain exogenously added sulfate acceptor substrate is the most appropriate blank for such assays.

Radioactively labeled sulfate acceptors have also been used for ST assays – particularly those in which steroid hormones are substrates. Those assays utilize nonradioactive PAPS and either ^{3}H- or ^{14}C-labeled sulfate acceptors (SINGER 1985). Obviously, assays of this type are only practical in situations in which the radioactively labeled sulfate acceptor is readily available. When steroids are used as substrates for such assays, unreacted radioactively labeled sulfate acceptor substrate is usually removed by organic solvent extraction, leaving the water-soluble, sulfated reaction product in the aqueous phase. An assay based on a similar principle has also been used to measure bile acid ST activity (BARNES et al. 1983). The development of sensitive assays capable of measuring the activities of ST enzymes was required to make it possible to purify and characterize these enzymes.

D. Purification of Sulfotransferase Enzymes

The general strategy used most frequently in the purification of ST enzymes was established over a decade ago, when Sekura and Jakoby set out to isolate and purify rat liver PSTs (SEKURA and JAKOBY 1979). An important aspect of that approach has been the use of anion exchange chromatography, usually performed with diethylaminoethanol (DEAE) cellulose or DEAE Sepharose CL-6B, to separate, at least partially, different ST activities. Anion exchange chromatography was used to separate rat liver PSTs I, II, III, and IV (SEKURA et al. 1979), and it was the technique used to separate human TL and TS PSTs – initially from blood platelet preparations (REITER et al. 1983). Other standard chromatographic techniques that have been used in the purification of ST enzymes include hydroxyapatite and gel filtration, almost always in combination with one or more of a variety of affinity chromatographic columns with varying degrees of specificity for ST enzymes. SEKURA and JAKOBY (1979) utilized Affi-Gel Blue and ATP agarose chromatography, and subsequent investigators have utilized heparin Sepharose (OTTERNESS et al. 1989; HERNÁNDEZ et al. 1992), adenosine diphosphate (ADP) agarose (COUGHTRIE and SHARP 1990), PAP agarose (HEROUX and ROTH 1988; FALANY et al. 1990), estradiol-17β Sepharose (TSENG et al. 1985), and p-hydroxyphenylacetic acid agarose (BORCHARDT and SCHASTEEN 1982) affinity columns to purify different ST enzymes. Previous reviews have described detailed protocols for the purification of specific STs (JAKOBY et al. 1980; SINGER 1985), and those reviews or the original publications should be consulted for detailed procedures. Investigators studying all of these enzymes have reported difficulty with stability of purified ST preparations, and most workers add sulfhydryl-reducing reagents such as dithiothreitol to buffers to help stabilize purified enzyme preparations. It has also been reported that the addition of glycerol and/or sucrose can help to stabilize purified STs (DUFFEL et al. 1991). The availability of purified ST enzymes made it possible to develop antibodies that could be used to screen cDNA expression libraries and also made it possible to determine partial amino acid sequences from these purified proteins that could be used to design oligonucleotide probes for use in screening cDNA libraries. Therefore, isolation and biochemical characterization of purified ST enzymes was required to make it possible to begin to apply the techniques of molecular biology to the study of these enzymes.

E. Molecular Cloning of Sulfotransferase Enzyme cDNAs

I. Introduction

ST cDNAs cloned to this time vary from 1000 to 1800 nucleotides in length, with open reading frames that range from 846 to 960 nucleotides. Therefore, the encoded proteins range from 282 to 320 amino acids – correlating well with the results of biochemical studies, which have usually shown that subunit molecular masses for cytoplasmic ST enzymes vary from 30 to 35 kDa. As cDNAs for these enzymes are cloned, it might be anticipated that confusion with regard to the number and properties of STs would decrease, but that is not a forgone conclusion. First, it is important that detailed information be provided with regard to the enzymes used to obtain the information required for cDNA cloning. Of equal importance is that each cDNA be expressed in vitro and that the biochemical properties of the expressed protein be determined and compared with those of well-characterized enzymes. Model substrates for each class of ST should be tested with each expressed protein. In addition, other biochemical properties should be studied, including thermal stability and the effects of inhibitors and activators. A striking example of the need for this degree of care is provided by attempts to characterize a PST cDNA cloned from rat liver, which are described below. The following paragraphs will briefly describe the molecular cloning of the ST cDNAs that have been reported up to now. The general properties of these cDNAs are summarized in Table 3.

II. Phenol Sulfotransferase cDNAs

The first cDNA for a PST was cloned from a Sprague-Dawley rat liver cDNA library (Ozawa et al. 1990; rPST in Tables 2, 3 and Fig. 5). This cDNA was cloned by screening an expression library with a polyclonal antibody to purified rat liver "4-nitrophenol ST." Unfortunately, no other characteristics of the enzyme used to generate the antibody were reported. Since 4-nitrophenol can serve as a substrate for rat liver PSTs I, II, and IV and, as will be described subsequently, for several other rat liver enzymes, the identity of the protein used to generate the antibody was unclear. Furthermore, the original authors did not express the cDNA in vitro, leaving the identity of the encoded protein ambiguous. Subsequently, three separate laboratories have studied this cDNA, and each group has reported that a different enzymatic activity is associated with the encoded protein. One group expressed the cDNA in COS-1 cells, a mammalian expression system, and reported that the enzyme was capable of catalyzing the sulfation of 4-nitrophenol and of minoxidil (Hirshey et al. 1992). They referred to the encoded enzyme as "minoxidil ST." A second group expressed the same cDNA in an *Escherichia coli* expression system, and the fusion protein that they obtained was capable of catalyzing the sulfation of *N*-hydroxy-2-acetylaminofluorene (Yerokun et al. 1992). Finally, a third group expressed the cDNA in an *E. coli* expression system and demonstrated that the expressed enzyme was capable of catalyzing the sulfation of 2-naphthol, 1-naphthalenemethanol and tyrosine methyl ester, implying that it represented rat liver PST IV (Chen et al. 1992). This confusing situation highlights the importance of characterizing as completely as possible the protein that serves as the basis for the cloning of a cDNA and, of equal importance, taking advantage of the knowledge gained during three decades of biochemical studies of ST enzymes to characterize thoroughly the protein encoded by that cDNA. The next PST cDNA cloned, that of human TS or P PST (see Table 1 and Fig. 4) offers an example of better use of this biochemical knowledge.

A cDNA for human TS PST was cloned by screening a human liver cDNA library with the rat liver PST clone described above (Wilborn et al. 1993; hTSPST in Tables 2, 3 and Fig. 5). The human liver cDNA cloned in this fashion was then expressed in COS-7 cells, and the expressed protein was capable of catalyzing the sulfation of μM concentrations of 4-nitrophenol, but it did not sulfate μM concentrations of dopamine, a model substrate for human TL or M PST. The expressed protein could also catalyze

Table 3. cDNAs for cytoplasmic sulfotransferase enzymes

cDNA	cDNA designation(s) by reporting authors	Activity name, abbreviation(s)	cDNA length, nucleotides	Encoded protein length, amino acids	cDNA library
hTSPST	P-PST-1	TS PST P PST	1206	295	Human liver
rPST	PST-1	AST PST	1028	291	Rat liver (S.D.)
rPST	Mx-STb	Mx-ST	1245	291	Rat liver (S.D.)
rPST	AST IV	AST IV	1127	285[a]	Rat liver (S.D.)
rPST	–	Tyrosine-ester ST	–	291	–
rEST	EST_r	EST	1309	295	Rat liver (F-344)
bEST	OST	OST	1812	295	Bovine placenta
gpEST	EST	EST	1192	296	Guinea pig adrenal
hDHEAST	DHEA ST A DHEA ST G	DHEA ST	1745 1050	285	Human liver
rHSST1	ST-20	STa	1028	284	Rat liver (S.D.)
rHSST2	ST-40	STa	1015	284	Rat liver (S.D.)
rSMP2	SMP-2	SMP-2	1040	282	Rat liver (S.D.)
fcFST3	pFST3	3-ST	1158	311	*Flaveria chloraefolia* terminal bud
fcFST4′	pFST4′	4′-ST	1242	320	*Flaveria chloraefolia* terminal bud

Trivial names for the enzyme activity and cDNA are listed as well as the length of the cDNA, the number of amino acids encoded by the open reading frame, the source of the cDNA library, and criteria used to classify the enzyme encoded by each cDNA.
TS, thermostable; ST, sulfotransferase; PST, phenol ST; EST, estrogen ST; HSST, hydroxysteroid

Table 3. *continued*

Evidence in support of classification					*References*
Comparison with amino acid sequences of native protein	Substrate specificity	Compounds not sulfated	Immunoreactive protein	Comigration on SDS-PAGE	
+	A-nitrophenol, minoxidil	Dopamine	+	+	WILBORN et al. (1993)
N.R.	N.R.	N.R.	+	N.R.	OZAWA et al. (1992)
+	A-nitrophenol, minoxidil	N.R.	+	+	HIRSHEY et al. (1992)
+	*N*-Hydroxy-2-acetylaminofluorene	N.R.	+	+	YEROKUN et al. (1992)
+	2-Naphthol, 1-naphthalenemethanol, tyrosine methyl ester	N.R.	+	+	CHEN et al. (1992)
+	Estradiol	N.R.	+	+	DEMYAN et al. (1992)
+	N.R.	N.R.	N.R.	N.R.	NASH et al. (1988)
+	Estradiol	Pregnenolone	+	+	OEDA et al. (1992)
+	DHEA	Dopamine, A-nitrophenol	N.R.	+	OTTERNESS et al. (1992)
+	N.R.	N.R.	+	N.R.	OGURA et al. (1989)
+	N.R.	N.R.	+	N.R.	OGURA et al. (1990)
N.R.	N.R.	N.R.	+	+	CHATTERJEE et al. (1987)
+	Quercetin, isorhamnetin, rhamnetin, kaempferol	Quercetin 3-sulfate, isorhamnetin 3-sulfate, tamarixetin 3-sulfate, kaempferol 3-sulfate	+	N.R.	VARIN et al. (1992)
–	Quercetin 3-sulfate, isorhamnetin 3-sulfate, kaempferol 3-sulfate	Quercetin, kaempferol, isorhamnetin, rhamnetin, tamarixetin 3-sulfate	+[b]	N.R.	VARIN et al. (1992)

ST; SMP, senescence marker protein; FST, flavonol ST; MxST, minoxidil ST; OST, oestrogen ST; AST, aryl ST; DHEA, dehydroepiandrosterone; S.D., Sprague-Dawley; F-344, Fischer 344; N.R., not reported.
[a] Truncated clone. [b] Antibody to 3-ST.

the sulfation of minoxidil, confirming reports that TS PST is the enzyme responsible for the sulfation of that drug in human tissue (FALANY and KERL 1990).

III. Estrogen Sulfotransferase cDNAs

The first EST cDNA was cloned from a bovine placental cDNA library (NASH et al. 1988; bEST in Tables 2, 3 and Fig. 5). These investigators had obtained partial amino acid sequence information from tryptic fragments of the bovine placental enzyme. That information was used to design degenerate oligonucleotides with which to screen the cDNA library. The protein encoded by the cDNA clone contained all of the amino acid sequences present in tryptic fragments of the native enzyme. Unfortunately, no expression data were reported. The subsequent isolation of a cDNA for guinea pig adrenal EST (gpEST in Tables 2, 3 and Fig. 5) utilized amino acid sequence information obtained from guinea pig adrenal EST to design degenerate oligonucleotide primers for use with the polymerase chain reaction (PCR) (OEDA et al. 1992). These primers were used to amplify a nondegenerate oligonucleotide probe that was then used to screen a guinea pig adrenal cDNA library. The deduced amino acid sequence of the protein encoded by this cDNA contained the sequences obtained from tryptic fragments of the native adrenal enzyme. Expression of this cDNA in COS-7 cells demonstrated that the encoded protein could catalyze the sulfation of estradiol-17β, but not that of pregnenolone. Finally, a cDNA for rat liver EST was isolated from a rat liver cDNA library by use of a monoclonal antibody to the purified rat liver protein (DEMYAN et al. 1992; rEST in Tables 2, 3 and Fig. 5). The deduced amino acid sequence included sequences obtained from a clostripain-generated peptide fragment of the native protein. Expression of this cDNA in COS-7 cells demonstrated that the encoded protein could catalyze the sulfation of estradiol-17β.

IV. Hydroxysteroid Sulfotransferase cDNAs

The first HSST cDNA cloned, and apparently the first cDNA cloned for any ST, was reported by CHATTERJEE et al. (1987). However, this cDNA was not cloned because of an interest in sulfate conjugation. These investigators were studying a rat liver protein that displayed age-dependent variation, the so-called SMP-2 (CHATTERJEE et al. 1981). Livers of mature female rats contained much higher quantities of this protein than did those of male animals. CHATTERJEE et al. (1987) took advantage of this sexual dimorphism and generated an SMP-2-enriched cDNA library that was subsequently probed with cDNAs from male and female rat liver. "Female-specific" clones were then used to isolate mRNA species, which were translated and immunoprecipitated with anti-SMP-2 antibody. Although the enzymatic activity of this cDNA clone (rSMP2 in Tables 2, 3 and Fig. 5) has never been determined, it appears to belong within the HSST family based on sequence homology with cDNAs cloned subsequently. Two HSST cDNAs were isolated by OGURA et al. (1989, 1990) from a rat liver cDNA expression library that was screened with polyclonal antibodies against purified female rat liver HSST (rHSST1 and rHSST2 in Tables 2, 3 and Fig. 5). The amino acid sequences of the proteins encoded by these two clones were 89.9% identical, and they each contained amino acid sequences present in the native rat protein. Unfortunately, neither enzymatic activity nor other biochemical properties of the proteins encoded by either of these clones were reported. Finally, human liver DHEA ST cDNA has been cloned (OTTERNESS et al. 1992; hDHEAST in Tables 2, 3 and Fig. 5). The cloning strategy took advantage of the areas of high homology shown in Fig. 5, although only three ST cDNAs had been cloned at that time. The sequences of these areas were used to design primers for PCR that were used to amplify a unique sequence from human liver cDNA. This PCR amplification product, in turn, was used to screen a human liver cDNA library. Two full-length cDNA clones were isolated that contained identical open reading frames. The predicted amino acid sequence for the encoded protein contained the amino acid sequences obtained from proteolytic fragments of the native human liver protein. Both of the cDNAs cloned were expressed in COS-1 cells, and both were capable of catalyzing the sulfation of DHEA, but not the sulfation of μM concentrations of 4-nitrophenol or dopamine, model substrates for the two forms of PST present in human liver (Table 1). Finally, the expressed DHEA ST activity had an (IC_{50}) value for inhibition by DCNP identical with that of human liver DHEA ST.

V. Flavonol Sulfotransferase cDNAs

Flavonols such as quercetin (see Fig. 1) can undergo sulfation at the 3 position, followed by sequential sulfation of the flavonol 3-sulfate at either the 3′ or 4′ positions (VARIN and IBRAHIM 1989). These reactions are catalyzed by separate cytoplasmic ST enzymes. Two unique FST cDNAs were cloned by screening a *F. chloraefolia* terminal bud cDNA expression library with polyclonal antibodies raised against FST-3 purified from *F. chloraefolia* terminal buds (VARIN et al. 1992; fcFST3 and fcFST4′ in Tables 2, 3 and Fig. 5). Partial FST-3 amino acid sequence information had been obtained, and those sequences were contained in the protein encoded by one of the cDNAs. Expression of these two cDNAs in an *E. coli* expression system demonstrated that the expressed fusion proteins had the same substrate and position specificities for the sulfation of flavonols as did FST-3 and FST-4′.

VI. Conclusions

Although several ST cDNAs have been cloned, characterization of the proteins that they encode has been variable. The substrate specificities of proteins encoded by nearly half of the reported cDNAs have not been determined, and, even in those that have, there has been a tendency to study only one or very few substrates. Enzyme properties other than ability to catalyze the sulfation of one or a limited number of substrates, substrates that are frequently known to serve as sulfate acceptors for more than one ST enzyme, have usually not been tested. In some cases, the degree of characterization of the protein to which antibodies have been developed for use in screening cDNA expression libraries has been so limited that it is virtually impossible to determine which ST enzyme might have been cloned. The data already obtained by the application of the techniques of molecular biology to study ST enzymes are exciting, but they also serve to emphasize that these techniques do not represent a panacea or a substitute for the careful characterization of the properties of proteins encoded by the cloned cDNAs. In the next section, a brief overview of these properties will be provided.

F. Properties of Sulfotransferase Enzymes

I. Introduction

A great deal has been learned during the past three decades with regard to the properties of cytoplasmic ST enzymes. Many, but not all, of these enzymes are homodimers, with monomeric molecular mass values that vary from approximately 30 to 35 kDa. The results of substrate kinetic analyses of reactions catalyzed by cytoplasmic ST enzymes are generally compatible with the conclusion that they are ordered bisubstrate reactions with PAPS as the leading substrate (Anhalt et al. 1982; Whittemore et al. 1985, 1986). This conclusion has been supported by the results of photoaffinity labeling experiments (Otterness et al. 1989, 1991). Finally, most of these enzymes exhibit profound substrate inhibition (Reiter et al. 1983; Campbell et al. 1987a; Sundaram et al. 1989a), an important practical issue that complicates attempts to "screen" enzyme preparations with only one or a few concentrations of substrate. The subsequent discussion will briefly outline selected properties of the PSTs, ESTs, HSSTs, and FSTs.

II. Phenol Sulfotransferase Properties

1. Human Phenol Sulfotransferase Properties

The first systematic studies of PST activity in human tissue were performed in the 1960s by Boström and Wengle (1964) with an assay procedure that required a PAPS-generating system. Therefore, the results that they obtained were qualitative rather than quantitative, but their demonstration of PST activity in human tissue served as a stimulus for subsequent investigators. In the late 1970s, it was reported that PST activity was present in an easily accessible human tissue, the blood platelet (HART et al. 1979), and it was subsequently shown that many, if not all, human tissues contain at least two forms of PST (REIN et al. 1981; REIN et al. 1982; REITER and WEINSHILBOUM 1982a; REITER et al. 1983). These observations stimulated a decade of intense study of the biochemistry, regulation, and functional significance of PSTs in human tissue. Every human tissue that has been studied in detail expresses both TS and TL PST activities (YOUNG et al. 1984; ANDERSON et al. 1986; BARAŃCZYK-KUŹMA and SZYMCZYK 1986; CAMPBELL et al. 1987a; SUNDARAM et al. 1989a). The general properties of these two enzymes are listed in Table 1 and are depicted in graphical form in Fig. 4. However, both the relative and absolute levels of the two activities vary dramatically from tissue to tissue and, within the brain, striking regional variations in both activities have been reported (YOUNG et al. 1984; BARAN and JELLINGER 1992). In tissues that have been studied in large numbers of subjects, e.g., liver, jejunum, and platelet, no gender- or age-dependent differences in TS or TL PST activities have been reported (CAMPBELL et al. 1987a; SUNDARAM et al. 1989a; PRICE et al. 1988, 1989). Individual variation in levels of TS PST activity in the platelet are highly correlated with individual differences in that enzyme activity in human cerebral cortex, liver, and jejunum (YOUNG et al. 1985; CAMPBELL and WEINSHILBOUM 1986; SUNDARAM et al. 1989b). However, variations in levels of human platelet TL PST activity are not significantly correlated with individual differences in TL PST activity in other organs (YOUNG et al. 1985; CAMPBELL and WEINSHILBOUM 1986; SUNDARAM et al. 1989b). These observation will take on additional importance during the subsequent discussion of PST pharmacogenetics.

Biochemically, TS and TL PST purified from human liver and platelet are both homodimers, with apparent monomer molecular masses of 32 kDa and 34 kDa, respectively (HEROUX and ROTH 1988; FALANY et al. 1990). TL PST preferentially catalyzes the sulfation of a large number of phenolic and catechol monoamines, including the important neurotransmitters dopamine, norepinephrine, and epinephrine (REIN et al. 1981; REITER et al. 1983). TS PST is capable of catalyzing the *O*-sulfation of simple phenolic compounds as well as the phenolic estrogens estrone and estradiol-17β (CAMPBELL et al. 1987b; HERNÁNDEZ et al. 1992). TS PST is also capable of catalyzing the *N*-sulfation of 2-naphthylamine (see Fig. 1) (HERNÁNDEZ et al. 1991), demonstrating that this enzyme does not merely catalyze *O*-sulfation.

2. Rat Phenol Sulfotransferase Properties

In 1979, SEKURA and JAKOBY separated three PSTs, I, II, and IV, from rat liver by the use of anion exchange chromatography. Like the PSTs in human tissue, these enzymes are homodimers, with molecular mass values for the dimers of approximately 64 kDa for PST I and II and 61 kDa for PST IV (SEKURA and JAKOBY 1979). The substrate specificities of these enzymes are pH dependent, but all three are capable of catalyzing the sulfation of 4-nitrophenol – with reported K_m values of 1.6 and 2.5 mM for PST I and II, respectively, while that for PST IV is 0.17 mM. Of the three isoforms, only PST IV is capable of catalyzing the sulfation of biogenic amines, and then only at the nonphysiologic pH of 9.0. PST IV can also catalyze the sulfation of tyrosine methyl ester, benzylic alcohols, and *N*-hydroxyarylamines (SEKURA and JAKOBY 1979; JAKOBY et al. 1980). It was against the background provided by the work of SEKURA and JAKOBY (1979) that subsequent investigators isolated additional isoforms of PST from rat tissue. One group used p-hydroxyphenylacetic acid agarose affinity chromatography to isolate a rat liver PST with a molecular mass of 69–70 kDa and a K_m value for 4-nitrophenol at pH 6.0 of 3.6 μM (BORCHARDT and SCHASTEEN 1982). This enzyme was capable of catalyzing the sulfate conjugation of catecholamines at pH 6.4. A rat liver acetaminophen ST with a pH optimum of 9.0 has also been reported (COUGHTRIE and SHARP 1990). The activity of this enzyme was twice as great in livers of male as in those of female animals. Finally, a rat liver minoxidil ST with a very low K_m for 4-nitrophenol, 0.5 μM, has been isolated (HIRSHEY and FALANY 1990). All of these investigators suggested that they had isolated isoforms of PST that differed from rat liver PSTs I, II, and IV. At this time, it is clear only that rat liver contains at least three and probably many more PST activities, the substrate specificities, function, and regulation of which remain to be determined. PSTs have also been studied in rat brain, stomach, and kidney (FOLDES and MEEK 1973; BARAŃCZYK-KUŹMA et al. 1981, 1985).

3. Properties of Phenol Sulfotransferase in Other Species

PST activities have been studied and characterized to varying degrees in bovine, porcine, canine, guinea pig, rhesus monkey, and marmoset tissue (BANERJEE and ROY 1968; ROMAIN et al. 1982; BARAŃCZYK-KUŹMA et al. 1992; BARAŃCZYK-KUŹMA and SZYMCZYK 1987; UEKI et al. 1989; BARAŃCZYK-KUŹMA and CISZEWSKA-PILCZYŃSKA 1989). When investigators have attempted to determine whether multiple isoforms of PST existed in several species, evidence for multiple forms has been found (ROMAIN et al. 1982; BARAŃCZYK-KUŹMA and CISZEWSKA-PILCZYŃSKA 1989; BARAŃCZYK-KUŹMA et al. 1992; UEKI et al. 1989). In the case of the marmoset, the argument has been made that this species might represent an experimental animal model system similar to humans (UEKI et al. 1989). However, it now seems likely that it will only be possible to sort out the relationships among PSTs in vertebrate species after the molecular cloning of cDNAs from these species, followed by functional studies of the proteins encoded by the cDNAs.

III. Estrogen Sulfotransferase Properties

EST activity has been studied primarily in placental, uterine, adrenal, and hepatic tissue. Included among the species in which ESTs have been studied are human, guinea pig, mouse, pig, cow, and rat (GREEN and SINGER 1983; TSENG et al. 1985; HOBKIRK et al. 1985, 1990; BROOKS et al. 1987; ADAMS 1991). Although early reports of molecular mass values for ESTs were quite varied, the bovine adrenal and placental enzymes were recently reported to be homodimers with monomeric molecular mass values of 35–36 kDa (MOORE et al. 1988; ADAMS 1991), and guinea pig adrenal EST was found to be a dimer with a monomer molecular mass of 35 kDa (HOBKIRK et al. 1990). The majority of reports have stressed that these enzymes catalyze the sulfation of estradiol-17β and estrone, but that DHEA and pregnenolone are either poor substrates or are not sulfate conjugated by ESTs. Attempts to purify ESTs have been plagued by the instability of the purified enzymes, although they can be partially stabilized by the addition of thiols (FREEMAN et al. 1983; HOBKIRK et al. 1985; TSENG et al. 1985). EST may be "activated" in the presence of 1–10 mM Mg^{2+} (FREEMAN et al. 1983). The regulation of EST activity by progesterone in some tissues will be discussed below when the regulation of STs is described.

IV. Hydroxysteroid Sulfotransferase Properties

In 1958, NOSE and LIPMANN succeeded in chromatographically separating rat liver enzymes that catalyzed the sulfation of DHEA, 4-nitrophenol, and estrone, indicating that HSSTs, those enzymes that sulfated nonphenolic steroids such as DHEA, might represent a class of STs separate from PSTs and ESTs. DHEA has been the substrate used most frequently to assay HSST activity. HSSTs have subsequently been characterized in human liver and adrenal, rat liver, porcine liver, and hamster epididymal tissue (MARCUS et al. 1980; COOKE et al. 1983; BOUTHILLIER et al. 1985; FALANY et al. 1989; COMER and FALANY 1992). HSSTs catalyze the sulfate conjugation of 3β-hydroxysteroids and – at least in human liver – of bile acids such as lithocholic acid (RADOMINSKA et al. 1990) as well as cholesterol (AKSOY et al. 1993a), estrone (HERNÁNDEZ et al. 1992), and even the cardiac glycoside digitoxin (SCHMOLDT et al. 1992). As described previously, HSST cDNAs have been cloned from human and rat liver (CHATTERJEE et al. 1987; OGURA et al. 1989, 1990; OTTERNESS et al. 1992). Although no bile acid ST cDNAs have been cloned other than human liver DHEA ST cDNA, partial N-terminal amino acid sequence information has been published for a rat liver bile acid ST (BARNES et al. 1989). These 34 amino acid residues differ from, but show high homology with, the sequences of rat liver HSSTs for which cDNAs have been cloned. In addition, rat liver bile acid ST, a protein with a subunit molecular mass of 30 kDa, can catalyze the sulfation of DHEA (BARNES et al. 1989). These observations may indicate that another line of investigation, gastroenterologic studies of bile acid biotransformation, may be merging into the broader stream of ST research.

Biochemical studies indicate that hepatic HSSTs from both humans and rats are homodimers with monomer molecular masses of approximately

35 kDa (MARCUS et al. 1980; FALANY et al. 1989; COMER and FALANY 1992). Human liver HSST activity is maximal in the presence of 0.3–10 mM Mg^{2+} (FALANY et al. 1989; HERNÁNDEZ et al. 1992). Both human and rat liver HSST can be separated into three different charged species during isoelectric focusing (HOMMA et al. 1991, 1992; OTTERNESS et al. 1992), raising the question of charge isoforms of HSST in these species, possibly as a result of post-translational modification. Gender- and age-dependent variation in rat liver HSST activity will be described in the course of the subsequent description of the regulation of ST activities.

V. Flavonol Sulfotransferase Properties

Flavonoids such as quercetin are thought to function as "stress metabolites" after exposure of plants to ultraviolet radiation or microbial attack (HAHLBROCK and SCHEEL 1989). These compounds can undergo sequential sulfation, beginning at the 3 position (see Fig. 1), followed by either 3′- or 4′-sulfate conjugation (VARIN and IBRAHIM 1989). Three FSTs have been isolated from *F. chloraefolia* shoot tips. One of these enzymes, FST-3, catalyzes the initial 3-sulfation of quercetin and other flavonols, while the other two, FST-3′ and FST-4′, catalyze subsequent conjugation of the 3-sulfated compounds (VARIN and IBRAHIM 1989). All three enzymes are monomeric cytoplasmic proteins with molecular masses of approximately 35 kDa. FST-3 can catalyze the sulfate conjugation of a large number of flavonols, but not flavonol 3-sulfates, while FST-3′ and FST-4′ catalyze the sulfation of a series of flavonol 3-sulfates (VARIN and IBRAHIM 1992). Highest activities for all three of these enzymes are found in terminal buds and the first pair of leaves of *Flaveria* species. FST activity is also present in mature flowers, but it is not detectable in plant roots (HANNOUFA et al. 1991).

G. Regulation of Sulfotransferase Enzymes

I. Introduction

Studies of ST enzymes performed during the past decade have usually focused on the biochemical characteristics and function of these enzymes. However, there are already reports that, at least in some species, the activities of these enzymes can be controlled by genetic and/or humoral factors. Studies of the pharmacogenetics of ST enzymes have been performed primarily with humans, while studies of the humoral regulation of ST enzymes have been performed predominantly with experimental animals. The subsequent discussion will briefly describe our current understanding of the role of inheritance in the regulation of individual variation in ST enzyme activity levels and other properties in humans. The role of hormonal factors in the regulation of these enzyme activities will then be addressed.

II. Sulfotransferase Enzyme Pharmacogenetics

The presence of TS and TL PST activities in an easily accessible human tissue, the blood platelet (HART et al. 1979), made it possible to initiate studies of the role of inheritance in the regulation of these enzyme activities. Initial experiments estimated the "heritability" of individual variation in PST activities in platelet samples from monozygotic and dizygotic twins (REVELEY et al. 1982/1983). The results indicated that the heritability of platelet TS PST activity varied from 0.83 to 0.96 (i.e., 83%–96% of the total variance in enzyme activity resulted from the effects of inheritance), while the heritability of platelet TL PST activity varied from 0.48 to 0.70 (REVELEY et al. 1982/1983). These data were confirmed and extended by studies of platelet TL PST activity in blood samples from 232 first-degree relatives in 49 nuclear families (PRICE et al. 1988) and studies of platelet TS PST activity performed with samples from 237 first-degree relatives in 50 nuclear families (PRICE et al. 1989). Family studies confirmed the high heritability of both platelet enzyme activities and raised the possibility of major gene (mendelian) effects on the inheritance of levels of both activities. Unfortunately, as mentioned previously, genetically determined levels of TL PST activity in the human platelet do not correlate significantly with those of TL PST in tissues such as the brain, liver, and jejunum (YOUNG et al. 1985; CAMPBELL and WEINSHILBOUM 1986; SUNDARAM et al. 1989b). However, there is a highly significant correlation between TS PST activity in platelets and these tissues (r_s, 0.94 for cerebral cortex, 0.79 for liver, and 0.85 for jejunal mucosa) (YOUNG et al. 1985; CAMPBELL and WEINSHILBOUM 1986; SUNDARAM et al. 1989b). Therefore, genetically regulated variation in TS PST activity in the platelet reflects individual differences in levels of this enzyme activity in other human tissues – including potential sites of drug and xenobiotic metabolism. Finally, TS PST in human hepatic and brain tissue samples exists as two separate isoforms that can be separated by anion exchange chromatography (WHITTEMORE et al. 1985; CAMPBELL et al. 1987a; WEINSHILBOUM 1988). Tissue from individual human subjects contains one, the other, or both of these isoforms of TS PST, indicating that they may represent allozymes, products of two different alleles at a single genetic locus (WEINSHILBOUM 1988, 1990).

Pharmacogenetic variation in PST activity may result in inherited differences among individuals in the sulfation of drugs, xenobiotics, neurotransmitters and hormones. Data in support of that possibility have already been reported. There is a significant correlation between genetically determined variation in platelet TS PST activity and individual differences in the sulfate conjugation of the drug acetaminophen after oral administration (REITER and WEINSHILBOUM 1982b; BONHAM-CARTER et al. 1983). Furthermore, individuals with low levels of platelet TS PST activity are at increased risk for the occurrence of diet-induced migraine headaches (LITTLEWOOD et al. 1982). The investigators who reported the latter data speculated that relative inability to catalyze the sulfate conjugation of as yet unidentified phenolic compounds in the diet might be related to this increased risk (LITTLEWOOD et al. 1982). The cloning of cDNAs and genes for TS and TL PST should eventually make it possible to determine the molecular mechanisms responsible for genetic regulation of these enzyme activities in humans.

III. Humoral Regulation of Sulfotransferase Enzymes

Evidence for hormonal regulation of ST activities comes predominantly from studies of rodents, experiments that have demonstrated gender-dependent differences in levels of ST enzyme activities, especially in hepatic tissue. It has already been noted that acetaminophen ST activity in male rat liver is twice as great as that in the livers of female rats (COUGHTRIE and SHARP 1990). There have also been reports that PST II activity is increased in the livers of male as compared with female rats (MATSUI and WATANABE 1982). These data raise the possibility of regulation of PST activity in rodent liver by sex hormones. However, it should be emphasized once again that no significant gender- or age-dependent differences in human TS or TL PST activities have been reported in studies of large numbers of hepatic, jejunal mucosal, or platelet samples (CAMPBELL et al. 1987a; SUNDARAM et al. 1989a; PRICE et al. 1988, 1989). Therefore, care must be taken not to assume that gender-dependent variations in these enzyme activities can be generalized among species, or even from organ to organ within a species. There have also been reports that ESTs and HSSTs are subject to humoral regulation.

Guinea pig uterine EST is detectable only during pregnancy, reaching a maximum between 47 and 55 days of gestation and then decreasing at term (63 days) (FREEMAN et al. 1983). These data are supported by observations that porcine endometrial EST can be detected only after ovariectomized animals are treated with both estrogens and progestational agents (BROOKS et al. 1987) and by the results of studies of cultured human endometrium in which EST activity was increased by exposure to progestational agents (CLARKE et al. 1982). Finally, as noted previously, the first ST for which a cDNA was cloned (SMP-2), was studied primarily because of a striking gender-dependent difference in the quantity of this protein in rat liver, with much higher concentrations in livers of female than in those of male rats (CHATTERJEE et al. 1981). Although the cDNA for SMP-2 has never been expressed enzymatically, this protein appears to belong within the HSST family on the basis of amino acid sequence homology (see Table 2 and Figs. 5 and 6). Western blot analyses of rat liver HSST protein levels have demonstrated much higher concentrations in hepatic tissue from mature female than in that of male animals (HOMMA et al. 1992). In males, HSST protein levels decrease from 20 to 60 days of age, and then increase once again during senescence, from 110 to 550 days of age. Northern blot analyses confirmed those observations and demonstrated four- to sixfold higher HSST mRNA levels in hepatic tissue of mature female than in that of mature male rats (RUNGE-MORRIS and WILUSZ 1991). Once again, caution must be exercised to avoid extrapolating these results to other species. A recent "population" study of the only known HSST in human liver, DHEA ST, failed to demonstrate significant male–female differences in level of enzyme activity in the 94 samples of hepatic tissue examined (AKSOY et al. 1993b). In summary, a great deal of information indicates that some ST enzyme activities can be regulated, at least in part, by hormonal factors. It is anticipated that our understanding of molecular mechanisms responsible for this regulation will increase when cDNAs and genomic DNAs for these enzymes become widely available for experimental use.

H. Conclusion

Knowledge of the function, biochemistry, and molecular biology of enzymes that catalyze sulfation has increased dramatically since Baumann first described the sulfate conjugation of exogenous compounds (BAUMANN 1876). It is now clear that tissues of eukaryotic organisms contain several different classes of cytoplasmic ST enzymes. These enzymes differ physically in their primary amino acid sequences and functionally in their substrate specificities and regulation. The cloning of cDNAs for ST enzymes should make it possible to develop a classification scheme based on amino acid sequence that will simplify communication with regard to these enzymes. Furthermore, the availability of molecular tools such as cDNAs should enhance the ability of investigators to study the function and regulation of these enzymes. However, exciting and useful as they are, the techniques of molecular biology represent only one approach to the study of ST enzymes. Merely observing that the protein encoded by a cDNA is capable of catalyzing a reaction does not eliminate the possibility that other enzymes might also be capable of doing so. In addition, such studies give little indication of the relative in vivo importance of any particular ST isoform. Ultimately, experiments performed with whole animals, cells in culture, tissue preparations, purified enzymes, and expressed cDNAs will all be required to characterize this metabolic pathway fully.

Our present understanding of ST enzymes has resulted from the convergence of several lines of research. Pharmacologists have studied sulfate conjugation because of interest in the biotransformation of drugs and xenobiotic compounds; neuroscientists have pursued the role of sulfate conjugation in the metabolism of neurotransmitters such as the catecholamines; endocrinologists have investigated these enzymes because of their role in the biotransformation of hormones, particularly steroid hormones; and gastroenterologists have been interested in the metabolism of bile acids. Each of these perspectives has enriched knowledge of this important group of enzymes. Rapid advancement in understanding of the molecular biology of STs will further clarify both the phylogenetic relationship among enzymes that catalyze this important pathway in the biotransformation of drugs, xenobiotic compounds, neurotransmitters, and hormones and make it possible for future investigators to explore their functional significance and regulation.

Acknowledgements. We thank Luanne Wussow for her invaluable assistance in the preparation of this manuscript. This work was supported in part by NIH grants GM 28157 and GM 35720.

References

Adams JB (1991) Enzymatic synthesis of steroid sulphates XVII. On the structure of bovine estrogen sulfotransferase. Biochim Biophys Acta 1076:282–288

Aksoy IA, Otterness DM, Weinshilboum RM (1993a) Cholesterol sulfation in human liver: catalysis by dehydroepiandrosterone sulfotransferase. Drug Metab Dispos 21:268–276

Aksoy IA, Sochorová V, Weinshilboum R (1993b) Human liver dehydroepiandrosterone sulfotransferase: nature and extent of individual variation. Clin Pharmacol Ther 54:498–506

Anderson RJ, Weinshilboum RM (1979) Phenolsulphotransferase: enzyme activity and endogenous inhibitors in human erythrocyte. J Lab Clin Med 94:158–171

Anderson RJ, Weinshilboum RM (1980) Phenolsulphotransferase in human tissue: radiochemical enzymatic assay and biochemical properties. Clin Chim Acta 103:79–90

Anderson RJ, Yoon JK, Sinsheimer EG, Jackson BL (1986) Human pituitary phenol sulfotransferase: biochemical properties and activities of the thermostable and thermolabile forms. Neuroendocrinology 44:117–124

Anhalt E, Holloway CJ, Brunner G, Trautschold I (1982) Mechanism of sulphate transfer from 4-nitrophenylsulphate to phenolic acceptors via liver cytosolic sulphotransferase. Enzyme 27:171–178

Banerjee RK, Roy AB (1968) Kinetic studies of the phenol sulfotransferase reaction. Biochim Biophys Acta 151:573–586

Baran H, Jellinger K (1992) Human brain phenolsulfotransferase. Regional distribution in Parkinson's disease. J Neural Transm 4:267–276

Barańczyk-Kuźma A, Ciszewska-Pilczyńska A (1989) Sulfation in male reproductive organs: bull and boar testis phenol sulfotransferase. Biochem Pharmacol 38: 4231–4236

Barańczyk-Kuźma A, Szymczyk T (1986) Lung phenol sulfotransferases: thermal stability of human and bovine enzymes. Biochem Pharmacol 35:995–999

Barańczyk-Kuźma A, Szymczyk T (1987) Extrahepatic sulfation of phenols: bovine lung and intestinal phenol sulfotransferase. Biochem Pharmacol 36:3141–3146

Barańczyk-Kuźma A, Borchardt RT, Schasteen CS, Pinnick CL (1981) Phenol sulfotransferase: purification and characterization of the rat brain enzyme. In: Sandler M, Usdin E (eds) Phenolsulfotransferase in mental health research. MacMillan, London, pp 55–73

Barańczyk-Kuźma A, Borchardt RT, Pinnick CL (1985) Phenol sulfotransferase: purification and characterization of the rat kidney and stomach enzymes. Acta Biochim Pol 32:35–45

Barańczyk-Kuźma A, Audus KL, Borchardt RT (1992) Properties of phenol sulphotransferase from brain of the monkey *Rhesus macaca*. Acta Biochim Pol 39: 153–158

Barnes S, Walchop R, Neighbors AS (1983) Alkaline butanol extraction of bile acids and steroid sulfate esters: application to the assay of sulfotransferases. Anal Biochem 133:470–475

Barnes S, Buchina ES, King RJ, McBurnett T, Taylor KB (1989) Bile acid sulfotransferase I from rat liver sulfates bile acids and 3-hydroxy steroids: purification, N-terminal amino acid sequence, and kinetic properties. J Lipid Res 30:529–540

Baumann E (1876) Ueber Sulfosäuren im Harn. Ber Dtsch Chem Ges 54–58

Bonham-Carter SM, Rein G, Glover V, Sandler M, Caldwell J (1983) Human platelet phenol sulphotransferase M and P: substrate specificities and correlation with in vivo sulphoconjugation of paracetamol and salicylamide. Br J Clin Pharmacol 15:323–330

Borchardt RT, Schasteen CS (1982) Phenol sulfotransferase: I. Purification of a rat liver enzyme by affinity chromatography. Biochim Biophys Acta 708:272–279

Borchardt RT, Barańczyk-Kuźma A, Pinnik CL (1983) An ecteola-cellulose chromatography assay for 3′-phosphoadenosine-5′-phosphosulfate: phenol sulfotransferase. Anal Biochem 130:334–338

Boström H, Wengle B (1964) Studies of ester sulphates: IXX. On sulphate conjugation in adult human liver extracts. Acta Soc Med Ups 69:41–63

Bouthillier M, Bleau G, Chapdelaine A, Roberts KD (1985) The purification of 3β-hydroxysteroid sulfotransferase of the hamster epididymis. J Steroid Biochem 22:733–738

Brooks SC, Battelli MB, Corombos JD (1987) Endocrine steroid sulfotransferases: porcine endometrial estrogen sulfotransferase. J Steroid Biochem 26:285–290

Burchell B, Nebert DW, Nelson DR, Bock KW, Iyanagi T, Jansen PLM, Lancet D, Mulden GJ, Chowdhury JR, Siest G, Tephly TR, Mackenzie PI (1991) The UDP glucuronosyltransferase gene superfamily: suggested nomenclature based on evolutionary divergence. DNA Cell Biol 10:487–494

Campbell NRC, Weinshilboum R (1986) Human phenol sulfotransferase (PST): correlation of liver and platelet activities. Can Soc Clin Invest 9 Suppl: A14

Campbell NRC, Van Loon JA, Weinshilboum RM (1987a) Human liver phenol sulfotransferase: assay conditions, biochemical properties and partial purification of isozymes of the thermostable form. Biochem Pharmacol 36:1435–1446

Campbell NRC, Van Loon JA, Sundaram RS, Ames MM, Hansch C, Weinshilboum R (1987b) Human and rat liver phenol sulfotransferase: structure–activity relationships for phenolic substrates. Mol Pharmacol 32:813–819

Chatterjee B, Nath TS, Roy AK (1981) Differential regulation of the messenger RNA for three major senescence marker proteins in male rat liver. J Biol Chem 256:5939–5941

Chatterjee B, Majumdar D, Ozbilen O, Murty CVR, Roy AK (1987) Molecular cloning and characterization of cDNA for androgen-repressible rat liver protein, SMP-2. J Biol Chem 262:822–825

Chen X, Yang Y-S, Zheng Y, Martin BM, Duffel MW, Jakoby WB (1992) Tyrosine-ester sulfotransferase from rat liver: bacterial expression and identification. Protein Expression Purification 3:421–426

Clarke CL, Adams JB, Wren BG (1982) Induction of estrogen sulfotransferase by progesterone in organ culture. J Clin Endocrinol Metab 55:70–75

Comer KA, Falany CN (1992) Immunological characterization of dehydroepiandrosterone sulfotransferase from human liver and adrenal. Mol Pharmacol 41: 645–651

Cooke GM, Ferguson SE, Rytina E, Gower DB (1983) Properties of porcine liver and testicular steroid sulphotransferases: reaction conditions and influence of naturally occurring steroids and steroid sulphates. J Steroid Biochem 19: 1103–1109

Coughtrie MWH, Sharp S (1990) Purification and immunochemical characterization of a rat liver sulfotransferase conjugating paracetamol. Biochem Pharmacol 40:2305–2313

Demyan WF, Song CS, Kim DS, Her S, Gallwitz W, Rao TR, Siomczynska M, Chatterjee B, Roy AK (1992) Estrogen sulfotransferase of the rat liver: complementary DNA cloning and age- and sex-specific regulation of messenger RNA. Mol Endocrinol 6:589–597

Devereux J, Haeberli P, Smithies O (1984) A comprehensive set of sequence analysis programs for the VAX. Nucleic Acids Res 12:387–395

Dodgson KS (1977) Conjugation with sulfate. In: Parke DV, Smith RL (eds) Drug metabolism from microbe to man. Francis, London, pp 91–104

Dodgson KS, Rose FA (1970) Sulfoconjugation and sulfohydrolysis. In: Fishman WF (ed) Metabolic conjugation and metabolic hydrolysis, vol 1. Academic, New York, pp 239–325

Duffel MW, Binder TP, Hoise L, Baden HA, Sanders JA, Knapp SA, Baron J (1991) Purification, immunochemical characterization, and immunohistochemical localization of rat hepatic aryl sulfotransferase IV. Mol Pharmacol 40:36–44

Falany CN (1991) Molecular enzymology of human liver cytosolic sulfotransferases. Trends Pharmacol Sci 12:255–259

Falany CN, Kerl EA (1990) Sulfation of minoxidil by human liver phenol sulfotransferase. Biochem Pharmacol 40:1027–1032

Falany CN, Vazquez ME, Kalb JM (1989) Purification and characterization of human liver dehydroepiandrosterone sulphotransferase. Biochem J 260:641–646

Falany CN, Vazquez ME, Heroux JA, Roth JA (1990) Purification and characterization of human liver phenol-sulfating phenol sulfotransferase. Arch Biochem Biophys 278:312–318

Feng D-F, Doolittle RF (1987) Progressive sequence alignment as a prerequisite to correct phylogenetic trees. J Mol Evol 25:351–360

Foldes A, Meek JL (1973) Rat brain phenolsulfotransferase – partial purification and some properties. Biochim Biophys Acta 327:365–374

Freeman DJ, Saidi F, Hobkirk R (1983) Estrogen sulfotransferase activity in guinea pig uterus and chorion. J Steroid Biochem 18:23–27

Green JM, Singer SS (1983) Enzymatic sulfation of steroids: XVIII. Study of the specific estradiol-17β sulfotransferase of rat liver cytosol that converts the estrogen to its 3-sulfate, and some elements of the endocrine control of its production. Can J Biochem Cell Biol 61:15–22

Hahlbrock K, Scheel D (1989) Physiology and molecular biology of phenylpropanoid metabolism. Annu Rev Plant Physiol Plant Mol Biol 40:347–369

Hannoufa A, Varin L, Ibrahim RK (1991) Spatial distribution of flavonoid conjugates in relation to glycosyltransferase and sulfotransferase activities in *Flaveria bidentis*. Plant Physiol 97:259–263

Hart RF, Renskers KJ, Nelson EB, Roth JA (1979) Localization and characterization of phenol sulfotransferase in human platelets. Life Sci 24:125–130

Hashimoto Y, Orellana A, Gil G, Hirschberg CB (1992) Molecular cloning and expression of rat liver N-heparan sulfate sulfotransferase. J Biol Chem 267: 15744–15750

Hernández JS, Powers SP, Weinshilboum RM (1991) Human liver arylamine N-sulfotransferase activity: thermostable phenol sulfotransferase catalyzes the N-sulfation of 2-naphthylamine. Drug Metab Dispos 19:1071–1079

Hernández JS, Watson RWG, Wood TC, Weinshilboum RM (1992) Sulfation of estrone and 17β-estradiol in human liver: catalysis by thermostable phenol sulfotransferase and by dehydroepiandrosterone sulfotransferase. Drug Metab Dispos 20:413–422

Heroux JA, Roth JA (1988) Physical characterization of a monoamine-sulfating form of phenol sulfotransferase from human platelets. Mol Pharmacol 34:194–199

Hirshey SJ, Falany CN (1990) Purification and characterization of rat liver minoxidil sulphotransferase. Biochem J 270:721–728

Hirshey SJ, Dooley TP, Reardon IM, Henrikson RL, Falany CN (1992) Sequence analysis, in vitro translation, and expression of the cDNA for rat liver minoxidil sulfotransferase. Mol Pharmacol 42:257–264

Hobkirk R, Glasier MA, Brown LY (1990) Purification and some characteristics of an oestrogen sulphotransferase from guinea pig adrenal gland and its non-identity with adrenal pregnenolone sulphotransferase. Biochem J 268:759–764

Hobkirk R, Girard LR, Durham NJ, Khalil MW (1985) Behavior of mouse placental and uterine estrogen sulfotransferase during chromatography and other procedures. Biochim Biophys Acta 828:123–129

Homma H, Sasaki T, Matsui M (1991) Properties of androsterone-sulfating sulfotransferase in female rat liver. Chem Pharm Bull (Tokyo) 6:1499–1503

Homma H, Nakagome I, Kamakura M, Matsui M (1992) Immunochemical characterization of developmental changes in rat hepatic hydroxysteroid sulfotransferases. Biochim Biophys Acta 1121:69–74

Honkasalo T, Nissinen E (1988) Determination of phenol sulfotransferase activity by high-performance liquid chromatography. J Chromatogr 424:136–140

Huttner WB (1982) Sulphation of tyrosine residues – a widespread modification of proteins. Nature 299:273–276

Jakoby WB, Sekura RD, Lyon ES, Marcus CJ, Wang JL (1980) Sulfotransferases. In: Jakoby WB (ed) Enzymatic basis of detoxication, vol 2. Academic, New York, pp 199–228

Johnson GA, Barshun KJ, McCall JM (1982) Sulfation of minoxidil by liver sulfotransferase. Biochem Pharmacol 31:2949–2954

Levy G (1986) Sulfate conjugation in drug metabolism: role of inorganic sulfate. Fed Proc 45:2235–2240

Littlewood J, Glover V, Sandler M, Petty R, Peatfield R, Rose FL (1982) Platelet phenolsulphotransferase deficiency in dietary migraine. Lancet 1:983–985

Marcus CJ, Sekura RD, Jakoby WB (1980) A hydroxysteroid sulfotransferase from rat liver. Anal Biochem 107:296–304

Matsui M, Watanabe HK (1982) Developmental alteration of hepatic UDP-glucuronosyltransferase and sulphotransferase towards androsterone and 4-nitrophenol in Wistar rats. Biochem J 204:441–447

Meisheri KD, Cipkus LA, Taylor CJ (1988) Mechanism of action of minoxidil sulfate-induced vasodilation: a role for increased K+ permeability. J Pharmacol Exp Ther 245:751–760

Moore SS, Thompson EOP, Nash AR (1988) Oestrogen sulfotransferase: isolation of a high specific activity species from bovine placenta. Aust J Biol Sci 41:333–341

Mulder GJ, Jakoby WB (1990) Sulfation. In: Mulder GJ (ed) Conjugation reactions in drug metabolism. Taylor and Francis, New York, pp 107–161

Mulder GJ, Krijgsheld KR (1981) The availability of inorganic sulfate for sulfate conjugation in vivo. In: Sandler M, Usdin E (eds) Phenolsulfotransferase in mental health research. Macmillan London, pp 127–144

Nash AR, Glenn WK, Moore SS, Kerr J, Thompson AR, Thompson EOP (1988) Oestrogen sulfotransferase: molecular cloning and sequencing of cDNA for bovine placental enzyme. Aust J Biol Sci 41:507–516

Nebert DW, Nelson DR, Coon MJ, Estabrook RW, Feyereisen R, Fujii-Kuriyama Y, Gonzalez FJ, Guengerich FP, Gunsalus IC, Johnson EF, Loper JC, Sato R, Waterman MR, Waxman DJ (1991) The P450 superfamily: update on new sequences, gene mapping and recommended nomenclature. DNA Cell Biol 10:1–14

Nomenclature Committee of the International Union of Biochemistry on the Nomenclature and Classification of Enzyme-Catalyzed Reactions (1984) Enzyme nomenclature 1984. Academic, New York, pp 266–268

Nose Y, Lipmann F (1958) Separation of steroid sulfokinases. J Biol Chem 233: 1348–1351

Oeda T, Lee YC, Driscoll WJ, Chen H-C, Strott CA (1992) Molecular cloning and expression of a full-length complementary DNA encoding the guinea pig adrenocortical estrogen sulfotransferase. Mol Endocrinol 6:1216–1226

Ogura K, Kajita J, Narihata H, Watabe T, Ozawa S, Nagata K, Yamazoe Y, Kato R (1989) Cloning and sequence analysis of a rat liver cDNA encoding hydroxysteroid sulfotransferase. Biochem Biophys Res Commun 165:168–174

Ogura K, Kajita J, Narihata H, Watabe T, Ozawa S, Nagata K, Yamazoe Y, Kato R (1990) cDNA cloning of the hydroxysteroid sulfotransferase STa sharing a strong homology in amino acid sequence with the senescence marker protein SMP-2 in rat livers. Biochem Biophys Res Commun 166:1494–1500

Otterness DM, Powers SP, Miller LJ, Weinshilboum RM (1989) Human liver thermostable phenol sulfotransferase: photoaffinity labeling with 2-iodo-4-azidophenol. Mol Pharmacol 36:856–865

Otterness DM, Powers SP, Miller LJ, Weinshilboum RM (1991) 3′-Phosphoadenosine-5′-phosphosulfate: photoaffinity ligand for sulfotransferase enzymes. Mol Pharmacol 39:34–41

Otterness DM, Wieben ED, Wood TC, Watson RWG, Madden BJ, McCormick DJ, Weinshilboum RM (1992) Human liver dehydroepiandrosterone sulfotransferase: molecular cloning and expression of cDNA. Mol Pharmacol 41:865–872

Ozawa S, Nagata K, Gong D, Yamazoe Y, Kato R (1990) Nucleotide sequence of a full-length cDNA (PST-1) for aryl sulfotransferase from rat liver. Nucleic Acids Res 18:4001

Price RA, Cox NJ, Spielman RS, Van Loon J, Maidak BL, Weinshilboum RM (1988) Inheritance of human platelet thermolabile phenol sulfotransferase (TL PST) activity. Genet Epidemiol 5:1–15

Price RA, Spielman RS, Lucena AL, Van Loon JA, Maidak BL, Weinshilboum RM (1989) Genetic polymorphism for human platelet thermostable phenol sulfotransferase (TS PST) activity. Genetics 122:905–914

Radominska A, Comer KA, Zimniak P, Falany J, Iscan M, Falany CN (1990) Human liver steroid sulphotransferase sulphates bile acids. Biochem J 272: 597–604

Rein G, Glover V, Sandler M (1981) Phenolsulphotransferase in human tissue: evidence for multiple forms. In: Sandler M, Usdin E (eds) Phenolsulfotransferase in mental health research. Macmillan, London, pp 98–126

Rein G, Glover V, Sandler M (1982) Multiple forms of phenolsulfotransferase in human tissues: selective inhibition by dichloronitropheol. Biochem Pharmacol 31:1893–1897

Reiter C, Weinshilboum RM (1982a) Acetaminophen and phenol: substrates for both a thermostable and a thermolabile form of human platelet phenol sulfotransferase. J Pharmacol Exp Ther 221:43–51

Reiter C, Weinshilboum R (1982b) Platelet phenol sulfotransferase activity: correlation with sulfate conjugation of acetaminophen in man. Clin Pharmacol Ther 32:612–621

Reiter C, Mwaluko G, Dunnette J, Van Loon J, Weinshilboum R (1983) Thermolabile and thermostable human platelet phenol sulfotransferase: substrate specificity and physical separation. Naunyn Schmiedebergs Arch Pharmacol 324:140–147

Reveley AM, Carter SMB, Reveley MA, Sandler M (1982/1983) A genetic study of platelet phenolsulfotransferase activity in normal and schizophrenic twins. J Psychiatr Res 17:303–307

Romain Y, Demassieux S, Carriére S (1982) Partial purification and characterization of two isoenzymes involved in the sulfurylation of catecholamines. Biochem Biophys Res Commun 106:999–1005

Roy AB (1981) Sulfotransferases. In: Mulder GJ (ed) Sulfation of drugs and related compounds. CRC, Boca Raton, pp 83–130

Runge-Morris M, Wilusz J (1991) Age- and gender-related gene expression of hydroxysteroid sulfotransferase-a in rat liver. Biochem Biophys Res Commun 175:1051–1056

Sakai D, Zachos M, Lingwood CA (1992) Purification of the testicular galactolipid: 3′-phosphoadenosine-5′-phosphosulfate sulfotransferase. J Biol Chem 267: 1655–1659

Schmoldt A, Blömer I, Johannes A (1992) Hydroxysteroid sulfotransferase and a specific UDP-glucuronosyltransferase are involved in the metabolism of digitoxin in man. Naunyn Schmiedebergs Arch Pharmacol 346:226–233

Sekura RD, Jakoby WB (1979) Phenol sulfotransferases. J Biol Chem 254: 5658–5663

Sekura RD, Jakoby WB (1981) Aryl sulfotransferase IV from rat liver. Arch Biochem Biophys 211:352–359

Sekura RD, Marcus CJ, Lyon EC, Jakoby WB (1979) Assay of sulfotransferases. Anal Biochem 95:82–86

Singer SS (1985) Preparation and characterization of the different kinds of sulfotransferases. In: Zakim D, Vessey DA (eds) Methodological aspects of drug metabolizing enzymes. Biochemical Pharmacology and Toxicology, vol 1. Wiley, New York, pp 95–159

Smith TF, Waterman MS (1981) Comparison of bio-sequences. Adv Appl Math 2:482–189

Sundaram RS, Szumlanski C, Otterness D, Van Loon JA, Weinshilboum RM (1989a) Human intestinal phenol sulfotransferase: assay conditions, activity levels and partial purification of the thermolabile (TL) form. Drug Metab Dispos 17:255–264

Sundaram RS, Van Loon JA, Tucker R, Weinshilboum RM (1989b) Sulfation pharmacogenetics: correlation of human platelet and small intestinal phenol sulfotransferase. Clin Pharmacol Ther 46:501–509

Toth LA, Kao G, Elchisak MA (1987) Factors influencing the recovery of dopamine sulfate in the assay of phenol sulfotransferase. Life Sci 40:473–480

Tseng L, Lee LY, Mazella J (1985) Estrogen sulfotransferase in human placenta. J Steroid Biochem 22:611–615

Ueki A, Willoughby J, Glover V, Sandler M (1989) Distribution of phenolsulophotransferase and monoamine oxidase in the common marmoset. Biochem Pharmacol 38:2383–2385

Varin L, Ibrahim RK (1989) Partial purification and characterization of three flavonol-specific sulfotransferases from *Flaveria chloraefolia*. Plant Physiol 90:977–981

Varin L, Ibrahim RK (1992) Novel flavonol 3-sulfotransferase: purification, kinetic properties, and partial amino acid sequence. J Biol Chem 267:1858–1863

Varin L, Barron D, Ibrahim RK (1987) Enzymatic assay for flavonoid sulfotransferase. Anal Biochem 161:176–180

Varin L, DeLuca V, Ibrahim RK, Brisson N (1992) Molecular characterization of two plant flavonol sulfotransferases. Proc Natl Acad Sci USA 89:1286–1290

Watabe T, Ishizuka T, Isobe M, Ozawa N (1982) A 7-hydroxymethylsulfate ester as an active metabolite of 7,12-dimethylbenz[a]anthracene. Science 215:403–405

Weinshilboum RM (1986a) Sulfate conjugation of neurotransmitters and drugs: an introduction. Fed Proc 45:2220–2222

Weinshilboum RM (1986b) Phenol sulfotransferase in humans: properties, regulation, and function. Fed Proc 45:2223–2228

Weinshilboum R (1988) Phenol sulfotransferase inheritance. Cell Mol Neurobiol 8:27–34

Weinshilboum R (1990) Sulfotransferase pharmacogenetics. Pharmacol Ther 45: 93–107

Wengle B (1964) Studies on ester sulphates: XVI. Use of ^{35}S-labelled inorganic sulphate for quantitative studies of sulphate conjugation in liver extracts. Acta Chem Scand 18:65–76

Whittemore RM, Roth JA (1985) A modified ecteola-cellulose assay for M and P phenol sulfotransferase. Biochem Pharmacol 34:1647–1652

Whittemore RM, Pearce LB, Roth JA (1985) Purification and kinetic characterization of a dopamine sulfating form of phenol sulfotransferase from human brain. Biochemistry 24:2477–2482

Whittemore RM, Pearch LB, Roth JA (1986) Purification and kinetic characterization of a phenol sulfating form of phenol sulfotransferase from human brain. Arch Biochem Biophys 249:464–471

Wilborn TW, Comer KA, Dooley TP, Reardon IM, Heinrikson RL, Falany CN (1993) Sequence analysis and expression of the cDNA for the phenol sulfating form of human liver phenol sulfotransferase. Mol Pharmacol 40:70–77

Yerokum T, Etheredge JL, Norton TR, Carter HA, Chung KH, Birckbichler PJ, Ringer DP (1992) Characterization of a complementary DNA for rat liver aryl sulfotransferase IV and use in evaluating the hepatic gene transcript levels of rat at various stages of 2-acetylaminofluorene-induced hepatocarcinogenesis. Cancer Res 52:4779–4786

Young WF Jr, Okazaki H, Laws ER Jr, Weinshilboum RM (1984) Human brain phenol sulfotransferase: biochemical properties and regional localization. J Neurochem 43:706–715

Young WF Jr, Laws ER Jr, Sharbrough FW, Weinshilboum RM (1985) Human phenol sulfotransferase: correlation of brain and platelet activities. J Neurochem 44:1131–1137

CHAPTER 3

Regulation of Expression of Rat Liver Glutathione S-Transferases: Xenobiotic and Antioxidant Induction of the Ya Subunit Gene

T.H. RUSHMORE, C.B. PICKETT, and A.Y.H. LU

A. Perspectives

The glutathione S-transferases (GSTs) are a family of proteins that conjugate glutathione, via the sulfur atom of cysteine, to various electrophiles (BOYLAND and CHASSEAUD 1969; CHASSEAUD 1979; JACOBY 1978; MANNERVIK 1985; MANNERVIK and DANIELSON 1988; PICKETT and LU 1989; COLES and KETTERER 1990; ARMSTRONG 1991; TSUCHIDA and SATO 1992). In addition to the conjugation of electrophiles, the GSTs bind with high affinity a variety of hydrophobic compounds such as heme, bilirubin, polycyclic hydrocarbons, and dexamethazone (LITWACK et al. 1971; ARIAS et al. 1976; BHARGAVA et al. 1980; HOMMA and LISTOWSKY 1985).

GSTs have now been purified and the genes encoding various enzymes have been cloned from many sources. Those found in the rat liver have been the most extensively studied and will be the focus of this review.

GSTs have been identified in both the cytosolic and particulate fractions of the liver cell. The cytosolic forms are homodimers or heterodimers of at least 13 subunits. The microsomal form has little sequence identity to any of the cytosolic GSTs and it exists most likely as a trimer (MORGENSTERN et al. 1988; LUNDQVIST et al. 1992; HIRATSUKA et al. 1990; MEYER et al. 1991; OGURA et al. 1991).

In the past few years, the application of molecular biological techniques to elucidate GST gene structure and function has begun to reveal the immense complexity of this multigene family. With the use of high-level expression systems in prokaryotic cells coupled with site-directed mutagenesis, significant advances have been made in the analysis of GST function and enzymatic mechanism(s). Within the past year, three GSTs have been crystallized and their structures presented.

The various subunits of GST have been shown to be induced in a tissue-specific manner by various xenobiotics (phenobarbitol, 3-methylcholanthrene, *trans*-stilbene oxide). Cloning of both the cDNA and genomic sequences of the GSTs has permitted the identification and analysis of several *cis*-acting sequences in the promoters that are required for their induction and regulation by different stimuli. From the detailed analysis of the Ya subunit gene, a unique *cis*-acting regulatory element, the antioxidant-responsive element (ARE), has been identifed and characterized (RUSHMORE et al. 1990).

In this review, we will focus our attention on the structure and regulation, including site-directed mutagenesis and crystal structures of genes encoding several of the rat liver GSTs. A brief discussion of nomenclature and a compilation of both cDNA and genomic clones of the rat GSTs will be presented. Mechanism(s) for the regulation of transcriptional activation of the alpha Ya1 subunit gene will be discussed, with emphasis on the mechanism(s) of regulation by planar aromatic compounds and phenolic antioxidants.

B. Occurrence and Structure

The majority of the rat liver GSTs are found in the cytosolic fraction of the cells. The soluble GSTs have all been shown to be dimeric holoenzymes (dimers) composed of either identical or nonidentical subunits. The relative molecular mass of the subunits ranges from 23 to 29 kDa. There are at least two membrane- or organelle-bound forms of GST that have been identified and/or purified; microsomal GST (Morgenstern et al. 1988; Lundqvist et al. 1992) and a second form that catalyzes synthesis of leukotriene C_4 (Piper 1984; Ford-Hutchinson 1990). In contrast to the cytosolic forms, the microsomal form of GST appears to be a trimer composed of identical 17-kDa subunits.

C. Nomenclature

The early nomenclature for the GSTs was based on the differences in their substrate utilization. Crudely separated or partially purified enzymes were identified as aryltransferase, epoxide transferase, alkyltransferase, or alkenetransferase. With further purification, the various transferases were shown to have considerable overlap in their substrate specificity.

The first comprehensive nomenclature for the GSTs was provided by Jacoby and Habig (1980), who suggested that the enzymes which had been identified in rat liver cytosol be named empirically as GST E, D, C, B, A, and AA, in order of their elution from a carboxymethylcellulose ion exchange matrix.

Structural analysis of these GSTs by electrophoretic separation indicated that the enzymes were in fact homo- and heterodimers of several different subunits. The various forms described above showed different substrate specificities that were apparently related to their subunit composition (Mannervik and Jenson 1982). This observation that the enzymatic properties of a protein dimer was dependent upon its constituent subunits led to the idea that the various forms of GST could be named based on their specific subunit composition. Therefore, a nomenclature was adopted that denoted each distinct protein subunit by an Arabic numeral (Jacoby et al.

1984). The active holoenzyme would be designated then as 1-1 or 2-2, etc. To date, at least 13 distinct subunits have been named.

An alternative system for naming the subunits of rat GSTs was based on their relative mobilities on a sodium dodecyl sulfate polycrylamino gel electrophoresis (SDS-PAGE) gel (BASS et al. 1977; BEALE et al. 1983; KITAHARA et al. 1984; HAYES and MANTLE 1986). The three major subunits identified in rat liver cytosol after Coomasie blue (Kenacid Blue) staining were designated Ya, Yb, and Yc in order of decreasing mobility on the SDS-PAGE gel (Ya being the fastest). Yp, a subunit originally identified in the placenta and in preneoplastic liver nodules, had a mobility slightly faster than Ya (ERIKSSON et al. 1983; SATO et al. 1984; SATOH et al. 1985).

A useful species-independent classification scheme was described by MANNERVIK et al. (1985), who recognized that the soluble GSTs could be separated into three unambiguous classes, alpha, mu, and pi (recently a new classification has been added, theta; HIRATSUKA et al. 1990; MEYER et al. 1991), based on differences in their structural, immunological, and enzymatic properties. Within the same isozyme class, these properties were highly conserved across the species. However, between isozyme class they diverged significantly, even within the same species. Therefore, including the microsomal enzymes, there are at least five classes of mammalian GSTs. Table 1 summarizes the classes and subunit designations for the rat GSTs.

D. cDNA and Genomic Clones of Rat Glutathione S-Transferases

I. cDNA Clones of the Alpha Gene Family (Subunits Ya1, Ya2, and Yc)

The first full-length cDNA clones coding for the complete amino acid sequence of the Ya subunit of rat liver GST were isolated by PICKETT (1984) and Tu and coworkers (LAI et al. 1984). Previously, KALINYAK and TAYLOR (1982) and DANIEL et al. (1983) had reported the isolation and sequence of partial cDNA clones of the Ya subunit of rat liver GST (ligandin).

The cDNA for the Ya subunit clone pGTB38 (PICKETT et al. 1984) is 950 nucleotides in length with an open reading frame encoding a polypeptide of 222 amino acids with a calculated molecular weight of 25547. The coding sequence is flanked by 39 nucleotides of 5′ untranslated region and 114 nucleotides of 3′ untranslated region. The cDNA for a second form of Ya subunit, clone pGTR261 (LAI et al. 1984), is 830 nucleotides in length with an open reading frame encoding a polypeptide of 222 amino acids with a calculated molecular weight of 25600. The coding sequence is flanked by 63 nucleotides of 5′ untranslated region and 100 nucleotides of 3′ untranslated region.

Table 1. Nomenclature for rat liver glutathione S-transferases: subunit name, cDNA clones, and genomic clones

Class	Subunit[a]	Nomenclature[b]	cDNA clones[c]	Genomic clones[d]
Alpha	Ya1	1	PGTB38	TELAKOWSKI-HOPKINS et al. (1986)
	Ya2	1	pGTR261	
	Yc	2	pGTB42	
	Yk	8	λGTRA8	
	Yl	10		
Mu	Yb1	3	pGTA/C44, pGST200	MORTON et al. (1990)
	Yb2	4	pGTA/C48, pGTR187C	LAI et al. (1988)
	Yb3	6	Yb3-cDNA	ABRAMOVITZ and LISTOWSKY (personal communication)
	Yn2	9		
	Yo	11		
	Yb4			LAI et al. (1988)
Pi	Yp	7	pGP5	OKUDA et al. (1987)
Theta	Yrs	?	theta-1	
		5		
		12		
		13		

[a] Nomenclature of BASS et al. (1977), BEALE et al. (1983), KITAHARA et al. (1984), and HAYES and MANTLE (1986).
[b] Nomenclature of JAKOBY et al. (1984).
[c] References for cDNA clones can be found in text.
[d] References for genomic cloning and analysis.

TELAKOWSKI-HOPKINS et al. (1985) have reported the isolation of a cDNA clone encoding the Yc subunit of rat liver. Clone pGTB42 is 900 nucleotides in length with an open reading frame encoding a polypeptide of 221 amino acids with a calculated molecular weight of 25322. The coding sequence is flanked by 44 nucleotides of 5′ untranslated region and 157 nucleotides of 3′ untranslated region.

Comparison of the nucleotide sequence of the Ya and Yc subunits revealed that the Ya and Yc mRNAs were very homologous. Over identical regions in both clones (nucleotides −39 to 780) there was a 66% nucleotide sequence homology. In the protein-coding region (nucleotides +1 to 662), the Ya and Yc mRNAs were 75% identical in nucleotide sequence. In contrast to the amino acid-coding region, the amino acid sequence of the Ya and Yc subunits have an overall homology of 68%. The first 74 N-terminal amino acids of the two subunits are 76% homologous, whereas the middle third and last third (carboxyl terminal domain) are only 68% and 60% homologous, respectively. The 5′ and 3′ untranslated regions show very little sequence homology.

Based upon the nucleotide sequence difference in the coding region of the Ya and Yc mRNAs along with the divergent 5′ and 3′ regions, the Ya and Yc subunits of rat liver GST were believed to be derived from two different genes (Telakowski-Hopkins et al. 1985; Tu et al. 1984).

Comparison of the sequence of the two Ya clones pGTB38 and pGST261 revealed a number of significant differences suggesting the possibility of microheterogeneity within the Ya gene family. The clones contained 15 nucleotide replacements in the amino acid-coding region that translated into eight amino acid changes. The 3′ untranslated regions of the two Ya mRNAs contained the most significant divergence, permitting the classification of at least two forms of Ya mRNA, Ya1 (pGTB38) and Ya2 (pGTR261), and supporting the idea that the two cDNA clones were derived from separate genes.

A fourth alpha class cDNA has been reported by Stenberg et al. (1992) that codes for subunit 8. The GST isozyme, designated GST 8-8, has a uniquely high activity with 4-hydroxyalkenal substrates. The cDNA clone, λGTRA8, contains 862 nucleotides encoding 222 amino acid residues. The sequence was identical to that previously determined for the isolated protein except for residues 18 and 48. The overall sequence homology to other rat alpha class subunits is 64%–66%.

II. cDNA Clones of the Mu Gene Family (Subunits Yb1, Yb2, Yb3, and Yb4)

At least three Yb subunit cDNA clones have been isolated and characterized to date; Yb1 (pGTA/C44, pGST200), Yb2 (pGTR187, pGTA/C48, pGTR187C), and Yb3 (Yb3-cDN). A fourth Yb type subunit, Yb4, has been identified and its amino acid sequence deduced from a genomic clone. It is not known if Yb4 is expressed in the rat.

The Yb1 cDNA clone pGTA/C44 (Ding et al. 1985) contains an open reading frame that encodes a polypeptide of 218 amino acids with a molecular weight of 25 919. The coding region is flanked by 37 nucleotides of 5′ untranslated region and 348 nucleotides of 3′ untranslated region. A second Yb1 cDNA clone, pGTR200, was isolated by Lai et al. (1986) that also contains an open reading frame encoding 218 amino acids with a molecular weight of 25 915, but differs from pGTBA/C44 in four nucleotides (two amino acids). The 5′ and 3′-untranslated regions of the two clones are essentially identical.

Two nearly full-length cDNA clones (pGTA/C48, pGTR187) have been isolated that are complementary to the Yb2 subunit of rat liver GST (Ding et al. 1986; Lai and Tu 1986b). Both clones are missing the entire 5′ untranslated region and the nucleotides coding for the first 24 and 32 amino acids, respectively.

Recently, Lai et al. (1988) have reported the isolation of a cDNA clone, λGTR187C, that contains the complete amino acid-coding region for the rat liver Yb2 subunit, 218 amino acids. The overall nucleotide sequence homology in the amino acid-coding region between the Yb1 and Yb2 subunits is 84%, whereas in the 3′ untranslated region there is only 32% homology. The amino acid sequence of the Yb1 and Yb2 subunits is 79% identical.

Abramovitz and Listowsky (1987) have isolated a cDNA clone for a third Yb type GST, Yb3, found predominantly in the rat brain. The clone, Yb3-cDNA, contains an open reading frame encoding a polypeptide of 218 amino acids with a molecular weight of 25549. The clone contains 18 nucleotides of 5′ untranslated region and 533 nucleotides of 3′ untranslated region. The nucleotide sequence of the amino acid-coding region is 80% homologous with the Yb1 and Yb2 cDNAs, while the 3′ untranslated regions are markedly divergent. The amino acid sequence derived from the cDNA of Yb3 was 78% identical to Yb1 and 80% identical to Yb2.

A fourth Yb type subunit from rat liver has been described by Lai et al. (1988), Yb4. The genomic DNA clone, λGTR4-1, contains the complete gene, from which the amino acid-coding sequence and protein sequence (218 amino acids in length) have been deduced. Again, it is not known whether the Yb4 subunit is expressed in the rat.

III. cDNA Clones of the Pi Gene Family (Subunit Yp)

Suguoka et al. (1985) have isolated cDNA clones complementary to the mRNA specific for the Yp subunit (subunit 7) of GST. The Yp cDNA clone, pGP5, contains an open reading frame that encodes 209 amino acids with a molecular weight of 23307. Comparison of the nucleotide sequence of the coding region of the Yp subunit with the Ya/Yc and Yb subunits revealed an amino acid sequence homology of 32% and 24%, respectively.

IV. cDNA Clones of the Theta Gene Family (Subunit Yrs)

Ogura et al. (1991) have isolated a cDNA clone containing the entire coding sequence for the subunit of GST Yrs-Yrs. This cDNA, designated theta-1, contains an open reading frame of 732 nucleotides encoding a polypeptide of 224 amino acids residues. The predicted molecular weight of the Yrs subunit is 27311.

The deduced AA sequence of the subunit protein Yrs shares a weak homology of less than 23% with the reported sequences of all the subunits proteins of alpha, mu, and pi class GSTs. This fact strongly suggested that GST Yrs-Yrs and the other putative theta class subunits, 5, 12, and 13, with extremely strong homology in their N-terminal amino acid sequences, are products from a new gene family that would differ from those for class alpha, mu, or pi (Meyer et al. 1991).

V. cDNA Clones of the Microsomal Gene Family

DEJONG et al. (1988) have isolated a cDNA clone for the subunit of rat liver microsomal GST. The clone contains an open reading frame that encodes 154 amino acids with a molecular weight of 17430. A number of amino acid differences were found in the deduced amino acid sequence from that originally obtained by protein-sequencing techniques (MORGENSTERN et al. 1988; LUNDQVIST et al. 1992; HIRATSUKA et al. 1990; MEYER et al. 1991; OGURA et al. 1991). The Southern blot analysis of genomic DNA suggests the presence of a single microsomal GST gene in the rat genome that is approximately 12 kbp long.

Leukotrienes and peptidoleukotrienes, such as LTD_4, have been shown to be important in the pathogenesis of diseases such as human bronchial asthma. The leukotrienes are derived from arachidonic acid that is released within the cell from the sn-2 position of membrane phospholipids probably through the action of a recently identified arachidonate-selective cytosolic phospholipase A_2 (PIPER 1984; FORD-HUTCHINSON 1990). The released arachidonate is converted to the unstable epoxide, leukotriene A_4, in a two-step reaction that is catalyzed by the cytosolic enzyme 5-lipoxygenase. Leukotriene A_4 can be further metabolized via one of two possible pathways. It is either hydrated by the cytosolic enzyme LTA_4 hydrolase, producing LTB_4, or it is conjugated to reduced glutathione by a membrane-bound enzyme to form the sulfidopeptide leukotriene C_4. The enzyme that conjugates GSH to LTA_4 is leukotriene C4 (LTC_4) synthase, a novel glutathione S-transferase (PIPER 1984; FORD-HUTCHINSON 1990).

Several studies have reported partial purifications of the leukotriene C_4 synthase from various sources such as mouse mastocytoma cells, RBL-1 cells and guinea pig lung (SÖDERSTRÖM et al. 1990; IZUMI et al. 1989). These studies concluded that the leukotriene C_4 synthase was localized in the microsomal fraction rather than in the cytosol, which contains the bulk of the GST activity. Recently, NICHOLSON et al. (1992a,b) have succeeded in purifying leukotriene C_4 synthase from differentiated U937 cells and the human monocyte cell line THP-1. The final enzyme preparation was greater than 10000-fold purified and contained three polypeptides with relative molecular masses of 37.1, 24.5, and 18.0 kDa, respectively. The 18-kDa polypeptide is thought to be associated with enzymatic activity, since it could be specifically labeled by a radioiodinated leukotriene C_4 photoaffinity probe.

E. Structure of Glutathione S-Transferase Genes

I. Glutathione S-Transferase Alpha Class Family

Genomic Southern blots of rat liver genomic DNA using the 5′ and 3′ regions of the Ya and Yc subunit cDNAs suggested the presence of at least five Ya type subunits and at least two Yc type subunits (ROTHKOPF et al. 1986). To date, only one of these genes, subunit Ya1, has been isolated and characterized (TELAKOWSKI-HOPKINS et al. 1986, 1988).

The Ya1 gene, clone λGTB45-15, contains seven exons and six introns and spans 10 kbp in length. A sequence similar to the Goldberg-Hogness promoter TATA box (TATTA) is located 32 base pairs upstream from the start of transcription.

Comparision of the Ya1 subunit amino acid sequence encoded by exon 3 with the cDNA sequence of the Yc subunit gene revealed the region that was most divergent between the Ya and Yc polypeptides. There was only a 36% amino acid sequence homology between the Ya and Yc polypeptides in this region, despite an overall identity of 66% between the two polypeptides. Similarly, exon 5 encoded an amino acid sequence that was very divergent between the Ya and Yc polypeptides. There was only a 51% amino acid sequence identity between the Ya and Yc polypeptides in this region.

Exons 2 and 4 encoded amino acid residues of the Ya1 subunit that were the most highly conserved in the Yc polypeptide. The amino acid sequences of the Ya polypeptide encoded by exons 2 and 4 are 86% and 91% identical, respectively, to the corresponding sequences in the Yc polypeptide. Exons 6 and 7 encode regions of the Ya polypeptide that have an amino acid sequence identity that was similar to the overall sequence homology of the Ya and Yc polypeptide (66%).

It would appear then that the genes encoding the Ya and Yc subunits are comprised of highly conserved as well as highly divergent exons that may impart both similar and unique functional properties to the two subunits. The divergent exons (exons 3 and 5) may encode amino acids responsible for substrate specificity, whereas the exons encoding amino acids that are highly conserved between the two subunits (exons 2 and 4) may form the glutathione-binding domain (see recent crystallographic data, REINEMER et al. 1991, 1992; LIU et al. 1992; JI et al. 1992).

II. Glutathione S-Transferase Mu Class Family

Genomic Southern blots of rat liver genomic DNA with a Yb probe revealed multiple bands in different restriction digests, indicating a multigene family encoding the GST Yb subunits (LAI et al. 1986). To date, three Yb type genes have been isolated and characterized, Yb1, Yb2, and Yb4 (LAI et al. 1988; MORTON et al. 1990).

Sequence analysis of the genes has demonstrated a great similarity in gene structure in the Yb family. All the genes contain eight exons and seven introns and span approximately 5 kbp. The exon–intron structure of the Yb genes are quite different from that of the Ya and Yp genes. The Yb genes span approximately 5 kbp and are segregated into eight exons and seven introns, whereas the Ya (10 kbp) and the Yp genes (3kbp) contain seven exons and six introns.

The 5′-flanking region of the Yb1 gene contains a sequence similar to the Goldberg-Hogness promoter TATA box located 29 nucleotides upstream from the start of transcription. The Yb2 gene also contains in its promoter two regulatory elements, the CCAAT box and the TATA (ATA) box. There are two copies of the CCAAT box (−84 to −80 bp and −76 to −72 bp) in the 5′-flanking region. The putative TATA box, TATCA (−28 to −24 bp) differs from the concensus TATA box (TATAA). The promoter of the Yb4 gene contains a TATA box sequence, TATAAT, at 59 nucleotides upstream of the ATG initiation codon (comparable with the position in the Yb2 gene). There is no CCAAT box sequence in the Yb4 gene, but the sequence GCAGT, which may be the best fit for the CCAAT box, lies 73 bp upstream of the TATA box.

Sequence homogeneity has been maintained within the Yb genes beginning with exon 3 through the end of exon 5 and again beginning with exon 6 through the end of exon 7. Diversion occurs near the 3′-end of exon 5 and extends through almost all of intron 5 and through most of exon 8. This pattern of maintaining sequence homogeneity in some parts and generating sequence diversity in others (as described for the Ya and Yc subunits) suggests an attractive model for the evolution of genes encoding multisubstrate enzymes.

III. Glutathione S-Transferase Pi Class Family

Okuda et al. (1987) have reported the isolation and characterization of the rat Yp gene. Sequence analysis indicates that the gene contains seven exons and six introns and spans approximately 3 kbp. The cap site maps 70 nucleotides upstream form the translation initiation site. The TATA box was found 27 bp upstream from the cap site. The hexanucleotide sequence GGGCGG was found at position −47 to −42. In addition to the Yp gene, Okuda et al. (1987) has reported the presence of several processed type pseudogenes, which most likely originated by reverse transcription followed by insertion at specific sites.

F. Structure–Function Analysis of Glutathione S-Transferases

I. Site-Directed Mutagenesis

The active site of the GSTs has been shown to contain two binding sites, one binding site for glutathione (G-site) and a second site for substrate binding (H-site). Since the GSTs display significant variation in their binding and conjugating activity with a number of chemically distinct substrates, the G-site is probably very similar in all of the reduced glutathione (GSH) transferase subunits, while the H-site is considered to be unique in each isozyme.

Prior to the solution of a three-dimensional structure for a GST, very little was known concerning the identity of the amino acid residues in the active site (G- and H-sites) of the functional enzyme. Experiments based on kinetic and chemical modification techniques suggested that the active site might contain either cysteine, histidine, tryptophan, arginine, or aspartic acid (RICCI et al. 1991; VAN OMMEN et al. 1988, 1989, 1991; AWASTHI et al. 1987; TAMAI et al. 1990; CHANG et al. 1991).

With the cloning of multiple cDNAs for the GSTs and the application of high-level expression of the GSTs in prokaryotic cell systems coupled with site-directed mutagenesis, significant advances in our understanding of GST structure and function has been possible. Using these techniques, several laboratories have identified residues within the GSTs that are essential for the GST activities of ligand binding and glutathione conjugation. The recent data will be briefly reviewed.

Mutagenic analysis of rat alpha, mu, and pi class isozymes and of the human mu and pi class enzymes has clearly shown that none of the cysteine residues in the GSTs are essential for catalysis (TAMAI et al. 1991; HSIEH et al. 1991; WIDERSTEN et al. 1991; WANG et al. 1991, 1992a). The histidine residues in rat GST 1-1 and 3-3 and in the human pi GSTs were substituted with several related and unrelated amino acids. Only mutations at His 159 produced a change in the specific activity of the rat 1-1 enzyme. A slight decrease in activity was seen when His 159 was changed to either Val, Tyr, or Lys, while a mutation to either Arg or Asp had no effect on the activity (TAMAI et al. 1991; HSIEH et al. 1991; WIDERSTEN et al. 1991; WANG et al. 1991, 1992a; ZHANG et al. 1991; KONG et al. 1991, 1992; MANOHARAN et al. 1992).

The role of tryptophan and aspartic acid in both catalysis and binding of heme was investigated by WANG et al. (1991, 1992b). Substitution of phenylalanine for the single tryptophan residue in rat alpha class 1-1 isozyme had no effect on catalysis or the binding of heme. Mutation of each of the four Asp residues to either Asn or Glu also had no effect on the catalytic activity. Substitution of Asp 101 or 157 with Asn did result in an increase in the ability of the mutant enzyme to bind GSH (WANG et al. 1992b). Mutation of Arg 13, 20, 69, and 187 to Ala (all four changed at the same time) in the human mu class GST (M1a-1a) produced a mutant with decreased specific activity (WIDERSTEN et al. 1991). The data from these mutation studies suggested that Cys, His, Trp, and Asp residues were not involved in the catalytic mechanism of the cytosolic GSTs.

II. Crystallographic Solution of Glutathione S-Transferases

Recently, the three-dimensional structure of two pi class GSTs complexed with the inhibitors glutathione sulfonate and S-hexylglutathione (REINEMER et al. 1991, 1992) and the rat 3-3 isozyme (LIU et al. 1992. JI et al. 1992) have been solved. In the following section we will briefly review several important points about the crystal structure of the GSTs.

The three-dimensional structure of the porcine pi homodimeric GST (Reinemer et al. 1991) revealed a globular protein with unit cell dimensions of 55Å × 52Å × 45Å. Each of the subunits in the homodimer was folded into two domains of different structures. The first domain, residues 1–74, consisted of a central four-stranded β-sheet flanked on one side by two α-helices and on the other side by a bent irregular helix structure. The second domain, residues 81–207, contained five α-helices. In the crystal structure, the dimeric GST binds two molecules of glutathione sulfonate at a site on domain I, the G-site. The side chains lining the G-site include Tyr 7, Gly 12, Arg 13, Trp 38, Lys 42, Gln 49, Pro 51, Gln 62, Ser 63, and Glu 95. Interestingly, no cysteine residue was shown to be part of the G-site. The sulfonate group of the inhibitor was shown interacting with Tyr 7, a residue that is conserved in the aligned amino acid sequences of the mammalian, *Schistosoma japonicum* and maize GSTs.

The three-dimensional structure of the human placental pi enzyme (Reinemer et al. 1992) closely resembled that of the porcine structure. Subunit folding, overall structure, and association are very similar when the structures are superimposed. Crystallization of the enzyme in the presence of the competitive inhibitor S-hexylglutathione allowed the identification of the binding regions for both glutathione (G-site) and electrophilic substrates (H-site). The specific interactions between the inhibitor, S-hexylglutathione, and the enzyme were very similar to those described for the porcine enzyme. The side chains lining the H-site include Tyr 7, Phe 8, Pro 9, Val 10, Val 35, Tyr 106, and Gly 203.

Although the rat class mu (rat 3-3 isozyme) and porcine class pi GSTs have only 31% sequence identity, the crystal structure of the rat enzyme shows that it adapts a similar folding topology (Ji et al. 1992). The class mu GST is globular in shape with dimensions of 53Å × 62Å × 56Å. The structure of the rat GST 3-3 can be divided into two domains. Domain I is comprised of residues 1–82 and contains four β-strands and three α-helices arranged in a $\beta\alpha\beta\alpha\beta\beta\alpha$ motif. Domain II is comprised of amino acid residues 90–217, which are arranged in five α helices. Like the pi class GST, domain I is the glutathione binding domain (G-site), whereas domain II represents the xenobiotic substrate-binding site. Even though the overall topology of the two GSTs are quite similar, significant differences also exist (Reinemer et al. 1991).

Based on the alignment of cDNA sequence and the crystallographic data described above, several groups have investigated changes in the amino acids involved in the formation of both the G- and H-sites of several GSTs. Tyrosine 6, conserved in at least 12 mammalian GSTs, was studied using site-directed mutagenesis by several groups. This conserved tyrosine residue was replaced by several amino acids in the rat 1-1 and 3-3 forms and the human A1-1 and pi P1-1 forms of GST (Manoharan et al. 1992; Wang et al. 1992b; Liu et al. 1992; Stenberg et al. 1991; Kolm et al. 1992). In all cases, mutation of the conserved tyrosine resulted in a decrease of at least 90% in specific activiy of the GST. These results demonstrated that the tyrosine residue at the G-site plays a critical role in catalysis.

G. Transcriptional Regulation of Glutathione S-Transferase Gene Expression

I. Pi Gene (Subunit Yp)

Using deletion analysis, Sakai et al. (1988) have identified two regions of the 5′-flanking regulatory region of the rat GST pi gene required for regulation of transcription. The two enhancing elements were found at 2.5 and 2.0 kbp upstream from the transcription start site and designated GPEI and GPEII (GST P enhancer I and II). A consensus sequence for the phorbol 12-O-tetradecanoate 13-acetate-responsive element, AP-1-binding site (TRE), was identified in GPEI and at −61 nucleotides upstream from the transcription start site. GPEII contained two SV40 enhancer core-like sequences and one polyoma core-like sequence. A silencing element was found 400 bp upstream of the transcription start site.

5′ and 3′ deletion analysis of GPEI narrowed the essential sequence for the enhancing effect to a region (approximately 30 nucleotides) that contained a TRE-like octanucleotide at the 3′-end. Further deletion and point mutation analysis indicated that the enhancing element was composed of two imperfect TPA-responsive elements (TREs). Each of the TRE-like sequences alone had no activity, but together they acted synergistically to form a strong enhancer (Okuda et al. 1989, 1990). More recently, Diccianni et al. (1992) have provided evidence which shows that novel transcription factors bind to the GPEI sequence and mediate transcription in the absence of *Jun* and *Fos*.

Further analysis of the silencer region revealed that it functions in an orientation-independent manner in several heterologous gene constructs when transfected into rat hepatoma and nonhepatoma cells as well as in human and mouse cell lines. These data suggest that the unit acts as a general negative regulator of basal gene expression. The functional silencer unit consists of several *cis*-acting elements that function cooperatively. Each element itself is not sufficient for full silencing activity. At least three proteins bind to the silencer, one of which, designated SF-A, has been identified as the *trans*-activator LAP-IL6-DBP (Imagawa et al. 1991a, 1991b).

II. Alpha Gene (Subunit Ya1)

Early studies concerning the induction of several phase II enzymes in the rat indicated that several GSTs isozymes were elevated in the livers of animals administered 3-methylcholanthrene or phenobarbital. With respect to the isozymes containing the Ya subunit, the increase in enzyme content and/or activity was paralled by an elevation in the translational activity of the Ya mRNA (DING and PICKETT 1985). Using in vitro translation systems and immunoprecipitation with specific antibodies raised against purified GST YaYc heterodimer, an increase in the translational activity of the Ya mRNA was detected as early as 4h after a single administration of 3-methylcholanthrene reaching maximal induction (five- to sevenfold) between 16 and 24h (PICKETT et al. 1983). RNA blot analysis using cDNA clones complementary to the Ya mRNA confirmed that the increase in the translational activity of the Ya mRNA was due to an accumulation in the steady state level of mRNA specific for the Ya subunit. Nuclear run-on experiments indicated that transcriptional activation of the Ya subunit gene was responsible for the mRNA accumulation (PICKETT et al. 1984).

1. Identification of Regulatory Elements

The original data reported by TELAKOWSKI-HOPKINS et al. (1986, 1988) showed that the promoter from the GST Ya subunit gene contained at least two regulatory elements between nucleotides −1651 and −663 of the flanking region. These regulatory elements, *cis*-acting sequences, were required for maximal basal and xenobiotic inducible expression of CAT activity. To more precisely localize these elements within the promoter, a series of chimeric genes using various lengths of the 5′-flanking region of rat liver GST Ya subunit gene fused to the structural gene encoding the bacterial enzyme chloramphenicol acetyl transferase (CAT) were constructed. The deletion constructs, spanning the entire 1717 bps of the flanking region, were transfected into HepG2 cells and the CAT activity monitored in the presence and absence of several inducers. Using this deletion strategy, we have identified five distinct regulatory elements in the rat Ya subunit gene's promoter (RUSHMORE et al. 1990, 1991; PAULSON et al. 1990). A summary of the data is presented in Fig. 6.

Two liver specific enhancer elements were identified in the promoter of the Ya gene that contributed toward the expression of the maximal basal level activity. The first element, nucleotides −860 to −850, contained a core DNA recognition sequence that was recognized by HNF 1 (hepatocyte nuclear factor 1; PAULSON et al. 1990). The second hepatocyte-specific enhancer, localized between nucleotides −775 and −755, contained a DNA sequence recognized by HNF 4 (PAULSON et al. 1990).

Computer-aided examination of the 5′-flanking sequence of the Ya gene promoter revealed the presence of two "potential" regulatory elements, a xenobiotic-responsive element (XRE) and a glucocorticoid-responsive element (GRE), that were not found during deletion analysis. An XRE core sequence (GCGTG) was identified upstream of the HNF1 sequence between nucleotides −908 and −899. The XRE, found in multiple copies in the 5′-flanking region of the cytochrome P-450 1AI structural gene, is recognized by the liganded Ah receptor complex (DENISON et al. 1988, 1989; FUJISAWA-SEHARA et al. 1988). A concensus GRE sequence was found between nucleotides −1609 and −1595 (RUSHMORE et al. 1990; PROUGH and RUSHMORE, personal observation). The GRE is found in many genes that respond to steroid hormone treatment and has been shown to be required for direct receptor-mediated activation by several steroid hormones.

The last *cis*-acting regulatory element in the flanking region of the Ya subunit gene, identified by its ability to mediate induction of the Ya subunit gene by β-naphthoflavone and 3-methylcholanthrene, shared no apparent sequence similarity to the XRE sequence (RUSHMORE et al. 1990, 1991; RUSHMORE and PICKETT 1990, 1991). Deletion analysis identified a 41 nucleotide sequence, nucleotides −722 to −682, that provided both basal (constitutive) and xenobiotic (β-naphthoflavone, 3-methylcholanthrene, or benzo(a)pyrene) inducibility to the Ya subunit gene. This regulatory element was designated the antioxidant-responsive element (ARE) based on data described below.

2. Sequence Requirements of the Antioxidant-Responsive Element for Basal and Xenobiotically Inducible Activity

Extensive deletion analysis of the 41 nucleotide ARE (Fig. 1) indicated that the enhancer element provided at least two transcriptional activities to the

CLONE	ARE DELETION SEQUENCE	CAT ACTIVITY pmoles $[^{14}C]$ Chloramphenicol Acetylated/hr/ug	
		BASAL	INDUCIBLE
-722CAT	gagcttggaaatggcattgctaatggtgacaaagcaacttt	31.9 ± 2.8	77.4 ± 4.6
-714CAT	aaatggcattgctaatggtgacaaagcaacttt	28.8 ± 3.6	74.5 ± 6.1
-708CAT	cattgctaatggtgacaaagcaacttt	17.7 ± 2.5	40.5 ± 4.9
-705CAT	tgctaatggtgacaaagcaacttt	18.0 ± 3.8	32.0 ± 3.9
-703CAT	ctaatggtgacaaagcaacttt	17.9 ± 2.9	37.5 ± 4.1
-702CAT	taatggtgacaaagcaacttt	18.0 ± 2.3	36.7 ± 5.5
-699CAT	tggtgacaaagcaacttt	10.4 ± 2.1	27.7 ± 3.9
-697CAT	gtgacaaagcaacttt	10.7 ± 1.8	25.7 ± 3.5
-696CAT	tgacaaagcaacttt	9.6 ± 2.0	9.3 ± 2.0
-693CAT	caaagcaacttt	9.9 ± 2.3	9.8 ± 2.5
-690CAT	agcaacttt	10.0 ± 1.8	9.9 ± 1.9
-687CAT	aacttt	10.1 ± 2.3	9.8 ± 2.0
-722(-685)CAT	gagcttggaaatggcattgctaatggtgacaaagcaac	29.5 ± 3.5	80.0 ± 5.5
-722(-688)CAT	gagcttggaaatggcattgctaatggtgacaaagc	32.0 ± 2.9	81.5 ± 6.1
-722(-697)CAT	gagcttggaaatggcattgctaatgg	9.9 ± 2.6	10.1 ± 2.8
-722(-704)CAT	gagcttggaaatggcattg	10.1 ± 3.0	10.3 ± 2.5
-164CAT		10.2 ± 2.6	10.5 ± 2.3

Fig. 1. Deletion analysis of the antioxidant-responsive element (*ARE*) HepG2 cells were transfected with the various deletion ARE-Ya CAT chimeric clones and left untreated or exposed to 50 u*M* β-naphthoflavone (β-NF) for 24 h. CAT activity was monitored as described previously (RUSHMORE et al. 1990). The experimental value for CAT activity is expressed as pmoles chloramphenicol acetylated/h/per μg cell lysate and is the mean ± S.D. of triplicate determinations. In addition, tert-butylhydroquinone (60 μ*M*) and hydrogen peroxide (500 μ*M*) were used in the experiments. The results, not shown, were identical to those shown for β-NF

Ya subunit gene, basal (constitutive) and xenobiotic inducible activity. Stepwise 5′-deletion of the ARE sequence from nucleotide −722 to nucleotide −697 gradually abolished the basal level expression present in the complete ARE. The remaining sequence was still capable of mediating the induction of CAT activity after exposure to phenolic antioxidants (see below) and planar aromatic hydrocarbons (PAHs). Deletions past nucleotide −697 abolished both the basal and inducible activity of the ARE. Similar deletions were carried out from the 3′-end of the ARE. Deletion past nucleotide −688 abolished both basal and xenobiotic inducible activities. The remaining sequence, 5′-GTGACAAAGC-3′, was subsequently shown to be the minimal sequence required for xenobiotic inducible activity (RUSHMORE et al. 1991).

A second approach for analyzing the essential nucleotides, point mutation analysis, was performed on the ARE to determine which nucleotides were required for either basal and/or inducible activities. The analysis, shown in Fig. 2, revealed that any change in the TGAC of the core sequence abolished both basal and inducible activities. Mutation of either the 3′ G or C (or both) of the core sequence abolished only the inducible activity. Point mutations in the AAA of the core sequence had no effect on either the basal or inducible activity (RUSHMORE et al. 1991).

3. Induction of the Ya Subunit Gene by Phenolic Antioxidants Through the Antioxidant-Responsive Element

During the deletion analysis of the Ya subunit gene promoter, we observed that removal of the XRE sequence did not abolish transcriptional activation of the chimeric CAT constructs by planar aromatic compounds. These results suggested that the XRE in the Ya subunit gene might not be essential for transcriptional activation of the Ya gene by planar aromatic compounds. Since the XRE was the only well-characterized *cis*-acting element through which these compounds could activate transcription, we thought that the ARE might be a second element that could mediate transcriptional activation by planar aromatic compounds. Based on this observation, we investigated in more depth the interrelationships between the XRE, the requirements for a functional Ah receptor and active cytochrome P-450 1AI and their relationship(s) to induction through the ARE.

In several reports by TALALAY and coworkers, data was presented suggesting that an Ah receptor-independent mechanism could account for the induction of several phase II drug-metabolizing enzymes by phenolic antioxidants such as tert-butylhydroquinone or 3,5-di-tert-butylcatechol (PROCHASKA et al. 1985; PROCHASKA and TALALAY 1988; DELONG et al. 1987; TALALAY et al. 1988). In a series of experiments using HepG2 and mutant mouse hepatoma cell lines, we showed that the Ya subunit gene was activated through the ARE and XRE after exposure to planar aromatic compounds (β-naphthoflavone, 3-methylcholanthrene, or benzo(a)pyrene) only in cells that contained or expressed functional Ah receptors and active cytochrome

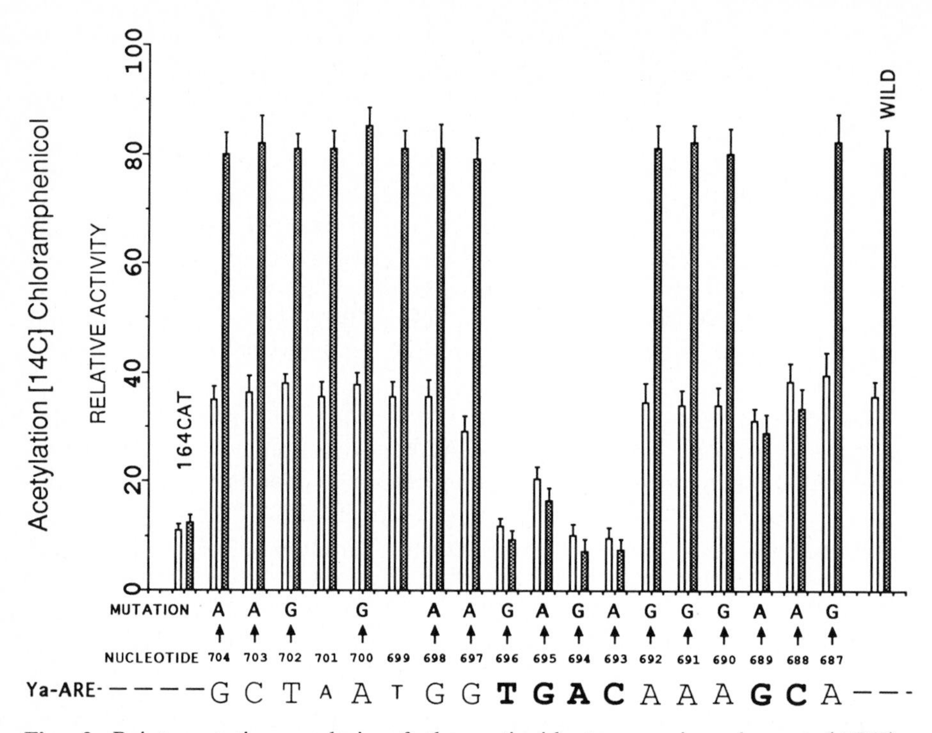

Fig. 2. Point mutation analysis of the antioxidant-responsive element (ARE). Oligonucleotides corresponding to the various ARE mutations were subcloned in front of expression clone −164CAT as described previously (RUSHMORE et al. 1991). The various clones were transfected into HepG2 cells with the β-galactosidase expression plasmid pCH110 and left untreated or exposed to 50 μM β-naphthoflavone (β-NF) for 24 h. Chloramphenicol acetyl transferase (CAT) and β-galactosidase activities were monitored as described. The experimental value for CAT is expressed as the relative activity, CAT activity divided by β-galactosidase activity, and is the mean ± S.D. of triplicate determinations All assays were done in triplicate. The subcloned AREs all contained the entire 41 nucleotide sequence from −722 to −682

P-450 1AI (RUSHMORE and PICKETT 1990, 1991; Fig. 3, 4). Cells deficient in either the Ah receptor or P-450 failed to increase transcription through the ARE or XRE when exposed to planar aromatic hydrocarbons. Exposure of the cells deficient in either the Ah receptor or cytochrome P-450 1AI to the phenolic antioxidants tert-butylhydroquinone or 3,5-di-tert-butylcatechol, resulted in activation of gene transcription through the ARE, but not the XRE (Fig. 4). These results clearly demonstrated, at the molecular level, a mechanism by which GST Ya subunit could be induced by phenolic antioxidants that was Ah receptor and cytochrome P-450 1AI independent.

FRILING et al. (1990, 1992) have also identified two sequences in the 5′-flanking region of a mouse GST Ya subunit gene that shows significant sequence homology to the ARE sequence we identified in the rat GST Ya

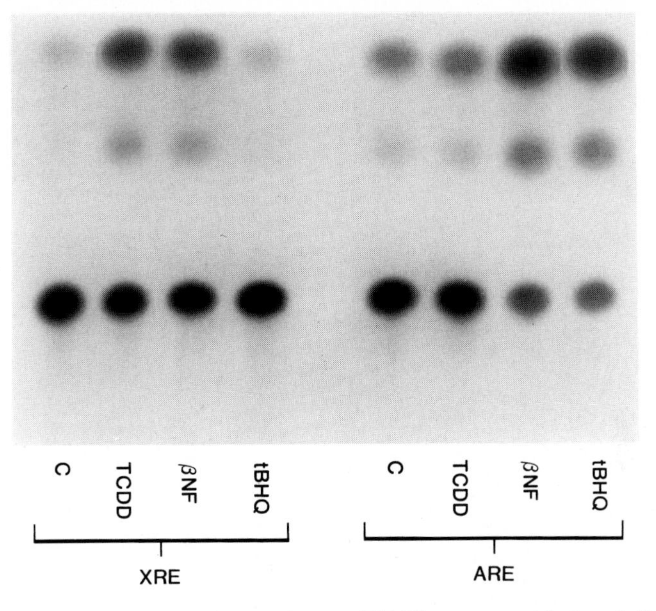

Fig. 3. Chloramphenicol acetyl transferase (CAT) assays with lysed HepG2 cells transfected with xenobiotic-responsive element (*XRE*)-164CAT and antioxidant-responsive element (ARE)-164CAT expression clones (RUSHMORE et al. 1990; RUSHMORE and PICKETT 1991). Transient assay were performed using 10 n*M* 2,3,7,8-tetrachlorodiberzo-*p*-dioxin (*TCDD*), 50 *μM* *β*-naphthoflavone (*β-NF*), or 60 *μM* tert-butylhydroquinone (tBHQ). *C* represents control transfections in the presence of dimethylsulfoxide. CAT activity was monitored by thin-layer chromatography followed by autoradiograph

subunit gene. They have shown induction with most of the compounds we have used to identify and classify the rat Ya ARE. They have named the mouse sequence the electrophile-responsive element (EpRE).

4. DNA Binding Studies

In vitro binding experiments and protection studies were carried out on the ARE sequence to determine whether any proteins could bind to the sequence and, if so, to identify those nucleotides to which the protein(s) had bound. The results of these experiments are shown in Fig. 5. The factor(s) appears to bind in the major groove and involve contact with the GpG dinucleotide and the G residue within the TGAC tetramer on the coding strand (Fig. 5A; NGUYEN and PICKETT 1992). In addition, DNase I protection analysis mapped an extended region, 5′ from the core sequence, that we had previously shown to be essential for full basal level expression (RUSHMORE et al. 1991). The *trans*-acting factor or factors were present in nuclear extracts from

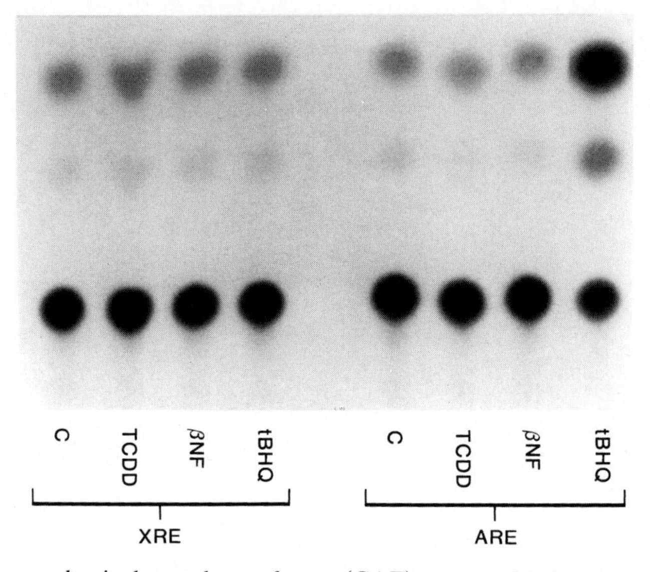

Fig. 4. Chloramphenicol acetyl transferase (CAT) assays with lysed mouse class II variant cells transfected with xenobiotic-responsive element (XRE)-164CAT and antioxidant-responsive element (ARE)-164CAT expression clones (RUSHMORE et al. 1990; RUSHMORE and PICKETT 1991). Transient assay were performed using 10 n*M* 2,3,7,8-tetrachlorodibenzo-*p*-dioxin (TCDD), 50 μ*M* β-naphtoflavone (β-NF), or 60 μ*M* tert-butylhydroquinone (*tBHQ*). *C* represents control transfections in the presence of dimethylsulfoxide. CAT activity was monitored by thin-layer chromatography followed by autoradiography

untreated and tert-butylhydroquinone-induced cells, suggesting a mechanism of induction other than an inducible DNA–protein interaction.

The ability of the ARE to form specific complexes with nuclear protein(s) was assessed by gel mobility shift assays (Fig. 5B). The results showed that a single specific complex was formed with the labeled probe. The specificity of binding was monitored by competition experiments in which an excess of unlabeled oligonucleotide was added to the binding reactions. The addition of 100-fold molar excess of unlabeled ARE abolished the formation of the binding complex, whereas addition of the same molar excess of an unrelated oligonucleotide did not interfere with the binding. Moreover, the presence of a 100-fold molar excess of an oligonucleotide containing the XRE core sequence had no effect on the formation of the complex.

To determine if the core sequence described above was required for the formation of the complex, we synthesized a 41-bp oligonucleotide in which the ARE core sequence, GTGACAAAGC, was mutated. The mutated ARE sequence was not able to compete for binding with the native ARE

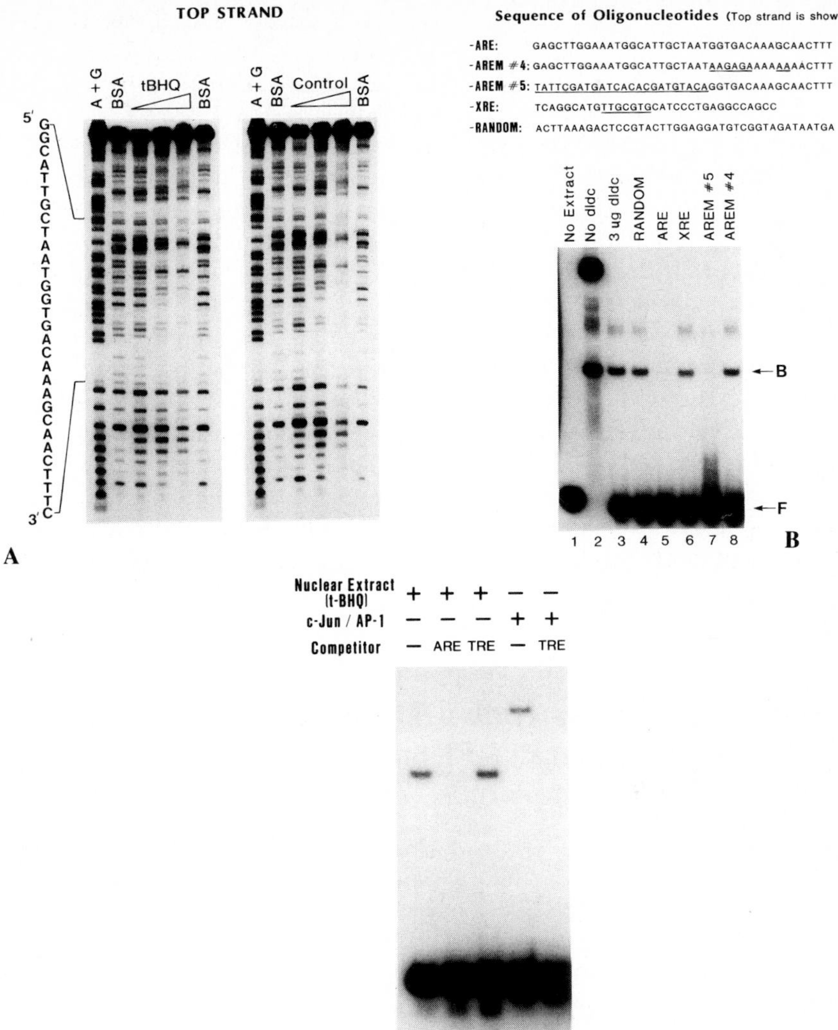

Fig. 5. A–C. Analysis of DNA–protein interactions at the antioxidant-responsive element (ARE). **A** DNase I protection assays. Uniquely end-labeled DNA fragments containing the ARE sequence were incubated with increasing amounts of nuclear extracts from control or tert-butylhydroquinone (tBHQ)-treated HepG2 cells. The DNA–protein complexes were subjected to limited digestion with DNase I and the reaction products analyzed on a 12% polyacrylamide-7 *M* urea gel. **B** Detection of ARE-binding activity in nuclear extracts by gel mobility shift assays. The synthetic double-stranded oligonucleotides were labeled with ^{32}P and incubated with nuclear extracts from control or tBHQ-treated HepG2 cells. Competitor DNA included in each binding reaction is indicated at the top. The *arrows* indicate the position of the bound (*B*) or free (*F*) DNA. **C** DNA–protein interaction between the ARE and c-Jun. Gel mobility shift assays were performed to assess the ability of human c-Jun protein to bind to the ARE. ^{32}P-labeled ARE probe was incubated with either nuclear extract from tBHQ-treated cells or pure c-Jun protein. Competitor DNA included in each binding reaction is indicated at the top. TRE; 5′-CTAGTGATGAGTCAGCCGGATC-3′

sequence. These data indicated that the gel shift obtained with the ARE probe was a specific protein–DNA interaction.

Comparision of the ARE core sequence with that from several other enhancer elements revealed a striking, though not perfect, similarity with the core recognition sequence for *c-Jun*, TGAC (ANGEL et al. 1987). This and the work presented by FRILING et al. (1992) prompted us to examine whether *c-Jun* was involved in the protein–DNA complex. As judged by gel mobility shifts, purified *c-Jun* did not bind to the rat ARE sequence (Fig. 5C). Only in the presence of excess *c-Jun* could any binding be demonstrated. However, in this case, the position of the shifted band in the presence of excess *c-Jun* was significantly different than that produced with nuclear extract from HepG2 cells. Furthermore, a consensus TRE sequence (AP-1 binding site) from the human collagenase gene did not compete for the binding of the ARE with nuclear factors from the hepatoma cells (ANGEL et al. 1987). Therefore, the identity of the *trans*-acting factor(s) which interact with the rat ARE and activate transcription by reactive oxygen species is most likely not *c-Jun* and consequently remains to be identified.

H. Transcriptional Activation Through the Antioxidant- and Xenobiotic-Responsive Element: A Study of Model Compounds

Several compounds were assayed for their potential as activators of transcription through the ARE and/or XRE in a cell-based assay system (RUSHMORE and PICKETT 1991). Briefly, HepG2 cells, transiently transfected with an expression clone containing either the ARE or XRE synthetic sequence inserted upstream of the Ya subunit minimal promoter, were exposed to the potential inducers for 24 h and the CAT activity monitored. Using this assay system, several classes of compounds have been screened for their ability to activate transcription through the ARE and/or XRE. The results of these induction experiments are compiled in Table 2.

Several planar aromatic compounds were tested in the assay. All of the compounds that were tested were capable of activating transcription through the XRE in cells that possessed a functional Ah receptor. TCDD was the most potent inducer of CAT constructs containing the XRE. All of the PAHs were active as inducers through the ARE except TCDD, a slowly metabolized PAH. This data is consistent with our previous demonstration of the requirement for prior metabolism of PAHs before these compounds or their metabolites activate transcription through the ARE (RUSHMORE and PICKETT 1990, 1991; Figs. 3, 4).

In order to define the minimal structure for a compound that could activate transcription through the ARE, a structure–activity study was carried out using the cell-based assay as described above. In these experi-

Table 2. Transcriptional activation of glulathione-S-transferase Ya gene via the antioxidant- and xenobiotic-responsive element sequences using a transactivation assay in HepG2 cells

Compound	Induction		References
	ARE[a]	XRE[b]	
Planar aromatic compounds			
TCDD	−	++++[c]	Rushmore and Pickett (1991)
Benzo(a)pyrene	++++	+++	Rushmore and Pickett (1992)
1,2-Benzanthracene	+++	+++	Prough and Rushmore (personal observation)
2,3-Benzanthracene	+++	+++	Prough and Rushmore (personal observation)
β-Naphthoflavone	++	++	Rushmore et al. (1990)
3-Methylcholanthrene	+++	+++	Rushmore et al. (1990)
Phenolic antioxidants			
Tert-butylhydroquinone	++	−	Rushmore et al. (1991)
3,5-Di-tert-butylcatechol	++	−	Rushmore et al. (1991)
Polyhydroxylated benzenes			
Resorcinol	−	−	Rushmore et al. (1991)
Catechol	++	−	Rushmore et al. (1991)
Hydroquinone	++	−	Rushmore et al. (1991)
Benzoquinone	++	+	Rushmore et al. (1991)
1,2,3-Benzenetriol	++	+	Rushmore et al. (1991)
1,2,4-Benzenetriol	++	−	Rushmore et al. (1991)
1,3,5-Benzenetriol	−	−	Rushmore et al. (1991)
Methyl-hydroquinone	++	−	Rushmore and Pickett (unpublished data)
3-Methylcatechol	+++	−	Rushmore and Pickett (unpublished data)
4-Methylcatechol	+++	−	Rushmore and Pickett (unpublished data)
Flavonoids			
Myricetin	+	−	Rushmore and Pickett (1992)
Quercetin	++	−	Rushmore and Pickett (1992)
Fisetin	++	−	Rushmore and Pickett (1992)
Flavone	++	+	Rushmore and Pickett (1992)
Flavanone (2,3-dihydroflavone)	++	−	Rushmore and Pickett (1992)
Pro-oxidative treatments			
Hydrogen peroxide	++	−	Rushmore et al. (1991)
Menadione	++	−	Rushmore and Pickett (1992)
Fe^{3+}/8-hydroxyquinoline	++	−	Rushmore and Pickett (unpublished data)

TCDD, 2,3,7,8-tetrachlorodibenzo-*p*-dioxin; ARE, antioxidant-responsive element; XRE, xenobiotic-responsive element; −, no induction; +, induction of 1- to 2.5-fold; ++, induction of 2.5- to fourfold; +++, induction of four to sixfold; ++++, induction greater than sixfold.

[a] ARE sequence previously identified in rat GST Ya subunit gene promoter, nucleotides −722 to −682 (Rushmore et al. 1990a).

[b] XRE represents dioxin (TCDD)-responsive element, nucleotides −908 to −899 in rat GST Ya subunit gene promoter (Rushmore et al. 1990a).

ments, we exposed cells transfected with the ARE expression clone to a series of polyhydroxylated benzenes and monitored for induction of CAT activity. The results are summarized in Table 2. Only those compounds that contained, minimally, a 1,2 or 1,4 hydroxylation (*ortho* and *para* substitutions) on the benzene ring (hydroquinone, catechol, 1,2,3-trihydroxybenzene, and 1,2,4-trihydroxybenzene) were capable of activating transcription through the ARE. Benzene and phenol were not inducers. Compounds containing a 1,3 substitution about the benzene ring, resorcinol or 1,3,5-trihydroxybenzene, were not active as inducers through the ARE or XRE. Within the series, only 1,2,3-trihydroxybenzene and benzoquinone were able to activate transcription through the ARE and the XRE (Rushmore et al. 1991).

A feature common to all of the polyhydroxylated compounds described above that activated transcription through the ARE was their ability to undergo or drive redox cycling with the potential to generate superoxide anion and hydrogen peroxide. Since hydrogen peroxide could be produced during exposure to these compounds, we added hydrogen peroxide to the assay system and showed a clear dose-dependent induction of CAT activity through the ARE, but not the XRE (Rushmore et al. 1991).

I. Mechanisms of Induction of Glutathione S-Transferase Ya1 Subunit Gene

Several mechanisms for transcriptional regulation of the Ya subunit gene are presented in simplified form in Fig. 6. As shown in Fig. 6, the Ya subunit gene contains a GRE. Binding of a steroid receptor–ligand complex to the GRE could activate transcription by a mechanism similar to that described for the Ah receptor and PAHs.

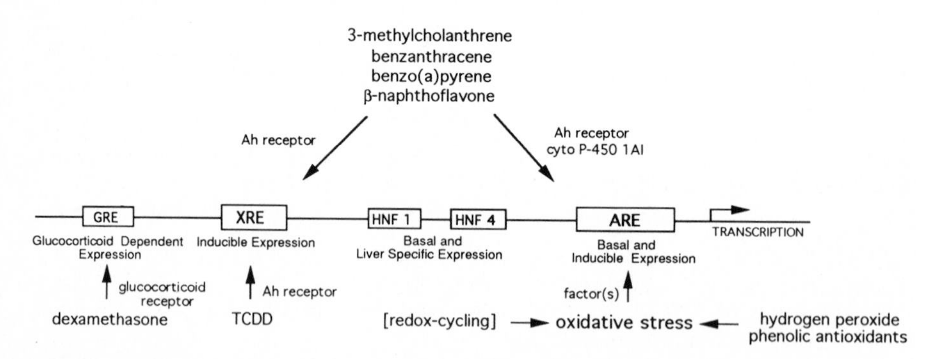

Fig. 6. Mechanisms for transcriptional regulation of the Ya subunit gene. *GRE*, glucocorticoid-responsive element; *XRE*, xenobiotic-responsive element; HNF, hepatocyte nuclear factor; *ARE*, antioxidant-responsive element

A second mechanism for transcriptional activation of the Ya subunit gene involves the Ah receptor–ligand complex. The Ah receptor can interact directly with one of several ligands (PAHs) such as TCDD and activate transcription after translocation of the complex (receptor–ligand) into the nucleus with subsequent binding to the XRE. This mechanism has been well documented for the mouse P450 IA1 gene (DENISON et al. 1988, 1989; FUJISAWA-SEHARA et al. 1988; NEUBOLD et al. 1989). In another mechanism involving an active Ah receptor, the Ah receptor–ligand complex can upregulate cytochrome P450 IA1, permitting metabolism of PAH(s) to metabolites that interact with the ARE and activate transcription. The "metabolites" could either interact directly with factor(s) activating the ARE – these factors are at present unknown – or they could react further to induce a pro-oxidative environment within the cell that, as described below, could activate transcription through the ARE. In the last mechanism described for transcriptional activation of the Ya subunit gene, phenolic antioxidants or pro-oxidative treatment of cells could create an "oxidative stress" within the cell that activates transcription through the ARE, no Ah receptor or P450 being required. The oxidative stress may be formed as a result of several processes such as exposure to hydrogen peroxide, iron loading, or through the process of redox cycling.

The results from our experiments are consistent with the model proposed by TALALAY and coworkers (PROCHASKA et al. 1985; PROCHASKA and TALALAY 1988; DELONG et al. 1987; TALALAY et al. 1988), who have suggested that phase II drug-metabolizing enzymes, such as the GSTs, are induced by tert-butylhydroquinone (phenolic antioxidants) and β-naphthoflavone (PAHs) by different mechanisms. Talalay proposed that phenolic antioxidants activate transcription by means of an electrophilic signal which operates independently of Ah receptors or induction of cytochrome P450 IA1. Our data supports this hypothesis and demonstrates that one DNA sequence through which phenolic antioxidants activate transcription is the antioxidant responsive element or ARE.

Finally, the ability of reactive oxygen species to activate gene transcription through the ARE sequence is most likely part of a signal transduction pathway through which eukaryotic cells respond to oxidative stress. The interaction of product(s) resulting from an oxidative stress with the ARE could lead to the induction of enzymes that protect the cells from endogenous and/or exogenous compounds that undergo redox cycling and form reactive oxygen species. Consistent with this hypothesis is the demonstration of a functional ARE sequence in the flanking regions of the rat (FAVREAU and PICKETT 1991) and human (JAISWAL 1991; LI and JAISWAL 1992) reduced nicotinamide adenine dinucleotide phosphate (NAD(P)H)-quinone reductase genes. This enzyme has been shown to be critical in protecting cells against reactive oxygen species due to redox cycling of exogenous and endogenous quinones (RILEY and WORKMAN 1992).

References

Abramovitz M, Listowsky I (1987) Selective expression of a unique glutathione S-transferase Yb3 gene in rat brain. J Biol Chem 262:7770–7773

Angel P, Imagawa M, Chiu R, Stein B, Imbra RJ, Rahmsdorf HJ, Jonat C, Herrlich P, Karin M (1987) Phorbol ester-inducible genes contain a common cis element recognized by a TPA-modulated transacting factor. Cell 49:729–739

Arias IM, Fleischner G, Kirsch R, Mishkin S, Gatmaitan Z (1976) On the structure, regulation, and function of ligandin. In: Arias IM, Jacoby WB (eds) Glutathione: metabolism and function. Raven, New York, pp 175–188

Armstrong RN (1991) Chem Res Toxicol 4:131–140

Awasthi YC, Bhatnagar A, Singh SV (1987) Evidence for the involvement of histidine at the active site of glutathione S-transferase pi from human liver. Biochem Biophys Res Commun 143:965–970

Bass NM, Kirsch RE, Tuffs SA, Marks I, Saunders SJ (1977) Ligandin heterogeneity: evidence that the two non-identical subunits are monomers of two distinct proteins. Biochim Biophys Acta 492:163–175

Beale D. Meyer DJ, Taylor JB, Ketterer B (1983) Evidence that the Yb subunits of hepatic glutathione transferases represent two different but related families of polypeptides. Eur J Biochem 137:125–129

Bhargava MM, Ohmi N, Listowski I, Arias IM (1980) Subunit composition, organic anion binding, catalytic and immunological properties of ligandin from rat testis. J Biol Chem 255:724–727

Boyland E, Chasseaud LF (1969) The role of glutathione and glutathione S-transferases in mercapturic acid biosynthesis. Adv Enzymol Relat Areas Mol Biol 32:173–219

Chang L, Wang L, Tam M (1991) The single cysteine residue on an alpha family chick liver glutathione S-transferase CL 3-3 is not functionally important. Biochem Biophys Res Comm 180:323–328

Chasseaud LF (1979) Role of glutathione and glutathione S-transferase in the metabolism of chemical carcinogens and other electrophilic agents. Adv Cancer Res 29:175–274

Coles B, Ketterer B (1990) The role of glutathione and glutathione transferases in chemical carcinogenesis. CRC Crit Rev Biochem Mol Biol 25:47–50

Daniel V, Sarid S, Bar-Nun S, Litwack G (1983) Rat ligandin mRNA molecular cloning and sequencing. Arch Biochem Biophys 227:266–271

DeJong JL, Morgenstern R, Jornvall H, DePierrre JW, Tu C-PD (1988) Gene expression of rat and human microsomal glutathione S-transferases. J Biol Chem 263:8430–8436

DeLong MJ, Santamaria AB, Talalay P (1987) Role of P1-450 in the induction of NAD(P)H: quinone reductase in a murine hepatoma cell line and its mutant. Carcinogenesis 8:1549–1553

Denison MS, Fisher JM, Whitlock JP Jr (1988) The DNA recognition site for the dioxin-Ah receptor complex. J Biol Chem 263:17221–17224

Denison MS, Fisher JM, Whitlock JP Jr (1989) Protein-DNA interactions at recognition sites for the dioxin-Ah receptor complex. J Biol Chem 264:16478–16482

Diccianni MB, Imagawa M, Muramatsu M (1992) The dyad palindromic glutathione S-transferase P enhancer binds multiple factors including AP1. Nucleic Acids Res 20:5153–5158

Ding GJ-F, Lu AYH, Pickett CB (1985) Rat liver glutathione S-transferases. Nucleotide sequence analysis of a Yb1 cDNA clone and prediction of the complete amino acid sequence of the Yb1 subunit. J Biol Chem 260:13268–13271

Ding GJ-F, Ding VD-H, Rodkey JA, Bennett CD, Lu AYH, Pickett CB (1986) Rat liver glutathione S-transferases. DNA sequence analysis of a Yb2 cDNA clone and regulation of the Yb1 and Yb2 mRNAs by phenobarbital. J Biol Chem 261:7952–7957

Ding VD-H, Pickett CB (1985) Transcriptional regulation of rat liver glutathione S-transferase genes by phenobarbital and 3-methylcholanthrene. Arch Biochem Biophys 240:553–559

Eriksson LC, Sharma RN, Roomi MW, Ho RK, Farber E, Murray RK (1983) A characteristic electrophoretic pattern of cytosolic polypeptides from hepatocyte nodules generated during liver carcinogenesis in several models. Biochem Biophys Res Commun 177:740–745

Favreau LV, Pickett CB (1991) Transcriptional regulation of the rat NAD(P)H: quinone reductase gene. Identification of regulatory elements controlling basal level expression and inducible expression by planar aromatic compounds and phenolic antioxidants. J Biol Chem 266:4556–4561

Ford-Hutchinson AW (1990) Leukotriene B4 in inflammation. Crit Rev Immunol 10:1–12

Friling RS, Bensimon A, Tichauer Y, Daniel V (1990) Xenobiotic-inducible expression of murine glutathione S-transferase Ya subunit gene is controlled by an electrophile-responsive element. Proc Natl Acad Sci USA 87:6258–6262

Friling RS, Bergelson S, Daniel V (1992) Two adjacent AP-1-like binding sites from the electrophilic responsive element of the murine glutathione S-transferase Ya subunit gene. Proc Natl Acad Sci USA 89:668–672

Fujisawa-Sehara A, Yamane M, Fujii-Kuriyama Y (1988) A DNA-binding factor specific for xenobiotic responsive elements of P450c gene exists as a cryptic form in cytoplasm: its possible translocation to nucleus. Proc Natl Acad Sci USA 85:5859–5863

Hayes JD, Mantle TJ (1986) Anomalous electrophoretic behaviour of the glutathione S-transferase Ya and Yk subunits isolated from man and rodents. Biochem J 237:731–740

Hiratsuka A, Sebata N, Kawashima K, Okuda H, Ogura K, Watabe T, Satoh K, Hatayama I, Tsuchida S, Ishikawa T, Sato K (1990) A new class of rat glutathione S-transferase Yrs-Yrs inactivating reactive sulfate esters as metabolites of carcinogenic arylmethanols. J Biol Chem 265:11973–11981

Homma H, Listowsky I (1985) Identification of Yb-glutathione-S-transferase as a major rat liver protein labeled with dexamethasone 21-methanesulfonate. Proc Natl Acad Sci USA 82:7165–7169

Hsieh JC, Huang SC, Chen WL, Lai YC, Tam MF (1991) Cysteine-86 is not needed for the enzymic activity of glutathione S-transferase 3-3. Biochemical J 278: 293–297

Imagawa M, Osada S, Koyama Y, Suzuki T, Hirom PC, Morimura S, Muramatsu M (1991a) SF-B that binds to a negative element in glutathione transferase P gene is similar or identical to trans-activator LAP/IL6-DBP. Biochem Biophys Res Comm 179:293–300

Imagawa M, Osada S, Okuda A, Muramatsu M (1991b) Silencer binding proteins function on multiple cis-elements in the glutathione transferase P gene. Nucleic Acids Res 19:5–10

Izumi T, Honda Z, Oshihi N, Kitamusa S, Seyama Y, Shimizu T (1989) Partial purification and characterization of leukotriene C4 synthase from guinea pig lung. Adv Prostaglandin Thromboxane Leukotriene Res 19:90–93

Jakoby WB (1978) The glutathione S-transferases: a group of multifunctional detoxification proteins. Adv Enzymol Relat Areas Mol Biol 46:383–414

Jacoby WB, Habig WH (1980) Detoxication enzymes. In: Jacoby WB (ed) Enzymatic basis of detoxication. Academic, New York, pp 63–94

Jacoby WB, Ketterer B, Mannervik B (1984) Glutathione transferases: nomenclature. Biochem Pharmacol 33:2539–2540

Jaiswal AK (1991) Human NAD(P)H: quinone oxioreductase (NQ01) gene structure and induction by dioxin. Biochemistry 30:10647–10653

Ji X, Zhang P, Armstrong RN, Gilliland GL (1992) The 3-dimensional structure of a glutathione S-transferase from the mu-gene class – structural analysis of the

binary complex of isoenzyme 3-3 and glutathione at 2.2-Angstrom resolution. Biochemistry 31:10169–10184
Kalinyak JE, Taylor JM (1982) Rat glutathione S-transferase. Cloning of double-stranded cDNA and induction of its mRNA. J Biol Chem 257:523–530
Kitahara A, Satoh K, Nishimura K, Ishikawa T, Ruike K, Sato K, Tsuda H, Ito N (1984) Changes in molecular forms of rat hepatic glutathione S-transferase during chemical hepatocarcinogenesis. Cancer Res 44:2698–2703
Kolm R, Sroga GE, Mannervik B (1992) Participation of the phenolic hydroxyl group of tyr-8 in the catalytic mechanism of human glutathione S-transferase P1-1. Biochem J 285:537–540
Kong KH, Inoue H, Takahashi K (1991) Non-essentiality of cystein and histidine residues for the catalytic activity of human class Pi glutathione S-transferase. Biochem Biophys Res Commun 181:748–755
Kong KH, Nishida M, Inuoe H, Takahashi K (1992) Tyrosine-7 is an essential residue for the catalytic activity of human class Pi glutathione S-transferase: chemical modification and site-directed mutagenisis. Biochem Biophys Res Commun 182:1122–1129
Lai H-C, Li N-Q, Weiss MJ, Reddy CC, Tu C-PD (1984) The nucleotide sequence of a rat liver glutathione S-transferase subunit cDNA clone. J Biol Chem 259:5536–5542
Lai H-CJ, Grove G, Tu C-PD (1986) Cloning and sequence analysis of a cDNA for a rat liver glutathione S-transferase Yb subunit. Nucleic Acids Res 14:6101–6114
Lai H-CJ, Tu C-PD (1986) Rat glutathione S-transferases supergene family. Characterization of an anionic Yb subunit cDNA clone. J Biol Chem 261:13793–13799
Lai H-CJ, Qian B, Grove G, Tu C-PD (1988) Gene expression of rat glutathione S-transferases. Evidence for gene conversion in the evolution of the Yb multigene family. J Biol Chem 263:11389–11395
Li Y, Jaiswal AK (1992) Regulation of human NAD(P)H:quinone oxidoreductase gene. Role of AP1 binding site combined within human antioxidant responsive element. J Biol Chem 267:15097–15104
Litwack G, Ketterer B, Arias IM (1971) Nature 234:466–467
Liu S, Zhang P, Ji X, Johnson WW, Gilliland GL, Armstrong RN (1992) Contribution of tyrosine 6 to the catalytic mechanism of isozyme 3-3 of glutathione S-transferase. J Biol Chem 267:4296–4299
Lundqvist G, Yucel-Lindberg T, Morgenstern R (1992) The oligometric structure of rat liver microsomal glutathione S-transferase studies by chemical cross-linking. Biochim Biophys Acta 1159:103–108
Mannervik B (1985) The isoenzymes of glutathione transferase. Adv Enzymol Relat Areas Mol Biol 57:357–417
Mannervik B, Danielson UH (1988) Glutathione transferases – structure and catalytic activity. CRC Crit Rev Biochem Mol Biol 23:283–337
Mannervik B, Jenson H (1982) Binary combinations of four protein subunits with different catalytic specificities explain the relationship between six basic glutathione S-transferases in rat liver cytosol. J Biol Chem 257:9909–9912
Mannervik B, Alin P, Guthenberg C, Jenson H, Tahir MK, Warholm M, Jornvall H (1985) Identification of three classes of cytosolic glutathione transferase common to several mammalian species: correlation between structural data and enzymatic properties. Prod Natl Acad Sci USA 82:7202–7206
Manoharan TH, Gulick AM, Puchalski RB, Servais AL, Fahl WE (1992) Structural studies on human glutathione S-transferase pi – substitution mutations to determine amino acids necessary for binding glutathione. J Biol Chem 267:18940–18945
Meyer DJ, Coles B, Pemble SE, Gilmore KS, Fraser GM, Ketterer B (1991) Theta, a new class of glutathione transferases purified from rat and man. Biochem J 274:409–414

Morgenstern R, Lundqvist G, Mosialou E, Andersson C (1988) Membrane-bound glutathione transferase: function and properties. In: Hayes JD, Pickett CB, Mantle TJ (eds) Glutathione S-transferases and drug resistance. Taylor and Francis, New York, pp 57–64

Morton MR, Bayney RM, Pickett CB (1990) Isolation and characterization of the rat glutathione S-transferase Yb1 subunit gene. Arch Biochem Biophys 277:56–60

Neubold LA, Shirayoshi Y, Ozato K, Jones JE, Nebert DW (1989) Regulation of mouse CYP1A1 gene expression by dioxin: requirement of two cis-acting elements during induction. Mol Cell Biol 9:2378–2386

Nguyen T, Pickett CB (1992) Regulation of rat glutathione S-transferase-Ya subunit gene expression – DNA-protein interaction at the antioxidant responsive element. J Biol Chem 267:13535–13539

Nicholson DW, Ali A, Klemba MW, Munday NA, Zamboni RJ, Ford-Hutchinson AW (1992a) Human leukotriene C4 synthase expression in DMSO-differentiated U937 cells. J Biol Chem 267:17849–17857

Nicholson DW, Klemba NW, Rasper DM, Metters KM, Zamboni RJ, Ford-Hutchinson AW (1992b) Purification of human leukotriene C4 synthase from DMSO-differentiated U937 cells. Eur J Biochem 209:725–734

Ogura K, Nishiyama T, Okuda T, Kajital J, Narihata H, Watabe T, Hiratsuka A, Watabe T (1991) Molecular cloning and amino acid sequencing of rat liver class theta glutathione S-transferase Yrs-Yrs inactivating reactive sulfate esthers of carcinogenic arylmethanols. Biochem Biophys Res Commun 181:1294–1300

Okuda A, Sakai M, Muramatsu M (1987) The structure of the rat glutathione S-transferase P gene and related pseudogenes. J Biol Chem 262:3858–3863

Okuda A, Imagawa M, Maeda Y, Sakai M, Muramatsu M (1989) Structural and functional analysis of an enhancer GPEI having a phorbol 12-O-tetradecanoate 13-acetate responsive element-like sequence found in the rat glutathione transferase P gene. J Biol Chem 264:16919–16926

Okuda A, Imagawa M, Sakai M, Muramatsu M (1990) Functional cooperativity between two TPA responsive elements in undifferentiated F9 embryonic stem cells. EMBO J 9:1131–1135

Paulson KE, Darnell JE Jr, Rushmore TH, Pickett CB (1990) Analysis of the upstream elements of the xenobiotic compound-inducible and positionally regulated glutathione S-transferase Ya gene. Mol Cell Biol 10:1841–1852

Pickett CB, Lu AYH (1989) Glutathione S-transferases: gene structure, regulation, and biological function. Annu Rev Biochem 58:743–764

Pickett CB, Jeter RL, Wang RN, Lu AYH (1983) Coordinate induction of multiple mRNAs specific for rat liver phenobarbitol inducible cytochrome P450. Arch Biochem Biophys 225:854–860

Pickett CB, Telakowski-Hopkins CA, Ding GJ-F, Argenbright L, Lu AYH (1984) Rat liver glutathione S-transferases. Complete nucleotide sequence of a glutathione S-transferase mRNA and the regulation of the Ya, Yb, and Yc mRNAs by 3-methylcholanthrene and phenobarbital. J Biol Chem 259:5182–5188

Piper PJ (1984) Physiol Rev 64:744–761

Prochaska HJ, Talalay P (1988) Regulatory mechanisms of monofunctional and bifunctional anticarcinogenic enzyme induction in murine liver. Cancer Res 48:4776–34782

Prochaska HJ, De Long MJ, Talalay P (1985) On the mechanism of induction of cancer-protective enzymes: a unifying proposal. Proc Natl Acad Sci USA 82:8232–8236

Reinemer P, Dirr HW, Ladenstein R, Schaffer J, Gallay O, Huber R (1991) The three-dimensional structure of class pi glutathione S-transferase in complex with glutathione sulfonate at 2.3 A resolution. EMBO J 10:1997–2005

Reinemer P, Dirr HW, Ladenstein R, Huber R, Lo Bello M, Federici G, Parker W (1992) Three-dimensional structure of class Pi glutathione S-transferase from human placenta in complex with S-hexylglutathione at 2.8 Å resolution. J Mol Biol 227:214–226

Ricci G, Del Boccio G, Pennelli A, Lo Bello M, Petruzzelli R, Caccuri AM, Barra D, Federici G (1991) Redox forms of human placenta glutathione transferase. J Biol Chem 266:21409–21415

Riley RJ, Workman P (1992) DT-diaphorase and cancer chemotherapy. Biochem Pharmacol 43:1657–1669

Rothkopf GS, Telakowski-Hopkins CA, Stotish RL, Pickett CB (1986) Multiplicity of glutathione S-transferase genes in the rat and association with a type 2 Alu repetitive element. Biochemistry 25:993–1002

Rushmore TH, Pickett CB (1990) Transcriptional regulation of the rat glutathione S-transferase Ya subunit gene. Characterization of a xenobiotic-responsive element controlling inducible expression by phenolic antioxidants. J Biol Chem 265: 14648–14653

Rushmore TH, Pickett CB (1991) Xenobiotic responsive elements controlling inducible expression by planar aromatic compounds and phenolic antioxidants. Methods Enzymol 206:409–420

Rushmore TH, Pickett CB (1992) Induction of the rat glutathione S-transferase Ya subunit gene through the antioxidant responsive element (ARE) by flavonoids. Proc Am Assoc Cancer Res 33:14

Rushmore TH, Morton MR, Pickett CB (1991) The antioxidant responsive element. Activation by oxidative stress and identification of the DNA consensus sequence required for functional activity. J Biol Chem 266:11632–11639

Rushmore TH, King RG, Paulson KE, Pickett CB (1990) Regulation of glutathione S-transferase Ya subunit gene expression: identification of a unique xenobiotic-responsive element controlling inducible expression by planar aromatic compounds. Proc Natl Acad Sci USA 87:3826–3830

Sakai M, Okuda A, Muramatsu M (1988) Multiple regulatory elements and phorbol 12-O-tetradecanoate 13-acetate responsiveness of the rat placental glutathione transferase gene. Proc Natl Acad Sci USA 85:9456–9460

Sato K, Kitahara A, Satoh K, Ishikawa T, Tatematsu M, Ito N (1984) The placental form of glutathione S-transferase as a new marker protein for preneoplasia in rat chemical hepatocarcinogenesis. Gann 75:199–202

Satoh K, Kitahara A, Soma Y, Knaba Y, Hatayama I, Sato K (1985) Purification, induction, and distribution of placental glutathione transferase: a new marker enzyme for preneoplastic cells in the rat chemical hepatocarcinogenesis. Proc Natl Acad Sci USA 82:3964–3968

Söderström M, Mannervik B, Hammarström S (1990) Leukotriene C4 synthase: characterization in mouse mastocytoma cells. Methods Enzymol 187:306–312

Stenberg G, Board PG, Mannervik B (1991) Mutation of an evolutionarily conserved tyrosine residue in the active site of a human class alpha glutathione S-transferase. FEBS Lett 293:153–155

Stenberg G, Ridderstrom M, Engstrom A, Pemble SE, Mannervik B (1992) Cloning and heterologous expression of a cDNA encoding class alpha rat glutathione S-transferase 8-8, an enzyme with high catalytic activity towards genotoxic alpha, beta unsaturated carbonyl compounds. Biochemical J 284:313–319

Suguoka Y, Kano T, Okuda A, Sakai M, Kitagawa T, Muramatsu M (1985) Cloning and the nucleotide sequence of rat glutathione S-transferase P cDNA. Nucleic Acids Res 13:6049–6057

Talalay P, DeLong MJ, Prochaska HJ (1988) Identification of a common chemical signal regulating the induction of enzymes that protect against chemical carcinogenesis. Proc Natl Acad Sci USA 85:8261–8265

Tamai K, Satoh K, Tsuchida S, Hatayama I, Maki T, Sato K (1990) Specific inactivation of glutathione S-transferases in class pi by SH-modifiers. Biochem Biophys Res Commun 167:331–338

Tamai K, Shen H, Tsuchida S, Hatayama I, Satoh K, Yasui A, Oikawa A, Sato K (1991) Role of cysteine residues in the activity of rat glutathione transferase P (7-7): elucidation by oligonucleotide site-directed mutagenesis. Biochem Biophys Res Commun 179:790–797

Telakowski-Hopkins CA, Rodkey JA, Bennett CD, Lu AYH, Pickett CB (1985) Rat liver glutathione S-transferases. Construction of a cDNA clone complementary to a Yc mRNA and prediction of the complete amino acid sequence of a Yc subunit. J Biol Chem 260:5820–5825

Telakowski-Hopkins CA, Rothkopf GS, Pickett CB (1986) Structural analysis of a rat liver glutathione S-transferase Ya gene. Proc Natl Acad Sci USA 83: 9393–9397

Telakowski-Hopkins CA, King RG, Pickett CB (1988) Glutathione S-transferase Ya subunit gene: identification of regulatory elements required for basal level and inducible expression. Proc Natl Acad Sci USA 85:1000–1004

Tsuchida S, Sato K (1992) Glutathione transferases and cancer. CRC Crit Rev Biochem Mol Biol 27:337–384

Tu C-PD, Lai H-CJ, Li N, Weiss MJ, Reddy CC (1984) The Yc and Ya subunits of rat liver glutathione S-transferases are the products of separate genes. J Biol Chem 259:9434–9439

Van Ommen B, den Besten C, Rutten ALM, Ploemen JHTM, Vos RME, Muller F, Van Bladeren PJ (1988) Active site-directed irreversible inhibition of glutathione S-transferases by the glutathione conjugate of tetrachloro-1, 4-benzoquinone. J Biol Chem 263:12939–12942

Van Ommen B, Ploemen JHTM, Ruven HJ, Vos RME, Bogaards JJP, Van Berkel WJH, Van Bladeren PJ (1989) Studies on the active site of rat glutathione S-transferase isoenzyme 4-4. Chemical modification by tetrachloro-1, 4-benzoquinone and its glutathione conjugate. Eur J Biochem 181:423–429

Van Ommen B, Ploeman JHTM, Bogaards JJP, Monks TJ, Gau SS, Van Bladeren PJ (1991) Irreversible inhibition of rat glutathione S-transferase 1-1 by quinones and their glutathione conjugates. Structure-activity relationship and mechanism. Biochem J 276:661–666

Wang RW, Newton DJ, Pickett CB, Lu AYH (1991) Site-directed mutagenesis of glutathione S-transferase YaYa: nonessential role of histidine in catalysis. Arch Biochem Biophys 286:574–578

Wang RW, Newton DJ, Huskey S-E, McKeever BM, Pickett CB, Lu AYH (1992a) Site-directed mutagenesis of glutathione S-transferase YaYa – important roles of tyrosine-9 and aspartic acid-101 in catalysis. J Biol Chem 267:19866–19871

Wang RW, Newton DJ, Pickett CB, Lu AYH (1992b) Site-directed mutagenesis of glutathione S-transferase YaYa – functional studies of histidine, cysteine, and tryptophan mutants. Arch Biochem Biophys 297:86–91

Widersten M, Holstrom E, Mannervik B (1991) Cystein residues are not required for the catalytic activity of human class mu glutathione S-transferase M1a-1a. FEBS Lett 293:156–159

Zhang P, Graminski GF, Armstrong RN (1991) Are the histidine residues of glutathione S-transferase important in catalysis? An assessment by 13C NMR spectroscopy and site-specific mutagenesis. J Biol Chem 266:19475–19479

CHAPTER 4

Human *N*-Acetyltransferases

K.P. VATSIS and W.W. WEBER

A. Introduction

Human variability in drug acetylation was discovered nearly four decades ago during the initial clinical trials of isoniazid as an antituberculosis drug (reviewed in WEBER 1987). Isoniazid was a remarkably effective therapeutic agent, but, despite its effectiveness, a high proportion (3.5%–17%) of treated patients developed a devastating, progressive nerve toxicity. Pharmacokinetic studies of isoniazid elimination in twins and in families revealed serum concentrations of tuberculostatic forms of the drug distributed into two (or three) genetically determined subgroups. This led to the proposal that persons with low blood levels be classified as "rapid" inactivators and those with high levels as "slow" inactivators of isoniazid (MITCHELL and BELL 1957). Later, after the genetic variability (polymorphism) in drug levels was attributed to differences in *N*-acetyltransferase (NAT)[1] activity (JENNE et al. 1961; JENNE 1965; EVANS and WHITE 1964), the term "inactivator" was supplanted by "acetylator." Since then, the two genetically distinct major phenotypes have usually been referred to as rapid and slow acetylators.

By the mid-1960s, the accumulated evidence indicated that isoniazid and a few other drugs, including sulfamethazine and hydralazine, underwent *N*-acetylation at remarkably different rates in vivo and in vitro, whereas *N*-acetylation of certain other drugs, such as *p*-aminosalicylate, *p*-aminobenzoate, and sulfanilamide, proceeded to the same extent among rapid and slow acetylators of isoniazid-sulfamethazine. It was hypothesized that acetylation of isoniazid and certain polycyclic amines in rapid and slow acetylators is mediated either by two related but separate NATs with different physicochemical and kinetic properties, or, alternatively, by an identical (rate-limiting) enzyme that varies in amount because of structural gene differences among individuals (polymorphic pathway with "widely differing acetylation capacity"). On the other hand, acetylation of *p*-aminosalicylate and other simple aromatic amines is largely effected by a different NAT species, the

---

[1] *N*-acetyltransferase proteins and genes are printed in regular type (NAT) and italics (*NAT*), respectively.

amount and catalytic activity of which are invariant (monomorphic pathway with "uniform capacity") (JENNE et al. 1961).

The association of acetylator status with drug toxicity was extended to several widely used therapeutic agents during the next few years. Acetylation polymorphism has thus attracted considerable attention as a significant predictive factor in the safe use of drugs and as a model for individual susceptibility to chemically induced disorders.

B. Biochemical and Immunochemical Studies on Liver Cytosolic *N*-Acetyltransferases

JENNE (1965) was the first investigator to isolate partially purified (approximately 300-fold) NATs from rapid and slow acetylators of isoniazid. The enzyme preparations had a number of physicochemical and kinetic properties in common – including column chromatographic behavior, temperature inactivation curves, pH profiles, as well as substrate affinity and K_i (inhibitor) constants – differing (by ten- to 20-fold) only in the V_{max} with isoniazid. Two peaks with comparable isoniazid activities were evident upon anion exchange chromatography of the enzyme from a rapid acetylator, but this observation was not discussed. A quarter of a century later, GRANT et al. (1989) also prepared partially purified (1000-fold) NAT from human liver cytosol with high sulfamethazine *N*-acetylation activity and similarly observed two elution peaks on a diethylaminoethyl (DEAE)-Sephacel anion exchange chromatography column. The earlier eluting activity peak exhibited a molecular mass (M_r) of 31 kDa upon sodium dodecyl sulfate polycrylamide gel electrophoresis (SDS-PAGE), and was judged by tryptic peptide mapping to be an NAT protein. Moreover, a rabbit antiserum raised against the earlier eluting peak recognized two bands of identical M_r (31 kDa) on immunoblots of the two DEAE-Sephacel peak fractions, indicating the presence of two highly similar NAT proteins in human liver cytosol. These were found to have different affinities for sulfamethazine and acetyl coenzyme A (CoA), respectively, and approximately a twofold difference in turnover number (GRANT et al. 1989), but their relationship was not clear at this time. Later expression studies showed that both of the 31-kDa proteins are products of the *NAT2* locus: the protein in the first peak fraction ostensibly represents the primary gene product (NAT2A), while that in the second peak fraction (NAT2B) appears to arise from NAT2A either by post-translational modification or as an artifact of the purification procedure (GRANT et al. 1991).

Low, intermediate, and high sulfamethazine *N*-acetylation activities in cytosol from 26 liver biopsy specimens correlated well with rates of caffeine elimination by the same subjects in vivo (GRANT et al. 1990), findings which corroborated those of EVANS and WHITE (1964) with isoniazid. Furthermore, the intensity of immunoreactive 31-kDa protein bands in partially purified cytosol from liver of phenotypically slow, intermediate, and rapid acetylators, respectively, increased in parallel with the V_{max} values for sulfamethazine, but there was no appreciable change in the substrate affinity constants determined with partially purified cytosol (Grant et al. 1990) or crude liver cytosol (Kilbane et al. 1991). The findings presented in this section collectively favor one of the aforementioned alternative explanations for "polymorphic" acetylation of isoniazid-sulfamethazine, namely, that activity differences between rapid and slow acetylators of these compounds most likely reflect "differences in amount of an identical enzyme molecule, representing a mutation in the genic mechanism controlling the rate of enzyme synthesis" (Jenne 1965).

C. Molecular Genetics of *N*-Acetyltransferases

I. Identification of *N*-Acetyltransferase Genes

1. Cloning and Chromosomal Mapping

The emergence of molecular genetics in the *N*-acetylation field was made possible by the reported amino acid composition of tryptic peptides of electrophoretically homogeneous liver NAT from rapid acetylator rabbits (Andres et al. 1987). These peptides were essential for the construction of oligonucleotide screening probes and isolation of chicken and rabbit NAT cDNAs (Ohsako et al. 1988; Blum et al. 1989; Sasaki et al. 1991), which eventually led to identification of human NAT cDNAs and genomic clones. The NAT cDNAs originated from Japanese subjects, and were obtained from libraries made with mRNA from two liver samples of undetermined acetylator phenotype (Ohsako and Deguchi 1990). Three loci containing NAT genes were identified by Blum et al. (1990) upon screening of a library constructed with leukocyte DNA from a Caucasian with a heterozygous acetylator phenotype; these were designated *NAT1*, *NAT2*, and *NATP*, and corresponded to *Eco*RI fragments of 1.3, 1.9, and 4.7 kb, respectively. Subsequently, the genes corresponding to the NAT cDNAs from Japanese were also isolated from libraries made with DNA from hepatic tissue of unreported acetylator phenotype (Ebisawa and Deguchi 1991). For the sake of simplicity, the terminology of Blum et al. (1990) will be adopted for the remainder of this review.

NAT1 and *NAT2* contain open reading frames of 870 bp that encode proteins with an estimated M_r of around 33.5 kDa; the coding exon of both genes is uninterrupted by introns. *NATP* had amassed several detrimental mutations in the coding region, and was considered to be a pseudogene (Blum et al. 1990). The coding regions of *NAT1* and *NAT2* have 87% nucleotide identity and 80% deduced amino acid similarity (Ohsako and Deguchi 1990; Blum et al. 1990; Ebisawa and Deguchi 1991).

The boundary of the 5′ untranslated region (UTR) of *NAT1* and *NAT2* has been inferred from the structure of the corresponding cDNA (OHSAKO and DEGUCHI 1990), but the real transcriptional start sites have not been mapped. Both genes contain a consensus sequence for a 3′ splice acceptor site 6 bp upstream from the initiator ATG codon, and in general display a great deal of identity in this region extending about 200 nucleotides 5′ to the initiator ATG. Interestingly, only *NAT2* utilizes this 3′ splice acceptor site, with the rest of the 5′ UTR located 8 kb upstream as a consequence of the intervening intron; the 5′ UTR of *NAT1* is free of introns (OHSAKO and DEGUCHI 1990; BLUM et al. 1990; EBISAWA and DEGUCHI 1991; DEGUCHI 1992). The nature of the 5′ UTR in the two genes has prompted the speculation that *NAT2* evolved from *NAT1* (EBISAWA and DEGUCHI 1991). The 3′ UTR of the two genes also exhibits substantial nucleotide identity.

Southern blot analysis of a number of human–rodent somatic cell hybrid DNAs has shown that *NAT1* and *NAT2* reside on chromosome 8 (BLUM et al. 1990), but the relative position and orientation of the two genes have not yet been determined.

2. Heterologous Expression

Transient expression of Caucasian *NAT1* and *NAT2* in monkey kidney COS-1 cells led to the following observations (BLUM et al. 1990): (a) the electrophoretic mobility of recombinant NAT2 was indistinguishable from that of liver cytosolic NAT2A and NAT2B (approximately 31 kDa), the content of which had previously been shown to vary (from negligible to significant) on immunoblots of liver cytosol with low, intermediate, and high sulfamethazine *N*-acetylation activity, respectively (GRANT et al. 1990). In contrast, expressed NAT1 migrated with an M_r of about 33 kDa, much closer to that estimated from the deduced amino acid sequence of both gene products (approximately 33.5 kDa). The reasons for the discrepancy between estimated and observed molecular mass for NAT2 have not been elaborated upon; (b) the deduced amino acid sequence of NAT2 contained six tryptic peptide sequences that had been determined for partially purified liver cytosolic NAT2A (GRANT et al. 1989); and (c) the expressed proteins had *N*-acetylation activity toward sulfamethazine, with an NAT2 to NAT1 activity ratio of 3.5. Expressed NATP possessed neither immunoreactivity nor catalytic activity, consistent with the view that *NATP* is a pseudogene. It was concluded from these data that *NAT1* and *NAT2* represent the monomorphic and polymorphic gene loci, respectively. Such a conclusion concerning *NAT1* was unwarranted, however, since a comprehensive structural characterization of the gene from different individuals was not attempted.

Transfection of Chinese hamster ovary (CHO) cells with NAT1 and NAT2 cDNAs from Japanese revealed: (a) the same electrophoretic mobility for NAT2 (approximately 31 kDa) as that displayed by the partially purified or crude liver cytosolic enzyme (GRANT et al. 1989, 1990, 1991; BLUM et al. 1990, 1991) and by NAT2 expressed in COS-1 cells (BLUM et al. 1990, 1991); (b) a decrease in the catalytic activity of expressed NAT2 from a mutant with a coding region base substitution (explained in Sect. D); (c) differences in the substrate selectivity profiles of NAT1 and NAT2; and (d) a *Kpn*I restriction fragment length polymorphism (RFLP) on blots of genomic DNA digested with *Kpn*I, *Bam*HI, or *Eco*RI and probed with NAT2 cDNA, but no RFLPs on similar blots probed with NAT1 cDNA. The conclusion that *NAT2* represented a polymorphic locus was reasonable, but, as noted above for the Caucasian genes and detailed in Sect. E, the data on *NAT1* were meager at best and did not by any means support the premise that this is a monomorphic locus (*NAT1* was isolated from just one genomic clone, and no characterization beyond sequencing was attempted).

II. Properties of Hepatic and Recombinant *N*-Acetyltransferases

1. Substrate Selectivity

The substrate selectivity profiles of NAT1 and NAT2 in partially purified liver cytosol and in crude cytosol from transfected mammalian cells are illustrated in Table 1. It should be pointed out at the outset that the large differences in absolute values between COS-1 and CHO cells merely reflect a difference in units: activities with COS-1 cells are given as "nmol/min per unit of immunoreactive protein" (determined by densitometric scanning of the protein bands on immunoblots), while those with CHO cells are presented as "nmol/min per mg cell cytosolic protein." It is quite apparent that hepatic and expressed NAT1 and NAT2 have overlapping catalytic activities, but a certain degree of selectivity is discernible upon consideration of the intrinsic clearance ($Cl_i = V_{max}/K_m$) values for the different substrates (not shown in Table 1). The NAT2 to NAT1 Cl_i ratio for sulfamethazine is 220 in liver cytosol and 13 in COS-1 cell cytosol, indicating that *N*-acetylation of this substrate is preferentially brought about by NAT2. Conversely, the NAT2 to NAT1 Cl_i ratios for *p*-aminosalicylic and *p*-aminobenzoic acids are in the range of less than 0.001 to less than 0.0001 in both preparations, implicating NAT1 as the main enzyme in *N*-acetylation reactions with these substrates. NAT1 and NAT2 seem to be equally effective with the carcinogen 2-aminofluorene, notwithstanding the incongruity in the NAT2 to NAT1 Cl_i ratio in liver (7.6) relative to COS-1 cell cytosol (0.4). Although *N*-acetylation of procainamide appears to be catalyzed primarily by NAT2, the affinity of NAT2 for this substrate (approximately 2.8 m*M*) is no better than that for the "NAT1 substrate" *p*-aminosalicylic acid (approximately 3.0 m*M*); in addition, there is a large disparity in the NAT2 to NAT1 Cl_i ratio with procainamide in COS-1 cells (0.6) relative to liver (12). By far the

Table 1. Substrate selectivity profiles of human N-Acetyltransferases[a]

Substrate	*N*-Acetylation activity[b]					
	Hepatic NATs		Expressed NATs			
	NAT1	NAT2A[c]	COS-1 cells		CHO cells	
			NAT1	NAT2	NAT1	NAT2
Sulfamethazine	0.4	5.5 (13.8)[d]	28	37 (1.3)	0.9	42.1 (46.8)
Procainamide	6.0	6.2 (1.0)	510	27 (0.05)	7.4	9.4 (1.3)
p-Aminosalicylic acid	14.8	2.6 (0.2)	1280	14 (0.01)	n.d.	n.d.
p-Phenetidine	n.d.	n.d.	n.d.	n.d.	150	33.7 (0.2)
p-Aminobenzoic acid	13.9	–[e]	1250	–[e]	608	0
2-Aminofluorene	16.4	11.4 (0.7)	1395	36 (0.03)	65.8	13.7 (0.2)

NAT, N-acetyltransferase; CHO, Chinese hamster ovary; n.d., not determined.
[a] The data with liver and recombinant NATs in COS-1 cells were obtained with tissue and NATs from Caucasians (GRANT et al. 1991). Proteins were expressed in CHO cells transfected with NAT cDNAs derived from Japanese subjects (OHSAKO and DEGUCHI 1990).
[b] Cytosol from liver with intermediate sulfamethazine *N*-acetylation activity and from COS-1 cells transfected with *NAT1* and *NAT2* from a heterozygote was applied to a diethylaminoethyl (DEAE)-Sephacel anion exchange chromatography column, and the proteins were eluted with a linear salt gradient from 50 to 200 m*M* KCl. Fractions eluting at relatively low KCl concentrations had activity with *p*-aminosalicylate but not with sulfamethazine, whereas the opposite was true for the fractions that eluted at higher KCl concentrations; all fractions exhibited activity with 2-aminofluorene. Kinetic studies were carried out with pooled peak fractions containing the partially purified hepatic proteins, and with crude COS-1 cell cytosol containing the recombinant NATs. The activities shown are V_{max} values, given as nmol *N*-acetylated product formed per min/mg protein for the hepatic proteins and as nmol/min per arbitrary unit of immunoreactive protein for the gene products in COS-1 cells (GRANT et al. 1991). Kinetic experiments were not performed with the proteins expressed in CHO cells, and the values shown (in nmol *N*-acetylated product formed per min/mg protein) are from activity determinations at a single substrate concentration (OHSAKO and DEGUCHI 1990).
[c] Two NAT2 peak fractions with sulfamethazine *N*-acetylation activity, designated NAT2A and NAT2B, were seen at relatively high KCl concentrations, whereas the product of *NAT2*-transfected COS-1 cells eluted as a single peak coincident with that of NAT2A. Both the activity and affinity of hepatic NAT2B were somewhat higher than those of NAT2A for the substrates shown.
[d] The numbers in parentheses are NAT2/NAT1 activity ratios.
[e] Recombinant NAT2 and hepatic NAT2A and NAT2B were apparently activated by *p*-aminobenzoate up to a concentration of 10 m*M*, beyond which enzyme destruction was seen. Determination of kinetic constants was not possible under these conditions (GRANT et al. 1991).

greatest affinity was that of NAT2 for 2-aminofluorene (1–2 μM) (GRANT et al. 1991). Somewhat puzzling is that isoniazid, the prototype compound for the "classical" *N*-acetylation polymorphism, was not examined with the hepatic or expressed proteins.

2. Stability

A significant attenuation (42%) in *p*-aminosalicylate but not in sulfamethazine *N*-acetylation activity has been observed upon overnight dialysis of liver cytosol at 4°C prior to DEAE-Sephacel anion exchange chromatography, suggesting that NAT1 may be more labile than NAT2. Support for this suggestion was obtained from transient expression of the proteins, which gave half-lives at 37°C of 3.5 h (NAT1) and 61 h (NAT2) when assayed with sulfamethazine as substrate (GRANT et al. 1991). Assessment of NAT1 stability with sulfamethazine is rather curious in light of the considerably greater selectivity of this protein for *p*-aminosalicylate (Table 1), raising the possibility that it could be the sulfamethazine *N*-acetylation activity of NAT1, and not NAT1 per se, that is thermolabile. Additionally, it is not known whether wild-type NAT1 or a structural variant of this protein might possess such intrinsic instability, since *NAT1* genotypes (Sect. E.I.) were not determined for the liver specimens submitted to column chromatography or the *NAT1* sample transfected in COS-1 cells (GRANT et al. 1991).

D. The *NAT2* Locus

I. Structural Heterogeneity

1. Coding Region Mutations

Five to six allelic variants with non-silent and silent nucleotide substitutions in the protein-coding region of *NAT2* have been identified in Caucasian and Japanese subjects of established acetylator phenotype (Fig. 1). The mutant alleles are characterized by one or two amino acid changes, accompanied in most cases by a silent substitution (bars 2, 3, 5, and 7). The various point mutations result in obliteration of a restriction site (bars 3, 5, and 6) or a pair of sites; in the latter instance, a *Fok*I site is eliminated together with a *Taq*I site (bar 2) or a *Bam*HI site (bar 7). Only the $A^{803}{\rightarrow}G$ transition leads to the creation of a new site (*Dde*I; bars 4 and 5). The alleles on bars 3–5 possess the same $T^{341}{\rightarrow}C$ mutation (I114T), and in addition exhibit either the $C^{481}{\rightarrow}T$ silent substitution (L161L) and concomitant eradication of the *Kpn*I site (bars 3 and 5), or the $A^{803}{\rightarrow}G$ transition associated with the conservative change (K268R) and appearance of the *Dde*I site (bars 4 and 5). The mutants on bars 6 and 7 share the *Bam*HI site mutation (G286E), differing only at position 282.

2. Far Downstream Mutations

Southern blot hybridization of *Kpn*I ± *Bam*HI-digested DNA (n = 86) indicated the presence of *Kpn*I sites about 5 and 5.5 kb downstream from

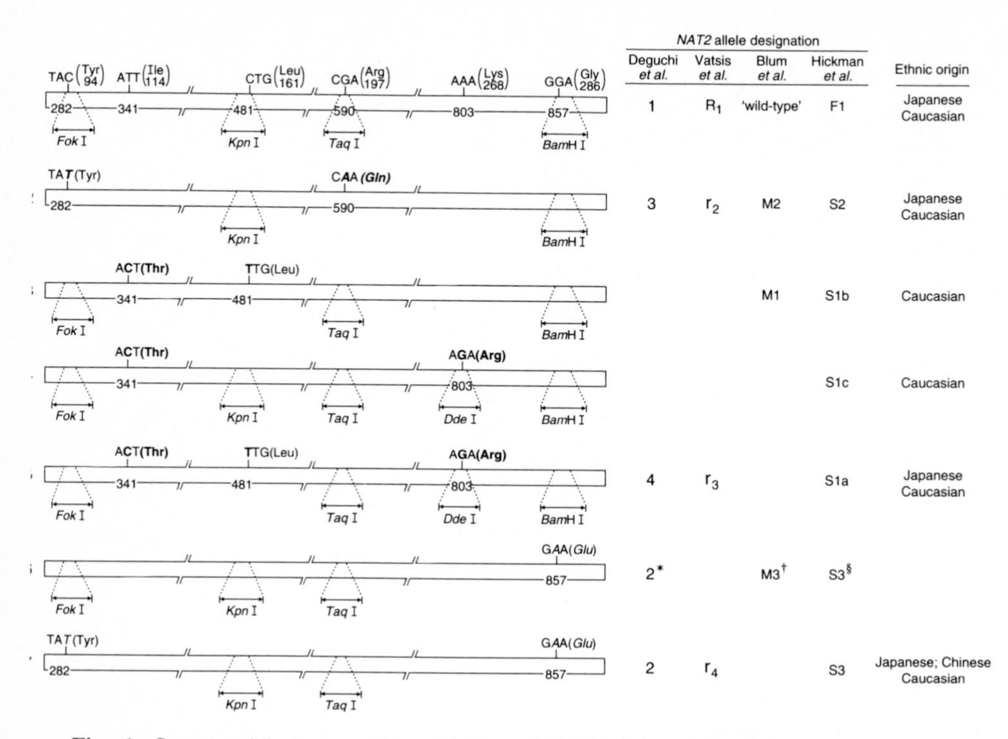

Fig. 1. Structural heterogeneity of human NAT2. Schematic illustration of 0.6-kb coding exon segments (nt 270–870; not drawn to scale) of normal (*bar 1*) and mutant (bars 2–7) *NAT2* alleles identified in different laboratories. *NAT2 from Japanese*: alleles 1 and 2* were detected by sequencing of cDNA and corresponding genomic clones (OHSAKO and DEGUCHI 1990; EBISAWA and DEGUCHI 1991). Allele 3 was identified by restriction fragment length polymorphism (RFLP) analysis of genomic DNA on Southern blots (DEGUCHI et al. 1990). The structure of genomic alleles 1, 2, and 3 was recently determined by sequencing (DEGUCHI 1992); the author commented that allele 4 was also determined by sequencing and found to be identical to variant r_3 originally reported by VATSIS et al. (1991). *NAT2 from Caucasians*: the structure of alleles R_1, r_2, r_3 (VATSIS et al. 1991), and r_4 (VATSIS et al. 1993) was determined by double-stranded sequencing of 1.3-kb fragments of polymerase chain reaction (PCR)-generated *NAT2*. The "wild-type" (BLUM et al. 1990) and mutant alleles M1 and M2 (BLUM et al. 1991) were detected by single-stranded sequencing, whereas allele M3 was visualized on agarose gels after amplification with allele-specific primers made solely to the *Bam*HI site ($G^{857}A$). Alleles F1, S2, S1 (now designated S1b, *bar 3*) and S3§ (*bar 6*) had been detected by endonuclease cleavage of PCR-generated *NAT2* (HICKMAN and SIM 1991); alleles S1b (previously designated S1; HICKMAN and SIM 1991), S1c, S1a, and S3 (*bar 7*) were most recently identified by RFLP analyses and limited sequencing of PCR-generated *NAT2* (HICKMAN et al. 1992).

*2**, DEGUCHI (1992) stated that repeated sequencing of the cDNA (OHSAKO and DEGUCHI 1990) corresponding to allele 2, which had originally shown only the $G^{857}A$ substitution (*bar 6*), now revealed both the $C^{282}T$ and $G^{857}A$ transitions (*bar 7*). It has not been established, however, that the "new" allele 2 (*bar 7*) occurs in Japanese to the exclusion of "old" allele 2* (*bar 6*; see text Sect. D.I.3.a for details).

M3†, Allele M3 was identified by agarose gel electrophoresis of *NAT2* fragments amplified with allele-specific primers bearing the wild-type and mutant bases at the coding region *Kpn*I site, respectively. Alleles 1 and 2 contained the 5.5-kb *Kpn*I fragment, whereas allele 3 had the 5.0-kb *Kpn*I fragment (DEGUCHI et al. 1990). A similar RFLP pattern was observed with Caucasian wild-type and mutant M2 alleles (fragment sizes of 5 and 4.4 kb, respectively), spurring the proposal that M2 is identical to allele 3 (BLUM et al. 1991). Such a relationship was not apparent, however, because allele 3 (unlike M2) had not yet been sequenced (DEGUCHI et al. 1990).

Definitive proof for the structural kinship of mutant alleles M2 and 3 was provided by the recent publication of 9.2-kb sequences for genomic clones from homozygotes of alleles 1, 2, and 3, respectively (DEGUCHI 1992), all three of which contain *Kpn*I sites 5.3 kb downstream from that present in the coding exon. Secondly, a T→G substitution in allele 3 results in the appearance of a new *Kpn*I site, located 4.7 kb 3′ to that in the coding exon. These far downstream *Kpn*I sites along with that in the coding region are responsible for the banding pattern differences in *Kpn*I-cleaved genomic DNA, and find a usefulness in *NAT2* genotype determination by Southern blot hybridization (OHSAKO and DEGUCHI 1990; DEGUCHI et al. 1990; BLUM et al. 1991; DEGUCHI 1992).

3. Allelic and Genotypic Frequencies

a) Japanese

*Kpn*I RFLP analysis with liver (n = 84) and leukocyte (n = 52) DNA has shown that allele 1 is by far the most prevalent in Japanese, representing 70% of all alleles. Allele 2 is minor (comprising 7%–8% of all alleles and 22%–25% of the mutant alleles), while allele 3 is a major allele, accounting for 21%–25% of all *NAT2* alleles and for 70%–78% of the mutant alleles in this ethnic group (DEGUCHI et al. 1990; DEGUCHI 1992). Allele 4 was not detected but was listed with a frequency of 1%, indicating that it is very rare in Japanese. Moreover, the identity of allele 2 was not demonstrated conclusively, as no *Fok*I digestions were performed together with *Bam*HI in a separate study on genotype determination with a large number of polymerase chain reaction (PCR)-generated *NAT2* samples (n = 145; DEGUCHI 1992). Stated differently, it was not ascertained whether allele 2 contained

---

position 857 only ($G^{857}A$), suggesting that the *Fok*I site mutation ($C^{282}T$) most likely went undetected (BLUM et al. 1991).

S3[§], This allele was originally described to be identical to M3; it was seen on agarose gels after cleavage of PCR-generated *NAT2* with *Bam*HI only, suggesting (as for M3 above) that the $C^{282}T$ mutation was not detected because cleavage with *Fok*I was not performed (HICKMAN and SIM 1991). Subsequent work in the same laboratory unmasked both the *Fok*I and *Bam*HI site mutations, and this allele (*bar* 7) was again denoted S3 (HICKMAN et al. 1992). The possible existence of S3 or M3 (*bar 6*) among Caucasians cannot be ruled out at this time only the $G^{857}A$ substitution (Fig. 1, bar 6), or both the $C^{282}T$ and $G^{857}A$ substitutions (Fig. 1, bar 7).

Approximately half (47%–56%) of the subjects (n = 86) were homozygous for allele 1, and another 34%–44% were heterozygotes of alleles 1 and 2 (11%–14%) and 1 and 3 (20%–33%). Homozygotes of mutant alleles 2 and 3, respectively, and compound heterozygotes (2/3) comprised only 9%–10% of the population examined. The same frequency was found in 29 unrelated persons, the acetylator phenotype of whom was determined with isoniazid in vivo. Genotype 1/1 was associated with a high *N*-acetylisoniazid to isoniazid plasma ratio (n = 10), genotypes 1/2 and 1/3 showed an intermediate plasma ratio of *N*-acetylated to unmetabolized isoniazid (n = 14), and genotypes 2/3 and 3/3 had a low plasma ratio (n = 3). *NAT2* genotypes correlated very well with acetylator phenotypes, except for two homozygotes of allele 1 who displayed an intermediate *N*-acetylisoniazid to isoniazid plasma ratio (DEGUCHI et al. 1990). Overall, 90% of the Japanese investigated had high and intermediate activities and only 10% had low activities, in accord with previous reports on acetylator phenotype frequency in this ethnic group (SUNAHARA et al. 1961).

The mean activity values for liver cytosolic *p*-phenetidine *N*-acetylation also correlated well with six genotypes (n = 42; 37 rapid, five slow), but the individual values for genotypes 1/1, 1/2, and 1/3 (n = 37) varied markedly, and there was considerable overlap in at least ten of the 37 values for these three genotypes (DEGUCHI 1992). Besides postmortem tissue changes and other factors that may in part be responsible for the discrepancy between *NAT2* genotypes and acetylator phenotypes determined with liver tissue in vitro (VATSIS et al. 1991; DEGUCHI 1992), the wide variation in *p*-phenetidine *N*-acetylation (DEGUCHI 1992) may also be a consequence of differences in the extent of NAT1 contribution to the overall catalytic activity, since expressed NAT1 is five times more active with this substrate than NAT2 (Table 1; OHSAKO and DEGUCHI 1990).

b) Caucasians

Initial computations of allelic frequencies for Caucasians were inconclusive because they failed to take into account allele r_3 (BLUM et al. 1991; HICKMAN and SIM 1991; SIM and HICKMAN 1991). These estimates had indicated that allele M1 (BLUM et al. 1991) or S1 (HICKMAN and SIM 1991), found to be structurally identical (Fig. 1, bar 3), represented 46%–61% of the mutant alleles. More thorough characterization of *NAT2* mutants after publication of variant r_3 (VATSIS et al. 1991) showed that the allele originally designated S1 (HICKMAN and SIM 1991) and subsequently assigned the notation S1b (HICKMAN et al. 1992; Fig. 1, bar 3) is actually rare, accounting for only 1.5% of the mutant alleles (HICKMAN et al. 1992). In contrast, variant r_3 (Fig. 1, bar 5) has turned out to be the preponderant allele in Caucasians, making up about 45% of all alleles and 55% of the mutant alleles (HICKMAN et al. 1992).

Preliminary estimates ($n = 48$) additionally show variant r_2 to be a major allele, variant r_4 a minor allele, and variant S1c (like S1b) to contribute little to the Caucasian *NAT2* allelic pool. Therefore, it seems that mutants r_2 and r_3 account for an astounding 75% of all alleles, or for about 90% of the mutant alleles in this ethnic group (HICKMAN et al. 1992). Furthermore, the overall contribution of Caucasian alleles r_2 (approximately 25%) and r_4 (approximately 5%) appears to be quite similar to that of the corresponding *NAT2* alleles in Japanese (3 and 2, respectively). The dramatic difference in the frequency of alleles R_1 and r_3 in Caucasians (R_1, 20%; r_3, 45%) relative to Japanese (R_1, 70%; r_3, 1%) has been suggested as a possible reason for the well-known acetylator phenotype differences in these ethnic groups (DEGUCHI 1992), with 90% of the Japanese but only about 55% of the Caucasians possessing the rapid phenotype (WEBER 1987).

II. Characterization of Mutants

1. mRNA and Protein Content in Genotypically Defined Liver Tissue

Similar findings were reported by two independent investigations on *N*-acetylation activities and NAT2 mRNA and protein steady state levels in genotypically defined liver tissue from Caucasians and Japanese. The liver specimens from Caucasians ($n = 5$) represented five of the six possible combinations of the wild-type allele and mutant alleles M1 and M2 (genotype M1/M2 was not examined; BLUM et al. 1991), and those from Japanese ($n = 42$) encompassed six genotypes with all possible combinations of alleles 1, 2, and 3 (DEGUCHI 1992). As with tissue of undetermined NAT2 genotype (GRANT et al. 1990), immunoreactive NAT2 followed a course parallel to that seen for *N*-acetylation activity: it was substantial in liver cytosol from wild-type/wild-type (1/1) homozygotes with high *N*-acetylation activity, present in lesser amounts in tissue from wild-type/M1, wild-type/M2 (1/3), and 1/2 heterozygotes with intermediate catalytic activity, but only marginally detectable or undetectable in tissue from mutant homozygotes and compound heterozygotes (2/3) with little or no activity. In contrast to the marked differences in activity and NAT2 content, the size and abundance of NAT2 message were comparable in all but one of the samples. Tissue from homozygotes of mutant allele 3 exhibited an appreciably weaker mRNA signal (DEGUCHI 1992), consistent with previous observations in the same laboratory (DEGUCHI et al. 1990) but contrary to the demonstration of ample transcript in liver from Caucasians with the corresponding genotype (M2/M2; BLUM et al. 1991). Further quantitative measurements of mRNA steady state levels by slot-blot hybridization gave comparable values for the NAT2 mRNA to β-actin mRNA ratio irrespective of genotype, suggesting that defective transcription may not be the "major" cause of low *N*-acetylation activity in mutant allele 3 (DEGUCHI 1992).

2. Transfection of Mammalian Cells with *NAT2* Alleles and Chimeric Gene Constructs

The results of experiments on transient expression of *NAT2* wild-type/wild-type, M1/M1, and M2/M2 genotypes in COS-1 cells (BLUM et al. 1991), and of 1/1, 2/2, and 3/3 genotypes in CHO cells (DEGUCHI 1992) essentially mirrored those with liver tissue described in the preceding section (heterozygous rapid and slow genotypes were not expressed). In this connection, the mutant alleles had no effect on total RNA content, but caused a precipitous fall in *N*-acetylation activity and a marked diminution or extinction of the NAT2 band on immunoblots of transfected cell culture cytosol. The M_r of NAT2 in CHO cells transfected with allele 1 was 34 kDa (DEGUCHI 1992), significantly different from the 31-kDa band detected in cytosol from the same cells transfected with the cDNA corresponding to allele 1 (OHSAKO and DEGUCHI 1990), in cytosol from COS-1 cells transfected with wild-type *NAT2* (BLUM et al. 1990, 1991; GRANT et al. 1991), and in crude or partially purified liver cytosol with relatively high *N*-acetylation activity (GRANT et al. 1989, 1990, 1991; BLUM et al. 1990, 1991).

Neither the K_m for the substrate nor that for the cofactor was altered in the expressed M1 and M2 proteins relative to the values obtained with wild-type NAT2 (BLUM et al. 1991). The K_m for sulfamethazine had also been found to be invariant in crude cytosol (KILBANE et al. 1991) and in partially purified cytosol from liver tissue with high, intermediate, and low sulfamethazine *N*-acetylation activity and NAT2 content (GRANT et al. 1990). It seems, therefore, that low *N*-acetylation activity (or slow acetylation) in humans is the result of a reduction in the liver cytosolic content of mutant NAT2, which, at least for the M1 and M2 proteins, appear to be kinetically indistinguishable from normal or wild-type NAT2 present in homozygous rapid acetylators or heterozygotes with intermediate activity.

The relative contribution of the individual mutations was assessed by expression of chimeric *NAT2* constructs in mammalian cells. Experiments with COS-1 cells (BLUM et al. 1991) showed that, for mutant M1, both the silent substitution (L161L) and the large hydropathy alteration resulting from the I114T change (VATSIS et al. 1991) were obligatory for the decrease in catalytic activity and immunoreactive M1 protein. The thermostability of the expressed wild-type and M1 proteins at 37°C was identical ($t_{1/2}$ = 22 h), suggesting that the mutations in M1 are deleterious to mRNA translational efficiency. In contrast to M1, replacement of a cationic by an uncharged polar residue (R197Q) in M2 is ostensibly sufficient for the parallel decreases in catalytic activity and M2 protein, which came out to be less stable at 37°C ($t_{1/2}$ = 6 h) than the wild-type and M1 enzymes. Expression of chimeric constructs in CHO cells (DEGUCHI 1992) demonstrated that the silent substitution common to alleles 2 and 3 (Y94Y) had no effect on catalytic activity, but the single amino acid change in allele 2 (G286E) or allele 3 (R197Q) resulted in *N*-acetylation activities that were 6% of control values. Transcript or protein levels were not examined with the chimeric constructs in CHO cells. It was suggested that the decreased catalytic activity in mutants 2 and 3 could be explained by rapid degradation of mutant NAT2 protein, but this possibility was not evaluated. In addition, no data were presented with allele 4, but it was stated that the I114T change in this allele was by itself responsible for the decline in catalytic activity of the expressed protein (DEGUCHI 1992). Allele 4 has one more point mutation ($A^{803}G$) than M1, but shares with M1 the nonsilent (I114T) and silent (L161L) substitutions at nucleotides (nt) 341 and 481, respectively (Fig. 1, bars 3 and 5), both of which were necessary for the decreased catalytic activity and amount of expressed M1 protein (BLUM et al. 1991). This discordance may be a consequence of the different mammalian cell culture systems in which alleles M1 (COS-1 cells) and 4 (CHO cells) were expressed, but there is as yet no definitive proof for this supposition.

In summary, the demonstration of *NAT2* allelic variants (OHSAKO and DEGUCHI 1990; DEGUCHI et al. 1990; VATSIS et al. 1991; BLUM et al. 1991; HICKMAN and SIM 1991; DEGUCHI 1992; HICKMAN et al. 1992) and reasonable correspondence of *NAT2* genotypes with acetylator phenotypes, ascertained with substrates that undergo widely different elimination rates in vivo, establish NAT2 as the locus for the human *N*-acetylation polymorphism typified by isoniazid-sulfamethazine. Studies with hepatic tissue and mammalian cell culture expression systems suggest that "slow" acetylation in the variants thus far examined may be attributable to impaired translational efficiency of mutant NAT2 mRNA or enhanced degradation of mutant protein, culminating in a significant decrease in cytosolic NAT2 content (OHSAKO and DEGUCHI 1990; BLUM et al. 1991; DEGUCHI 1992) evidently without alteration of the kinetic properties of the enzyme (BLUM et al. 1991). The precise mechanism(s) underlying the effects of the mutations in NAT2 variant alleles have not been unraveled.

E. The *NAT1* Locus

I. Structural Heterogeneity

A systematic survey of *NAT1* genotypes in Caucasians, initiated over 2 years ago (VATSIS and WEBER 1991) and concluded recently (VATSIS and WEBER 1993), unequivocally shows *NAT1* to be a polymorphic locus, as detailed in the ensuing sections.

1. Allelic Variants of Caucasian *NAT1*

Direct sequencing of both strands of 1.6-kb fragments of *NAT1* from Caucasian subjects revealed three distinct alleles, the structures of which are shown in Fig. 2. The changes in variant allele v_2 entail two point mutations

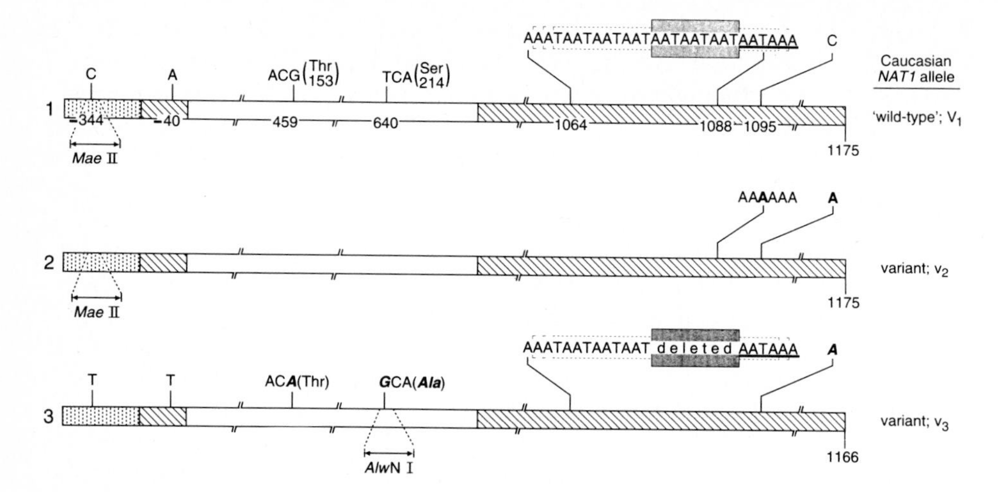

Fig. 2. Genetic variability at the Caucasian *NAT1* locus. The 1.6-kb fragments (nt −440 to 1175) of wild-type (*bar 1*) and variant (*bars 2 and 3*) *NAT1* alleles from Caucasians have been identified by direct sequencing and arbitrarily assigned the indicated *letters* and *numbers*. The 5′ flanking area is shown by the *stippled bar*, the 5′ and 3′ UTR by the *hatched bars*, and the coding exon by the *open bar*. A 3′ UTR sequence (nt 1064–1091) containing the consensus polyadenylation signal (AATAAA; *underlined*) is depicted on *bar 1*. The element $(AAT)_3$ highlighted by the *gray shaded frame (bar 1)* is shown as "deleted" from variant v_3 (*bar 3*), but this is actually intended to point out one such potential deletion site (alternative deletion sites are depicted by the *dashed lines* above and below this segment; see text for explanation). (Adapted from VATSIS and WEBER 1993)

in the 3′ UTR (nt 1088 and 1095), the more notable of which is the $T^{1088}\rightarrow A$ transversion that results in obliteration of the consensus polyadenylation signal (AATAAA→AAAAAA; bar 2). Nucleotide substitutions that alter the highly conserved AATAAA element, like those seen in the human α- and β-globin genes, lead to production of elongated and unstable transcripts (THEIN et al. 1988; ORKIN et al. 1985). Point mutations occur in all regions of *NAT1* variant v_3 (bar 3), including silent (T153T) and nonsilent (S214A) substitutions in the coding exon, and the same $C^{1095}\rightarrow A$ transversion also seen in the 3′ UTR of variant v_2. Two of the five point mutations in v_3 are at hypermutable CpG dinucleotides (nt −344 and 459), but it is not yet known whether these are mutational "hotspots" in Caucasian *NAT1*. Besides the point mutations, variant v_3 is also characterized by a nonanucleotide deletion from the segment extending from nt 1065 to 1090 in the 3′ UTR. This 26-bp segment consists of eight iterative AAT, ATA, and TAA triplets, giving rise to 18 nonanucleotide combinations (six each for the $(AAT)_3$, $(ATA)_3$, and $(TAA)_3$ motifs) as potential deletion sites (indicated by the dashed lines above and below this segment; bars 1 and 3). Elimination of each of these nonanucleotide elements results in the same sequence for allele v_3, thereby precluding determination of the precise location of the deletion site. The polyadenylation signal remains intact in homozygotes of allele v_3, but V_1v_3 and v_2v_3 heterozygotes have duplicate A/T bands at the sixth position of the consensus signal (AATAA*A*/AATAA*T*). Of particular significance is the fact that all three *NAT1* alleles exhibit Mendelian inheritance characteristics in three members of a two-generation family (VATSIS and WEBER 1993).

The nucleotide substitutions at positions −344 (5′ flank) and 640 (coding exon) in variant v_3 result in elimination of a *Mae*II site and formation of an *Alw*NI site, respectively (Fig. 2, bars 1 and 3). These rather unusual restriction sites are not ordinarily included in routine screening for gene polymorphism by RFLP analysis. None of the most widely investigated restriction sites is extinguished or generated by the mutations in variants v_2 and v_3, indicating that banding pattern differences would not have been observed upon cleavage of *NAT1* with the common restriction endonucleases. The negative results reported by two laboratories bear directly on this point: (a) no RFLPs were evident on Southern blots of three different samples of liver DNA digested with *Kpn*I, *Bam*HI, or *Eco*RI and probed with NAT1 cDNA, whereas a *Kpn*I RFLP was apparent on blots probed with NAT2 cDNA (OHSAKO and DEGUCHI 1990), and (b) a 920-bp *NAT1* fragment amplified by PCR with leukocyte DNA from three individuals gave the same banding pattern on agarose gels after digestion with eight different restriction endonucleases (WARD et al. 1992). It is fair to say, therefore, that the absence of banding pattern differences was not sufficient evidence against structural heterogeneity of *NAT1* (OHSAKO and DEGUCHI 1990), and, secondly, no technique can substitute for direct sequencing in initial investigations of allelic variation at any gene locus.

2. Ethnic Differences in Wild-Type *NAT1*

Significant differences exist between Caucasian *NAT1* allele V_1 and a putative wild-type allele from Japanese (Fig. 3). Of the eight nucleotide dissimilarities, five are in the coding exon and involve replacement of two Arg residues and one Glu residue (top) by three uncharged polar residues (bottom), representing a net loss of two positive charges and a negative charge in Japanese relative to Caucasian NAT1. Dissimilarities are also seen in the 3′ UTR, namely, a transversion (nt 884) and deletion of two bases (nt 976 and 1105) from this region of *NAT1* from Japanese.

II. Functional Aspects of Allelic Heterogeneity

Given the profound structural variability at the human *NAT1* locus, it is pertinent to ask whether NAT1 participates in an acetylation polymorphism distinct from that involving NAT2. The answer appears to be affirmative, but the evidence is indirect in that NAT1 phenotypic determinations have not been carried out with established *NAT1* genotypes. By far the majority

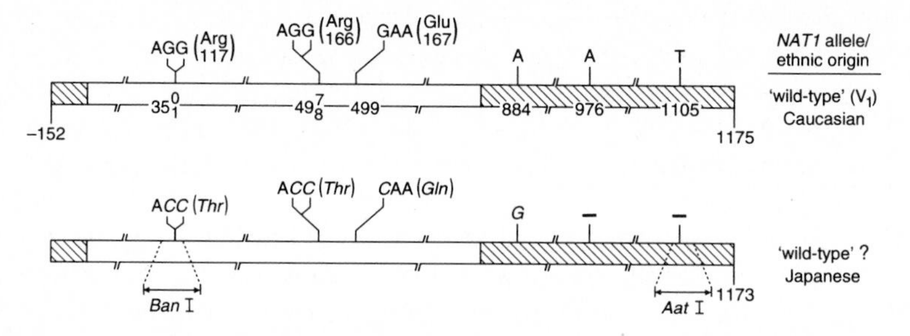

Fig. 3. Ethnic differences in *NAT1* structure. Caucasian "wild-type" NAT1 (*upper bar*; BLUM et al. 1990; VATSIS and WEBER 1993) is compared to a supposedly wild-type NAT1 cDNA (OHSAKO and DEGUCHI 1990) and corresponding genomic allele (EBISAWA and DEGUCHI 1991) from Japanese (*lower bar*). The various *NAT1* regions are marked as in Fig. 2 (1.3-kb fragments are shown here, since the 5′ flanking region of *NAT1* from Japanese has not been reported). It is not certain that the Japanese *NAT1* shown on the *lower bar* is the wild-type allele, since only one cDNA and one genomic clone have been sequenced and no structural variants have been described to date. *Ban*I and *Aat*I sites are generated in Japanese *NAT1* as a result of the nucleotide changes at positions 350/351 and 1105, respectively. Deletions are shown with a dash (*lower bar*)

of these investigations were conducted from the 1960s to the late 1980s, or at a time when the existence and substrate selectivity of NAT1 were unknown, and the notion of "monomorphic" *N*-acetylation of certain drugs pervaded the field. It is instructive, therefore, to bring the older literature into focus vis a vis new developments, some of which will be described first.

Human liver contains both NAT1 and NAT2 (GRANT et al. 1991). In mononuclear leukocytes, however, Eadie-Hofstee plots for *N*-acetylation of *p*-aminobenzoate and sulfamethazine are monophasic, and the two activities are highly correlated ($r = 0.94$). It is surmised that, unlike liver, mononuclear leukocytes have a single NAT that brings about *N*-acetylation of these substrates, albeit at significantly different rates (*p*-aminobenzoate to sulfamethazine V_{max} ratio = 21; CRIBB et al. 1991). Furthermore, the data in Table 1 and additional results with mononuclear leukocytes have demonstrated a selectivity of NAT1 for *p*-aminobenzoate and *p*-aminosalicylate (GRANT et al. 1991; CRIBB et al. 1991). These compounds along with sulfanilamide were labeled "monomorphic substrates" because they undergo *N*-acetylation in vitro and in vivo that is unrelated to the acetylator phenotype determined with isoniazid-sulfamethazine and other NAT2 substrates. Secondly, two population studies had shown a normal (unimodal) frequency distribution for *p*-aminobenzoate and *p*-aminosalicylate *N*-acetylation activities in vitro (MOTULSKY and STEINMANN 1962) and for *p*-aminosalicylate clearance in vivo (EVANS 1963). It was postulated from these observations that the human acetylation pathway for *p*-aminosalicylate and other simple aromatic amines has "uniform capacity" (JENNE 1965).

The findings that have fueled and propagated the concept of "monomorphic" or genetically invariant *N*-acetylation must now be scrutinized for the following reasons: (a) NAT1 has unambiguously been shown to be a polymorphic gene locus (Figs. 2, 3; VATSIS and WEBER 1993); (b) when compared to activities grouped into the two categories of "rapid" and "slow" acetylation of isoniazid-sulfamethazine, the mean activity values with NAT1 substrates are comparable whether obtained in vivo (JENNE et al. 1961; JENNE 1965; PETERS et al. 1965; DU SOUICH and ERILL 1976) or in vitro (GLOWINSKI et al. 1978; MCQUEEN and WEBER 1980; CRIBB et al. 1991; WEBER and VATSIS 1993); when the individual catalytic activity values are examined, however, differences become readily apparent, and these are often as extensive as those with sulfamethazine and other NAT2 substrates; (c) in certain instances, the sample number is very small (JENNE et al. 1961; JENNE 1965; PETERS et al. 1965), and only a few population studies have been undertaken (MOTULSKY and STEINMANN 1962; EVANS 1963; GRANT et al. 1992; WEBER and VATSIS 1993); (d) product detection methods have greatly improved in sensitivity and accuracy, e.g., high-pressure liquid chromatography (HPLC); and (e) the lack of correspondence between acetylator status (ascertained with NAT2 substrates) and catalytic activities with NAT1 substrates is now much better understood in light of our current knowledge concerning the occurrence of two NAT genes and substrate selectivity of the proteins which they encode, the allelic variation at both gene loci, and the recent realization supported by several independent criteria that *NAT1* and *NAT2* are independently expressed. The literature on these subjects will now be reviewed at some length.

1. Individual Variation in *N*-Acetylation of NAT1 Substrates In Vivo

Very early work (JENNE et al. 1961) had shown a twofold variation in the plasma half-lives for the elimination of *p*-aminosalicylate ($n = 11$), and a later investigation from the same laboratory (JENNE 1965) showed an approximately fourfold variation in the 12-h urinary ratio of *N*-acetylated to parent *p*-aminosalicylate ($n = 11$). Similar results were obtained for the 24-h urinary ratio of *N*-acetylated to unmetabolized sulfanilamide (values ranged from 0.6 to 1.3, $n = 6$; PETERS et al. 1965), and the amount of *N*-acetylated *p*-aminobenzoate excreted in the urine in 6 h was found in a different study to vary from 0.25 to 5.75 mg ($n = 20$; DU SOUICH and ERILL 1976). More recently, a sixfold variation was observed in the values for *N*-acetylated to unacetylated *p*-aminosalicylate measured in the urine by HPLC ($n = 9$; CRIBB et al. 1991). In addition, a population study ($n = 130$) from the same laboratory showed a high degree of variability in the urinary ratio of *N*-acetylated to unmetabolized *p*-aminosalicylate (GRANT et al. 1992), in agreement with the huge (over 40-fold) variability in this ratio demonstrated 30 years earlier ($n = 52$; EVANS 1963). More importantly, the frequency distribution of the clearance values in the study by GRANT et al. (1992) showed strong evidence for bimodality, which sharply contrasts to the unimodal pattern observed by EVANS (1963). The reasons for this disagreement are unclear, but the two studies differed in the total number of subjects examined (52 vs. 130), the dose administered (160 mg/kg vs. 500 mg!), and the method for detection of unacetylated and *N*-acetylated *p*-aminosalicylate (Bratton-Marshall vs. HPLC).

2. Individual Variation in *N*-Acetylation of NAT1 Substrates In Vitro

As with the studies in vivo, the original observation for a variation in rates of *p*-aminosalicylate *N*-acetylation in vitro was made three decades ago with human autopsy liver (JENNE 1965). Since that time, the following results have been collected with tissue preparations of undetermined *NAT1* genotype: (a) a fourfold variation in rates of *p*-aminobenzoate *N*-acetylation by liver cytosol (n = 7; GLOWINSKI et al. 1978); (b) a twofold variation in *p*-aminobenzoate *N*-acetylation activity in lymphocyte lysates (n = 39); the thermostability of lymphocyte NAT (NAT1) at 44°C was also assessed with *p*-aminobenzoate as substrate, and the first-order inactivation rate constant was found to vary from 0.034 to 0.183 min^{-1} (n = 39). The conclusion consistent with several pieces of evidence was that "a structural gene difference" was most likely responsible for the differential heat stability (MCQUEEN and WEBER 1980); (c) a dramatic (almost 90-fold) variation in V_{max} values for *p*-aminobenzoate *N*-acetylation by liver cytosol (n = 20; KILBANE et al. 1991); (d) at least a 25-fold difference in *p*-aminosalicylate and *p*-aminobenzoate *N*-acetylation by liver cytosol (n = 39), with a high degree of correlation (r = 0.98) for these activities (GRANT et al. 1991); (e) a sevenfold variability in rates of *p*-aminobenzoate *N*-acetylation (n = 23) and about a threefold difference in rates of *p*-aminosalicylate *N*-acetylation (n = 9) by the cytosolic fraction of mononuclear leukocytes; as in liver, a significant correlation existed between these activities in mononuclear leukocytes, as well as between *p*-aminosalicylate and *p*-aminobenzoate *N*-acetylation in vitro and *p*-aminosalicylate clearance in vivo (r = 0.67 and 0.87, respectively; CRIBB et al. 1991); (f) a threefold difference in V_{max} values for *p*-aminobenzoate *N*-acetylation by erythrocyte cytosol (n = 20; WARD et al. 1992); and (g) a three- to sixfold variation in *p*-aminobenzoate *N*-acetylation activity in whole blood hemolysates (n = 200; WEBER and VATSIS 1993). Finally, a normal distribution was obtained several years ago for *p*-aminobenzoate and *p*-aminosalicylate *N*-acetylation activities in erythrocytes, but neither the individual values nor the population size was reported (MOTULSKY and STEINMANN 1962). On the other hand, a more recent population study on *p*-aminobenzoate *N*-acetylation by whole blood from 200 individuals revealed a frequency distribution with a tendency toward bimodality (WEBER and VATSIS 1993).

It is obvious from the foregoing that substantial evidence exists for NAT1 phenotypic variation, which runs counter to the proposal of a *p*-aminosalicylate *N*-acetylation pathway with "uniform capacity" in humans (Jenne 1965). The corollary is that the structural heterogeneity at the *NAT1* locus (Figs. 2, 3; Vatsis and Weber 1993) could be the genetic basis for the appreciable *N*-acetylation activity differences observed with *p*-aminobenzoate and *p*-aminosalicylate in vivo and in vitro. The data thus support the tentative conclusion that NAT1 may participate in a discrete acetylation polymorphism that involves *p*-aminobenzoate, *p*-aminosalicylate, sulfanilamide, and possibly the carcinogen 2-aminofluorene, which is also effectively *N*-acetylated by NAT1 (Table 1). Indisputable evidence for this possibility must await further experimentation with established NAT1 phenotypes (Grant et al. 1991, 1992; Cribb et al. 1991; Weber and Vatsis 1993) and genotypes (Vatsis and Weber 1993).

F. Independent Expression of *NAT1* and *NAT2*

During the course of identification of *NAT1* allelic variants, it was noticed that the isoniazid-sulfamethazine acetylator phenotypes and *NAT2* genotypes were interspersed with *NAT1* genotypes (Vatsis and Weber 1993). These results, coupled with the absence of correspondence recently described for acetylator phenotypes/*NAT2* genotypes and *p*-aminobenzoate/*p*-aminosalicylate *N*-acetylation activities in different tissues (Grant et al. 1991; Cribb et al. 1991; Ward et al. 1992), indicate that *NAT1* and *NAT2* are independently expressed. Inspection of the literatute shows that the evidence for a lack of correlation between *N*-acetylation activities with NAT2 substrates that display the classical isoniazid-sulfamethazine acetylation polymorphism and NAT1 substrates that potentially could participate in a different acetylation polymorphism (Sect. E) has existed for many years. Specifically, a lack of correlation exists between: (a) the isoniazid-sulfamethazine acetylator phenotype determined in vivo and *p*-aminobenzoate, *p*-aminosalicylate, and sulfanilamide clearance in vivo (Jenne et al. 1961, $n = 11$; Jenne 1965, $n = 11$; Peters et al. 1965, $n = 6$; Du Souich and Erill 1976, $n = 20$; Grant et al. 1992, $n = 130$); (b) isoniazid-sulfamethazine acetylator phenotype determined in vivo and *p*-aminobenzoate/*p*-aminosalicylate *N*-acetylation activities in lymphocytes (McQueen and Weber 1980, $n = 33$; Cribb et al. 1991, $n = 9$), erythrocytes (Ward et al. 1992, $n = 17$), and whole blood (Weber and Vatsis 1993, $n = 49$) in vitro; and (c) sulfamethazine and *p*-aminobenzoate/*p*-aminosalicylate *N*-acetylation activities in liver cytosol (Glowinski et al. 1978, $n = 7$; Grant et al. 1991, $n = 39$). Only on one occasion was there a direct correspondence in V_{max} values for liver cytosolic *N*-acetylation of sulfamethazine and *p*-aminobenzoate ($r = 0.96$, $n = 18$; Kilbane et al. 1991), which, in view of the considerable evidence to the contrary, is a surprising result that remains to be explained.

In summary, it is clear that the isoniazid-sulfamethazine acetylator phenotypes and *NAT2* genotypes do not correlate with *p*-aminobenzoate/*p*-

aminosalicylate activities and *NAT1* genotypes in humans, which contrasts to the reciprocal relationship of these parameters in rabbits (SZABADI et al. 1978). The findings support the premise that *NAT1* and *NAT2* are independently expressed in humans, but it is not yet known whether the two genes are coordinately regulated.

Acknowledgement. Work in the authors' laboratory was supported by Grant GM-44965 from the National Institutes of Health, U.S. Department of Health and Human Services.

References

Andres HH, Vogel RS, Tarr GE, Johnson L, Weber WW (1987) Purification, physicochemical, and kinetic properties of liver acetyl CoA:arylamine N-acetyltransferase from rapid acetylator rabbits. Mol Pharmacol 31:446–456

Blum M, Grant DM, Demierre A, Meyer UA (1989) Nucleotide sequence of a full-length cDNA for arylamine N-acetyltransferase from rabbit liver. Nucleic Acids Res 17:3589

Blum M, Grant DM, McBride W, Heim M, Meyer UA (1990) Human arylamine N-acetyltransferase genes: isolation, chromosomal localization, and functional expression. DNA Cell Biol 9:193–203

Blum M, Demierre A, Grant DM, Heim M, Meyer UA (1991) Molecular mechanism of slow acetylation of drugs and carcinogens in humans. Proc Natl Acad Sci USA 88:5237–5241

Cribb AE, Grant DM, Miller MA, Spielberg SP (1991) Expression of monomorphic arylamine N-acetyltransferase (NAT1) in human leukocytes. J Pharmacol Exp Ther 259:1241–1246

Deguchi T (1992) Sequence and expression of alleles of polymorphic arylamine N-acetyltransferase of human liver. J Biol Chem 267:18140–18147

Deguchi T, Mashimo M, Suzuki T (1990) Correlation between acetylator phenotypes and genotypes of polymorphic arylamine N-acetyltransferase in human liver. J Biol Chem 265:12757–12760

Du Souich P, Erill S (1976) Patterns of acetylation of procainamide and procainamide-derived *p*-aminobenzoic acid in man. Eur J Clin Pharmacol 10: 283–287

Ebisawa T, Deguchi T (1991) Structure and restriction fragment length polymorphism of genes for human liver arylamine N-acetyltransferases. Biochem Biophys Res Commun 177:1252–1257

Evans DAP (1963) Pharmacogenetics. Am J Med 34:639–662

Evans DAP, White TA (1964) Human acetylation polymorphism. J Lab Clin Med 63:394–403

Glowinski IB, Radtke H, Weber WW (1978) Genetic variation in N-acetylation of carcinogenic arylamines by human and rabbit liver. Mol Pharmacol 14:940–949

Grant DM, Lottspeich F, Meyer UA (1989) Evidence for two closely related isozymes of arylamine N-acetyltransferase in human liver. FEBS Lett 244:203–207

Grant DM, Mörike K, Eichelbaum M, Meyer UA (1990) Acetylation pharmacogenetics: the slow acetylator phenotype is caused by decreased or absent arylamine N-acetyltransferase in human liver. J Clin Invest 85:968–972

Grant DM, Blum M, Beer M, Meyer UA (1991) Monomorphic and polymorphic human arylamine N-acetyltransferases: a comparison of liver isozymes and expressed products of two cloned genes. Mol Pharmacol 39:184–191

Grant DM, Vohra P, Avis Y, Ima A (1992) Detection of a new polymorphism of human arylamine N-acetyltransferase NAT1 using *p*-aminosalicylic acid as an in vivo probe. J Basic Clin Physiol Pharmacol Suppl 3:244

Hickman D, Sim E (1991) N-acetyltransferase polymorphism: comparison of phenotype and genotype in humans. Biochem Pharmacol 42:1007–1014

Hickman D, Risch A, Camilleri JP, Sim E (1992) Genotyping human polymorphic arylamine N-acetyltransferase: identification of new slow allotypic variants. Pharmacogenetics 2:217–226

Jenne JW (1965) Partial purification and properties of the isoniazid transacetylase in human liver. Its relationship to the acetylation of *p*-aminosalicylic acid. J Clin Invest 44:1992–2002

Jenne JW, MacDonald FM, Mendoza E (1961) A study of the renal clearances, metabolic inactivation rates, and serum fall-off interaction of isoniazid and para-aminosalicylic acid in man. Am Rev Respir Dis 84:371–378

Kilbane AJ, Petroff T, Weber WW (1991) Kinetics of acetyl CoA:arylamine N-acetyltransferase from rapid and slow acetylator human liver. Drug Metab Dispos 19:503–507

McQueen CA, Weber WW (1980) Characterization of human lymphocyte N-acetyltransferase and its relationship to the isoniazid acetylator polymorphism. Biochem Genet 18:889–904

Mitchell RS, Bell JC (1957) Clinical implications of isoniazid blood levels in pulmonary tuberculosis. N Engl J Med 257:1066–1070

Motulsky AG, Steinmann L (1962) Arylamine acetylation in human red cells. J Clin Invest 41:1387

Ohsako S, Deguchi T (1990) Cloning and expression of cDNAs for polymorphic and monomorphic arylamine N-acetyltransferases from human liver. J Biol Chem 265:4630–4634

Ohsako S, Ohtomi M, Sakamoto Y, Uyemura K, Deguchi T (1988) Arylamine N-acetyltransferase from chicken liver: II. Cloning of cDNA and expression in Chinese hamster ovary cells. J Biol Chem 263:7534–7538

Orkin SH, Cheng T-C, Antonarakis SE, Kazazian HH (1985) Thalassemia due to a mutation in the cleavage-polyadenylation signal of the human β-globin gene. EMBO J 4:453–456

Peters JH, Gordon GR, Brown P (1965) The relationship between the capacities of human subjects to acetylate isoniazid, sulfanilamide and sulfamethazine. Life Sci 4:99–107

Sasaki Y, Ohsako S, Deguchi T (1991) Molecular and genetic analyses of arylamine N-acetyltransferase polymorphism of rabbit liver. J Biol Chem 266:13243–13250

Sim E, Hickman D (1991) Polymorphism in human N-acetyltransferase – the case of the missing allele. Trends Pharmacol Sci 12:211–213

Sunahara S, Urano M, Ogawa M (1961) Genetical and geographic studies on isoniazid inactivation. Science 134:1530–1531

Szabadi RR, McQueen CA, Drummond GS, Weber WW (1978) N-acetylation of drugs. A genetically controlled reciprocal relationship between drug N-acetylating enzymes of rabbit liver and peripheral blood cells. Drug Metab Dispos 6:16–20

Thein SL, Wallace RB, Pressley L, Clegg JB, Weatherall DJ, Higgs DR (1988) The polyadenylation signal mutation in the α-globin gene cluster. Blood 71:313–319

Vatsis KP, Martell KJ, Weber WW (1991) Diverse point mutations in the human gene for polymorphic N-acetyltransferase. Proc Natl Acad Sci USA 88:6333–6337

Vatsis KP, Weber WW (1991) Genetic variation in human N-acetyltransferase at the *NAT1* and *NAT2* loci. Am J Hum Genet 49 Suppl: 112

Vatsis KP, Weber WW (1993) Structural heterogeneity of Caucasian N-acetyltransferase at the NAT1 gene locus. Arch Biochem Biophys 301:71–76

Vatsis KP, Rodgers L, Weber WW (1993) Human N-acetyltransferase variant r_4 at the *NAT2* gene locus. The Pharmacologist 35:204

Ward A, Hickman D, Gordon JW, Sim E (1992) Arylamine N-acetyltransferase in human red blood cells. Biochem Pharmacol 44:1099–1104

Weber WW (1987) The acetylator genes and drug response. Oxford University Press, Oxford

Weber WW, Vatsis KP (1993) Individual variability in *p*-aminobenzoic acid N-acetylation by human N-acetyltransferase (NAT1) of peripheral blood. Pharmacogenetics 3:209–212

CHAPTER 5

Genetic Regulation of the Subcellular Localization and Expression of Glucuronidase

R.T. SWANK, E.K. NOVAK, and L. ZHEN

A. Introduction

This is a propitious time to summarize information on the genetic regulation of the subcellular localization and expression of glucuronidase as exciting experimental results have appeared in these areas within the past 3 years. This review includes recent studies on the genetics and molecular mechanisms of glucuronidase subcellular localization, induction of glucuronidase by hormones, a new glucuronidase with unusual catalytic activity and inherited glucuronidase deficiency states. In particular we have stressed experimental results which have appeared since the comprehensive review by PAIGEN (1989) on the genetics, molecular biology, and cell biology of mammalian glucuronidase. Subcellular aspects of the regulation of mammalian glucuronidase including formation of the complex of glucuronidase and the accessory protein egasyn and the mechanism by which the complex is retained within the endoplasmic reticulum (ER) are emphasized.

Several reviews have summarized information on these and related subject areas. They include reviews on glucuronidase subcellular localization (LUSIS and PAIGEN 1977; SKUDLAREK et al. 1984), androgen-mediated induction in kidney (SWANK et al. 1978; BERGER and WATSON 1989), metabolic and genetic regulation (WAKABAYASHI 1970; PAIGEN 1979; LUSIS 1982), and deficiency states in humans (NEUFELD and MOENZER 1989).

B. Endoplasmic Reticulum Glucuronidase

I. Background

The earlier literature describing the evidence for microsomal glucuronidase has been clearly and exhaustively dealt with in the review by LUSIS and PAIGEN (1977). Some salient features of the system are as follows: Glucuronidase is an unusual "lysosomal" enzyme in that 30%–50% of total liver enzyme is in fact not found in the lysosome, but rather is in a "microsomal" fraction. Evidence that glucuronidase has a dual subcellular location originated in the pioneering experiments of DEDUVE et al. (1955). Later experiments (BEAUFAY et al. 1974; BROWN et al. 1987) showed that "microsomal" glucuronidase was in fact located in a fraction of microsomes identical with the ER. Essentially the same glucuronidase polypeptide, differing only in certain post-translational modifications, is present in both subcellular locations. Native glucuronidase in both lysosomes and microsomes is a tetramer composed of four subunits of 71–75 kDa.

Evidence that ER glucuronidase was complexed with from one to four (with the maximum of four set by the glucuronidase tetramer structure) molecules of an accessory protein egasyn and that complex formation was necessary for the accumulation of ER glucuronidase accrued from a wide variety of experiments in the laboratory of Dr. Ken Paigen (reviewed in LUSIS and PAIGEN 1977). Crucial to these experiments was the discovery of the *Eg*° mutation in the YBR inbred mouse strain (GANSCHOW and PAIGEN 1967). Mice containing this chromosome 8 mutation had no microsomal glucuronidase. The finding that microsomal glucuronidase existed in normal, but not *Eg*°, mice as a series of enzyme "M" forms of regularly increasing molecular weight (SWANK and PAIGEN 1973) spawned the notion that retention of glucuronidase within the ER required interaction with an accessory protein encoded by the *Eg* locus. That ER glucuronidase indeed existed in a stable physical complex with egasyn was established by coimmunoprecipitation of egasyn with specific glucuronidase antiserum (TOMINO and PAIGEN 1975). The absence of egasyn in *Eg*° mutant mice results in the concomitant absence of ER glucuronidase. Egasyn was characterized as a 64-kDa glycoprotein which was localized to microsomes (LUSIS et al. 1976).

II. Species Distribution of Liver Endoplasmic Reticulum Glucuronidase

Significant microsomal or ER glucuronidase is present in livers of mice, rats, rabbits, cows, humans, and tadpoles (LUSIS and PAIGEN 1977; PAIGEN 1989). No ER glucuronidase has been detected in liver homogenates of several chickens or ducks (TAKEUCHI and SWANK, unpublished). Thus far, only mice and rats have been carefully examined for the presence of an associated egasyn-like protein. Whether ER glucuronidase is associated with an egasyn-like protein in humans is uncertain, because adequate quantities of fresh human livers are not readily available for analysis. Also, human glucuronidase does not readily separate into defined microsomal and lysosomal components on nondenaturing gels. The availability of cloned egasyn cDNA has enabled a test of species specificity in formation of the glucuronidase complex (NOVAK et al. 1991). When cloned egasyn cDNA was transfected into mouse L cells, a cell type that does not normally contain egasyn and therefore does not form egasyn–glucuronidase complexes, complex formation between transfected egasyn and endogenous glucuronidase was readily detected. However, no complexes were detected when mouse egasyn cDNA was transfected into human HepG2 cells or monkey COS-1 cells, despite ample synthesis and ER insertion of egasyn. Therefore, the signal (see below) for retention of egasyn in the ER is species independent, while the signal for association of egasyn with glucuronidase is species restricted. As discussed below, the carboxyl terminal propeptide of glucuronidase is important in complex formation with egasyn, and the sequences of this peptide differ at four of 30 amino acid positions when mouse and human glucuronidases are compared. These differences and/or differences in the structures of mouse and human egasyns likely explain the above results.

III. Organ and Cellular Distribution of the Endoplasmic Reticulum Glucuronidase–Egasyn Complex

Earlier studies (LUSIS and PAIGEN 1977) established that liver and kidney have relatively high concentrations of ER glucuronidase, while lesser amounts are present in lung. In liver, ER glucuronidase is present in hepatocytes (DEIMLING 1988), while it is likely that kidney ER enzyme is present in proximal tubule cells, though this has not been directly demonstrated. In liver, appearance of the glucuronidase complex is developmentally regulated with a large increase immediately after birth. The appearance of the complex is likely regulated by the concomitant upregulation of egasyn (LUSIS and PAIGEN 1977).

The recent identification of egasyn as esterase-22 (see below) together with the finding that esterase-22 is present in tongue and submandibular gland (EISENHARDT and DEIMLING 1982) strongly suggest that the ER glucuronidase–egasyn complex is present in these organs, since glucuronidase is constitutively expressed in all tissues (except red blood cells). The relatively small amount of esterase-22 in these organs likewise predicts that the complex is at low concentrations. The exact cellular location of the complex in lung, submandibular gland, and tongue is unknown. Finally, LAZZARINO and GABEL (1990) have made the interesting observation that 40%–50% of total glucuronidase activity of mouse lymphoma cells is found in the microsomal fraction and have suggested that these cells contain egasyn or an egasyn-like protein that associates with β-glucuronidase in the microsomal compartment. No ER glucuronidase complex has been detected in spleen, brain, or heart. The lack of detectable esterase-22 in erythrocytes, testis, and skin (EISENHARDT and DEIMLING 1982) indicates that these cells lack ER glucuronidase.

IV. Subcellular Distribution of the Complex

1. Background

As discussed above, 30%–50% of rat liver glucuronidase is found in the ER fraction when liver homogenates are fractionated by rate zonal or equilibrium density gradient centrifugation (BEAUFAY et al. 1974) or osmotic shock (PAIGEN 1961) techniques. Further proof that the complex is found in the

ER is the fact that oligosaccharides of both egasyn (ZHEN et al. 1993) and glucuronidase bound to egasyn (SWANK et al. 1986) are sensitive to cleavage with endoglycosidase H. Also, recent confocal microscopic experiments have shown that egasyn is specifically distributed in a reticular ER-like pattern in cells transfected with egasyn cDNA (NOVAK et al. 1991).

Histochemical procedures (DEIMLING et al. 1988) have shown that liver ER glucuronidase is detectable only in hepatocytes, not in nonhepatocyte cells such as Kupffer's cells. Nonhepatocyte cells contribute a major fraction (43%) of total liver lysosomes (BLOUIN et al. 1977). Therefore, the true fraction of hepatocyte glucuronidase in the ER is undoubtedly considerably higher than 30%–50%, since the latter figures were derived from analyses on whole liver homogenates.

2. Glucuronidase is Located Within the Lumen of the Endoplasmic Reticulum

Studies from several laboratories have shown that ER proteins are found at two major locations, either attached to the ER membrane or free within the ER lumen (i.e., the interior space of ER vesicles). Surprisingly, ER luminal proteins are not secreted, even though they occupy the same space as newly synthesized secretory proteins.

When microsomes from mouse liver were treated with graded concentrations of the detergent Triton X-100 (BROWN et al. 1987), it was found that the ER glucuronidase–egasyn complex was released at low Triton X-100 concentrations along with other ER luminal markers. Furthermore, egasyn which was not complexed with glucuronidase also behaved as an ER luminal component. Complementary procedures such as release of luminal components by increasing time of sonication yielded similar results. Also, ER glucuronidase was protected from proteinases added to microsomal membranes. Thus, the ER glucuronidase–egasyn complex and free egasyn are luminal components.

The luminal location of ER glucuronidase likely has important consequences for its function. The active site of uridine diphosphate (UDP) glucuronyl transferase is thought to be on the luminal face of the ER (BERRY et al. 1975). The glucuronides it produces would be luminal and thus directly exposed to the action of ER glucuronidase. As described below, recent evidence has implicated ER glucuronidase in the hydrolysis of bilirubin glucuronides of hepatocytes.

V. Lysosomal Glucuronidase was Associated with Egasyn During Subcellular Transit

An interesting question is whether, in egasyn-positive tissues, glucuronidase in the lysosomal compartment interacted with ER egasyn on its subcellular journey to the lysosome or whether a separate subcellular route independent of egasyn was used. The experiments of SWANK et al. (1986) and PFISTER et al. (1988) showed that the former scenario holds. The physical properties of the great majority of lysosomal glucuronidase were found to be quite different, in terms of the degree of modification of oligosaccharide side chains, when liver enzyme from egasyn-negative and egasyn-positive mice were compared. Lysosomal glucuronidase from egasyn-negative mice was highly modified with complex sugars such as sialic acid and galactose, while minimal modification occurred in the same enzyme from egasyn-positive mice. This result might be due to shielding of glucuronidase oligosaccharides from Golgi sugar transferases by attached egasyn. Alternatively, egasyn attachment might signal a different subcellular route to the lysosome, bypassing the sugar transferases of the Golgi apparatus. In either case, it appears that, at least in liver of egasyn-positive mice, precursor glucuronidase, including the majority of that destined for lysosomes, forms a complex with egasyn. This precursor remains in a relatively stabile (half-life of 2–3 days; SMITH and GANSCHOW 1978) complex with egasyn within the ER. The precursor slowly dissociates from egasyn and is directed to the lysosome, presumably by mannose-6-phosphate dependent mechanisms (CREEK and SLY 1984). Whether egasyn remains attached to glucuronidase throughout the subcellular pathway up to and including insertion into lysosomes is uncertain. Presumably, such transport of egasyn to the lysosome would be an inefficient process because of competitive binding of egasyn to the HTEL receptor (see below). It is known that little or no egasyn is detectable in lysosomes, but whether this is due to lack of transport to or rapid degradation within lysosomes is unknown.

VI. Egasyn is an Esterase

1. Background

One of the more surprising, and fruitful, findings regarding ER glucuronidase was that the accessory protein egasyn is actually an active enzyme, an esterase. The location of the egasyn (Eg) gene within a cluster of esterases on mouse chromosome 8 (KARL and CHAPMAN 1974) together with similarities to esterases in molecular weight, isoelectric point, and subcellular location prompted us to test whether egasyn has esterase activity.

Indeed it was found (MEDDA and SWANK 1985) that a defined liver esterase reacted positively to specific antiserum to mouse egasyn. This same esterase was absent in three inbred mouse strains known to lack egasyn and was present in all egasyn positive strains. Also, when liver ER glucuronidase was isolated with glucuronidase antibody, the esterase copurified. The enzyme is a typical carboxyl esterase (HEYMANN 1980) in that it reacts with substrates such as α-napthyl acetate and is inhibited by organophosphorus compounds.

The detailed primary structure of egasyn is now available with the cloning of the cDNA for egasyn (Ovnic et al. 1991a). It predicts a protein of 562 amino acids with striking sequence conservation with known carboxylesterases. Histidine and serine residues are found at the amino acid positions expected for these active site residues in carboxyl esterases.

2. Identity of Egasyn Esterase

Thus far, 25 genetically distinct esterases have been identified in the mouse. In fact, at least 11 mouse carboxylesterases are encoded by genes in two chromosome 8 clusters which are thought to have arisen by repeated duplication of a single gene and subsequent diversification (Peters 1982; Ceci and Lusis 1992). A variety of genetic, cell biological, biochemical, and immunological approaches (Medda et al. 1986) established that egasyn is identical to mouse esterase-22. Esterase-22 is a member of esterase cluster 1 on mouse chromosome 8, along with Es-1, Es-N, Es-28, Es-6, and Es-9.

Glucuronidase also exists within the ER as a complex with an egasyn-like protein in rat liver (Medda et al. 1987b). Rat egasyn is likewise a carboxylesterase, in this case identical with rat esterase-3. The rat complex appears similar to that of the mouse in most important respects. It contains a large portion of total liver glucuronidase activity, is a 61–63 kDa glycoprotein, and is luminal. Egasyn-positive (90 total) and -negative (13 total) rat strains exist, and strains which lack egasyn lack ER glucuronidase, indicating that stabilization of glucuronidase in rat ER requires egasyn. The ability of mouse esterase-22 and rat esterase-3 to complex with ER glucuronidase was apparently acquired before evolutionary divergence of the rat and mouse, i.e., at least 10^7 years ago.

A difference between the complexes in the two species is that the rat complex is considerably more labile in vitro in that it is easily dissociated by relatively mild treatments such as extraction with Triton X-100 or by relatively low temperatures and is also much more readily dissociated in vivo by injection of organophosphorus compounds.

VII. The Egasyn–Glucuronidase Interaction is Highly Specific

An interesting question is whether egasyn which is not attached to glucuronidase is attached to other proteins, possibly serving to stabilize these proteins within the ER. Previous experiments had established that only 10% of total liver egasyn is complexed with glucuronidase. Taking advantage of the esterase activity of egasyn (Medda and Swank 1985), it was found that essentially all egasyn is attached to glucuronidase or is a free monomer of 60–65 kDa. This was true even when very mild conditions of extraction and electrophoresis were used. Thus, interaction of glucuronidase and egasyn is highly specific; egasyn does not serve as an accessory peptide to stabilize other proteins within the ER. It remains possible that egasyn interacts with other proteins for a much shorter time or much more weakly than it does with the glucuronidase precursor.

Additionally, glucuronidase is not bound to esterases other than egasyn (MEDDA and SWANK 1985). The propeptide portion of glucuronidase, which is critical in its interaction with egasyn (see below), does not interact with other esterases (MEDDA et al. 1989). The fact that glucuronidase is not bound to other esterases is consistent with the fact that the various liver carboxylesterases exhibit considerable substrate specificity in in vitro tests (HEYMANN 1980).

VIII. The Esterase-Active Site of Egasyn is Involved in Complex Formation

The above findings that egasyn is an esterase together with older observations that injection of organophosphorus inhibitors of esterases into rats causes a rapid and massive release of liver ER glucuronidase into plasma (WILLIAMS 1969; MANDELL and STAHL 1977; see below) prompted us to hypothesize that the esterase-active site of egasyn binds ER glucuronidase.

In fact, it was found (MEDDA et al. 1987a) that organophosphorus compounds caused a rapid dissociation of the high molecular weight egasyn–glucuronidase complex when administered in vivo or when added in vitro to microsomal suspensions. As predicted by the hypothesis, the egasyn esterase-active site was less accessible to substrates and to inhibitors when egasyn was complexed to β-glucuronidase. Also, dissociation of the complex by in vivo administration of organophosphorus compounds was followed by rapid and massive secretion of ER glucuronidase, but not egasyn, into plasma.

Together, this data indicates that the esterase-active site of egasyn binds egasyn to ER glucuronidase. This binding in turn compartmentalizes glucuronidase within the ER (summarized in Fig. 1). A quite unique aspect of this system is that the mechanism of subcellular compartmentalization of one protein involves the enzyme-catalytic site of a second protein. Also, these results show that the mysterious rapid and massive secretion of glucuronidase into plasma upon treatment of rats with organophosphorus insecticides occurs because the insecticides dissociate the glucuronidase–egasyn complex (Fig. 2). Since egasyn is bound only to glucuronidase, these results explain the specificity of the release (other lysosomal enzymes are not released). Whether assay of plasma glucuronidase activity of rats living in dumps, agriculture areas, etc., is an appropriate test for unacceptable environmental levels of organophophorous insecticides remains to be determined.

IX. The Propeptide Portion of the Glucuronidase Precursor is Involved in Complex Formation

Like many other lysosomal enzymes, glucuronidase is initially synthesized as a high molecular weight precursor (SKUDLAREK et al. 1984). Trimming of

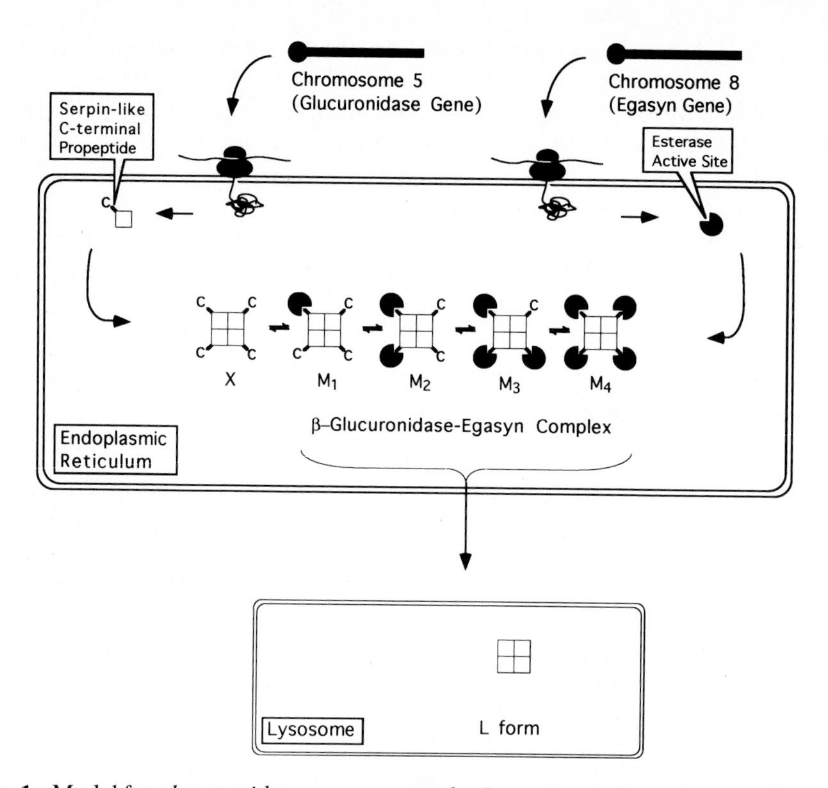

Fig. 1. Model for *glucuronidase–egasyn complex* formation in liver of normal (egasyn-positive mice). The glucuronidase precursor tetramer *X* combines with one to four molecules of egasyn within the lumen of the *endoplasmic reticulum.* M_1–M_4 complex formation occurs by interaction of the *serpin (serine proteinase inhibitor)-like carboxyl (C)-terminal propeptide* of X-glucuronidase with the *esterase-active site* of egasyn. The majority of precursor glucuronidase interacts with egasyn before entering *lysosomes* to produce *L-form* glucuronidase. Whether egasyn accompanies glucuronidase to lysosomes is unknown. In egasyn-negative mice, X-form glucuronidase directly enters lysosomes

precursor glucuronidase (subunit relative molecular mass (M_r) of 75 kDa) to the lower molecular weight mature form (subunit M_r of 72 kDa) is effected by proteinases in the lysosome or in prelysosomal organelles (BROWN and SWANK 1983). The glucuronidase propeptide is at the carboxyl terminus (ERICKSON and BLOBEL 1983). Although the exact point of cleavage is unknown, it appears from the molecular weight differences of precursor and mature forms that the size of the propiece is about 30 amino acids. Cleavage of the propiece is not necessary for enzymatic activation as it is for lysosomal cathepsins (ERICKSON 1989).

A wide variety of proteinases appear capable of hydrolyzing proglucuronidase to a form similar in size to the mature lysosomal form (BROWN et al. 1987). This suggests that the carboxyl terminal propeptide exists in an

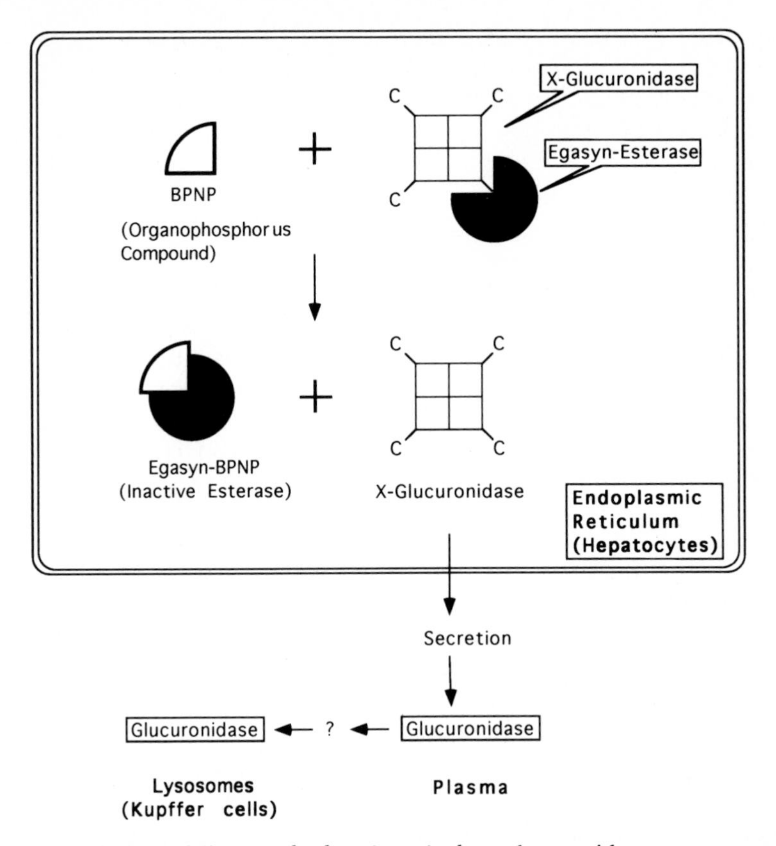

Fig. 2. Dissociation of liver *endoplasmic reticulum* glucuronidase–egasyn complex by *organophosphorus compounds* (adapted from MEDDA et al. 1987a). Injected organophosphorus compounds such as bis *p* nitrophenyl phosphate (*BPNP*) compete with the serpin-like C-terminal propeptide of precursor glucuronidase X for binding to the *egasyn–esterase*-active site. BPNP covalently binds to the active site, thus displacing glucuronidase and forming inactive egasyn–esterase. The dissociated M complexes yield X-form glucuronidase, which is rapidly secreted into plasma. Secreted *hepatocyte* glucuronidase likely undergoes uptake into *Kupffer's cells* (MANDELL and STAHL 1977), though a fraction may be directly transferred to lysosomes of hepatocytes (BELTRAMINI-GUARINI et al. 1984)

extended conformation, readily accessible to modifying enzymes and, by extension, to more permanent interaction with egasyn. The propiece of glucuronidase is likewise a logical candidate for the portion of glucuronidase which interacts with egasyn, since the form of glucuronidase complexed to egasyn is the high molecular weight precursor form rather than the processed form found within lysosomes.

The elucidation (reviewed in PAIGEN 1989) of the complete sequences of cDNAs of glucuronidase from several species enabled the synthesis of peptide reagents identical in sequence to defined regions of glucuronidase which might interact with egasyn. A 30-mer peptide corresponding to the carboxyl terminal 30 amino acids of proglucuronidase was synthesized and, in turn, a polyclonal antibody to the peptide was produced (MEDDA et al. 1989). This antibody interacted with proenzyme glucuronidase–egasyn complexes in which one, two, or three egasyn molecules were bound to the glucuronidase tetramer, but not with those complexes (M_4) which contained four egasyn molecules. This indicates that all available carboxyl termini of the glucuronidase proenzyme tetramer are complexed with, and therefore shielded by, egasyn in the M_4 complexes.

Since previous data had indicated that the esterase active site of egasyn interacted with glucuronidase in complex formation, it was predicted that the 30-mer propeptide would inhibit egasyn esterase activity. Indeed, the synthetic 30-mer is a specific and potent inhibitor (50% inhibition at $1.3\,\mu M$) of the esterase activity of purified egasyn (MEDDA et al. 1989). This same peptide exhibited little inhibitory activity toward other purified esterases.

Finally, there is in vivo data consistent with a role for the carboxyl terminal propeptide in complex formation. A congenic mouse mutant with an altered glucuronidase structural gene, the so called W26 mutant, was found (LI et al. 1990) to have an abnormally low content of ER glucuronidase, and that which was present was less avidly bound to egasyn. The mutant has a glycine residue substituted for an arginine at amino acid position 7 from the carboxyl terminus of the glucuronidase propeptide.

Together, these data describe a potent interaction of the exposed carboxyl terminal propeptide of glucuronidase with the esterase catalytic site of egasyn, which in turn results in the specific localization of glucuronidase within the lumen of the ER (Fig. 1). That egasyn interacts with the carboxyl terminus of glucuronidase rather than with other portions of glucuronidase strongly suggests that the interaction between these proteins is a post-translational, rather than a cotranslational event. Whether egasyn interacts with nascent glucuronidase subunits or only with completed glucuronidase tetramers in the ER is uncertain. However, interaction with egasyn is not necessary for formation of glucuronidase tetramers, since this process occurs normally in egasyn-deficient mice and in tissues which lack egasyn.

X. Sequence Similarity of the Glucuronidase Propeptide with Portions of the Reactive Site Region of the Serpin Superfamily

The catalytic sites of carboxyl esterases have striking similarities to those of serine proteinases (MYERS et al. 1988). Both types of catalytic sites have an invariant serine with a three in eight match in the sequence of a consensus octapeptide. They share inhibitor specificity in that diisopropyl flurophosphate (DFP) inactivates both by irreversible binding to the active site serine. Organophosphates and carbamates inhibit both. Also, they have overlapping substrate specificity.

We investigated, therefore, whether the mechanism of complex formation used by the egasyn–glucuronidase system is related to that of serine proteinases and their serpin (serine proteinase inhibitor) inhibitors (LI et al. 1990). Indeed, inspection of the amino acid sequences of the carboxyl terminal propeptides of mouse, rat, and human glucuronidases revealed sequence similarities to portions of the reactive site region of the serpin superfamily (Fig. 3). The five-amino acid sequence (RPFLF), located to the P′ side or toward the carboxyl terminal side, of the serpin-reactive site is conserved among the majority of serpins. Four amino acids (RPFXF) identical to this sequence are likewise found at the extreme carboxyl terminus of the pro-form of both rat and mouse glucuronidase. A closely related sequence is found at the carboxyl terminus of human glucuronidase. Also, a serine residue (enclosed) is present immediately to the carboxyl side (i.e., at the P_1' site) of the reactive center, as it is in the majority of serpins. The

Protein	Reactive site region	Carboxyl terminus
α_2-AP	G V E A A A A T S I A M S R ↓ M S L S L	F S V D R P F L F
α_1-PI	G T E A A G A M F L E A I P M S I P P E	V K F N K P F V F
α_1-Achy	G T G A S A A T A V K I T L L S A L V E T R T I	V R F N R P F L M
Contrapsin	G T E A A A A T G V I G G I R K A I L P A	V H F N R P F L F
AT III	G S E A A A S T A V V I A G R S L N P N R V T	F K A N R P F L F
β-PAI	G T V A S S S T A V I V S A R M A P E E	I I M D R P F L F
C1Inh	G V E A A A A S A I S V A R T L L V	F E V Q Q P F L F
HCII (hLS2)	G T Q A T T V T T V G F M P L S T Q V R	F T V D R P F L F
bpZ	G T E A G A A T V A M G V A M S M P L K V D L V D	F Y A N H P F L F
Ovalbumin	G R E V V G S A E A G V D A A S V S E E F R	D H P F L F
Ang (rat)	G E E E Q P T E S A Q Q P G S P E V L D	V T L S S P F L F
Ang (human)	D E E R E P T E S T Q Q L N K P E V L E	V T L N R P F L F
Glucuronidase (rat)	R E R Y W R I A N E T R G T G S V P R T Q	C M G S R P F T F
Glucuronidase (mouse)	R E R Y W R I A N E T G G H G S G P R T Q	C F G S R P F T F
Glucuronidase (human)	R E R Y W K I A N E T R Y P H S V A K S Q	C L E N S P F T

Fig. 3. Sequence similarity of the carboxyl terminus of the glucuronidase propeptide with the reactive site region of the serpin superfamily (adapted from LI et al. 1990). The reactive site sequences of the serpin superfamily were taken from SHIEH and TRAVIS (1987). The placements of gaps in the serpin sequences have been arbitrarily chosen and are required due to the different lengths of the reactive site loops. The placement of gaps in the glucuronidase propeptides was also arbitrary. *α_2-AP*, α_2-antiplasmin; *α_1-PI*, α_1-proteinase inhibitor; *α_1-Achy*, α_1-antichymotrypsin; *AT III*, antithrombin III; *β-PAI*, β-plasminogen activator inhibitor; *ClInh*, complement 1 inhibitor; *HCII*, heparin cofactor II; *hLS2*, human leuserpin; *bpZ*, barley protein 2; *Ang*, angiotensinogen. The *arrow* indicates the P_1-P_1' reactive center of the reactive sites of the serpins where cleavage of serpins occurs after complexing with specific serine proteinases. Conserved regions are *boxed*

other major region of sequence similarity among the serpins upstream of the reactive site (Fig. 3) is not found within the glucuronidase carboxyl terminus. The remainder of the glucuronidase sequence, outside of the carboxyl terminus, has no obvious regions similar in sequence to the serpins or in fact to other proteins, with the exception of *Escherichia coli* β-galactosidase.

Several considerations suggest that the serpin sequence similarity is likely functionally significant in terms of egasyn–glucuronidase complex formation. The first consideration is the above-mentioned similarities in the catalytic sites of serine proteinases and carboxylesterases. Second, as discussed above, the region of glucuronidase which is important in complex formation is in fact the carboxyl terminal propeptide. Third, the interaction of the glucuronidase propeptide with egasyn results in inhibition of egasyn esterase activity (MEDDA et al. 1989), just as serpins inhibit their target proteinases. Additional molecular approaches, including expression of specifically modified glucuronidase constructs, will be required to rigorously test the importance of the serpin-like regions of the propeptide region in complex formation.

The functional consequence of complex formation between serpins and serine proteinases is the control of proteolytic activity. The consequences in the glucuronidase–egasyn system are first that a considerable portion of glucuronidase is compartmentalized within the ER; second, in analogy to the serpin–serine proteinase system, it is possible that the inhibition of egasyn esterase activity which occurs upon complex formation with glucuronidase is physiologically important. Inhibition by the glucuronidase propeptide of all egasyn esterase activity likely occurs in organs which have high ratios of glucuronidase to egasyn, including kidney proximal tubule cells of male mice, lung, submandibular gland, and tongue.

It is of interest that a portion of the above RPFXF sequence is shared by a pentapeptide domain of α_1 antitrypsin–protease complexes (JOSLIN et al. 1991). This pentapeptide is recognized by a receptor on human hepatoma cells and monocytes. Receptor recognition in turn results in rapid clearance and degradation of complexes and increase in synthesis of α_1 antitrypsin.

XI. Endoplasmic Reticulum Retention Signal of Egasyn

A recurring theme in modern cell biology is that proteins destined for a particular subcellular site contain a specific sequence of amino acids that serve as a signal for targeting of that protein to the specific site. As examples, mitochondrial proteins have a sequence of basic residues at the amino terminus (PFANNER and NEUPERT 1990), nuclear proteins have a short internal sequence of basic amino acids (DINGWALL and LASKEY 1991), and peroxisomal proteins have an SKL carboxyl terminal-targeting sequence (GOULD et al. 1989). Typically, these signals are a short contiguous set of amino acids, and the signal is recognized by a specific receptor within the membrane of the target vesicle or an intermediate vesicle which shuttles to the target vesicle.

From the cDNA sequence of egasyn (OVNIC et al. 1991a) it was apparent that there is a typical signal sequence at the amino terminus which would cause nascent egasyn to traverse the ER membrane and enter the secretory pathway. Moreover, there is an HTEL sequence at the carboxyl terminus of egasyn. This sequence is similar to the carboxyl terminal KDEL sequence which retains other proteins such as BIP and protein disulfide isomerase within the lumen of the ER (PELHAM 1989). To determine whether the HTEL sequence acts as an ER retention signal, HTEL-deleted egasyn was expressed in mammalian cell lines (ZHEN et al. 1993). The majority of HTEL-deleted egasyn was secreted, while wild-type egasyn was retained in the ER. Furthermore, the HTEL sequence, when added to the carboxyl terminus of α_1-acid glycoprotein, a secretory protein, caused retention of this protein within the ER. Thus, the carboxyl terminal HTEL sequence of egasyn is both necessary and sufficient for retention of egasyn within the ER.

It was also found that this sequence, like the KDEL sequence, must be at the carboxyl terminus to serve as an efficient ER retention sequence. Addition of even one extra carboxyl terminal amino acid, lysine, completely abolished the ER retention ability of the HTEL sequence. Also, the sequence HTLE was not efficient in ER retention, indicating that the order of the EL terminal amino acids cannot be switched if the ER retention function is to be maintained.

XII. Endoplasmic Reticulum Retention Signals of Other Esterases

In similar experiments (ROBBI and BEAUFAY 1991; MEDDA and PROIA 1992; ZHEN et al. 1993), the possible ER retention role of other C-terminal sequences naturally occurring on various esterases was investigated. It was found that the C-terminal sequences HTEL, HIEL, HVEL, and HDEL are ER retention signals. On the other hand, C-terminal HTEHT and HTEHK, found on two cloned esterases, are not ER retention signals. From these results, it is possible to predict whether newly cloned members of the esterase family will be secretory or ER-bound enzymes. For instance, esterases which bear the H(X)EL (HTEL, HIEL, and HVEL) carboxyl terminal sequences are likely true ER proteins in vivo, while a rat liver carboxyl esterase with C-terminal HTEHT (LONG et al. 1988) is probably a secretory (plasma) protein. Among known esterases, pI 6.1 esterase (ROBBI and BEAUFAY 1991) and egasyn with C-terminal HVEL and HTEL, respectively, are corroborated ER components. Also, other esterases with either C-terminal HIEL or HTEL are cellular and predictably located in the ER, though their exact subcellular locations have not yet been verified.

The aforementioned duplication of esterase genes during evolution is the likely origin of the shared H(X)EL system among esterases. Egasyn and another carboxylesterase EsN (OVNIC et al. 1991b) are now known to be located within cluster 1. EsN is a secretory esterase (ZHEN et al. 1993) with the carboxyl terminal sequence HTELK. These facts indicate there is not a strong evolutionary pressure to maintain a constant type of esterase (i.e., ER or secreted) within a given cluster.

Evidence has been presented that a receptor recognizes proteins containing the carboxyl terminal KDEL signal in the *cis* Golgi apparatus or the salvage compartment (a compartment between the ER and *cis* Golgi apparatus) and shuttles these proteins back to the ER lumen, where they are released (PELHAM 1989). In this way, KDEL proteins are maintained within the ER. Whether the H(X)EL system found on egasyn and other esterases uses the same receptor and other subcellular components as the KDEL/HDEL system is unknown. However, it is likely that a shuttling system similar to that used by the KDEL system maintains the glucuronidase–egasyn complex within the ER (see Fig. 4).

XIII. Is Complexation with Other Proteins a General Function of Endoplasmic Reticulum Esterases?

Interesting data from the laboratory of Dr. Stephen Macintyre has revealed that the glucuronidase–esterase system is not the only example in which an ER esterase forms a complex with another protein, resulting in ER retention of that protein.

In this case, the other protein is rabbit C-reactive protein (CRP), which is synthesized in hepatocytes and secreted to plasma during acute phase response to tissue injury (KUSHNER 1982). Its rate of synthesis is increased several hundredfold in the acute phase. Unlike other acute phase proteins, its half-time for secretion is markedly (more than tenfold) prolonged when unstimulated hepatocytes are compared to hepatocytes prepared from rabbits undergoing the acute phase response.

By several types of subcellular fractionation experiments (MACINTYRE 1992), CRP of unstimulated hepatocytes is, like the glucuronidase–egasyn complex, an ER resident. In vitro experiments with detergent-permeabilized microsomes of unstimulated rabbits and labeled CRP established that CRP is bound to the lumenal side of the ER membrane. Binding was to two components, one of low affinity and a second high-affinity site. Microsomes from stimulated rabbits exhibited only the low-affinity component. By western blotting, radioiodinated CRP clearly binds to a 60-kDa protein of unstimulated microsomes. In contrast, there is no detectable binding to microsomes of stimulated hepatocytes. Direct binding of the 60-kDa protein to CRP has been detected in situ by chemically cross-linking microsomes followed by immunoprecipitation with anti-CRP (MACINTYRE, personal communication).

More recent experiments (MACINTYRE, personal communication) have established that the low- and high-affinity components are esterases. On

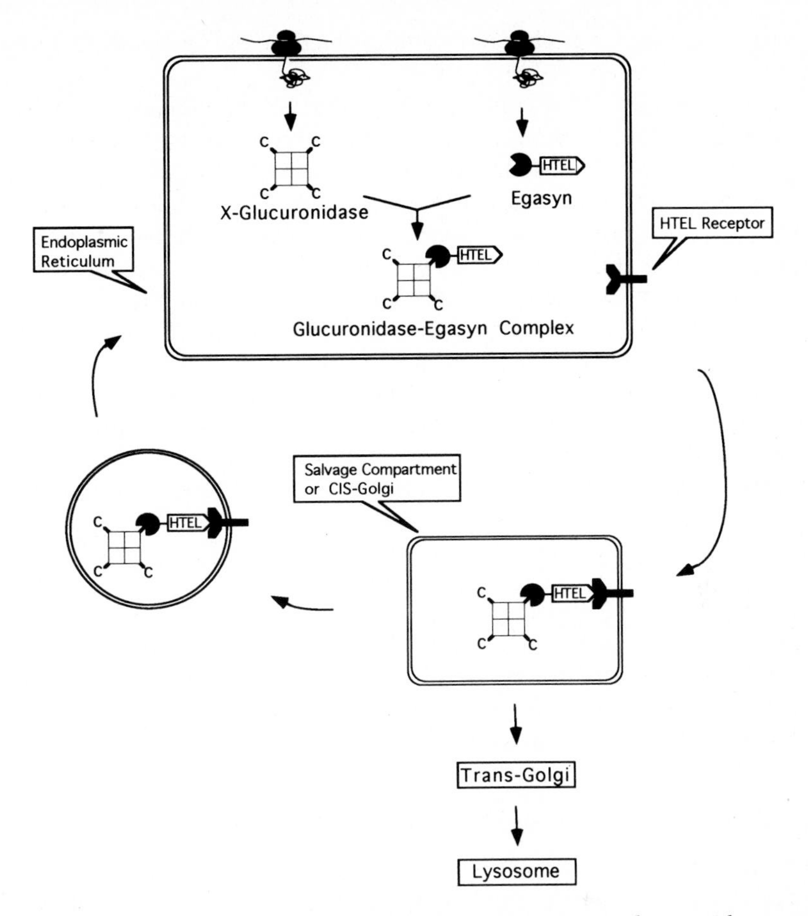

Fig. 4. Model for *endoplasmic reticulum* (ER) retention of *glucuronidase–egasyn complex* (adapted from PELHAM 1989). The C-terminal HTEL sequence on ER egasyn, which is complexed with glucuronidase, interacts with an *HTEL receptor*. The ER glucuronidase–egasyn complex together with an ER HTEL receptor (not bound to the HTEL sequence of egasyn) are shuttled by vesicles to the *cis Golgi* complex, where the HTEL receptor binds to the C-terminal HTEL sequence on egasyn. The glucuronidase–egasyn–HTEL receptor complex is then shuttled, by vesicles, back to the ER, where the glucuronidase–egasyn complex dissociates from the HTEL receptor. In this way, the rate of escape from the ER of the glucuronidase–egasyn complex is greatly reduced. A small amount of glucuronidase does escape and continues through the *trans Golgi* complex to the lysosome

nondenaturing gels, both have esterase activity. By partial amino acid sequencing of purified components, the low- and high-affinity components appear identical in fact to rabbit microsomal esterases forms 1 and 2, previously characterized by OZOLS (1989). Unlike the glucuronidase–egasyn system, the esterase catalytic site does not appear critical for complex formation with CRP, since phenylmethane sulfonylfluoride (PMSF) abolishes the esterase activity, but does not diminish binding of CRP to the esterase in blot assays.

There are interesting comparisons in control of subcellular routing of proteins in the two systems. In both, ER localization is modulated by regulation of expression of an accessory esterase. In the case of CRP, the accessory esterase is downregulated by the acute phase response and CRP is secreted. In the glucuronidase system, the acessory esterase is genetically downregulated in *Eg*$^{o/o}$ mice (LUSIS and PAIGEN 1977), and the resulting absence of egasyn expression results in redirection of stabile ER glucuronidase to the lysosome. A similar downregulation of egasyn and rerouting of glucuronidase to the lysosome occurs in organs such as brain, heart, and spleen (BEAUFAY et al. 1974). Likewise, when egasyn enzyme activity is "downregulated" by injection of organophosphorus compounds, ER glucuronidase is redirected to the secretory pathway and to lysosomes (Fig. 2). An opposite upregulation of liver egasyn occurs during development and after treatment of mice with phenobarbital (LUSIS and PAIGEN 1977), resulting in ER sequestration of a portion of glucuronidase formerly destined for the lysosome.

Finally, GRASSEL and HASILIK (1992) have reported that the precursor form of lysosomal cathepsin D forms a complex with a 60-kDa glycoprotein within the ER. Since the subcellular location, size, and glycosylation of the binding protein are consistent with those of ER esterases, it will be interesting to learn if it also is an accessory esterase.

XIV. Physiological Role of Endoplasmic Reticulum Glucuronidase

The defined role of lysosomal glucuronidase is in the degradation of glycosaminoglycans including dermatan, heparin, and chrondroitin sulfates. Its absence results in a typical lysosomal storage disease, mucopolysaccharidosis VII (MPS VII; NEUFELD and MUENZER 1989).

The role of ER glucuronidase is less certain. However, evidence is accumulating that it modulates the degree of glucuronidation of endogenous and xenobiotic substrates. The location of ER glucuronidase in microsomes of liver and kidney, which are principal organs involved in glucuronide conjugation reactions, makes ER glucuronidase particularly well suited for this task. Also, since ER glucuronidase is located within the lumen of the ER, probably in close proximity to the reactive site of UDP glucuronyltransferase, nascent glucuronides are likely to be readily accessible to the enzyme for deconjugation. Furthermore, glucuronidase maintains considerable activity at the neutral pH expected within the endoplasmic reticulum.

Several studies indicate that ER glucuronidase is capable of deglucuronidating endogenous and xenobiotic substrates. For example, BELINSKY et al. (1984) found that the production of *p*-nitrophenyl glucuronide by perfused livers was increased by removal of calcium from the perfusion fluid. This effect was associated with decreased microsomal glucuronidase activity (SOKOLOVE et al. 1984) with no effect on lysosomal glucuronidase. The authors suggest that elevation of cytosolic calcium concentrations resulting from activation of α-adrenergic receptors causes calcium-mediated activation of microsomal β-glucuronidase and decreased net glucuronide production. The hydrolysis of xenobiotics such as benzopyrene glucuronide was similarly stimulated by calcium activation of microsomal glucuronidase (WHITTAKER et al. 1985). SCHOLLHAMMER et al. (1975) have suggested that conjugation–deconjugation–reconjugation cycles naturally occur in the metabolism of glucuronides.

The results of recent studies utilizing normal mice and congenic mice lacking ER glucuronidase indicate that ER glucuronidase is likewise operative in deconjugation reactions in vivo (WHITING et al. 1993). The concentrations of bilirubin and its glucuronide metabolites were determined by high-pressure liquid chromatography (HPLC) in bile of normal C57BL/6J and congenic mutant mice lacking ER glucuronidase. A significant increase was observed in the relative amounts of bilirubin monoglucuronide and total glucuronides in mutant mice. No difference between normal and mutant mice was observed in the rates of synthesis of bilirubin glucuronides. These results suggest that levels of ER glucuronidase have implications for the initiation of pigment and cholesterol gallstones and for the biliary excretion of endogenous and xenobiotic substrates which undergo biliary glucuronidation.

As mentioned, an interesting additional function of ER glucuronidase may be to modulate the esterase activity of egasyn via binding to the egasyn esterase-catalytic site.

XV. Physiological Role of Endoplasmic Reticulum Esterases

The ER carboxylesterases are a large group of enzymes capable of hydrolyzing an extremely wide variety of substrates in vitro (HEYMANN 1980, 1982; MENTLEIN and HEYMANN 1984). These substrates include simple and complex esters, thioesters, carbamates, and amides. These groups in turn involve both naturally occurring substrates such as coenzyme (CoA) esters and monoglycerides together with xenobiotics such as drugs, antibiotics, herbicides, and insecticides. The in vivo role of individual carboxylesterases has been more difficult to fully establish, in part because of overlapping substrate specificity among the many esterases. This phenomenon results in no obvious physiological effect when a given esterase is absent in particular inbred strains of mice (PETERS 1982). However, it is reasonable to assume that, as a group, the ER esterases serve to hydrolyze the above compounds in vivo.

As described above, an additional function of one esterase (egasyn) is to maintain glucuronidase within the ER and there is evidence that another esterase serves a similar function for C-reactive protein.

XVI. Abnormal Subcellular Distribution of Glucuronidase in the *Gus*ⁿ Mouse

The *Gus*ⁿ mouse is an example of an inherited alteration in the subcellular distribution of a two-site enzyme. In this case, the ratio of ER and lysosomal glucuronidase is altered (SWANK et al. 1987). An alteration in the structural gene of glucuronidase yields glucuronidase with a more basic isoelectric point and a loss of one oligosaccharide side chain (NOVAK and LI, unpublished). In liver homogenates, the ratio of ER to lysosomal glucuronidase is 1.3, as opposed to a value of 0.5 in normal C57BL/6J mice. The altered ratio is entirely accounted for by a threefold decrease in the lysosomal component; ER glucuronidase concentrations are normal. The latter fact indicates that egasyn–glucuronidase interactions are not dependent upon sugar side chain structure of glucuronidase.

BRACEY and PAIGEN (1989) found that the lowered glucuronidase concentrations in various tissues of this mutant result from either an increase in the rate of glucuronidase protein degradation, a lowering of the rate of glucuronidase synthesis, or both. Decreases in rates of protein synthesis were not due to decreases in glucuronidase mRNA levels. Rather, the amount of mature enzyme synthesized per message molecule, or translational yield (the efficiency with which the message is translated and/or the fraction of newly made polypeptides that are incorporated into glucuronidase tetramers), was less for these tissues. It is likely that the increased rate of degradation of mutant lysosomal glucuronidase is caused by the oligosaccharide deficiency, since it is well known that oligosaccharide side chains protect glycoproteins from the actions of proteinases.

No obvious physiological consequences arise as a result of this altered subcellular distribution. It is likely that the reduced lysosomal glucuronidase is at adequate concentrations to prevent lysosomal storage disease (see below).

C. Regulation of Expression of Glucuronidase

I. Androgen-Regulated Genetic Elements

Kidney proximal tubule cells of male mice are notably hypertrophied when compared to female mice. This is an androgen-mediated effect, since androgen treatment of females or castrated males results in enlargement of these same cells. Accompanying this hypertrophy is a significant induction of several enzymes including D-amino acid oxidase, alcohol dehydrogenase, and β-glucuronidase (reviewed in SWANK et al. 1978; PAIGEN 1989; BERGER and WATSON 1989).

The induction of kidney glucuronidase activity varies from 20- to 50-fold in most inbred strains. High-inducing haplotypes include the *Gus*ᵃ type, low-inducing strains include the *Gus*[b] or *Gus*[h] types, and a noninducing haplotype is *Gus*[or]. The time course of glucuronidase induction is rather slow when compared with other hormone-responsive enzyme systems. Detectable increase in glucuronidase activity does not occur until 24 h later for *Gus*[a] mice and 48 h later for *Gus*[b] or *Gus*[h] mice, and maximal induction is not obtained until 3 weeks later.

The experiments of LUND et al. (1991) strongly indicate that androgen inducibility of kidney glucuronidase is regulated by elements within the proximal end of intron 9 of the glucuronidase structural gene. Two elements within this intron are likely candidate regions which interact with factors important in the induction process. These elements are altered in mice with differing induction phenotypes.

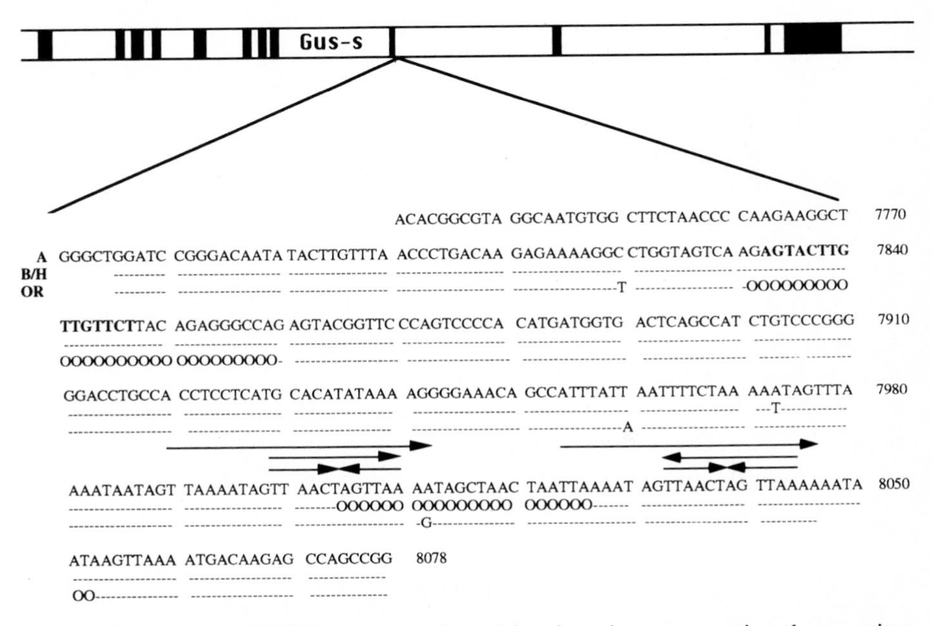

Fig. 5. Comparison of DNA sequence from inbred strains representing three major GUS androgen-response phenotypes (adapted from LUND et al. 1991). The *Gus*-s structural gene is depicted above. *Filled areas* represent each of the 12 exons of the 14-kb gene. The *expanded area* represents the region of interest in intron 9. Sequence numbering commences at the transcription initiation site of *Gus-s*. *Dashes* indicate nucleotide identities with those of the published *Gus*[a] DNA sequence, and a *zero* indicates that a nucleotide is missing relative to the *Gus*[a] sequence. An area of complex dyad symmetry is depicted by *arrows* between residues 7990 and 8046. The 23-bp direct repeat is indicated by the two *long arrows* (7990–8012 and 8024–8046); the 12-bp inverted repeat, contained within the direct repeat, is designated by the *arrows* spanning positions 7999–8010 and 8033–8044. Palindromic sequences within this inverted repeat are indicated by the *adjacent arrows* at positions 7999–8004 and 8005–8010 and again at positions 8033–8038 and 8039–8044. A consensus glucocorticoid-responsive element (GRE) sequence is indicated in *bold type* and spans positions 7833–7847

First, a consensus glucorticoid-responsive element (GRE) was found at nucleotide positions 7833–7847 (Fig. 5). That this is a critical region in androgen responsiveness is suggested by the fact that it is totally deleted in mice of the *Gus*^{or} haplotype, which have no detectable kidney glucuronidase induction after androgen administration. GRE-like sequences have been identified within and upstream of several steroid-inducible genes (Ham et al. 1988; Denison et al. 1989). Second, a nuclease-hypersensitive site was found at a closely linked (approximately 130 base pairs) region downstream of the GRE in a 57-base pair region of complex dyad symmetry. The importance of this region in glucuronidase induction is indicated by the fact it is partially deleted (Fig. 5) in several inbred strains of the *Gus*^{b} and *Gus*^{h} haplotypes. Furthermore, two proteins were identified which bound specifically to the region of complex dyad symmetry, and the levels of these proteins were dramatically higher in extracts of androgen treated than in those of untreated mice. It is of interest that these proteins are still induced in hypophysectomized mice, indicating that growth hormone, which is required for glucuronidase induction, acts through other factors. The authors propose a model in which the GRE-like sequence may interact with the androgen receptor to generate the accessibility needed for androgen-inducible binding factors in kidney to bind at the region of complex dyad symmetry and regulate the degree of induction of glucuronidase.

Androgens induce glucuronidase in submaxillary gland, with induction more pronounced in mice of the glucuronidase N haplotype (Bracey and Paigen 1988). Interestingly, the mechanism of induction is quite different from that of kidney in that there is no concomitant increase in glucuronidase mRNA levels. Rather, the induction is a function of translational yield. From an analysis of induction in mice containing various glucuronidase haplotypes, it was concluded (Bracey and Paigen 1988) that the DNA sequences determining the submaxillary gland response are distinct from those determining the androgen induction of glucuronidase mRNA in kidney.

II. Estrogen-Specific (*Gus*-e) Genetic Elements

As emphasized by Jaussi et al. (1992), genes may respond to a balance of multiple hormones in vivo. In the case of glucuronidase, its androgen-mediated induction in kidney is strongly antagonized by estrogen (Fishman 1951). Jaussi et al. (1992) found that this antagonistic effect is mediated at the level of glucuronidase mRNA concentration. The effect on mRNA concentration in turn was mediated mainly at the level of mRNA synthesis, with smaller effects on mRNA stability. Estrogen had no effect on the ability to concentrate androgen receptor in the nucleus. The effects of sex steroids on seven other genes known to be testosterone-responsive in kidneys of mice were also studied. A wide variety of responses to estrogen, ranging from antagonism to additive induction, were noted. The authors propose that each gene interacts with both the androgen receptor complex and the estrogen receptor complex with the ultimate outcome dependent on each gene's regulatory structure.

WATSON et al. (1992) have described an estrogen locus (*Gus*-e) within the glucuronidase gene complex which is apparently separate from androgen response loci of the complex. When the estrogen-mediated suppression of the induction of kidney glucuronidase by androgens was measured in congenic mice of differing glucuronidase gene haplotypes, two classes emerged. The first class (haplotypes B, H, and N) was suppressed to a high degree (about 75%) by estrogen, and the second class (haplotypes A, CL, and CS) was suppressed to a lesser extent (about 50%). Separation into these classes was independent of the degree of induction of glucuronidase by androgens in the same strains. Furthermore, the estrogen effect was *cis*-acting. These facts indicate that androgen and estrogen act on separate response elements within the glucuronidase gene complex. As in the case of androgens, estrogens acted mainly at the transcriptional level. Kinetic studies indicated that estrogen increases the rate of gene deactivation rather than decreasing the rate of gene activation. The authors suggest that estrogen alters the nature, or effectiveness, of androgen receptor bound to specific response elements. It seems likely that the combined genetic–molecular approach used successfully in elucidating the nature of the glucuronidase androgen response elements will be successful in defining these interesting estrogen response elements.

III. Tissue-Specific (*Gus*-u) and Temporal (*Gus*-t) Genetic Elements

The *cis*-active systemic regulator, designated *Gus*-u, uniformly regulates glucuronidase levels in all tissues throughout development. A *trans*-acting developmental regulator, designated *Gus*-t regulates glucuronidase activity in certain tissues after the 12th postnatal day in certain tissues (reviewed in PAIGEN 1989). Mice of common inbred strains fall into different Gus-u and Gus-t haplotypes. Strains of the $[Gus]^h$ haplotype are typified by inbred strain C3H/HeJ, while mice of the $[Gus]^a$ and $[Gus]^b$ haplotypes are typified by inbred strains A/J and C57BL/6J. Typically, all tissues of C3H/HeJ mice exhibit a threefold lower glucuronidase activity prior to the 12th postnatal day (the *Gus*-u effect). Afterwards, glucuronidase activity levels are reduced a further three- to fourfold in C3H/HeJ liver (the *Gus*-t effect). The *Gus*-t effect is particularly fascinating, since it is the only example of a *trans*-active genetic element which is tightly linked to the gene over which it exerts control.

An interesting recent finding is that these genetic elements have no effect on the levels of glucuronidase mRNA in the affected tissues (WAWRZYNIAK et al. 1989a). The data suggest that tissue-specific and temporal effects on glucuronidase activity levels are exerted following the accumulation of processed glucuronidase mRNA transcripts. BRACEY and PAIGEN (1987) investigated differences in glucuronidase expression between tissues and likewise found they arise primarily from alterations in translational yield. Glucuronidase tissue concentrations are therefore largely regulated by methods other than transcriptional mechanisms, the common mode in mammals. A post-transcriptional mechanism indicates that sequences within glucuronidase exons are responsible and that the *Gus*-u and *Gus*-t elements must encode a recognition site on the processed glucuronidase transcript or on the glucuronidase protein product. As pointed out by WAWRZYNIAK et al. (1989a), there are examples (LEE et al. 1983) where differences between transcripts involving primary sequences and/or secondary structure around initiation codons alter rates of attachment to ribosomes and/or other stages of translation initiation. It is also possible that *Gus*-t may act via the glucuronidase polypeptide itself to regulate its own synthesis by autoregulation.

Sequencing of glucuronidase cDNA from inbred strains containing the various glucuronidase haplotypes has revealed the molecular basis of the *Gus*-u regulatory element (WAWRZYNIAK et al. 1989b). The mRNA of glucuronidase of C3H/HeJ mice was found to differ from that of C57BL/6J by a single base at position 272. This predicts an isoleucine at residue 87 of the second exon in the H polypeptide versus threonine in the B polypeptide. This change must, therefore, be the basis of the inherited differences in tissue levels of glucuronidase (the *Gus*-u effect) between these types of mice. This same amino acid change must likewise be responsible for the known increase in heat lability of glucuronidase in tissues of C3H mice. In fact, several algorithms predict that this amino acid change would cause significant changes in the secondary structure of glucuronidase (WAWRZYNIAK et al. 1989b).

D. An Exoglucuronidase Acting on Nonsulfated Glycosaminoglycans

NAKAMURA et al. (1990) have described a new exoglucuronidase from rabbit liver acting only on nonsulfated glycosaminoglycans such as chondroitin. The native enzyme has a molecular weight of 130000, considerably less than that of classical glucuronidase, which has a molecular weight of about 300000. Attempts to identify a subunit molecular weight on denaturing gels proved inconclusive. However, the new exoglucuronidase appears to have a unique antigenic structure, since it does not cross-react with antibody raised against glucuronidase which hydrolyzes *p*-nitrophenyl-β-D-glucuronide. The new enzyme is less stable, is more sensitive to high ionic strength, and has a higher pH optimum than classical glucuronidase. Both enzymes are equally inhibited by saccharo-1,4, lactone. The new enzyme acts only on nonsulfated chondroitin, is actually inhibited by sulfated chondroitin, and does not hydrolyze synthetic *p*-nitrophenyl-β-glucuronide substrate.

It will be interesting to identify the subcellular location and tissue specificities of the new enzyme and to determine whether the enzyme is androgen regulated. The authors suggest that the new exoglucuronidase is probably involved in catabolism of glycosaminoglycans rather than in detoxification reactions, while previously characterized β-glucuronidase probably is involved in both pathways. A related question is whether deficiency of the enzyme leads to a new lysosomal storage disease.

It should also be emphasized that a large number of endoglucuronidases active on various glycosaminoglycans have been reported (TAKAGAKI et al. 1988). These have no exoglucuronidase activity and are almost certainly enzymes different from classical glucuronidase.

E. Inherited β-Glucuronidase Deficiency States

A deficiency in the classical exoglucuronidase which cleaves synthetic *p*-nitrophenyl-β-D-glucuronide substrates results in the lysosomal storage disease MPS VII. Recent studies have identified animal models of this disease, which has provided insights into potential therapies.

I. Mucopolysaccharidosis VII in Humans

MPS VII in humans is a recessively inherited disease caused by a severe deficiency of β-glucuronidase, resulting in accumulation of undegraded glycosaminoglycans in lysosomes (NEUFELD and MOENZER 1989). Like other lysosomal storage diseases, symptoms include facial and skeletal deformities, growth and mental retardation, hepatosplenomegaly, corneal clouding, metachromatic granules in blood leukocytes, accumulation of undegraded glycosaminoglycans in lysosomes, and their excretion into urine. About 20 patients have been described with symptoms ranging from mild chronic disease to severe, in which preadolescent death occurs. Although bone marrow transplantation therapy has been reported for some patients with lysosomal storage disease, it has not been applied to MPS VII.

TOMATSU et al. (1990) have reported the molecular defect in the β-glucuronidase cDNA isolated from fibroblasts of a 6-year-old girl with MPS VII. Although mRNA is expressed at equal intensity in normal and mutant cells, the amount of β-glucuronidase activity using synthetic substrates was 2% of normal. By sequence analysis, a C→T substitution results in a replacement of alanine 619 with valine. The mutation occurs in a hydrophobic region highly conserved in β-glucuronidase from *E. coli*, rat, and man, suggesting that maintaining structural integrity in this region is necessary for maintaining enzyme activity.

More recently, glucuronidase from two additional MPS VII patients has been sequenced (TOMATSU et al. 1991). Fibroblasts from both patients had normal concentrations of glucuronidase mRNA. A 24-year-old male had the identical mutation as found in the 6-year-old girl above. The other patient, a 7-year-old female, had 2 C→T substitutions resulting in arginine 382 replacement with cysteine and proline 649 replacement with leucine. To test whether either of these mutations affected β-glucuronidase activity, glucuronidase cDNA was altered by in vitro mutagenesis and transfected into COS cells. The Pro^{649}→Leu construct had normal enzyme activity. However, the constructs with Ala^{619}→Val or Arg^{382}→Cys produced little or no enzyme activity. The Arg^{382}→Cys, similar to the Ala^{619}→Val, is found in a conserved domain present in human, rat, mouse, and *E. coli* glucuronidase. The authors suggest cysteine forms new intramolecular or intermolecular disulfide bonds, resulting in an altered structure and a loss of catalytic activity.

II. Animal Models of Mucopolysaccharidosis VII

The first animal model for MPS VII was described in the dog (SCHUCHMAN et al. 1989; HASKINS et al. 1991). Liver β-glucuronidase, using synthetic substrates, was 2% of normal and was associated with vacuolated cytoplasm and the presence of undegraded glycosaminoglycans in urine. The dogs presented an autosomal recessive pattern of inheritance. Interestingly, 35% of β-glucuronidase from normal liver was soluble without the addition of detergents, while 78% of β-glucuronidase from MPS VII livers was soluble. This may indicate that accumulated glycosaminoglycans cause an increase in lysosomal fragility.

Until recently, the only small animal model for MPS VII available was the C3H mouse, which has 10% of normal C57BL β-glucuronidase in many tissues and presents mild symptoms. Young mice (2–3 months old) are asymptomatic, while older mice (12 months) present with twofold more liver glycosaminoglycans than normal Swiss Webster mice (YATZIV et al. 1978). HOOGERBRUGGE et al. (1987) have shown that C3H bone marrow recipients from C57BL normal marrow have increased β-glucuronidase in bone marrow-derived tissues. Less increase was found in kidney and lung, and no increase in enzyme activity was observed in the central nervous system.

More recently, BIRKENMEIER et al. (1989) and VOGLER et al. (1990) have described a mouse model for MPS VII which presents with less than 1% of normal β-glucuronidase activity. The mouse has a shortened life span (one fifth of normal) and has the structural abnormalities and cytoplasmic inclusions typical of human MPS VII. In contrast to the MPS VII human cases described above, glucuronidase mRNA is 200-fold less than that of normal mice. However, the β-glucuronidase mRNA is androgen inducible in kidney as it is in normal mice.

It has been demonstrated that lowered β-glucuronidase activity was solely responsible for the symptoms of MPS VII in this mouse by construction of a mutant mouse bearing the human β-glucuronidase transgene (KYLE et al. 1990). Mice homozygous for MPS VII bearing the human β-glucuronidase transgene had ten times the normal mouse β-glucuronidase activity. The glycosaminoglycan accumulation in tissues was corrected, as was the secondary elevation of other lysosomal enzymes. No morphological evidence of lysosomal storage disease and no other symptoms (dwarfism, gait disturbance, limb deformities) associated with mouse MPS VII were evident. Interestingly, an adipose deficiency associated with mouse MPS VII, but not the human disease, was also corrected in the transgenic mouse.

The MPS VII mouse has been used to evaluate bone marrow transplantation as a possible mode of therapy for this disease. When 7-week-old MPS VII mice received syngeneic bone marrow transplants from normal donors (Birkenmeier et al. 1991), their life span returned to near normal. The β-glucuronidase activity increases ranged from 10% of normal in brain to normal values in thymus. Accumulation of glycosaminoglycans was corrected in spleen, but not in kidney or liver. However, morphologically, Kupffer's cells and hepatocytes did not contain cytoplasmic inclusions. In the kidney, only glomerular mesangial cells were corrected for β-glucuronidase. Lysosomal storage deficiency persisted in neurons, and skeletal abnormalities were not corrected. Thus, bone marrow transplantation may be useful for treatment of MPS VII, but many lysosomal storage disease symptoms are not corrected. Perhaps bone marrow transplantation at an earlier age will result in even more successful therapy.

Animal models of MPS VII are being used to evaluate gene therapy in somatic cells. Glucuronidase was transformed by retrovirus-mediated gene transfer into cells cultured from MPS VII dogs. These include bone marrow cells, retinal pigment epithelium (Wolfe et al. 1990), and muscle cells (Smith et al. 1990). Both glucuronidase enzyme activity and functional ability to degrade glycosaminoglycans were restored in the transduced cells.

The novel experiments of Wolfe et al. (1992) have raised the possibility of delivering β-glucuronidase to the central nervous system in MPS VII. These researchers placed the β-glucuronidase gene under the control of the latency-associated transcript (LAT) promoter in the neurotropic herpesvirus (HSV-1). The LAT transcript is the only gene expressed by HSV-1 during latency. After infection, β-glucuronidase was expressed in a few cells of neuronal tissues, trigeminal ganglia, and brain stem. Thus, it may be possible to deliver enzymes to the central nervous system to augment bone marrow transplantation therapy or somatic gene therapy.

Recently, another mouse model for MPS VII (Chapman et al., personal communication) has become available. This mouse has about 2%–5% normal β-glucuronidase activity (synthetic substrate activity) in most tissues. However, this minimal amount of activity is enough to keep young animals apparently healthy. It is unknown whether MPS symptoms appear as the animals age.

None of the normal or mutant β-glucuronidase-deficient humans, dogs, or mice have been tested for the presence of the new exoglucuronidase (Nakamura et al. 1990) or endoglucuronidase (Takagaki et al. 1988) activities which act only on natural substrates. It will be interesting to determine whether deficiencies of the new enzymes lead to new lysosomal storage diseases. Human MPS VII is a heterogeneous disease. This heterogeneity likely arises from different polymorphisms at the glucuronidase gene. However, it is also possible that differences in activities of these new glucuronidases contribute to the clinical heterogeneity.

Acknowledgements. We thank Cynthia Bates for excellent secretarial assistance. Also, we thank Stephen Macintyre, Roger Ganschow, Ken Paigen, and Gordon Watson for providing papers and preprints describing their recent research.

References

Beaufay H, Amar-Costesec A, Thines-Sempoux D, Wibo M, Robbi M, Berthet J (1974) Analytical study of microsomes and isolated subcellular membranes from rat liver. Subfractionation of the microsomal fraction by isopycnic and differential centrifugation in density gradients. J Cell Biol 61:213–231

Belinsky SA, Kauffman FC, Sokolove PM, Tsukuda T, Thurman RG (1984) Calcium-mediated inhibition of glucuronide production by epinephrine in the perfused rat liver. J Biol Chem 259:7705–7711

Beltramini-Guarini P, Gitzelmann R, Pfister K (1984) Presence and absence of the microsomal β-glucuronidase in mice correlates with differences in the processing of the lysosomal enzyme. Eur J Cell Biol 34:165–170

Berger F, Watson G (1989) Androgen-regulated gene expression. Annu Rev Physiol 51:51–65

Berry C, Stellon A, Hallinan T (1975) Guinea pig liver microsomal UDP-glucuronyltransferase: compartmented or phospholipid-constrained. Biochim Biophys Acta 403:335–344

Birkenmeier EH, Davisson MT, Beamer WG, Ganschow RE, Vogler CA, Gwynn B, Lyford K, Maltais LM, Wawrzyniak CJ (1989) Murine mucopolysaccharidosis type VII characterization of a mouse with β-glucuronidase deficiency. J Clin Invest 83:1258–1266

Birkenmeier EH, Barker JE, Vogler CA, Kyle JW, Sly WS, Gwynn B, Levy B, Pegors C (1991) Increased life span and correction of metabolic defects in murine mucopolysaccharidosis type VII after syngeneic bone marrow transplantation. Blood 72:3081–3092

Blouin A, Bolender RP, Weibel ER (1977) Distribution of organelles and membranes between hepatocytes and non-hepatocytes in the rat liver parenchyma. J Cell Biol 72:441–455

Bracey LT, Paigen K (1987) Changes in translational yield regulate tissue-specific expression of β-glucuronidase. Proc Natl Acad Sci USA 84:9020–9024

Bracey LT, Paigen K (1988) Androgen induction of β-glucuronidase translational yield in submaxillary gland of B6.N mice. Mol Endocrinol 2:701–705

Bracey LT, Paigen K (1989) The N haplotype of the murine β-glucuronidase gene is altered in both its systemic regulation and its response to androgenic induction. Biochem Genet 27:1–15

Brown JA, Swank RT (1983) Subcellular redistribution of newly synthesized macrophage lysosomal enzymes: correlation between delivery to lysosomes and maturation. J Biol Chem 258:15323–15328

Brown JA, Novak EK, Takeuchi K, Moore K, Medda S, Swank RT (1987) Lumenal location of the microsomal β-glucuronidase-egasyn complex. J Cell Biol 105: 1571–1578

Ceci JD, Lusis AJ (1992) Mouse chromosome 8. Mammal Genome 3:S121–S135

Creek KE, Sly WS (1984) The role of the phosphomannosyl receptor in the transport of acid hydrolases to lysosomes. In: Dingle JT, Dean RD, Sly W (eds) Lysosomes in biology and pathology, vol 7. Elsevier, Amsterdam, pp 63–82

DeDuve C, Pressman BC, Gianetto R, Wattiaux R, Appelmans F (1955) Tissue fractionation studies. VI. Intracellular distribution patterns of enzymes in rat liver tissue. Biochem J 60:604–617
Deimling OV, Budde R, Katz N, Schaefer HE, Swank RT (1988) Zytochemie der β-Glucuronidase in der Rattenleber: Darstellung einer genetischen Variation in Inzuchtstämmen. Acta Histochem (Jena) 36:305–310
Denison SH, Sands A, Tindall DJ (1989) A tyrosine aminotransferase glucocorticoid response element also mediates androgen enhancement of gene expression. Endocrinology 124:1091–1093
Dingwall C, Laskey RA (1991) Nuclear targetting sequences – a consensus? Trends Biochem Sci 16:478–481
Eisenhardt E, Deimling OV (1982) Interstrain variation of esterase-22, a new isozyme of the house mouse. Comp Biochem Physiol 73B:719–724
Erickson AH (1989) Biosynthesis of lysosomal cathepsins. J Cell Biochem 40:117–127
Erickson AH, Blobel G (1983) Carboxyl-terminal proteolytic processing during biosynthesis of the lysosomal enzymes β-glucuronidase and cathepsin D. Biochemistry 22:5201–5205
Fishman WH (1951) β-Glucuronidase and the action of steroid hormones. Ann NY Acad Sci 54:548–551
Ganschow RE, Paigen K (1967) Separate genes determining the structure and intracellular location of hepatic glucuronidase. Proc Natl Acad Sci USA 58: 938–945
Gould SJ, Keller G-A, Hosken N, Wilkinson J, Subramani S (1989) A conserved tripeptide sorts proteins to peroxisomes. J Cell Biol 108:1657–1664
Grassel S, Hasilik A (1992) Human cathepsin D precursor is associated with a 60 kDa glycosylated polypeptide. Biochem Biophys Res Commun 182:276–282
Ham JA, Thompson M, Webb NP, Parker M (1988) Characterization of response elements for androgens, glucocorticoids and progestins in mouse mammary tumor virus. Nucleic Acids Res 16:5263–5276
Haskins ME, Aguirre GD, Jezyk PF, Schuchman EH, Desnick RJ, Patterson DF (1991) Animal model of human disease mucopolysaccharidosis VII (Sly syndrome). Am J Pathol 138:1553–1555
Heymann E (1980) Carboxyl esterases and amidases. In: Jakoby WB (ed) Enzymatic basis of detoxification, vol 2. Academic, New York, pp 291–323
Heymann E (1982) Hydrolysis of carboxylic esters and amides. In: Jakoby WB, Bend JR, Caldwell J (eds) Metabolic basis of detoxification. Academic, New York, pp 229–245
Hoogerbrugge PM, Poorthuis JHM, Mulder AH, Wagemaker G, Dooren LJ, Vossen JMJJ, van Bekkum DW (1987) Correction of lysosomal enzyme deficiency in various organs of β-glucuronidase-deficient mice by allogeneic bone marrow transplantation. Transplantation 43:609–614
Jaussi R, Watson G, Paigen K (1992) Modulation of androgen-responsive gene expression by estrogen. Mol Cell Endocrinol 86:187–192
Joslin G, Fallon RJ, Bullock J, Adams SP, Perlmutter DH (1991) The SEC receptor recognizes a pentapeptide neodomain of α_1-antitrypsin-protease complexes. J Biol Chem 266:11282–11288
Karl TR, Chapman VM (1974) Linkage and expression of the EG locus controlling inclusion of β-glucuronidase into microsomes. Biochem Genet 11:367–372
Kushner I (1982) The phenomenon of the acute phase response. Ann NY Acad Sci 389:39–48
Kyle JW, Birkenmeier EH, Gwynn B, Vogler C, Hoppe PC, Hoffman JW, Sly WS (1990) Correction of murine mucopolysaccharidosis VII by a human β-glucuronidase transgene. Proc Natl Acad Sci USA 87:3914–3918
Lazzarino D, Gabel CA (1990) β-Glucuronidase is transported slowly to lysosomes in BW5147 mouse lymphoma cells: evidence that the prelysosomal enzyme is not restricted to the endoplasmic reticulum. Arch Biochem Biophys 282:100–109

Lee KAW, Guertin D, Sonnenberg N (1983) mRNA secondary structure as a determinant in cap recognition and initiation complex formation. J Biol Chem 247:3622–3629

Li H, Takeuchi KH, Manly K, Chapman V, Swank RT (1990) The propeptide of β-glucuronidase: further evidence of its involvement in compartmentalization of β-glucuronidase and sequence similarity with portions of the reactive site region of the serpin superfamily. J Biol Chem 265:14732–14735

Long RM, Satoh H, Martin BM, Kimura S, Gonzalez FJ, Pohl LR (1988) Rat liver carboxylesterase: cDNA cloning, sequencing and evidence for a multigene family. Biochem Biophys Res Commun 156:866–873

Lund SD, Gallagher PM, Wang B, Porter SC, Ganschow RE (1991) Androgen responsiveness of the murine β-glucuronidase gene is associated with nuclease hypersensitivity, protein binding, and haplotype-specific sequence diversity within intron 9. Mol Cell Biol 11:5426–5434

Lusis AJ (1982) Genetic regulation of expression of mammalian lysosomal enzymes. In: Varina RS, Varma R (eds) Glycosaminoglycans and proteoglycans in physiological and pathological processes of body systems. Karger, Basel, pp 55–71

Lusis A, Paigen K (1977) Mechanisms involved in the intracellular localization of mouse glucuronidase. In: Rattazzi MC, Scandalios JG, Whitt GS (eds) Isozymes. Current topics in biological and medical research, vol 2. Liss, New York, pp 63–106

Lusis AJ, Tomino S, Paigen K (1976) Isolation, characterization and radioimmunoassay of murine egasyn, a protein stabilizing glucuronidase membrane binding. J Biol Chem 251:7753–7760

Macintyre SS (1992) Regulated export of a secretory protein from the ER of the hepatocyte: a specific binding site retaining C-reactive protein within the ER is downregulated during the acute phase response. J Cell Biol 118:253–265

Mandell B, Stahl P (1977) Effect of diisopropyl phosphofluoridate on rat liver microsomal and lysosomal β-glucuronidase. Biochem J 164:549–556

Medda S, Proia RL (1992) The carboxylesterase family exhibits C-terminal sequence diversity reflecting the presence or absence of endoplasmic reticulum retention sequences. Eur J Biochem 206:801–806

Medda S, Swank RT (1985) Egasyn, a protein which determines the subcellular distribution of β-glucuronidase, has esterase activity. J Biol Chem 260: 15802–15808

Medda S, Deimling OV, Swank RT (1986) Identity of esterase-22 and egasyn, the protein which complexes with microsomal β-glucuronidase. Biochem Genet 24:229–243

Medda S, Stevens AM, Swank RT (1987a) Involvement of the esterase active site of egasyn in compartmentalization of β-glucuronidase within the endoplasmic reticulum. Cell 50:301–310

Medda S, Takeuchi K, Devore-Carter D, Deimling OV, Heymann E, Swank RT (1987b) An accessory protein identical to mouse egasyn is complexed with rat microsomal β-glucuronidase and is identical to rat esterase-3. J Biol Chem 262:7248–7253

Medda S, Chemelli RM, Martin JL, Pohl LR, Swank RT (1989) Involvement of the carboxyl-terminal propeptide of β-glucuronidase in its compartmentalization within the endoplasmic reticulum as determined by a synthetic peptide approach. J Biol Chem 264:15824–15828

Mentlein R, Heymann E (1984) Hydrolysis of ester- and amide-type drugs by the purified isoenzymes of nonspecific carboxylesterase from rat liver. Biochem Pharmacol 33:1243–1248

Myers M, Richmond RC, Oakeshott JG (1988) On the origins of esterases. Mol Biol Evol 5:113–119

Nakamura T, Takagaki K, Majima M, Kumura S, Kubo K, Endo M (1990) A new type of exo-β-glucuronidase acting only on non-sulfated glycosaminoglycans. J Biol Chem 265:5390–5397

Neufeld EF, Moenzer J (1989) The mucopolysaccharidoses. In: Scriver CR, Beaudet AL, Sly WS, Valle D (eds) The metabolic basis of inherited disease, vol 11. McGraw-Hill, New York, pp 1565–1587
Novak E, Baumann H, Ovnic M, Swank RT (1991) Expression of egasyn-esterase in mammalian cells. J Biol Chem 266:6377–6380
Ovnic M, Swank RT, Fletcher C, Zhen L, Novak EK, Baumann H, Heintz N, Ganschow RE (1991a) Characterization and functional expression of a cDNA encoding egasyn (esterase-22): the endoplasmic reticulum targetting protein of β-glucuronidase. Genomics 11:956–967
Ovnic M, Tepperman K, Medda S, Elliott RW, Stephenson DA, Grant SG, Ganschow RE (1991b) Characterization of a murine cDNA encoding a member of the carboxyl-esterase multigene family. Genomics 9:344–354
Ozols J (1989) Isolation, properties and the complete amino acid sequence of a second form of 60-kDa glycoprotein esterase. J Biol Chem 264:12533–12545
Paigen K (1961) The effect of mutation on the intracellular location of β-glucuronidase. Exp Cell Res 25:286–301
Paigen K (1979) Acid hydrolases as models of genetic control. In: Roman HL, Campbell A, Sandler LM (eds) Annual reviews genetics. Annual Reviews, Palo Alto, pp 417–466
Paigen K (1989) Mammalian β-glucuronidase: genetics, molecular biology and cell biology. In: Cohn WE, Moldave K (eds) Progress in nucleic acid research and molecular biology, vol 37. Academic, New York, p 155
Pelham HRB (1989) Control of protein exit from the endoplasmic reticulum. Annu Rev Cell Biol 5:1–23
Peters J (1982) Nonspecific esterases of *Mus musculus*. Biochem Genet 20:585–606
Pfanner N, Neupert W (1990) The mitochondrial protein import apparatus. Annu Rev Biochem 59:331–353
Pfister K, Bosshard N, Zopfi M, Gitzelmann R (1988) Egasyn affects the processing of β-glucuronidase in mouse liver. Biochem J 255:825–832
Robbi M, Beaufay H (1991) The COOH terminus of several liver carboxylesterases targets these enzymes to the lumen of the endoplasmic reticulum. J Biol Chem 266:20498–20503
Schollhammer I, Poll DS, Brokel MH (1975) Liver microsomal β-glucuronidase and UDP-glucuronyl transferase. Enzyme 20:269–276
Schuchman EH, Toroyan TK, Haskins ME, Desnick RJ (1989) Characterization of the defective β-glucuronidase activity in canine mucopolysaccharidosis type VII. Enzyme 42:174–180
Shieh B-H, Travis J (1987) The reactive site of human α_2-antiplasmin. J Biol Chem 262:6055–6059
Skudlarek MD, Novak EK, Swank RT (1984) Processing of lysosomal enzymes in macrophages and kidney. In: Dingle JT, Dean RT, Sly (eds) Lysosomes in biology and pathology, vol 7. Elsevier, Amsterdam, pp 17–43
Smith BF, Hoffman RK, Giger U, Wolfe JH (1990) Genes transferred by retroviral vectors into normal and mutant myoblasts in primary cultures are expressed in myotubes. Mol Cell Biol 10:3268–3271
Smith K, Ganschow RE (1978) Turnover of murine β-glucuronidase. J Biol Chem 253:5437–5442
Sokolove PM, Wilcox MA, Thurman RG, Kauffman FC (1984) Stimulation of hepatic microsomal β-glucuronidase by calcium. Biochem Biophys Res Commun 121:987–993
Swank RT, Paigen K (1973) Biochemical and genetic evidence for a macromolecular β-glucuronidase complex in microsomal membranes. J Mol Biol 77:371–389
Swank RT, Paigen K, Davey R, Chapman V, Labarca C, Watson G, Ganschow R, Brandt EJ, Novak EK (1978) Genetic regulation of mammalian glucuronidase. In: Greep RO (ed) Recent progress in hormone research, vol 34. Academic, New York, pp 401–436

Swank RT, Pfister K, Miller D, Chapman V (1986) The egasyn gene affects the processing of oligosaccharides of lysosomal β-glucuronidase in liver. Biochem J 240:445–454

Swank RT, Moore K, Chapman VM (1987) Abnormal subcellular distribution of β-glucuronidase in mice with a genetic alteration in enzyme structure. Biochem Genet 25:161–174

Takagaki K, Nakamura T, Majima M, Endo M (1988) Isolation and characterization of a chondroitin sulphate-degrading endo-β-glucuronidase from rabbit liver. J Biol Chem 263:7000–7006

Tomatsu S, Sukigawa K, Ikedo Y, Fakuda S, Yamada Y, Sasaki T, Okamoto H, Kuwabara T, Orii T (1990) Molecular basis of mucopolysaccharidosis type VII. Replacement of Ala 619 in β-glucuronidase with Val. Gene 89:283–287

Tomatsu S, Fakuda S, Sukegawa K, Ikedo Y, Yamada S, Yamada Y, Sasaki T, Okamoto H, Kuwakara T, Yamaguchi S, Kiman T, Shintaku H, Isshiki G, Orii T (1991) Mucopolysaccharidosis type VII. Characterization of mutations and molecular heterogeneity. Am J Hum Genet 48:89–96

Tomino S, Paigen K (1975) Egasyn, a protein complexed with microsomal glucuronidase. J Biol Chem 250:1146–1148

Vogler C, Birkenmeier EH, Sly WS, Levy B, Pegors C, Kyle JW, Beamer WG (1990) A murine model of mucopolysaccharidosis VII. Gross and microscopic findings in β-glucuronidase-deficient mice. Am J Pathol 136:207–216

Wakabayashi M (1970) β-Glucuronidases in metabolic hydrolysis. In: Fishman WH (ed) Metabolic conjugation and metabolic hydrolysis. Academic, New York, pp 519–601

Watson G, Jaussi R, Tabron D, Paigen K (1992) The *Gus-e* locus regulates of estrogen repression of androgen-induced β-glucuronidase expression in mouse kidney. Biochem Genet 31:155–166

Wawrzyniak CJ, Meredith SA, Ganschow RE (1989a) Two genetic elements regulate murine β-glucuronidase synthesis following transcript accumulation. Genetics 121:119–124

Wawrzyniak CJ, Gallagher PM, D'Amore MA, Carter JE, Rinchik EM, Ganschow RE (1989b) DNA determinants of structural and regulatory variation within the murine β-glucuronidase gene complex. Mol Cell Biol 9:4074–4078

Whiting JF, Narciso JP, Chapman V, Ransil BJ, Swank RT, Gollan JL (1993) Deconjugation of bilirubin-1X_{α} Glucuronides: a physiological role of hepatic microsomal β-glucuronidase. J Biol Chem 268:23197–23201

Whittaker M, Sokolove PM, Thurman R, Kauffman FC (1985) Stimulation of 3-benzo[a]pyrenyl glucuronide hydrolysis by calcium activation of microsomal β-glucuronidase. Cancer Lett 26:145–152

Williams CH (1969) β-Glucuronidase activity in serum and liver of rats administered pesticides and hepatoxic agents. Toxicol Appl Pharmacol 14:283–292

Wolfe JH, Schuchman EH, Stramm LE, Concaugh EA, Haskins ME, Aquirre GD, Patterson DF, Desnick RJ, Gilboa E (1990) Restoration of normal lysosomal function in mucopolysaccharidosis type VII cells by retroviral vector-mediated gene transfer. Proc Natl Acad Sci USA 87:2877–2881

Wolfe JH, Deshmane SL, Fraser NW (1992) Herpes vector gene transfer and expression of β-glucuronidase in the central nervous system of MPS VII mice. Nature Genetics 1:379–384

Yatziv S, Erickson RP, Sandman R, Robertson WVB (1978) Glycosaminoglycan accumulation with partial deficiency of β-glucuronidase in the C3H strain of mice. Biochem Genet 16:1079–1084

Zhen L, Baumann H, Novak EK, Swank RT (1993) The signal for retention of the egasyn-glucuronidase complex within the endoplasmic reticulum. Arch Biochem Biophys 304:402–414

CHAPTER 6

Microsomal Amidases and Carboxylesterases

C.Y. WANG

A. Introduction

Deacylation is an important biological reaction which affects the efficacy and toxicity of chemotherapeutic amides and the carcinogenicity of aryl and heterocyclic amides. It is catalyzed by amidases, a group of nonspecific hydrolytic enzymes which are present mainly in microsomes. Amidases also have carboxylesterase activities and in this sense are identical to carboxylesterases. However, not all carboxylesterases have amidase activities. Thus, "amidases/carboxylesterases" refer to those which have both activities. This group of enzymes can catalyze the *O*-deacylation of *O*-acylhydroxamic acids (WANG et al. 1981), *N*-deacylation and *N*,*O*-acyltransfer of hydroxamic acids, *N*-acetylation of arylamines, and *O*-acetylation of hydroxylamines with acetyl coenzyme A (CoA; Fig. 1). They also catalyze the hydrolysis of thioesters, such as phenylthiolactate and butylthiocholine (MENTLEIN et al. 1984). Although they hydrolyze the esters of fatty acids, such as palmitoyl-L-carnitine, 1-palmitoyl glycerol, and oleoyl cholesterol, the physiological role of amidases/carboxylesterases is not yet clear (MENTLEIN et al. 1988).

Microsomal amidases/carboxylesterases can be inhibited by organophosphates and are B-esterases (ALDRIDGE 1952). They have been named either according to the type of chemical bonds they cleave or to a genetic nomenclature. Thus, they are carboxylesterases (EC 3.1.1), thioesterases (EC 3.1.2), and amidases (EC 3.5.1). In genetic nomenclature, each esterase is termed "Es" followed by an Arabic number, providing that there is sufficient proof for the coding of this esterase by a separate gene (MENTLEIN et al. 1987). Therefore, the pI 5.0, 5.5, 6.0, and 6.5 rat hepatic microsomal amidase/carboxylesterase are named as Es-15, Es-3, Es-10, and Es-4, respectively. However, the same enzyme may have been reported with varying pI values, due to differences in the charge of the protein under different experimental conditions. To circumvent these problems, the amidases/carboxylesterases reviewed here are identified according to species, pI values, and other characteristics, such as N-terminal amino acid sequence and molecular weight. Genetic nomenclature is given only when the identity of the enzyme is certain. Microsomal carboxylesterases/amidases have been reviewed earlier by HEYMANN (1980). Most of the material reviewed in this chapter has been published since then.

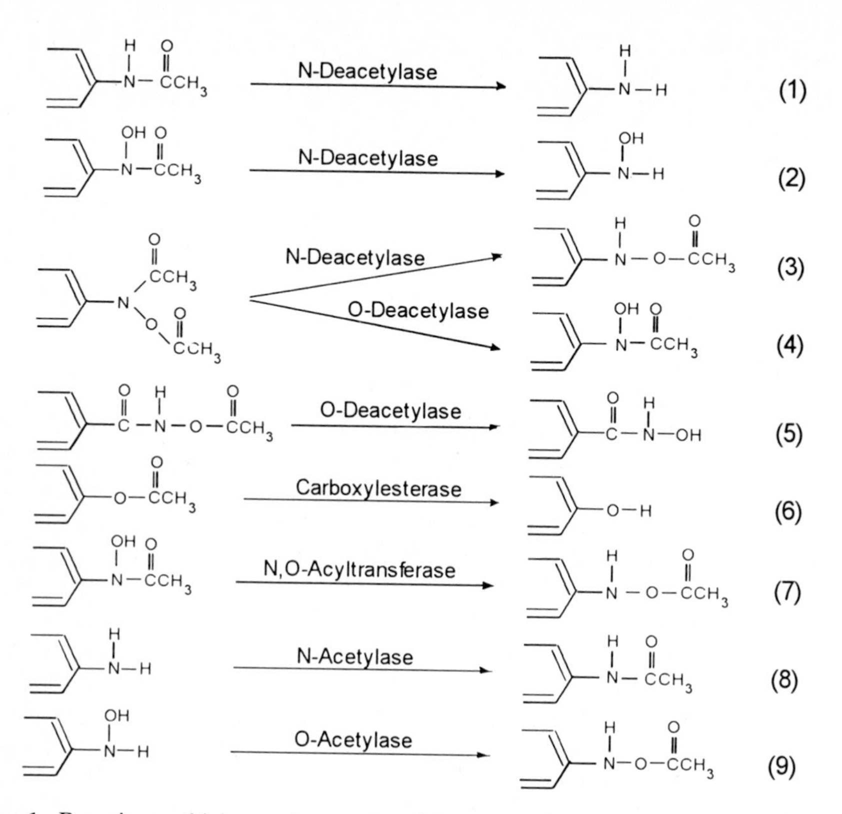

Fig. 1. Reactions which can be catalyzed by amidases/carboxylesterases. Due to these catalytic activities, these enzymes are also named after the reactions they catalyze, e.g., *N*-deacetylase. *N,O*-Acyltransferase catalyzes the internal acyltransfer of the hydroxamic acid (*reaction 7*). *N*- and *O*-acetylases utilize acetyl CoA as an acetyl donor

B. Distribution of Microsomal Amidases/Carboxylesterases

Deacetylation of arylacetamides can be demonstrated in various species of animals both in vitro and in vivo. The in vitro studies suggest that there may be a number of different deacetylating enzymes. They also show a variation in species and tissue location and a differing tissue specificity. Although amidases/carboxylesterases are found in microsomes, some are also found in other subcellular fractions. For example, pig liver microsomes deacetylate acetanilide and phenacetin (FRANKLIN et al. 1971). Chicken kidney enzymes of mitochondrial origin deacetylate N^4-acetylsulfanilamide, acetanilid, 4-acetamidobenzoate, and a number of other substituted acetanilids (FRANKLIN et al. 1971). Liver and kidney of the rat, rabbit, mouse, and guinea pig deacetylate 4-acetamidobenzoate. The activity is particularly high in the cytosol of rat kidney, but is not present in rat brain, blood, or skeletal muscle. This cytosolic activity is activated by Mn^{2+} and inhibited by 4-chloromercuribenzoate (FRANKLIN et al. 1971). Rat brain contains an arylamidase that can be inhibited by serotonin; rat liver arylamidases, on the other hand, cannot be inhibited by serotonin (FUJIMOTO 1974).

Liver homogenates of guinea pig, human, rat, rabbit, mouse, and dog deformylate the antimalarial agent 4,4′-diformamidodiphenyl sulfone (CHIOU 1971). The activity is particularly high in guinea pig and human livers and is very low in dog livers. This reaction is also catalyzed by the plasma of mouse, rat, guinea pig, and rabbit, but not by that of dog or human (GLEASON and VOUGH 1971). The plasma activities are inhibited by paraoxon, suggesting the involvement of a serine-esterase type enzyme.

The deacylation of amidothiazoles is more stringent with regard to specificity. Liver and small intestine homogenates of mice, hamsters, and guinea pigs and small intestine and stomach homogenates of rats deformylate the carcinogen *N*-[4-(5-nitro-2-furyl)-2-thiazolyl]formamide, but stomach homogenates of mouse and hamster can not. However, *N*-[4-(5-nitro-2-furyl)-2-thiazolyl]acetamide and formic acid 2-[4-(5-nitro-2-furyl)-2-thiazolyl]hydrazide are resistant to hydrolysis by homogenates of these organs (WANG and BRYAN 1974).

While several organs of rats and guinea pigs catalyze the *N*–deacetylation of *N*-hydroxy-*N*-acetyl-2-aminofluorene (N-OH-AAF; IRVING 1966), the deacetylase activities are particularly high in the ear ducts of rats and livers of guinea pigs (IRVING 1979). Liver microsomes of guinea pig, rat, hamster, mouse, rabbit, and dog also catalyze the *N*-deacetylation of N-OH-AAF, *N*-acetoxy-*N*-acetyl-2-aminofluorene (N-AcO-AAF), and *N*-hydroxy-*N*-acetyl-3,2′-dimethyl-4-aminobiphenyl (N-OH-DMAABP) and the *O*-deacetylation of N-AcO-AAF and N-AcO-DMAABP (Table 1); hepatic microsomes of these species also catalyze the *N*,*O*-acyltransfer of N-OH-AAF and *N*-hydroxy-*N*-formyl-2-aminofluorene (N-OH-FAF). Additionally, hepatic microsomes from rats, mice, hamsters, guinea pigs, rabbits, pigs, cow, dogs, and humans catalyze the deacylation of butanilicaine, isocarboxazid, 4-nitrophenyl acetate (4-NPA), and malathion (Table 1).

Hepatic microsomes of dogs, rats, mice, hamsters, and guinea pigs deacetylate the carcinogenic arylacetamides *N*-acetyl-4-aminobiphenyl, *N*-acetyl-2-aminonaphthalene, and *N*-acetyl-2-aminofluorene (2-AAF; LOWER and BRYAN 1976). Human liver and urinary bladder epithelial cells possess microsomal activities for the *N*-deacetylation and *N*,*O*-acetyltransfer of N-OH-AAF and *O*-acetylation of *N*-hydroxy-3,2′-dimethyl-4-aminobiphenyl (N-OH-DMABP; LAND et al. 1989).

The skins of rats and humans have a carboxylesterase of pI 6.0, which is likely to be identical to liver microsomal pI 6.0 amidase/carboxylesterase (Es-10; CLARK et al. 1992). Two carboxylesterases, referred to as R11 and R12, have been isolated from rat intestinal mucosa (SATOH et al. 1992). These two enzymes share a common antigenicity with rat liver pI 5.5 amidase (Es-3); however, their pIs have not yet been reported.

Table 1. *N*- and *O*-deactylation and *N*,*O*-acyltransfer activities of hepatic microsomes of various species

Species	Enzyme activity (nmol/min per mg protein)[a]									
	O-Deacetylation				*N*-Deacetylation				*N, O*-Acyltransfer	
	N-AcO-AAF[b]	N-AcO-DMAABP[b]	4-NPA[c]	Malathion[c]	N-OH-AAF[d]	N-OH-DMAABP[b]	Butanilicaine[c]	Isocarboxazid[c]	N-OH-AAF[d]	N-OH-FAF[d]
Guinea pig	2497 ± 275	601 ± 49	19000 ± 4600	41.4 ± 3.5	86.8 ± 3.2	1.20 ± 0.37	0.04 ± 0.01	885 ± 77	0.01 ± 0.01	0.32 ± 0.09
Rat	362 ± 39	49 ± 2	1930 ± 100	74.6 ± 9.2	3.3 ± 0.1	0.48 ± 0.06	0.12 ± 0.03	60 ± 12	0.017 ± 0.002	0.176 ± 0.08
Hamster	1160 ± 102	2347 ± 89	14900 ± 1100	26.4 ± 3.4	56.3 ± 3.5	3.19 ± 0.14	0.58 ± 0.07	249 ± 30	0.25, 0.65	0.14, 0.38
Mice	1588 ± 226[e]	736 ± 115[e]	8520 ± 500[f]	14.0 ± 2.4[f]	12.8 ± 0.9[e]	1.10 ± 0.13[e]	0.10 ± 0.10[g]	78.8 ± 6.4[g]	0.012, 0.027[e]	0.089, 0.084[e]
	1598 ± 331[h]	711 ± 60[h]			11.4 ± 0.8[h]	0.80 ± 0.11[h]			0.046, 0.016[i]	0.20, 0.21[i]
Rabbit	1373 ± 139	592 ± 76	10300	59.9	16.1 ± 1.8	1.42 ± 0.15	1.08	197	0.08	0.17
Dog	89, 73	107, 110	2420	26.7	3.2, 2.6	1.2, 1.0	1.06	68.8	0.003 ± 0.001	0.049 ± 0.01
Pig			10900	28.8			1.62	125		
Cow			8770	<0.002			1.11	48.3		
Monkey			4370 ± 320	42.5 ± 2.5			<0.005	169 ± 23		
Human			1060	<0.002			0.07	19.0		

N-AcO-AAF, *N*-acetoxy-*N*-acetyl-2-aminofluorene; N-AcO-DMAABP, *N*-acetoxy-*N*-acetyl-3,2′-dimethyl-4-aminobiphenyl; 4-NPA, 4-nitrophenyl acetate; N-OH-AAF, *N*-hydroxy-*N*-acetyl-2-aminofluorene; N-OH-DMAABP, *N*-hydroxy-*N*-acetyl-3,2′-dimethyl-4-aminobiphenyl; N-OH-FAF, *N*-hydroxy-*N*-formyl-2-aminofluorene.

[a] The data are expressed either as mean + S.D. from multiple determinations or as a mean from individual determination.
[b] Yamada et al. (1988).
[c] Hosokawa et al. (1990).
[d] Glowinski et al. (1993).
[e] BALB/c mouse.
[f] ICR mouse.
[g] A/J mouse.
[h] C3H mouse.
[i] C57 BL/J.

C. Purification of Microsomal Amidases/Carboxylesterases from Different Species

Amidases/carboxylesterases are glycoproteins that loosely bind to the luminal surface of endoplasmic reticulum. Therefore, the first step of the purification procedure is to release the protein from the microsomal particles. Ultrasonication (JARVINEN et al. 1971; GLOWINSKI et al. 1983; YAMADA et al. 1988), 1% saponin (HEYMANN and MENTLEIN 1981; HOSOKAWA et al. 1990), and 0.2%–0.25% Triton X-100 (ROBBI and BEAUFAY 1983; YAMADA et al. 1988; SONE et al. 1991; WANG et al. 1992) are frequently used to release the enzymes. Treatment with proteinase reduces some amidase and esterase activities (MENTLEIN et al. 1988); the use of this method is therefore not advisable. The released proteins can be fractionated by precipitation with ammonium sulfate, gel filtration and ion exchange column chromatography, and isoelectric focusing (HEYMANN and MENTLEIN 1981). Other schemes have included fractionation with acetone and chromatography on a Con A-Sepharose affinity column (ROBBI and BEAUFAY 1983), an immunoaffinity column (SATOH et al. 1989), and a hydrophobic column (PROBST et al. 1991). High-pressure liquid chromatography (HPLC) chromatofocusing and ion exchange have been successfully used for purification of amidases/carboxylesterases (HOSOKAWA et al. 1990; WANG et al. 1992; SONE et al. 1992). Some amidases/carboxylesterases are somewhat hydrophobic and tend to bind to the matrix during column chromatography or HPLC. This problem can be minimized by adding Triton X-100 to the elution solutions.

Amidases/carboxylesterases purified from various species can be classified into: (a) those with homology to rabbit form 1 amidase/carboxylesterase, (b) those with homology to rabbit form 2 amidase/carboxylesterase, and (c) those without homology to either one. The physical, chemical, and immunological properties of these enzymes are summarized in Tables 2–4.

I. Rabbit

Two forms of amidase/carboxylesterase (forms 1 and 2) have been purified from rabbit hepatic microsomes to electrophoretic homogeneity (OZOLS 1987, 1989). Their masses are approximately 60 kDa, but they differ in N-terminal amino acid sequences (Fig. 2). HOSOKAWA et al. (1990) also purified an amidase/carboxylesterase from rabbit liver. Its pI is 5.5, and mass 62 kDa. The N-terminal amino acid sequence of this enzyme is very similar to that of form 1 rabbit enzyme (Table 2).

II. Rat

Rat hepatic microsomes contain four amidases/carboxylesterases; they are Es-15 (pI 5.0), Es-3 (pI 5.5), Es-10 (pI 6.0), and Es-4 (pI 6.5; MENTLEIN et

Table 2. Physical and catalytic properties and N-terminal sequences of purified amidases/carboxylesterases of various species

Species	pI[a]	Subunit weight (kDa)	N Termini
Rat	5.0 (Es-15)	60	
	5.2 (Es-15)	60	
	5.0 (Es-15)	57–60	
	5.5 (Es-3)	61	
	5.6 (Es-3)	60	
	5.5 (Es-3)	61	X-P-S-X-P-P-V-V-N-X-V-K-G-K-V-L-G-K-Y-V-
	5.5 (Es-3)	57–60	
	5.35–5.79 (Egasyn)	61–63	
	6.0 (Es-10)	59 (trimer)	
	6.0 (Es-10)	59 (trimer)	Y-P-S-X-P-P-V-V-N-X-V-K-G-K-V-L-G-K-Y-V-
	6.0 (Es-10)	60 (trimer)	
	6.1 (Es-10)	57–60 (trimer)	
	5.7 (Es-10)	59 (trimer)	Y-P-S-S-P-P-V-V-N-T-V-K-G-K-V-L-G-D-Y-V-N-L-
	cDNA (Es-10)		Y-P-S-S-P-P-V-V-N-T-V-K-G-K-V-L-G-K-Y-V-N-L-
	5.8[b]	60 (trimer)	Y-P-S-S-P-P-V-V-D-T-V-K-G-K-V-L-G-K-
	6.5 (Es-4)	60	
	6.5 (Es-4)	61	D-P-S-X-P-P-V-V-D-T-V-K-G-K-V-L-G-K-Y-V-S-L-
	6.4, 6.2 (Es-4)	60	
	6.4 (Es-4)	57–60	
Mouse	5.9	60	
	4.67–5.40 (Es-22)[c]	64	H-P-S-S-P-P-M-V-D-T-V-Q-G-K-V-L-G-K-Y-I-S-L-
	Es-N cDNA		H-S-L-L-P-P-V-V-D-T-T-Q-G-K-V-L-G-K-Y-
Hamster	5.7	58	S-P-S-X-P-X-V-V-N-X-V-
	6.0	58 (trimer)	A-P-S-S-P-P-V-V-N-X-V-K-G-K-V-L-G-
	5.4	60	D-S-P-S-P-I-R-N-T-H-T-G-Q-V-R-G-L-V-H-K-
Guinea pig	5.3	57	
	5.9	64	X-X-P-S-X-P-X-V-V-D-X-K-V-G-K-V-L-G-K-Y-
Dog	5.0	60	Y-P-S-X-P-P-V-V-N-X-V-K-G-K-V-L-G-K-Y-V-
	5.6	60 (trimer)	Y-P-S-L-P-P-V-V-D-T-V-Q-G-K-V-
Pig	5.2–5.4	58–62	G-E-P-A-V-P-P-V-V-D-T-A-Q-G-X-X-L-G-K-Y-
	–[d]	58 (trimer)	G-Q-P-A-V-P-S-V-V-D-T-A-Q-G-R-V-L-G-R-Y-V-S-L-
	cDNA		G-Q-P-A-S-P-P-V-V-D-T-A-Q-G-R-V-L-G-K-Y-
Cow	6.0	64	L-A-V-S-P-P-I-V-D-X-A-Q-G-X-V-L-G-K-L-V-
Rabbit	Form 1	60	H-P-S-A-P-P-V-V-D-T-V-K-G-K-V-L-G-K-F-V-S-L-
	Form 2	60	Q-D-S-A-S-P-I-R-N-T-H-T-G-Q-V-R-G-S-L-V-H-V-
	5.5	62	H-P-S-X-P-P-V-V-N-X-V-K-G-K-V-L-G-K-Y-V-
Monkey	4.7	63	K-S-A-S-P-X-V-
	5.5	60	G-P-S-S-P-P-V-V-D-D-V-K-G-K-V-L-G-K-
Human	–	45	G-M-K-S-L-Y-L-L-I-V-G-I-L-I-A-Y-Y-I-Y-T-
	5.4	61	
	5.6	61	G-P-P-S-P-P-V-V-D-D-T-X-G-K-X-L-
	–[e]	60	G-H-P-S-S-P-P-V-V-D-T-V-H-G-K-V-L-G-

2-AAF, *N*-acetyl-2-aminofluorene; N-OH-AAF; *N*-hydroxy-N-acetyl-2-aminofluorene; 4-NPA, 4-nitrophenyl acetate; 2-AF, 2-aminofluorene.

[a] Unless specified otherwise, the enzymes are from liver microsomes. cDNA is indicated when the N-terminal sequences are deduced from the cDNA. In general, the identity of the enzyme expressed by this cDNA cannot be ascertained.

Table 2. (*Continued*)

Substrates	References
2-AAF, N-OH-AAF, 4-NPA	Wang et al. (1992)
Acetanilide	Mentlein and Heymann (1984)
4-NPA, 1-naphthylacetate	Robbi and Beaufay (1983)
2-AAF, N-OH-AAF, 4-NPA	Wang et al. (1992)
Butanilicaine, phenacetin, acetanilide, octanoylamide, aspirin	Mentlein and Heymann (1984)
Isocarboxazid, acetanilide, 4-NPA	Hosokawa et al. (1989, 1990)
4-NPA, 1-naphthylacetate	Robbi and Beaufay (1983)
Acetanilide, isobutyl propionate, methyl butyrate	Medda et al. (1987)
2-AAF, N-OH-AAF, 4-NPA	Wang et al. (1992)
Batanilicaine, isocarboxazid, malathion, acetanilide, 4-NPA	Hosokawa et al. (1987, 1990), Satoh et al. (1989)
Butanilicaine, octanoylamide, aspirin, clofibrate	Mentlein and Heymann (1984)
4-NPA, 1-naphthylacetate	Robbi and Beaufay (1983)
Acetanilide, 4-NPA	Takagi et al. (1988), Harano et al. (1988), Long et al. (1988)
	Robbi et al. (1990)
Butanilicaine, 4-NPA	Gaustad et al. (1991b)
2-AFF, N-OH-AAF, 4-NPA	Wang et al. (1992)
4-NPA, malathion	Hosokawa et al. (1990)
Octanoylamide, aspirin, clofibrate, butyl thicholine	Mentlein and Heymann (1984)
4-NPA, 1-naphthylacetate	Robbi and Beaufay (1983)
Butanilicaine, isocarboxazid, 4-NPA, malathion	Hosokawa et al. (1990)
1-Naphthylacetate	Ovnic et al. (1991a)
	Ovnic et al. (1991b)
Butanilicaine, isocarboxazid, 4-NPA, malathion	Hosokawa et al. (1990)
Butanilicaine, isocarboxazid, 4-NPA, malathion	Hosokawa (1990)
N-OH-AAF, 4-NPA	Sone et al. (1992)
Butanilicaine, isocarboxazid, 4-NPA, malathion	Hosokawa et al. (1990)
Butanilicaine, isocarboxazid, 4-NPA, malathion	Hosokawa et al. (1990)
Butanilicaine, isocarboxazid, 4-NPA, malathion	Hosokawa (1990)
2-AAF, N-OH-AAF, 4-NPA, 2-AF	Sone et al. (1994)
Butanilicaine, isocarboxazid, 4-NPA, malathion	Hosokawa (1990)
Aminoacyl 2- naphthylamides	Takahashi et al. (1989)
	Matsushima et al. (1991)
Butanilicaine, isocarboxazid, 4-NPA, malathion	Hosokawa (1990)
	Ozols (1987), Korza and Ozols (1987)
	Ozols (1989)
Butanilicaine, isocarboxazid, 4-NPA, malathion	Hosokawa et al. (1990)
Isocarboxazid, 4-NPA, malathion	Hosokawa et al. (1990)
Butanilicaine, isocarboxazid, 4-NPA, malathion	Hosokawa et al. (1990)
2-AAF, 4-NPA	Probst et al. (1991)
Butanilicaine, isocarboxazid, 4-NPA, malathion	Hosokawa (1990)
Butanilicaine, isocarboxazid, 4-NPA, malathion	Hosokawa (1990)
4-Nitrophenyl valerate	Munger et al. (1991)

[b] The enzyme is from rat lung.
[c] The N-terminal sequence is deduced from a cDNA believed to encode this enzyme.
[d] The enzyme is from intestinal mucosa.
[e] The enzyme is from human alveolar macrophage. The N-terminal sequence is deduced from a cDNA clone.

Table 3. Potential glycosylation and active sites of amidases/carboxylesterases

Species	Isozymes	Glycosylation sites (asparaginyl residues)	Active sites		References
			Serine residues	Histidine residues	
Rat	cDNA of a 59-kDa enzyme	61, 256, 458	203	435	LONG et al. (1988)
	cDNA of pI 6.0 (Es-10)	61, 471	203	448	ROBBI et al. (1990)
Rabbit	Form 1	61, 363	195	441	KORZA and OZOLS (1988)
	Form 2	249	201	430	OZOLS (1989)
Mouse	Egasyn cDNA (Es-22)	61, 257, 471	203	448	OVNIC et al. (1991a)
	Es-N cDNA	61, 256, 286, 359, 460	203	427	OVNIC et al. (1991b)
Human	cDNA of a 59-kDa enzyme	61	203	450	LONG et al. (1991)
	Macrophage esterase cDNA	62	204	451	MUNGER et al. (1991)

Table 4. Antigenicities of purified hepatic amidases/carboxylesterases. (Reproduced from HOSOKAWA 1990)

Species	pI[a]	Antibody[b]										
		RL1	RL2	RH1	H1	RB1	D1	P1	B1	MK1	MK2	HU1
Rat	6.5 (RL1)	+++	−	−	−	−	−			+	−	+
	5.5 (RL2)	−	+++	−	−	−	±			+	−	+
	6.0 (RH1)	−	−	+++	++	+	++	+++	+++	+++	−	+++
Mouse	5.9 (M1)	++	−	+								
Hamster	5.7 (H1)	−	−	+++	+++	+++				+++		+++
Guinea pig	5.9 (GPL1)	−	−	+	++	++				++		++
	5.3 (GPH1)	−	−	+	++	++				++		++
Rabbit	5.5 (RB1)	−	−	+++	+	+++				+++		+++
Dog	5.0 (D1)	−	−	+++			+++	++	++	+++		+++
Pig	5.2–5.4 (P1)	−	−	+++				+++				+++
Cow	6.0 (B1)	−	±	+++					+++			+++
Monkey	5.5 (MK1)	−	−	+++	+	+++				+++		+++
	4.7 (MK2)	−	−	−	−	−				−	+++	−
Human	5.6 (HU1)	−	−	+++			+++			+++	−	+++

[a] The enzymes are identified with their pI values. The designated names of the enzymes by the author are shown in the parentheses.
[b] Polyclonal antibodies against the enzymes are used.

```
                                   10                                      20                                     30
His-Pro-Ser-Ala-Pro-Pro-Val-Val-Asp-Thr-Val-Lys-Gly-Lys-Val-Leu-Gly-Lys-Phe-Val-Ser-Leu-Glu-Gly-Phe-Ala-Gln-Pro-Val-Ala-
Gln-Asp-Ser-Ala-Ser-Pro-Ile-Arg-Asn-Thr-His-Thr-Gly-Gln-Val-Arg-Gly-Ser-Leu-Val-His-Val-Glu-Gly-Thr-Asp-Ala-Gly-Val-His-

                                   40                                      50                                     60
Val-Phe-Leu-Gly-Val-Pro-Phe-Ala-Lys-Pro-Pro-Leu-Gly-Ser-Leu-Arg-Phe-Ala-Pro-Pro-Gln-Pro-Ala-Glu-Ser-Trp-Ser-His-Val-Lys-
Thr-Phe-Leu-Gly-Ile-Pro-Phe-Ala-Lys-Pro-Pro-Leu-Gly-Pro-Leu-Arg-Phe-Ala-Pro-Pro-Glu-Pro-Ala-Glu-Ala-Trp-Ser-Gly-Val-Arg-

                                   70                                      80                                     90
Asn-Thr-Thr-Ser-Tyr-Pro-Pro-Met-Cys-Ser-Ser-Asp-    Ala-Val-Ser-Gly-His-    -Met-Leu-Ser-Glu-Leu-Phe-Thr-Asn-Arg-Lys-Glu-
Asp-Gly-Thr-Ser-Leu-Pro-Ala-Met-Cys-Leu-Gln-Asn-Leu-Ala-Ile-Met-Asp-Gln-Asp-Val-Leu-Leu-Leu-His-Phe-Thr-Pro-Pro-

                                   100                                     110                                    120
Asn-Ile-Pro-Leu-Lys-Phe-Ser-Glu-Asp-Cys-Leu-Tyr-Leu-Asn-Ile-Tyr-Thr-Pro-Ala-Asp-Leu-Thr-Lys-Arg-Gly-Arg-Leu-Pro-Val-Met-
Ser-Ile-Pro-Met-        Ser-Glu-Asp-Cys-Leu-Tyr-Leu-Asn-Ile-Tyr-Ser-Pro-Ala-His-Ala-Arg-Glu-Gly-Ser-Asp-Leu-Pro-Val-Met-

                                   130                                     140                                    150
Val-Trp-Ile-His-Gly-Gly-Gly-Leu-Met-Val-Gly-Gly-Ala-Ser-Thr-Tyr-Asp-Gly-Leu-Ala-Leu-Ser-Ala-His-Glu-Asn-Val-Val-Val-Val-
Val-Trp-Ile-His-Gly-Gly-Gly-Leu-Thr-Met-Gly-Met-Ala-Ser-Met-Tyr-Asp-Gly-Ser-Ala-Leu-Ala-Ala-Phe-Glu-Asp-Val-Val-Val-Val-

                                   160                                     170                                    180
Thr-Ile-Gln-Tyr-Arg-Leu-Gly-Ile-Gly-Gly-Phe-Gly-Phe-Asn-Ile-Asp-Glu-Leu-                                -Phe-Leu-    Val-
Thr-Ile-Gln-Tyr-Arg-Leu-Gly-Val-Leu-Gly-Phe-    Phe-Ser-Thr-Gly-Asp-Gln-His-Ala-Thr-Gly-Asn-His-Gly-Tyr-Leu-Asp-Gln-Val-

                                   190                                     200                 *                  210
Ala-Val-Asn-Arg-Trp-Val-Gln-Asp-Asn-Ile-Ala-Asn-Phe-Gly-Gly-Asp-Pro-Gly-Ser-Val-Thr-Ile-Phe-Gly-Glu-Ser-Ala-Gly-Gly-Gln-
Ala-Ala-Leu-Arg-Trp-Val-Gln-Lys-Asn-Ile-Ala-His-Phe-Gly-Gly-Asn-Pro-Gly-Arg-Val-Thr-Ile-Phe-Gly-Glu-Ser-Ala-Gly-Gly-Thr-

                                   220                                     230                                    240
Ser-Val-Ser-Ile-Leu-Leu-Leu-Ser-Pro-Leu-Thr-Lys-Asn-Leu-Phe-His-Arg-Ala-Ile-Ser-Glu-Ser-Gly-Val-Ala-Leu-Leu-Ser-Ser-Leu-
Ser-Val-Ser-Ser-His-Val-Leu-Ser-Pro-Met-Ser-Gln-Gly-Leu-Phe-His-Gly-Ala-Ile-Met-Glu-Ser-Leu-Val-Ala-Leu-Leu-Pro-Gly-Leu-

                                   250                                     260                                    270
Phe-Arg-Lys-Asn-Thr-Lys-Ser-Leu-Ala-Glu-Lys-Ile-Ala-Ile-Glu-Ala-Gly-Cys-Lys-Thr-Thr-Thr-Ser-Ala-Val-Met-Val-His-Cys-Leu-
Ile-Thr-Ser-Ser-Ser-Glu-Val-Val-Ser-Thr-Val-Val-Ala-Asn-Leu-Ser-Arg-Cys-Gly-Gln-Val-Asp-Ser-Glu-Thr-Leu-Val-Arg-Cys-Leu-

                                   280                                     290                                    300
Arg-Gln-Lys-Thr-Glu-Glu-Glu-Leu-Met-Glu-Val-Thr-Leu-Lys-Met-Lys-Phe-Met-Ala-Leu-Asp-Leu-Val-Gly-Asp-Pro-Lys-Glu-Asn-Thr-
Arg-Ala-Lys-Ser-Glu-Glu-Glu-Met-Leu-Ala-Ile-Thr-    -Gln-Val-    Phe-Met-            Leu-Ile-Pro-Gly-

                                   310                                     320                                    330
Ala-Phe-Leu-Thr-Thr-Val-Ile-Asp-Gly-Val-Leu-Leu-Pro-Lys-Ala-Pro-Ala-Glu-Ile-Tyr-Glu-Glu-Lys-Lys-Tyr-Asn-Met-Leu-Pro-Tyr-
                    Val-Val-Asp-Gly-Val-Phe-Leu-Pro-Arg-His-Pro-Glu-Glu-Leu-Leu-Ala-Leu-Ala-Asp-Phe-Gln-Pro-Val-Pro-Ser-

                                   340                                     350                                    360
Met-Val-Gly-Ile-Asn-Gln-Gln-Glu-Phe-Gly-Trp-Ile-Ile-Pro-Met-Gln-Met-Leu-Gly-Tyr-Pro-Leu-Ser-Glu-Gly-Lys-Leu-Asp-Gln-Lys-
Ile-Ile-Gly-Ile-Asn-Asn-Asp-Glu-Tyr-Gly-Trp-Ile-Ile-Pro-Lys-Leu-Leu-Leu-Ala-Ile-Asp-Pro-Gln-Glu-Glu-Arg-    Asp-Arg-Gln-

                                   370                                     380                                    390
Thr-Ala-Thr-Glu-Leu-Leu-Trp-Lys-Ser-Tyr-Pro-Ile-Val-Gln-Val-Ser-Lys-Glu-Leu-Thr-Pro-Val-Ala-Thr-Glu-Lys-Tyr-Leu-Gly-Gly-
Ala-Met-Arg-Glu-Ile-Met-His-Gln-Ala-Thr-Lys-Gln-Leu-Met-Leu-Pro-Pro-Ala-Leu-Gly-Asp-Leu-Leu-Met-Asp-Glu-Tyr-Met-Gly-Ser-

                                   400                                     410                                    420
Thr-Asp-Asp-Pro-Val-Lys-Lys-Lys-Asp-Leu-Phe-Leu-Asp-Met-Leu-Ala-Asp-Leu-Leu-Phe-Gly-Val-Pro-Ser-Val-Asn-Val-Ala-Arg-His-
Asn-Glu-Asp-Pro-Lys-His-Leu-Met-Ala-Gln-Phe-Gln-Glu-Met-Met-Ala-Asp-Ala-Met-Phe-Val-Met-Pro-Ala-Leu-Arg-Val-Ala-His-Leu-

                                   430                                     440                                    450
His-Arg-Asp-Ala-Gly-Ala-Pro-Thr-Tyr-Met-Tyr-Glu-Tyr-Arg-Tyr-Arg-Pro-Ser-Phe-Ser-Ser-Asp-Met-Arg-Pro-Lys-Thr-Val-Ile-Gly-
Gln-Arg-Ser-His-    Ala-Pro-Thr-Tyr-Phe-Tyr-Glu-Phe-Gln-His-Arg-Pro-Ser-Phe-Thr-Lys-Asp-Leu-Arg-Pro-Pro-His-Val-Arg-Ala-

    *                              460                                     470                                    480
Asp-His-Gly-Asp-Glu-Ile-Phe-Ser-Val-Leu-Gly-Ala-Pro-Phe-Leu-            Lys-Glu-Gly-Ala-Thr-Glu-Glu-Glu-Ile-Lys-Leu-Ser-Lys-
Asp-His-Gly-Asp-Glu-Val-Val-Phe-Val-Phe-Arg-Ser-His-Leu-Phe-Gly-Ser-Lys-Val-Pro-Leu-Thr-Glu-Glu-Glu-Glu-Leu-Leu-Ser-Arg-

                                   490                                     500                                    510
Met-Val-Met-Lys-Tyr-Trp-Ala-Asn-Phe-Ala-Arg-Asn-Gly-Asn-Pro-Asn-Gly-Glu-Gly-Leu-Pro-Gln-Trp-Pro-Ala-Tyr-Asp-Tyr-Lys-Glu-
Arg-Val-Met-Lys-Tyr-Trp-Ala-Asn-Phe-Ala-Arg-Asn-Arg-Asn-Pro-Asn-Gly-Glu-Gly-Leu-Ala-His-Trp-Pro-Leu-Phe-Asp-Leu-Asp-Gln-

                                   520                                     530                                    540
Gly-Tyr-Leu-Gln-Ile-Gly-Ala-Thr-Thr-Gln-Ala-Ala-Gln-Lys-Leu-Lys-Asp-Lys-Glu-Val-Ala-Phe-Trp-Thr-Glu-Leu-Trp-Ala-Lys-Glu-
Arg-Tyr-Leu-Gln-Leu-Asn-Met-Gln-Pro-Ala-Val-Gly-Gln-Ala-Leu-Lys-Ala-Arg-Arg-Leu-Gln-Phe-Trp-Thr-His-Thr-Leu-Pro-Gln-Arg-

                                   550
Ala-Ala-Arg-Pro-Arg-Glu-Thr-Glu-        His-Ile-Glu-Leu.
Val-Gln-Glu-Leu-Arg-Gly-Thr-Glu-Gln-Lys-His-Thr-Glu-Leu.
```

Fig. 2. Comparison of amino acid sequences of rabbit liver forms 1 and 2 amidase/carboxylesterase. The sequence of form 1 is from Korza and Ozols (1988). The diisopropylphosphofluoridate (DFP)-binding seryl and histidyl residues are denoted by an *asterisk* (Reproduced from Ozols 1989) al. 1987). With the exception of Es-10, which is a trimer (~60 kDa subunit weight), the enzymes are monomers of approximately 60 kDa (Table 2).

Although we have purified all four enzymes (WANG et al. 1992) and HOSOKAWA et al. (1987) have purified the pI 6.5, pI 6.0, and pI 5.5 enzyme to electrophoretic homogeneity, ROBBI and BEAUFAY (1983) found microheterogeneity for the pI 5.0 enzyme and MENTLEIN et al. (1980, 1984, 1987) found the pI 5.5 and pI 5.0 enzyme to be heterogeneous. This microheterogenicity may be due to allelic heterozogosity of the gene (MENTLEIN et al. 1987) or to variation in the oligpsaccharide component of these enzymes (SONE et al. 1994).

The pI 6.0 amidase/carboxylesterase has also been purified from rat liver microsomes by SATOH et al. (1989) and HARANO et al. (1988), and from rat lung by GAUSTAD et al. (1991b). The lung enzymes is a 180-kDa protein (subunit relative molecular mass of 60 kDa), and its pI is 5.8.

Egasyn, which binds noncovalently to microsomal β-glucuronidase and stabilizes this enzyme, is a 61- to 63-kDa protein and its pI is 5.35–5.79. It catalyzes the hydrolysis of methyl butyrate, isobutyl propionate, and acetanilid. It is believed to be related to pI 5.5 amidase/carboxylesterase (Es-3; MEDDA et al. 1987).

The physical and enzymatic properties of the rat microsomal amidases/carboxylesterases which have been purified are compared in Table 2. The N-terminal amino acid sequences of these enzymes are homologous to those of rabbit form 1 amidase/carboxylesterase (Table 2).

III. Mouse

Mouse liver microsomes may contain as many as five carboxylesterases. Their pI values are 8.2–8.4, 5.6–5.8, 4.9–5.0, 4.6–4.7, and 4.2–4.3 (WU and MARLETTA 1988). No information is available regarding their amidase activities. Purified mouse hepatic microsomal egasyn is a 64-kDa protein. It has esterase activities and is identical to Es-22 (OVNIC et al. 1991a). Its N-terminal amino acid sequence, deduced from a cDNA clone, is homologous to that of rabbit form 1 enzyme (Table 2). Another amidase/carboxylesterase has been purified to electrophoretic homogeneity from mouse hepatic microsomes (HOSOKAWA et al. 1990). Its pI is 5.9, and subunit weight is 60 kDa.

IV. Hamster

Gel filtration resolves hamster hepatic microsomal proteins into two groups of amidases. While the *N*-deacetylation of 2-AAF and N-OH-AAF and the *O*-deacetylation of 4-NPA are catalyzed by both 180-kDa and 60-kDa proteins, the *N,O*-acetyltransfer of N-OH-AAF is primarily catalyzed by the smaller enzymes (Fig. 3). A purified 60-kDa enzyme (pI 5.4) is capable of *O*-deacetylation of 4-NPA (SONE et al. 1992). Its N-terminal amino acid sequence is homologous to that of rabbit form 2 amidase/carboxylesterase (Table 2).

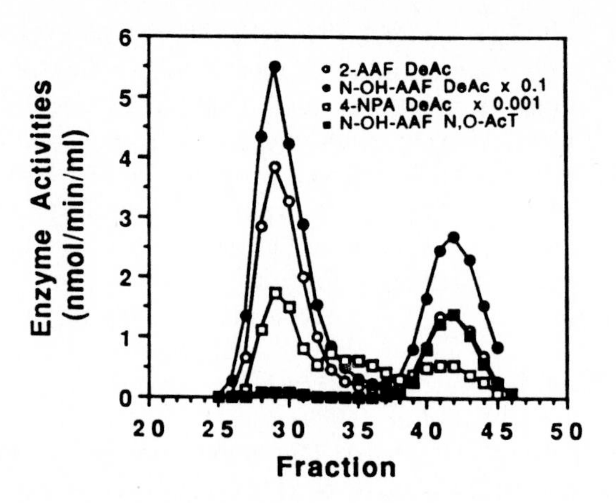

Fig. 3. Separation of hamster hepatic microsomal amidases/carboxylesterases with Sephacryl S-200 column chromatography. The relative molecular masses of these two fractions of enzymes are approximately 180 and 60 kDa. *N*-acetyl-2-aminofluorene (*2-AAF*) and 4-nitrophenyl acetate (*4-NPA*) deacetylase activities are primarily due to the larger enzyme(s). *N*-hydroxy-*N*-acetyl-2-aminofluorene (*N-OH-AAF*) deacetylase activities and *N*,*O*-acyltransferase activities are mainly due to the smaller enzyme(s). Note: the activities for N-OH-AAF deacetylation are reduced by ten times and that of 4-NPA deacetylation by 1000 times

Two additional amidases/carboxylesterases, pI 5.7 and 58 kDa (Hosokawa et al. 1990) and pI 6.0 and approximately 180 kDa (58-kDa subunit) (Hosokawa 1990), respectively, have been purified from hamster hepatic microsomes. The N-terminal amino acid sequences of these two enzymes are homologous to that of rabbit form 1 amidase/carboxylesterase (Table 2).

V. Guinea pig

Guinea pig hepatic microsomes are capable of the *N*-deacetylation of N-OH-AAF and 2-AAF and the *O*-deacetylation of N-AcO-AAF and *N*-acetoxy-*N*-acety-3,2′-dimethyl-4-aminobiphenyl (N-AcO-DMAABP; Glowinski et al. 1983; Yamada et al. 1988). Gel filtration resolves the microsomal enzymes into two different molecular weight groups. The *N*-deacetylation of N-OH-AAF and the *O*-deacetylation of N-AcO-AAF and N-AcO-DMAABP are mainly due to larger molecular weight enzymes, and the *N*-deacetylation of 2-AAF is mainly due to smaller molecular weight enzymes. These two enzymes also catalyze the *N*,*O*-acyltransfer of N-OH-AAF and N-OH-FAF, with the former being catalyzed mainly by the smaller enzymes and the latter by the larger enzymes.

Chromatofocusing of guinea pig liver microsomal proteins resolves them into at least three carboxylesterases characteristic of pI 5.6, 5.1, and 4.6

(GAUSTAD et al. 1991a). No further characteristics of these enzymes have been reported.

Two guinea pig hepatic microsomal amidases/carboxylesterases have been purified to electrophoretic homogeneity (HOSOKAWA et al. 1990). Their subunit weights and pIs are 64 and 57 kDa and pI 5.9 and pI 5.3, respectively. The N-terminal amino acid sequence of one of the enzymes is homologous to that of rabbit form 1 enzyme (Table 2).

VI. Dog

Dog liver microsomes are capable of the *N*-deacetylation of 2-AAF and N-OH-AAF, the *N*,*O*-acyltransfer of N-OH-AAF and N-OH-FAF, and *N*-acetylation of 2-aminofluorene (2-AF) with acetyl CoA (SONE et al. 1991). Gel filtration resolves the microsomal enzymes into three groups with masses of approximately 700 or more (enzyme II), 180 (enzyme I), and 60 kDa (Enzyme III; Fig. 4). The *N*-deacetylation of 2-AAF is primarily catalyzed by enzyme II. This enzyme also is primarily responsible for the *N*-acetylase activity of dog hepatic microsomes (SONE et al. 1991). Its pI is approximately 4.9, and subunit weight is 60 kDa (our unpublished observation). The *N*,*O*-acyltransfer activity is primarily carried out by enzyme I. Enzyme III catalyzes the *N*-deacetylation of N-OH-AAF. The subunit weight of enzyme I is 60 kDa and its pI is approximately 5.6 (SONE et al. 1994). Its N-terminal amino acid sequence is homologous to that of rabbit form 1 enzyme

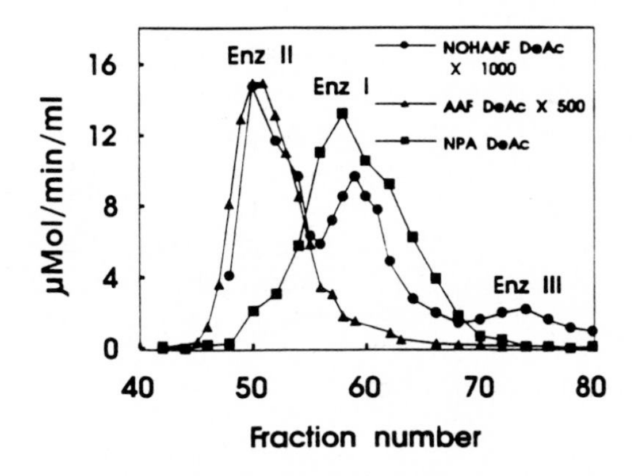

Fig. 4. Separation of dog hepatic microsomal amidases/carboxylesterases with Sephacryl S-200 column chromatography. The relative molecular mass of the largest enzyme(s) is greater than 700 kDa, the middle one is approximately 180 kDa, and the smallest one is approximately 60 kDa. The amidase and *N*,*O*-acyltransferase activities of the microsomes are primarily due to the largest and the middle mass enzymes, respectively (SONE et al. 1991). Note: the activities of *N*-hydroxy-*N*-acetyl-2-aminofluorene (*N-OH-AAF*) deacetylation and *N*-acetyl-2-aminofluorene (*2-AAF*) deacetylation have been multiplied by 1000 and 500 times, respectively

(Table 2). The other two amidases/carboxylesterases of dog liver have yet to be purified.

HOSOKAWA (1990) has purified a carboxylesterase from dog liver microsomes. The pI is 5.0, and its subunit weight is approximately 60 kDa. Its N-terminal amino acid sequence is homologous to that of rabbit form 1 enzyme (Table 2). It is not known whether this enzyme is identical to the pI 4.9 enzyme we have studied.

VII. Human

Human carboxylesterases may exist as several isozymes that are encoded by multiple genes (LONG et al. 1991). HOSOKAWA (1990) purified an amidase/carboxylesterase from human liver; the N-terminal amino acid sequence of this enzyme is homologous to that of rabbit form 1 amidase/carboxylesterase (Table 2).

KETTERMAN et al. (1989) have observed that human liver has three carboxylesterases (pI 6.8–8.1, 5.2–5.8, and 4.2–4.8). The purified pI 5.2–5.8 and pI 4.2–4.8 enzymes have molecular weights of 173 and 71 kDa, respectively. The N-terminal amino acid of the 5.2–5.8 pI enzyme is blocked and the N-terminal amino acid sequence of the 4.2–4.8 pI enzyme is different from that of forms 1 and 2 rabbit amidase/carboxylesterase. Neither enzyme has amidase activity. PROBST et al. (1991) purified a different type of amidase/carboxylesterase from human liver. It is a 45-kDa protein and catalyzes the hydrolysis of 2-AAF and 4-NPA. Its N-terminal amino acid sequence is not homologous to that of either form of the rabbit enzymes (Table 2).

It has been reported that monocytes in human blood contain as many as four carboxylesterase isozymes with pI values between 7.5 and 7.8. One of them has been purified (SABOORI and NEWCOMBE 1990). It is a trimer (60 kDa subunit weight), and its pI is 7.5–7.8; it does not hydrolyze either 2-AAF or N-OH-AAF. Another 60-kDa carboxylesterase, which may be different from the one just described, has been purified from human alveolar macrophages (MUNGER et al. 1991). Its N-terminal amino acid sequence (Table 2) is homologous to that of human liver enzyme purified by HOSOKAWA (1990), and its partial cDNA sequence is similar to that of a cDNA of human liver carboxylesterase (LONG et al. 1991).

VIII. Monkey

Two different amidases/carboxylesterases have been purified to electrophoretic homogeneity (HOSOKAWA et al. 1990). Their pIs and subunit weights are 5.5 and 4.7, and 60 and 63 kDa, respectively. Their N-terminal amino acid sequences are homologous to that of rabbit form 1 enzyme (Table 2).

IX. Pig

Hosokawa (1990) and Matsushima et al. (1991) have purified an amidase/carboxylesterase from pig liver, and Takahashi et al. (1989) have purified another enzyme from pig intestinal mucosa. The N-terminal amino acid sequences of these enzymes are homologous to that of rabbit form 1 enzyme (Table 2). The intestinal enzyme is a trimer (58-kDa subunit weight). It is a glycoprotein, and the subunit contains three residues each of mannose and N-acetylglucosamine (Takahashi et al. 1989). The liver enzyme has a pI of 5.2–5.4 and a subunit weight of 58–62 kDa (Hosokawa 1990).

X. Cow

An amidase/carboxylesterase purified from cow liver has a pI of 6.0 and a subunit weight of 64 kDa (Hosokawa 1990). Its N-terminal amino acid sequence is homologous to that of rabbit form 1 enzyme (Table 2).

D. Physical and Chemical Characteristics of Amidases/Carboxylesterases

I. Amino Acid Compositions and Amino Acid Sequences

Most of the amidases/carboxylesterases purified so far are homologous to either form 1 or form 2 enzymes of rabbit liver (Table 2), and the amino acid compositions of these enzymes purified from various species are very similar (Mentlein et al. 1980; Hosokawa et al. 1990).

Amino acid sequences have been derived either directly from protein or deduced from cDNA sequences. The amino acid sequences of rabbit forms 1 and 2 amidase/carboxylesterases are derived from the sequences of their tryptic peptides (Korza and Ozols 1988; Ozols 1989). Forms 1 and 2 enzymes have 539 and 532 amino acid residues, respectively (Ozols 1989). Their amino acid sequences are 50% identical, and their N-terminal sequences are different (Fig. 2).

cDNAs have been cloned for rat liver pI 6.0 amidase/carboxylesterase (Es-10; Robbi et al. 1990), a rat liver 59-kDa amidase/carboxylesterase (Long et al. 1988; Takagi et al. 1988), mouse egasyn (Es-22; Ovnic et al. 1991a) and Es-N esterase (Ovnic et al. 1991b), a pig liver amidase (Matsushima et al. 1991), human liver pI 6.0 carboxylesterase (Long et al. 1991), and a human alveolar macrophage carboxylesterase (Munger et al. 1991). Amino acid sequences have been deduced from the DNA sequences of these clones. Their N-terminal amino acid sequences are shown in Table 2.

The C-terminal amino acid sequences are: (a) -EHIEL for rabbit form 1 (Korza and Ozols 1988); (b) -HTEL for rabbit form 2 (Ozols 1989);

(c) -HTEHT for rat 59-kDa carboxylesterases (LONG et al. 1988; TAKAGI et al. 1988); (d) -HVEL (ROBBI et al. 1990) for rat liver pI 6.0; (e) -HAEL for a pig liver enzyme (MATSUSHIMA et al. 1991); and (f) -EHIEL for human liver pI 6.0 and an alveolar macrophage esterase (LONG et al. 1991; MUNGER et al. 1991). The motif -HXEL is a signal for the retention of these enzymes by endoplasmic reticulum, and the -HTEHT end indicates that the enzyme is to be secreted out of the cells (ROBBI and BEAUFAY 1992). Since the C termini of the cDNA clones of LONG et al. (1988) and TAKAGI et al. (1988) signify secreted esterases for these two clones, these two cDNA may not encode the mRNA of Es-10 (pI 6.0) amidase/carboxylesterase.

Transfection of COS cells with the cDNA clones which encode carboxylesterases results in the expression of active carboxylesterases (ROBBI and BEAUFAY 1992; OVNIC et al. 1991a).

II. Glycosylation Sites

Concanavalin A binds to pI 5.0, 6.0, and 6.5 rat liver amidases/carboxylesterases, suggesting these enzymes are polymannose type proteins (ROBBI and BEAUFAY 1983). This property has been utilized for the purification of many amidases/carboxylesterases with a con A column (HOSOKAWA 1990; TAKAHASHI et al. 1989). Treatment with endo-β-N-acetylglucosaminidase H decreases the mass weight of rat liver pI 6.5 (ROBBI and BEAUFAY 1988) and rabbit liver form 2 (OZOLS 1989), and the subunit weight of dog pI 5.6 (SONE et al. 1994) by 2 kDa. A pig amidase/carboxylesterase contains 3 mol each of mannose and glucosamine in each subunit (TAKAHASHI et al. 1989).

The glycosylation sites of esterases have an amino acid motif of N-X-S/T. This motif is found in the protein sequences of rabbit amidase/carboxylesterase forms 1 and 2 (Fig. 2) and in the sequences deduced from cDNA of other species. The asparaginyl residues of potential glycosylation sites in these proteins are shown in Table 3.

III. Active Sites

Organic phosphates, such as diisopropylphosphofluoridate (DFP) and bis(4-nitrophenyl)phosphate (BPNP), bind to serine and histidine residues of amidases/carboxylesterases and deactivate these enzymes. This allows for the identification of active sites of these enzymes. The amino acid sequences of the active sites are identical for enzymes prepared from different species. The sequences are as follows (the active sites are in boldface): V-T-I-F-G-E-**S**-A-G-G-, D-**H**-G-D-E-. The locations of these serine and histidine residues in rabbit forms 1 and 2 enzymes (Fig. 2) and in cDNA deduced sequences in other species are listed in Table 3. It is interesting to note that the 45-kDa amidase/carboxylesterase of human liver lacks an active site -G-X-S-X-G- motif (PROBST et al. 1991).

IV. Antigenicities

Amidases/carboxylesterases share a certain degree of cross-species antigenicity (Table 4). The polyclonal antibodies against rat pI 6.0 enzyme react with all the enzymes from other species, with the exception of monkey MK2 enzyme. The antibodies raised against the enzymes from other species, with the exception of the one raised against monkey MK2 enzyme, react with the enzymes from other species and with rat pI 6.0 enzyme. Thus, these carboxylesterases may be analogous to rat pI 6.0 enzyme. A polyclonal antibody raised against rat pI 6.0 enzyme (LONG et al. 1989) reacts with dog pI 5.6 enzyme and, conversely, a monoclonal antibody against dog pI 5.6 enzyme also reacts with the rat pI 6.0 enzyme (SONE et al. 1994).

E. Catalytic Properties

I. Catalytic Activities

Substrates that can be hydrolyzed by the amidases/carboxylesterases are listed in Table 2. Most of the enzymes can catalyze *N*- and *O*-deacylation. Since hepatic microsomes from various species are capable of *N*,*O*-acyltransfer (GLOWINSKI et al. 1983), their amidases/carboxylesterases may also be able to catalyze the same reaction. Purified amidases/carboxylesterases from the liver of rat (Table 5), dog (Table 6), and hamster (SONE et al. 1992) can catalyze *N*,*O*-acyltransfer. Amidases/carboxylesterases of dog liver also catalyze *N*-acetylation (Table 6), whereas that of rat liver cannot (WANG et al. 1992). The ability of *N*-acetylation of hepatic microsomes in species other than rat and dog has not been investigated.

Table 5. Catalytic activities of purified rat hepatic microsomal amidases/carboxylesterases (WANG et al. 1992)

	O-Deacetylation of 4-NPA[a]		*N*,*O*-Acyltransfer of N-OH-FAF[b]		2-AAF deacetylation[b] (nMol/min per mg protein)	N-OH-AFF deacetylation[b] (nMol/min per mg protein)
	K_m (m*M*)	V_{max} (nMol/min per mg protein)	K_m (m*M*)	V_{max} (nMol/min per mg protein)		
pI 5.0	0.10	670	0.01	0.57	4.4	143
pI 5.5	0.10	840	0.02	5.94	22.4	5.1
pI 6.0	0.06	5300	0.06	1.18	0.1	14.8
pl 6.5	0.28	15200	0.02	6.32	3.8	15.7

4-NPA, 4-nitrophenyl acetate; N-OH-FAF; *N*-hydroxy-*N*-formyl-2-aminofluorene; 2-AAF, *N*-acetyl-2-aminofluorene; N-OH-AAF, *N*-hydroxy-*N*-acetyl-2-aminofluorene; K_m, Michaelis constant; V_{max}, maximum velocity.
[a] Determined at 24°C.
[b] Determined at 37°C.

Table 6. Catalytic activity of partially purified dog hepatic microsomal amidases/carboxylesterases (SONE et al. 1991)

Enzyme	2-AF acetylation (nMol/min per mg protein)	2-AAF deacetylation (nMol/min per mg protein)	N-OH-AAF deacetylation (nMol/min per mg protein)	N-OH-AFF *N,O*-acetyltransfer (pMol/min per mg protein)	4-NPA deacetylation (μMol/min per mg protein)
Enzyme I (pI 5.6)	3.51	8.33	40.74	875.93	13.33
Enzyme II (pI 4.9)	2.07	4.11	1.37	23.68	0.08
Enzyme III	0.39	1.21	12.2	99.3	7.0

2-AF, 2-aminofluorene; 2-AAF, *N*-acetyl-2-aminofluorene; N-OH-AAF, *N*-hydroxy-*N*-acetyl-2-aminofluorene; 4-NPA, 4-nitrophenyl acetate.

II. Reaction Mechanisms

N- and *O*-deacylation and transacylation probably involve the same active sites of amidases/carboxylesterases. These reactions have been postulated to proceed through an acyl–enzyme intermediate (GOLDBERG and FRUTON 1970; GREENZAID and JENCKS 1971), followed by a nucleophilic attack resulting in deacylation or transacylation (BOYER and PETERSON 1992).

The first step involves the production of an acyl–enzyme intermediate from the ester group. BOYER and PETERSON (1992) stated that this step requires first nucleophilic attack of the active serine hydroxyl on the carbonyl carbon of the ester, which results in a transient tetrahedral intermediate that quickly collapses to yield an alcohol and the acyl–enzyme intermediate. They further stated that the second step, cleavage of the acyl–enzyme intermediate, involves nucleophilic attack of either water (hydrolysis) or an alcohol (transesterification), with the participation of histidine and the carboxylic acid residue in a concerted proton shuttle. The transition state passes through another tetrahedral intermediate, which collapses to yield the transesterified product. It has been postulated that there are two basic rate-determining steps in the transesterification reaction. These include the formation of the acyl–enzyme intermediate and partitioning of the intermediate between water and the alcohol. In addition to alcohol, amines have been demonstrated to act as nucleophiles. In order for the transesterification reaction to proceed, a mechanism must exist that enhances the molar reactivity of alcohols relative to water. This mechanism has been suggested to involve a hydrophobic alcohol-binding domain near the active site that appears to be saturable and inhibitable by competitive, nonreactive compounds such as acetone and dioxane.

Although this mechanism has been proposed for *O*-deacylation and transesterification, the same mechanism could conceivably proceed for *N*-deacylation and transamidation.

III. Enzyme Inhibition

1. Substrate Inhibition

High concentrations of acetylcholine are known to inhibit its hydrolysis by acetylcholinesterase (KRUPKA and LAIDLER 1961). In a kinetic study of the hydrolysis of 4-NPA by purified rat liver enzymes, we found that the pI 6.0 enzyme, but not other rat enzymes, is inhibited by increased concentrations of 4-NPA (Fig. 5). Limited solubility of the substrates N-OH-FAF and acetylated aminobiphenyls may preclude the observation of substrate inhibition of *N,O*-acyltransfer of N-OH-FAF and *N*-deacetylation of arylamides (SERTKAYA and GORROD 1988). Binding of the substrate to the alcohol-binding site of the acyl–enzyme intermediate, due to a high concentration of the substrate, may retard the release of the acyl group from the acyl–enzyme complex (KRUPKA and LAIDLER 1961). In contrast to 4-NPA, isoarecaidine propylester shows substrate activation at high concentrations of this substrate for the pI 6.0 enzyme (MENTLEIN and HEYMANN 1984).

2. Inactivation of Active Sites

Organophosphorus compounds which can phosphorylate the active site serine residue irreversibly inhibit amidases/carboxylesterases. These include paraoxon, soman, DFP, and BPNP (GAUSTAD et al. 1991a). BPNP and bis(4-cyanophenyl)phosphate are rather specific for liver amidases/carboxylesterases, exhibit a low toxicity, and can be used for in vivo experiments. BPNP shows a preference for the pI 5.5 amidase/carboxylesterase (HEYMANN and MENTLEIN 1981). The *N*-deacetylation activities of mouse liver microsomes are inhibited by BPNP treatment both in vitro and in vivo (LAI et al. 1988).

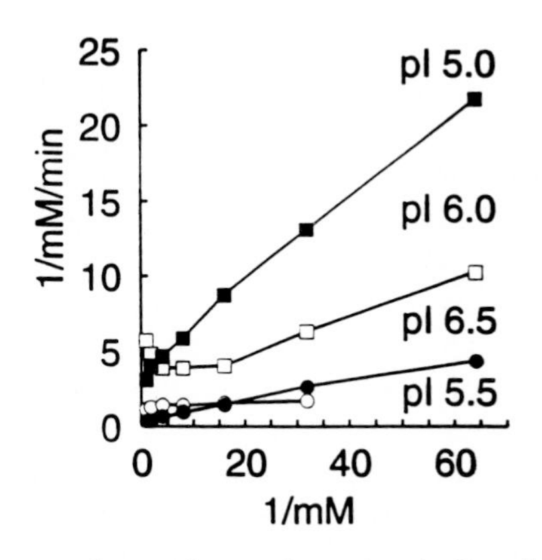

Fig. 5. Lineweaver-Burk plots of rat hepatic 4-nitrophenyl acetate (4-NPA) deacetylases. Substrate inhibition is found only for the pI 6.0 (Es-10) amidase/carboxylesterase

Contradictory results have been reported with regard to the involvement of cysteines in the active sites of amidases/carboxylesterases. 4-Chloromercuribenzoate (HEYMANN 1980) and iodoacetamide (SONE et al. 1991) do not inhibit amidases/carboxylesterases, suggesting that cysteine residues may not be involved in the catalytic activity of these enzymes. On the other hand, 4-chloromercuribenzoate has been reported to inhibit the deacetylation of N-OH-AAF and N-OH-FAF by guinea pig hepatic microsomes (GLOWINSKI et al. 1983). Additionally, the hydrolysis of *N*-hydroxy-*N*-2-monochloroacetylaminofluorene by guinea pig microsomes is inhibited by this substrate (WEEKS et al. 1980). These results suggest that cysteine residues may be involved. A histidine residue has been suggested to be involved in the active site of these enzymes. Acetyl leucine chloromethyl ketone reacts with the histidine residue of acylpeptide hydrolase, a serine hydrolase, and irreversibly inhibits this enzyme (SCALONI et al. 1992). This compound has yet to be investigated for inhibition of amidases/carboxylesterases.

F. Regulation of Expression of Amidases/Carboxylesterases

I. Regulation by Amidase/Carboxylesterase Genes

A locus map of the mouse, with comparative map points of human on mouse, has been compiled by HILLYARD et al. (1992). Esterase gene foci form two major clusters (Es-1, Es-28, Es-N, Es-6, Es-22, and Es-9; Es-2, Es-11, Es-23, and Es-7) in chromosome 8 of the mouse. Other esterase genes are scattered in chromosomes 3, 7, 8, 9, 11, 12, 14, and 19. Human esterase genes are mainly clustered in chromosome 16 (Es-1, Es-28, Es-6, Es-22, Es-9, Es-2, Es-11, and Es-23), although other esterase genes are located in chromosomes 3, 6, 11, 13, and 19. In contrast to these two species, rat esterase genes map into linkage group V (LG V) in chromosome 19 (HEDRICH and VON DEIMLING 1987; PRAVENEC et al. 1992).

Fifteen esterases have been reported for the rat, 12 of which are carboxylesterases that map into LG V (PRAVENEC et al. 1992). These esterase genes form two clusters in LG V. Es-2, Es-3, Es-4, Es-7, Es-8, Es-9, and Es-10 are located at cluster 1, and Es-1, Es-14, Es-15, Es-16 and Es-18 are located at cluster 2 (HEDRICH and VON DEIMLING 1987). Each gene is represented by only a small number of different alleles (HEDRICH and VON DEIMLING 1987). Rat liver amidase/carboxylesterase pI 5.0, pI 5.5, pI 6.0, and pI 6.5 are expressed by Es-15, Es-3, Es-10, and Es-4, respectively (MENTLEIN et al. 1987, 1988). The expression of these enzymes in different strains of rats is primarily regulated by the alleles of these genes. This is evidenced by the observation that liver carboxylesterase activities in different strains of rats are related to the genotype of egasyn (Es-3; NAKAMURA et al. 1989).

II. Regulation by Hormones

1. Regulation by Sex Hormones

The total carboxylesterase activity of liver microsomes is very low in 3-day-old rats, but increases considerably when the animals reach puberty. This occurs in both male and female rats. The pI 5.0 (Es-15) enzyme increases similarly in both male and female until puberty; afterwards, it levels off in females and decreases markedly in males (Robbi and Beaufay 1983). In adult rats, there is more pI 5.5 (Es-3) enzyme in female than in male rats (Hosokawa et al. 1987). In contrast, there are more pI 6.0 (Es-10) and 6.5 (Es-4) enzyme in male than in female rats (Robbi and Beaufay 1983; Hosokawa et al. 1987). Furthermore, castration decreases the pI 6.0 and 6.5 enzyme in the liver of male rats, but increases these enzymes in the liver of female rats. Castration decreases liver pI 5.5 enzyme in female rats, but does not affect that of male rats (Hosokawa et al. 1987). These results suggest that Es-10 and Es-4 may be positively regulated by testosterone, while Es-3 and Es-15 may be positively regulated by estrogen.

2. Regulation by Pituitary Hormones

Pituitary hormones regulate rat liver amidases/carboxylesterases. Removal of pituitary gland in the male rat reduces pI 6.5 amidase/carboxylesterase, but it has no effect on the pI 6.0 and pI 5.5 amidases/carboxylesterases. Human growth hormone reduces all three enzymes, and prolactin reduces the pI 6.5 and 6.0 enzymes in hypophysectomized rat (Hosokawa and Satoh 1988).

3. Regulation by Pancreatic Hormones

Insulin increases and glucagon reduces the amount of hepatic microsomal esterases. It has been suggested that while both hormones reduce the turnover of esterases, glucagon decreases the de novo synthesis of esterases (Heymann et al. 1979).

III. Enzyme Induction

Phenobarbital induces rat hepatic microsomal amidase (Raftell et al. 1977), *N*,*O*-acyltransferase, and carboxylesterase (Wang et al. 1992). This appears to be due to an increase in the amount of pI 5.0 (Robbi and Beaufay 1983), pI 5.5, and 6.0 (Hosokawa et al. 1987) amidases/carboxylesterases. The induction of these enzymes occurs in both male and female rats (Robbi and Beaufay 1983; Hosokawa et al. 1987).

Hydrocortisone and its derivatives induce hepatic microsomal esterase and amidase in the rat (Kaur et al. 1991), whereas 3-methylcholanthrene and benzo[a]pyrene do not (Ali et al. 1985). Aminopyrine induces the pI

5.5 and pI 6.5, but not pI 6.0, enzymes in male rats. The pI 5.5, but not pI 6.0 or 6.5, enzyme in male rats is induced by *trans*-stilbene oxide and Aroclor 1254. Clofibrate induces the pI 5.5, 6.0, and 6.5 enzymes (HOSOKAWA et al. 1988).

G. Role of Amidase/Carboxylesterase in Arylacetamide Toxicities and Carcinogenicities

With the exception of the dog, which has only a limited capacity of acetylation of arylamines, mammals are capable of both acetylation of arylamines and deacetylation of arylamides. Thus, arylamine levels following exposure to either an arylamine or arylamide are likely to be dependent on the overall capacities of these two enzyme systems.

I. Toxicity of Phenacetin and Acetaminophen

Phenacetin is known to be nephrotoxic, hepatotoxic, and carcinogenic. It also causes hemolytic anemia and methemoglobinemia. Production of methemoglobin in the rat by phenacetin is inhibited by BPNP and by 4-aminobenzoic acid. The latter is a substrate of *N*-acetylase and is likely to be an inhibitor of the reacetylation of phenetidine. *N*-Hydroxyphenetidine, a metabolite of deacetylated phenacetin, produces methemoglobin and hemolysis. These findings suggest that *N*-deacetylation is critical for the hematotoxicity of phenacetin (JENSEN and JOLLOW 1991).

The analgesic drug acetaminophen, a de-ethylated metabolite of phenacetin, is nephrotoxic in the rat and mouse. BPNP inhibits in vitro binding of acetaminophen to rat kidney microsomal protein and reduces the nephrotoxicity of acetaminophen in vivo in the rat (NEWTON et al. 1985). However, the nephrotoxicity and hepatotoxicity of acetaminophen in the mouse are not inhibited by either BPNP or tri-*O*-tolyl-phosphate. Immunochemical analysis of kidneys from acetaminophen-treated mice demonstrates covalently bound acetylated metabolite of acetaminophen. Thus, the nephrotoxicity of both phenacetin and acetaminophen is probably not related to deacetylation (HART et al. 1991).

II. Carcinogenicity of Arylamines

Arylamines are known to induce tumors of the urinary bladder in humans and tumors of this organ as well as others in experimental animals (GARNER et al. 1984). Evidence has been presented which indicates that this class of carcinogens is activated by the esterification of the arylhydroxylamine metabolites (MILLER and MILLER 1981). Acetylation of arylhydroxylamines and internal acetyltransfer of arylacetohydroxamic acids occur in the target organs of arylamines/arylamides, and the reactions are carried out by cytosolic enzymes (KING 1974). Therefore, cytosolic acetyltransferases play a role in the tumor induction by these carcinogens (KING 1985). The dog, which is sensitive to the carcinogenicity of arylamines/arylamides, lacks the cytosolic enzymes (LOWER and BRYAN 1973). Thus, the activation of this class of carcinogens in the dog appears to be due to the acetyltransfer activity of microsomal amidases/carboxylesterases which are present in dog bladder epithelial cells, the target of the carcinogens (WANG et al. 1985; SONE et al. 1991).

Deacetylation may also be important in the activation of arylamides in the liver of rat and mouse. Paraoxon and BPNP inhibit the deacetylation of 2-AAF and the incorporation of this carcinogen to the DNA in cultured rat hepatocytes. These organophosphates inhibit the deacetylation, but they do not inhibit the incorporation of the carcinogen into the DNA of cultured human hepatocytes (MONTEITH and STROM 1990). It is believed that the activation of 2-AAF in human hepatocytes is by *N,O*-acyltransferase (MONTEITH 1992). Thus, deacetylation appears to be important for the activation of arylamides in rat hepatocytes, but may not be important in human cells.

Preincubation of liver microsomes from infant male $B6C3F_1$ mice with BPNP or paraoxon reduces the deacetylation activity of the microsomes for N-OH-AAF. Pretreatment of the infant mice with BPNP before the administration of N-OH-AAF reduces the hepatic N-(deoxyguanosine-8-yl)-AF adduct levels. However, this pretreatment does not affect the levels of the acetylated adduct, N-(deoxyguanosine-8-yl)-AAF. The initiation of liver tumors by N-OH-AAF is also inhibited by this organophosphate pretreatment. On the other hand, pretreatment with BPNP does not affect the levels of hepatic DNA-N-(deoxyguanosine-8-yl)-AF adduct or the liver tumor initiation by N-OH-AF. These results demonstrate that deacetylation of N-OH-AAF to *N*-hydroxyl-2-aminofluorene is essential for the metabolic activation and liver tumor initiation in infant male $B6C3F_1$ mice by N-OH-AAF (LAI et al. 1988).

References

Aldridge WN (1952) Two types of esterase (A and B) hydrolyzing *p*-nitrophenyl acetate, propionate and butyrate and a method for their determination. Biochem J 53:110–117

Ali B, Kaur S, James EC, Parmar SS (1985) Identification and characterization of hepatic carboxylesterases hydrolyzing hydrocortisone esters. Biochem Pharmacol 34:1881–1886

Boyer CS, Petersen DR (1992) Enzymatic basis for the transesterification of cocaine in the presence of ethanol: evidence for the participation of microsomal carboxylesterases. J Pharmacol Exp Ther 260:939–946

Chiou CY (1971) Deformylation of 4,4′-diformamidodiphenyl sulfone (DFD) by mammalian liver homogenates. Biochem Pharmacol 20:2401–2408

Clark NWE, Scott RC, Foster J, Blain PG, Williams FM (1992) Esterase distribution in human and rat skin. Toxicol Lett Suppl 125

Franklin MR, Bridges JW, Williams RT (1971) The enzymic deacetylation of 4-acetamidobenzoic acid by rat tissues and the effect of manganese ions. Xenobiotica 1:121–130

Fujimoto D (1974) Serotonin-sensitive aryl acylamidase in rat brain. Biochem Biophys Res Commun 61:72–74

Garner RC, Martin CN, Clayson DB (1984) Carcinogenic aromatic amines and related compounds. In: Searles CE (ed) Chemical carcinogens, vol 1. American Chemical Society, Washington, pp 175–276

Gaustad R, Johnsen H, Fonnum F (1991a) Carboxylesterases in guinea pig. A comparison of the different isoenzymes with regard to inhibition by organophosphorus compounds in vivo and in vitro. Biochem Pharmacol 42:1335–1343

Gaustad R, Sletten K, Lovhaug D, Fonnum F (1991b) Purification and characterization of carboxylesterases from rat lung. Biochem J 274:693–697

Gleason LN, Vough BP (1971) Deformylation of 4,4′-diformamidodiphenyl sulfone (DFD) by plasma of certain mammals. Biochem Pharmacol 20:2409–2416

Glowinski IB, Savage L, Lee M-S, King CM (1983) Relationship between nucleic acid adduct formation and deacetylation of arylhydroxamic acids. Carcinogenesis 4:67–75

Goldberg MI, Fruton JS (1970) Kinetics of acyl transfer by beef liver esterase. Biochemistry 9:3371–3378

Greenzaid P, Jencks WP (1971) Pig liver esterase. Reactions with alcohols, structure-reactivity correlations, and the acyl-enzyme intermediate. Biochemistry 10:1210–1222

Harano T, Miyata T, Lee S, Aoyagi H, Omura T (1988) Biosynthesis and localization of rat liver microsomal carboxylesterase E1. J Biochem 103:149–155

Hart SGE, Beierschmitt WP, Bartolone JB, Wyand DS, Khairallah EA, Cohen SD (1991) Evidence against deacetylation and for cytochrome P450-mediated activation in acetaminophen-induced nephrotoxicity in the CD-1 mouse. Toxicol Appl Pharmacol 107:1–15

Hedrich HJ, von Deimling O (1987) Re-evaluation of LG V of the rat and assignment of 12 carboxylesterases to two gene clusters. J Hered 78:92–96

Heymann E (1980) Carboxylesterases and amidases. In: Jacoby WB (ed) Enzymatic detoxification, vol 2. Academic, New York, pp 291–323

Heymann E, Mentlein R (1981) Carboxlyesterases–amidases. Methods Enzymol 77:333–344

Heymann E, Mentlein R, Schmalz R, Schwabe C, Wagenmann F (1979) A method for the estimation of esterase synthesis and degradation and its application to evaluate the influence of insulin and glucagon. Eur J Biochem 102:509–519

Hillyard AL, Doolittle DP, Davisson MT, Roderick TH (1992) Locus map of mouse with comparative map points of human on mouse. Jackson Laboratory, Bar Harbor

Hosokawa M (1990) Differences in the functional roles of hepatic microsomal carboxylesterase isozymes in various mammals and humans. Xenobiotic Metab Dispos 5:953–963

Hosokawa M, Satoh T (1988) Effects of hypophysectomy and pituitary hormones on hepatic microsomal carboxylesterase isozymes in male rats. Res Commun Chem Pathol Pharmacol 62:279–288

Hosokawa M, Maki T, Satoh T (1987) Multiplicity and regulation of hepatic microsomal carboxylesterases in rats. Mol Pharmacol 31:579–584

Hosokawa M, Maki T, Satoh T (1988) Differences in the induction of carboxylesterase isozymes in rat liver microsomes by xenobiotics. Biochem Pharmacol 37:2708–2711

Hosokawa M, Maki T, Satoh T (1990) Characterization of molecular species of liver microsomal carboxylesterases of several animal species and humans. Arch Biochem Biophys 277:219–227

Irving CC (1966) Enzymatic deacetylation of *N*-hydroxy-2-acetylaminofluorene by liver microsomes. Cancer Res 26:1390–1396

Irving CC (1979) Species and tissues variations in the metabolic activation of aromatic amines. In: Griffin AC, Shaw CR (eds) Carcinogens: identification and mechanisms. Raven, New York, pp 211–227

Jarvinen M, Santti RSS, Hopsu-Havu VK (1971) Partial purification and characterization of two enzymes from guinea-pig liver microsomes that hydrolyze carcinogenic amides 2-acetylaminofluorene and *N*-hydroxy-2-acetylaminofluourene. Biochem Pharmacol 20:2971–2982

Jensen CB, Jollow DJ (1991) The role of *N*-hydroxyphenetidine in phenacetin-induced hemolytic anemia. Toxicol Appl Pharmacol 111:1–12

Kaur S, Khanna P, Parmar SS, Ali B (1991) Selective stimulation of carboxylesterases metabolizing charged steroid esters by hydrocortisone. Biochem Pharmacol 41:476–478

Ketterman AJ, Bowles MR, Pond SM (1989) Purification an characterization of two human liver carboxylesterases. Int J Biochem 21:1303–1312

King CM (1974) Mechanism of reaction, tissue distribution and inhibition of arylhydroxamic acid acyltransferase. Cancer Res 34:1503–1515

King CM (1985) Metabolism and the "initiation" of tumors by chemicals. In: Marnett LJ (ed) Arachidonic acid metabolism and tumor initiation. Nijhoff, Boston, pp 1–37

Korza G, Ozols J (1988) Complete covalent structure of 60-kDa esterase isolated from 2,3,7,8,-tetrachlorodibenzo-*p*-dioxin-induced rabbit liver microsomes. J Biol Chem 263:3486–3495

Krupka RM, Laidler KJ (1961) Molecular mechanisms for hydrolytic enzyme action. II. Inhibition of acetylcholinesterase by excess substrate. J Am Chem Soc 83:1448–1454

Lai CC, Miller EC, Miller JA, Liem A (1988) The essential role of microsomal deacetylase activity in the metabolic activation, DNA-(deoxyguanosin-8-yl)-2-aminofluorene adduct formation and initiation of liver tumors by *N*-hydroxy-2-acetylaminofluorene in the livers of infant male B6C3F_1 mice. Carcinogenesis 9:1295–1302

Land SJ, Zukowski K, Lee M-S, Debiec-Rychter M, King CM, Wang CY (1989) Metabolism of aromatic amines: relationships of *N*-acetylation, *O*-acetylation, *N,O*-acetyltransfer and deacetylation in human liver and bladder. Carcinogenesis 10:727–731

Long RM, Satoh H, Martin BM, Kimura S, Gonzales FJ, Pohl LR (1988) Rat liver carboxylesterase: cDNA cloning, sequencing, and evidence for a multigene family. Biochem Biophys Res Commun 156:866–873

Long RM, Calabrese MR, Martin BM, Pohl LR (1991) Cloning and sequencing of a human liver carboxylesterase isoenzyme. Life Sci 48:PL-43–PL-49

Lower GM Jr, Bryan GT (1973) Enzymatic *N*-acetylation of carcinogenic aromatic amines by liver cytosol of species displaying different organ susceptibilities. Biochem Pharmacol 22:1581–1588

Lower GM Jr, Bryan GT (1976) Enzymic deacetylation of carcinogenic arylacetamides by tissue microsomes of the dog and other species. J Toxicol Environ Health 1:421–432

Matsushima M, Inoue H, Ichinose M, Tsukada S, Miki K, Kurokawa K, Takahashi T, Takahashi K (1991) The nucleotide and deduced amino acid sequences of porcine liver proline-β-naphthylamidase. FEBS Lett 293:37–41

Medda S, Takeuchi K, Devore-Carter D, von Deimling O, Heymann E, Swank RT (1987) An accessory protein identical to mouse egasyn is complexed with rat microsomal β-glucuronidase and is identical to rat esterase-3. J Biol Chem 262:7248–7253

Mentlein R, Heymann E (1984) Hydrolysis of ester- and amide-type drugs by the purified isoenzymes of nonspecific carboxylesterase from rat liver. Biochem Pharmacol 33:1243–1248

Mentlein R, Heiland S, Heymann E (1980) Simultaneous purification and comparative characterization of six serine hydrolases from rat liver microsomes. Arch Biochem Biophys 200:547–559

Mentlein R, Suttorp M, Heymann E (1984) Specificity of purified monoacylglycerol lipase, palmitoyl-CoA hydrolase, palmitoyl-carnitine hydrolase, and nonspecific carboxylesterase from rat liver microsomes. Arch Biochem Biophys 228:230–246

Mentlein R, Rix-Matzen H, Heymann E (1988) Subcellular localization of nonspecific carboxylesterases, acylcarnitine hydrolase, monoacylglycerol lipase and palmitoyl-CoA hydrolase in rat liver. Biochim Biophys Acta 964:319–328

Mentlein R, Ronai A, Robbi M, Heymann E, von Deimling O (1987) Genetic identification of rat liver carboxylesterases isolated in different laboratories. Biochim Biophys Acta 913:27–38

Miller EC, Miller JA (1981) Mechanisms of chemical carcinogenesis. Cancer 47: 1055–1064

Monteith DK (1992) Inhibition of sulfotransferase in primary cultures of human hepatocytes affecting metabolism and binding of 2-acetylaminofluorene. Cancer Lett 64:109–115

Monteith DK, Strom SC (1990) A comparison of the inhibition of deacetylase in primary cultures of rat and human hepatocytes effecting metabolism and DNA-binding of 2-acetylaminofluorene. Cell Biol Toxicol 6:269–284

Munger JS, Shi G-P, Mark EA, Chin DT, Gerard C, Chapman HA (1991) A serine esterase released by human alveolar macrophages is closely related to liver microsomal carboxylesterase. J Biol Chem 266:18832–18838

Nakamura T, Satoh T, Horie T, Segami F, Tagaya O (1989) Strain differences of rat liver carboxylesterase activities related to the phenotype difference of esterase-3 (egasyn). Res Commun Chem Pathol Pharmacol 66:451–459

Newton JF, Kuo C-H, DeShone DM, Hoffle D, Bernstein J, Hook JB (1985) The role of *p*-aminophenol in acetaminophen-induced nephrotoxicity: effect of bias(*p*-nitrophenyl)phosphate on acetaminophen and *p*-aminophenol nephrotoxicity and metabolism in Fischer 344 rats. Toxicol Appl Pharmacol 81:416–430

Ovnic M, Swank RT, Fletcher C, Zhen L, Novak EK, Baumann H, Heintz N, Ganschow RE (1991a) Characterization and functional expression of a cDNA encoding egasyn (esterase-22): the endoplasmic reticulum-targeting protein of β-glucuronidase. Genomics 11:956–967

Ovnic M, Tepperman K, Medda S, Elliott RW, Stephenson DA, Grant SG, Ganschow RE (1991b) Characterization of a murine cDNA encoding a member of the carboxylesterase multigene family. Genomics 9:344–354

Ozols J (1987) Isolation and characterization of a 60-kilodalton glycoprotein esterase from liver microsomal membranes. J Biol Chem 262:15316–15321

Ozols J (1989) Isolation, properties, and the complete amino acid sequence of a second form of 60-kDa glycoprotein esterase. J Biol Chem 264:12533–12545

Pravenec M, Simonet L, Kren V, St Lenzin E, Levan G, Szpirer J, Szpirer C, Kurtz T (1992) Assignment of rat linkage group V to chromosome 19 by single strand conformation polymorphism analysis of somatic cell hybrids. Genomics 12:350–356

Probst MR, Jeno P, Meyer UA (1991) Purification and characterization of a human liver arylacetamide deacetylase. Biochem Biophys Res Commu 177:453–459

Raftell M, Berzins K, Blomberg F (1977) Immunochemical studies on a phenobarbital-inducible esterase in rat liver microsomes. Arch Biochem Biophys 181:534–541

Robbi M, Beaufay H (1983) Purification and characterization of various esterases from rat liver. Eur J Biochem 137:293–301

Robbi M, Beaufay H (1988) Immunochemical characterization and biosynthesis of pI-6.4 esterase, a carboxylesterase of rat liver microsomal extracts. Biochem J 254:51–57

Robbi M, Beaufay H (1992) Topogenesis of carboxylesterases: a rat liver isoenzyme ending in -HTEHT-COOH is a secreted protein. Biochem Biophys Res Commun 183:836–841
Robbi M, Beaufay H, Octave J-N (1990) Nucleotide sequence of cDNA coding for rat liver pI 6.1 esterase (ES-10), a carboxylesterase located in the lumen of the endoplasmic reticulum. Biochem J 269:451–458
Saboori AM, Newcombe DS (1990) Human monocyte carboxylesterase. Purification and kinetics. J Biol Chem 265:19792–19799
Satoh H, Martin BM, Schulick AH, Christ DD, Kenna JG, Pohl LR (1989) Human anti-endoplasmic reticulum antibodies in sera of patients with halothane-induced hepatitis are directed against a trifluoroacetylated carboxylesterase. Proc Natl Acad Sci USA 86:322–326
Satoh T, Kushida H, Sato G (1992) Metabolism of lipids and xenobiotics by carboxylesterases from rat intestinal mucossal membrane. Toxicol Lett Suppl 125
Scaloni A, Jones WM, Barra D, Pospischil M, Sassa S, Popowicz A, Manning LR, Schneewind O, Manning JM (1992) Acylpeptide hydrolase: inhibitors and some active site residues of the human enzyme. J Biol Chem 267:3811–3818
Sertkaya NN, Gorrod JW (1988) In vitro deacetylation studies with isomeric acetamidobiphenyls using selective carboxylesterase inhibitors. Anticancer Res 8:1345–1350
Sone T, Zukowski K, Land SJ, King CM, Wang CY (1991) Acetylation of 2-aminofluorene derivatives by dog hepatic microsomes. Carcinogenesis 12: 1887–1891
Sone T, Zukowski K, Land SJ, King CM, Martin BM, Pohl LR, Wang CY (1994) Characteristics of a purified dog hepatic microsomal *N,O*-acyltransferase. Carcinogenesis 15:in press
Sone T, Yamaguchi T, Isobe M, Takabatake E, Adachi T, Hirano K, Wang CY (1992) Purification and characterization of hamster hepatic microsomal *N,O*-acetyltransferase. Chem Pharm Bull (Tokyo) 40:2857–2859
Takagi Y, Morohashi K-I, Kawabata S-I, Go M, Omura T (1988) Molecular cloning and nucleotide sequence of cDNA of microsomal carboxylesterase E1 of rat liver. J Biochem 104:801–806
Takahashi T, Ikai A, Takahashi K (1989) Purification and characterization of proline-β-naphthylamidase, a novel enzyme from pig intestinal mucosa. J Biol Chem 264:11565–11571
Wang CY, Bryan GT (1974) Deacylation of carcinogenic 5-nitrofuran derivatives by mammalian tissues. Chem Biol Interact 9:423–428
Wang CY, Linsmaier-Bedner EM, Lee M-S (1981) Mutagenicity of the *O*-esters of *N*-acylhydroxylamines for Salmonella. Chem Biol Interact 34:267–278
Wang CY, Morton KC, Lee M-S (1985) Repair synthesis of DNA induced by the urinary *N*-hydroxy metabolites of carcinogenic arylamines in urotherlial cells of susceptible species. Cancer Res 45:221–225
Wang CY, Sone T, Zukowski K, Land S, King CM (1991) Purification of a dog hepatic microsomal *N,O*-acetyltransferase. Proc Am Assoc Cancer Res 32:119
Wang CY, Zukowski K, Lee M-S, Sone T (1992) Purification and characterization of rat hepatic *N,O*-acyltransferases. Carcinogenesis 13:2017–2020
Weeks CE, Allaben WT, Tresp NM, Louie SC, Lazear EJ, King CM (1980) Effects of structure of *N*-acyl-*N*-2-fluorenylhydroxylamines on arylhydroxamic acid acyltransferase, sulfotransferase, and deacylase activities, and on mutations in *Salmonella typhimurium* TA 1538. Cancer Res 40:1204–1211
Wu S-E, Marletta MA (1988) Carboxylesterase isozyme specific deacylation of diacetoxyscripenol (anguidine). Chem Res Toxicol 1:69–73
Yamada H, Lee M-S, Wang CY (1988) *N*- and *O*-deacetylation of *N*-acetoxy-*N*-arylacetamides by mammalian hepatic microsomes. Carcinogenesis 9:1995–2002

CHAPTER 7

O-, *N*-, and *S*-Methyltransferases

C.R. CREVELING and D.R. THAKKER

A. Introduction

The existence of methylation as a metabolic conjugation reaction was first established over a century ago when *N*-methylpyridinium metabolite was detected by HIS (1887) in dog urine after administration of pyridine. Since then, methyl transfer has been shown as one of the most widely utilized conjugation reactions in nature. A wide variety of endogenous molecules as well as xenobiotics are metabolically transformed by methyl transfer reactions; these molecules include proteins, nucleic acids, phospholipids, catecholamines, steroids, alkyl- and arylamines, and thiols. The transfer of a methyl group to a variety of heteroatoms, such as oxygen, nitrogen, and sulfur, is catalyzed by many methyltransferase enzymes with varying degree of substrate selectivity. It is interesting to note that despite a diversity of enzymes catalyzing the methyl transfer reaction, a common methyl donor is shared by all these enzymes, i.e., *S*-adenosyl-L-methionine (AdoMet). The *O*-methylation (THAKKER and CREVELING 1990; BOUDIKOVA et al. 1990; CREVELING 1993; KLEIN et al. 1992), *N*-methylation (ANSHER and JAKOBY 1990), and *S*-methylation (STEVENS and BAKKE 1990; HOFFMAN 1993) reactions have been discussed in recent comprehensive reviews. In this chapter, we will discuss recent developments in the molecular and structural biology of a few representative methyltransferases, i.e., catechol *O*-methyltransferase (COMT, EC 2.1.1.6), hydroxyindole *O*-methyltransferase (HIOMT, EC 2.1.1.4), phenethanolamine *N*-methyltransferase (PNMT, EC 2.1.1.28), histamine *N*-methyltransferase (HMT, EC 2.3.3.8), and *S*-methyltransferases. The reactions catalyzed by these enzymes are shown in Fig. 1. Important new information regarding the amino acid sequences, existence of isozymes, and tissue distribution of these enzymes has been developed by many investigators in the past 3 years. We have reviewed these studies in context of the metabolic, pharmacological, and toxicological importance of the *O*-, *N*-, and *S*-methylation reactions catalyzed by these enzymes.

B. The Methyl Transfer Reaction

While the catalytic mechanisms of various methyltransferases may differ, they all catalyze the reaction by bringing the methyl acceptor substrate,

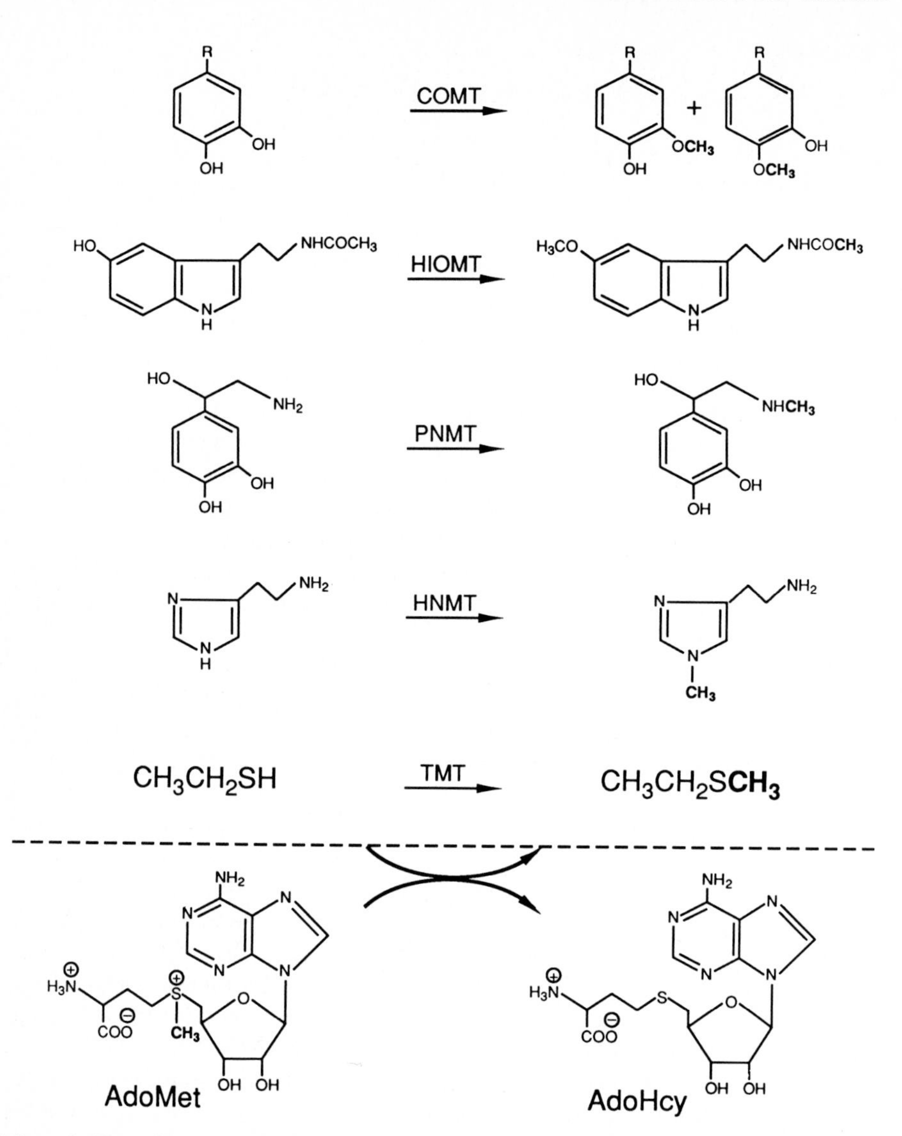

Fig. 1. Reactions catalyzed by *S*-adenosyl-L-methionine (*AdoMet*)-dependent methyltransferases. The methyltransferases shown are only representative members of this class of enzymes and do not constitute an exhaustive list of methyltransferases. *AdoHcy*, *S*-adenosylhomocysteine

specifically the heteroatom being methylated, in proximity of the electrophilic methyl group of AdoMet. This is exemplified in Fig. 2 by the methylation of a catechol substrate at the active site of COMT. In the case of the reaction catalyzed by COMT, the transfer of the methyl group to the phenolic oxygen occurs by a SN_2 mechanism. This was originally proposed by HIGAZI et al. (1976), based on an inverse α-deuterium secondary isotope

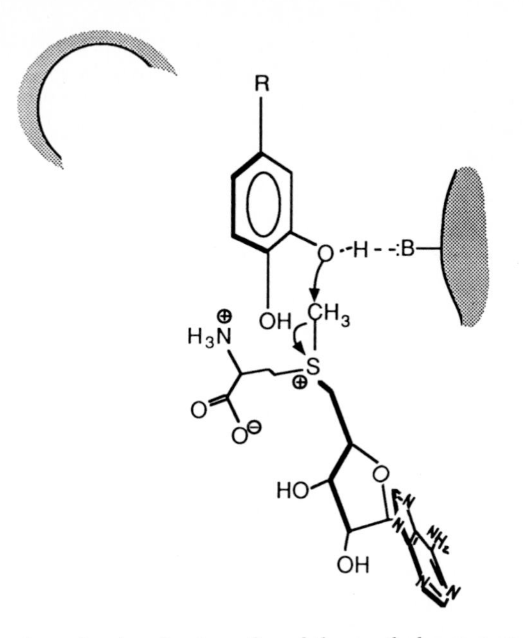

Fig. 2. The proposed mechanism for transfer of the methyl group at the active site of catechol *O*-methyltransferase (COMT) from *S*-adenosyl-L-methionine to phenolic hydroxyl group(s) of a catechol substrate. Evidence for direct methyl transfer by a SN_2 reaction has been obtained for COMT and histamine *N*-methyltransferase. It is reasonable to speculate that methyl transfer catalyzed by many other methyltransferases occurs by a similar mechanism

effect ($V_{max}H/V_{max}D = 0.832$) during methyl transfer to 3,4-dihydroxyacetophenone. Later, elegant studies by WOODWARD et al. (1980) and FLOSS and WOODWARD (1982) showed that when AdoMet with a chiral, double-labeled *S*-methyl group containing hydrogen, deuterium, and tritium was used as a methyl donor in a COMT-catalyzed reaction, the methyl group was transferred to the catechol substrate with an inversion of the configuration. This provided unequivocal evidence for a direct transfer of the methyl group from AdoMet to the catechol substrate by a SN_2 reaction. Similar studies with HMT also showed that the methyl group is directly transferred from AdoMet to histamine with concurrent inversion of configuration (ASANO et al. 1984). The kinetic studies with partially purified HMT (guinea pig brain) imply that the methyl transfer occurs via a methylated enzyme intermediate (THITHAPANDHA and COHN 1978); however, this has not been confirmed by more direct studies.

C. *S*-Adenosyl-L-Methionine

AdoMet, the methyl donor cosubstrate of most methyltransferases, was discovered by CANTONI in 1953. The critical role played by AdoMet in the regulation of a variety of critical cell functions by participating in transmethylation or transalkylation reactions has been reviewed extensively (see BORCHARDT et al. 1986). AdoMet is enzymatically synthesized from adenosine triphosphate (ATP) and L-methionine by ATP: L-methionine *S*-adenosyltransferase (EC 2.5.1.6). The diastereomer formed has *S* configuration at the chiral sulfonium center (DE LA HABA et al. 1959; CORNFORTH et al. 1977). AdoMet can also be formed by methylation of *S*-adenosylhomocysteine (AdoHcy) by N^5-methyltetrahydrofolate; however, L-methionine is the key precursor of this important cosubstrate of many methyltransferases. Administration of L-methionine intraperitonially or orally results in increased levels of AdoMet in several tissues (see MULDER and KRIJGSHELD 1984; BORCHARDT et al. 1986 for review of AdoMet biosynthesis and metabolism). In rats, the enzyme L-methionine *S*-adenosyltransferase is present in highest levels in liver, with almost 180-fold lower activity found in heart and brain. Despite this wide range of enzyme activity, the levels of AdoMet vary over a narrow range from 25 nmol/g tissue in brain to 68 nmol/g tissue in liver (ELORANTA 1977). Drugs and xenobiotics that are methylated by AdoMet-dependent methyltransferases can alter the tissue levels of AdoMet (GULDBERG and MARSDEN 1975; FULLER et al. 1983), although such effects on the levels of AdoMet are believed to be transient. Methionine analogs, such as ethionine or methionine sulfoximine, inhibit transmethylation reactions in vivo, presumably by inhibiting the biosynthesis of AdoMet (SHULL et al. 1966; VILLA-TREVINO et al. 1966; GRIFFITH et al. 1979; KREDICH and HERSHFIELD 1980; TISDALE 1980; TSUKUDA et al. 1980; ZIMMERMAN et al. 1980). Because *S*-adenosyl-L-homocysteine (AdoHcy) is a competitive inhibitor of AdoMet-dependent methyltransferase reactions (BORCHARDT et al. 1974), an alteration in the ratio of AdoMet to AdoHcy may play at least as important a role in modulating the methylation of substrates as do the absolute levels of AdoMet in various tissues.

Only the diastereomer with *S*-sulfonium center acts as a methyl donor cosubstrate in all the transmethylation reactions (DE LA HABA et al. 1959; ZAPIA et al. 1969; BORCHARDT et al. 1976b). The studies by BORCHARDT et al. (1976b) showed that even small changes in the base, sugar, or amino acid moieties caused large increases in the K_m values for many of the methyltransferases. AdoMet is converted to its demethylated product AdoHcy as a result of the transmethylation reactions (Fig. 1). AdoHcy competes for the AdoMet-binding site on many of the methyltransferases and thus is a potent inhibitor of AdoMet-dependent methyltransferases (BORCHARDT et al. 1974). It has been established that the amino and carboxylate groups on homocysteine, the six-amino group on the adenine moiety, and the 2′-hydroxyl group of the ribose moiety are required for binding of AdoHcy (and AdoMet) at the methyl donor active site of methyltransferases (COWARD et al. 1972, 1974; COWARD and SWEET 1972; COWARD and SLISZ 1973; BORCHARDT and WU 1974, 1975; BORCHARDT et al. 1974, 1976a).

D. *O*-Methylation

I. Overview

The *O*-methylation reaction, exemplified by methylation of catechols, hydroxyindoles, and carboxy groups of proteins, plays pivotal physiological, metabolic, and toxicological roles in mammalian systems. The methylation of *N*-acetylserotonin is a critical step in the biosynthesis of melatonin, a hormone implicated in the synchronization of reproductive cycles in some mammals and in affective diseases in humans (see EVERED and CLARK 1985; KARSCH et al. 1991). *O*-Methylation of aspartic and glutamic acid residues in proteins plays an important role in regulating the function of several proteins. This reaction is catalyzed by the enzyme protein carboxy *O*-methyltransferase (EC 2.1.1.24). Methylation of negatively charged amino acids at critical sites on proteins can significantly affect the three-dimensional structure of the proteins and consequently their function. Methylation and demethylation (ester formation and hydrolysis of the esters) may serve as switches to reversibly affect the structure and function of proteins (see USDIN et al. 1982 for review of carboxymethylation of proteins).

O-Methylation of catechols and catecholamines, catalyzed by the enzyme COMT, is probably the most extensively examined methyl transfer reaction (see THAKKER and CREVELING 1990 for a recent review). Since its discovery by AXELROD and TOMCHICK (1958), the primary function attributed to COMT was metabolic inactivation of circulating catecholamines. However, with advances in our understanding of the cellular localization of the soluble and the membrane-bound forms of COMT and with the availability of modern analytical techniques to detect and measure COMT activity, it has become apparent that COMT plays a very important and wide-ranging physiological, metabolic, and toxicological role in humans and in other mammlian species. In the central nervous system, in the cardiovascular system, and in several peripheral organs and tissues, COMT plays an important role in the metabolic inactivation of the catecholamine neurotransmitters and hormones. Methylation of one of the phenolic hydroxyl groups of catecholamines results in loss of their neurotransmitter or hormone function. However, it should be recognized that other enzymes such as monoamine oxidase or phenol sulfotransferase can also play a role in the inactivation of catecholamines.

COMT is widely distributed in animal tissues, with the highest tissue levels present in liver and kidney. In addition to hepatocytes, the predominant cellular localization of COMT is in virtually all epithelial cells and centrally in ependymal and glial cells (see CREVELING and HARTMAN 1982; THAKKER and CREVELING 1990; INOUE and CREVELING 1991). A very important physiological and pharmacological role of the *O*-methylation reaction is to provide metabolic barriers to control and modulate the passage of catechols to and from various organs and tissues. A few examples follow: the choroid plexus actively takes up catechols and metabolizes them to the pharmacologically inactive *O*-methylated derivatives. This barrier at the blood–cerebrospinal fluid (CSF) interphase prevents the passage of circulating catechols into the CSF. The presence of COMT in the ciliary body of eye probably serves a similar function in eye. Presence of elevated levels of COMT activity in the epithelial cells in the vas deferens and oviduct, in the ductal cells of breast, and in the luminal epithelium of uterus is clearly suggestive of the role of *O*-methylation in the reproductive process. A dramatic increase in the COMT activity in uterus during pregnancy in rats (see THAKKER and CREVELING 1990) further substantiates this role of *O*-methylation. It appears that the *O*-methylation reaction is used by nature to control and modulate the availability of catechol estrogens in the target organs during the reproductive processes. It is of particular interest to note that COMT is present in extremely high levels in certain tumor tissues, i.e., adenocarcinomas of breast tissue in women (ASSICOT et al. 1977; HOFFMAN et al. 1979; LONGCOPE 1983) as well as in mouse and rat (AMIN et al. 1983), and in β-islet insulinomas of rat and hamster (FELDMAN et al. 1979).

A variety of drugs and xenobiotics with the catechol functionality are subject to *O*-methylation catalyzed by COMT. These include catechols ranging in complexity from 1,2-dihydroxybenzene to complex polycyclic catechols of plant origin. Many pharmacological agents such as isoprenaline, epinephrine, dopa, a α-methyl dopa, carbidopa and benserazide are subject to metabolic inactivation by *O*-methylation. The inactivation by COMT of the catecholic drugs can have significant effect on the delivery of the drug molecules at the target site. This is well illustrated by comparing the behavioral effects of the isomeric d opamine agonists, i.e., the 5,6- and 6,7-dihydroxy derivatives of 2-amino-1,2,3,4-tetrahydronaphthalene, in mice. Between the two dopamine agonists, the 6,7-dihydroxy isomer was much less potent because of significantly lower brain concentrations achieved with this isomer. Indeed, this isomer is a much better substrate for COMT and, thus, is *O*-methylated more effectively than is the 5,6-dihydroxy isomer (HORN et al. 1981; YOUDE et al. 1984). While many of the drugs subject to metabolic inactivation are either central nervous system (CNS) or cardiovascular drugs, examples of the drugs that are metabolically inactivated by *O*-methylation can also be found in a variety of other therapeutic areas. For example, β-lactam antibiotics containing 3,4-dihydroxybenzoyl functionality are inactivated by COMT. Even drug molecules that contain a single phenolic moiety which is not subject to *O*-methylation, can become substrates of COMT after hydroxylation by cytochrome P450-dependent monooxygenases in the *ortho* position to the phenolic group. Many phenolic steroids, phenethylamines, and hydroxyindoles are metabolized by successive oxidation and *O*-methylation (see THAKKER and CREVELING 1990 and references therein).

II. Catechol *O*-Methyltransferase

1. Enzymology

COMT, a magnesium-dependent enzyme, catalyzes transfer of the methyl group on the sulfonium moiety of AdoMet to one of the phenolic hydroxyl groups of catechol substrates of a wide structural diversity. The products of these enzymatic reactions are an *O*-methylated catechol and AdoHcy. The pH optimum for the enzyme is over a pH range of 7.3–8.2. A second pH optimum reported near pH 9 may represent ionization of the phenolic group being methylated. Both ordered and rapid equilibrium random kinetic mechanisms have been proposed for different preparations of COMT (see THAKKER and CREVELING 1990). Based on the studies with functional group reagents and affinity-labeling agents using partially purified enzyme preparations, presence of two essential nucleophilic functional groups at the active site has been postulated (see THAKKER and CREVELING 1990). At least one of these groups is believed to be a sulfhydryl group. As indicated in Sect. B, it has been shown that the methyl transfer proceeds via a direct nucleophic attack by one of the phenolic groups of catechol substrates on the electron-deficient methyl group of AdoMet (see Fig. 2; HIGAZI et al. 1976; WOODWARD et al. 1980; FLOSS and WOODWARD 1982). The requirement for the catechol functionality is very stringent, if not absolute. L-Ascorbic acid (BLASCHKO and HERTTING 1971) is one of the very few examples of a noncatecholic substrate of COMT. The *O*-methylation reaction catalyzed by COMT exhibits differential regioselectivity toward different classes of catechol substrates. For catecholamine substrates such as norepinephrine and dopamine, the predominant site of *O*-methylation is the *meta*-hydroxyl group, giving rise to normetanephrine and 3-*O*-methyl dopamine; however, with catechol steroids and many xenobiotic catechols, the products are a mixture of the two possible *O*-methyl ethers (THAKKER et al. 1986). With the use of strategically monofluorinated derivatives of norepinephrine, an active site model for COMT has been postulated that explains the regioselectivity of the COMT substrates (THAKKER et al. 1986).

2. Inhibitors

As we have already indicated in a recent review (THAKKER and CREVELING 1990), there are three classes of compounds that inhibit COMT: (1) analogs of AdoHcy, (2) isosteres of catechol substrates, and (3) divalent and trivalent metal cations. Among these, only the isosteres of catechol substrates can inhibit COMT selectively without affecting other methyltransferases or other metal-dependent enzymes. Selective in vivo inhibitors of COMT can be quite useful in protecting catechol drugs, such as L-dopa, from metabolic inactivation. However, in vivo inhibitors of COMT with sufficient potency and selectivity to be useful as therapeutic agents or as pharmacological tools were not available until a novel class of in vitro and in vivo inhibitors of COMT was introduced in 1988 (Mannisto et al. 1988; Backstrom et al. 1989; Borgulya et al. 1989). These inhibitors, primarily derivatives of 3-nitropyrocatechol, compete with other catechols and interact with such high affinity to the catechol-binding site in COMT that they can be considered virtually irreversible (Taskinen et al. 1989). The most active of these compounds are extremely potent, with IC_{50} (concentration inhibiting response by 50%) values in vitro of 3–6 nM, several orders of magnitude lower than that known for COMT inhibitors such as U-0521 (3,4-dihydroxy-2-methylpropiophenone: IC_{50}, 6000 nM; Backstrom et al. 1989). A structure–activity analysis using computational chemistry and multivariate partial least squares (PLS) modeling of COMT inhibition (Lotta et al. 1992) by 99 1,5-disubstituted 3,4-dihydroxybenzenes confirmed the importance of two structural features for the inhibitory activity: (1) presence of an electron-withdrawing group, such as a nitro group, at C-5 and (2) presence of a carbonyl group at C-1, conjugated with the aromatic ring directly or through a carbon–carbon double bond (Backstrom et al. 1989). A similar quantum chemical analysis of COMT inhibition was reported by Shinagawa (1992), which included both the 1,5-disubstituted 3,4-dihydroxybenzene series (Backstrom et al. 1989) and the 3-hydroxy-4-methyoxybenzene series (Nikodejevic et al. 1970). In both series, the electron density on the oxygen atom of the hydroxyl group and the superdelocalizability at the C-5 position of the aromatic ring appeared to be important for activity as inhibitors of COMT.

Initial in vivo studies with the 3-nitropyrocatechols in mice indicated a high therapeutic index for the inhibitors Ro 41-0960 (2′-fluoro-3,4-dihydroxy-5-nitrobenzophenone), OR-462 (nitecapone, 3-(3,4-dihydroxy-5-nitrobenzylidine)-2,4-pentanedione), and OR-611 (entecaride, N,N-diethyl-2-cyano-3-(3,4-dihydroxy-5-nitrophenyl)acrylamide (Tornwall and Mannisto 1991). COMT activity in duodenum, liver, and red blood cells were examined after oral administration of OR-462 and OR-486 (3,4-dinitropyrocatechol), both highly effective inhibitors in vitro (IC_{50}, 10 and 14 nM, respectively). OR-462 (10 mg/kg, po) inhibited duodenal COMT for 5 h, while OR-486 (3 mg/kg, po) effectively inhibited COMT in peripheral tissues for 12 h and caused a modest inhibition of striatal COMT (35%) for 5 h (Nissinen et al. 1988b). OR-462 was administered to 12 healthy, male vounteers in increasing single oral doses from 1 to 100 mg. It was rapidly absorbed with peak plasma concentrations achieved in 45 min. Inhibition of COMT activity in red blood cells (50%) was proportional to plasma levels up to a dose of 150 mg. Maximal inhibition (70%) of gastroduodenal COMT was achieved after 1 h, with 44% inhibition persisting for over 3 h. No acute toxicity was observed up to a dose of 300 mg (Schultz et al. 1991). Zurcher et al. (1990) also report that Ro 40-7592 produces long-lasting inhibition of red blood cell COMT and is well tolerated by normal volunteers up to a dose of 800 mg. However, a possible and as yet unexplored untoward effect of effective inhibition of *O*-methylation is the potential reduction of the COMT-catalyzed inactivation and clearance of estrogen-derived 2- and 4-hydroxyestradiols. Accumulation of 4-hydroxyestradiol may play an essential role in estrogen-induced tumor formation, possibly by redox cycling, resulting in the generation of active radicals and DNA damage (Roy et al. 1990). Further, an additional cautionary proviso is suggested regarding the unknown effects of effective COMT inhibition on the physiological role of catecholestrogens during the peri-implantation period and the successful establishment of pregnancy (Chakraborty et al. 1990).

3. Role of Catechol *O*-Methyltransferase in the Therapy of Parkinson's Disease

An important clinical application for an effective inhibitor of COMT is in the symptomatic therapy of Parkinson's disease to increase the bioavailability of L-dopa in CNS. Parkinson's disease is characterized by a progressive degeneration of nigrostriatal dopaminergic pathways and a loss of the ability to synthesize and retain neuronal dopamine. Current dopamine replacement therapy involves the oral co-administration of L-dopa and a peripheral dopa decarboxylase inhibitor, leading to transport of L-dopa from plasma to the CNS, central decarboxylation of L-dopa, and thus the replenishment of striatal dopamine. Peripherally acting decarboxylase inhibitors, which prevent rapid peripheral decarboxylation of L-dopa, unfortunately promote the formation of large amounts of 3-*O*-methyl dopa catalyzed by COMT. A major fraction of this *O*-methylation occurs at the intestinal uptake site for L-dopa (Nissinen et al. 1988a; Schultz 1991). 3-*O*-Methyl dopa, with a half-life many times greater than that of L-dopa, may compete with L-dopa for the saturable large neutral amino acid transporter at the blood–brain barrier (Wade and Katzman 1975). Clearly, effective inhibition of both periperal and central COMT would reduce the formation of 3-*O*-methyl dopa, perhaps enhance the transport of L-dopa into brain, and thus increase the bioavailability of L-dopa in the CNS. The rationale for the use of COMT inhibitors in conjuction with L-dopa in the treatment of Parkinson's disease has been explored by several groups (Mannisto and Kaakkola 1990; Da Prada 1990, 1991; Nic a'Bhaird et al. 1990). Experimental studies with peripherally and centrally active new COMT inhibitors have been carried out in conjunction with L-dopa and peripheral decarboxylase inhibitors. These include studies in the rat (Nissinen et al. 1988b; Linden et al. 1988; Zurcher et al. 1990; Brannan et al. 1992; Acquas et al. 1992; Mannisto et al. 1992), mouse (Maj et al. 1992; Tornwall and Mannisto 1990), monkey (Cedarbaum et al. 1990, 1991), and rabbit (Friedgen et al. 1993; Halbrugge et al. 1993). The results clearly show a remarkable and long-lasting decrease in the formation of 3-methoxy dopa, an increase in the bioavailability of L-dopa in the striatum, and a shift in the metabolism of central dopamine, suggesting that more dopamine is made available in the striatum.

The initial clinical studies in man (KAAKKOLA et al. 1990; SCHULTZ et al. 1991; TASKINEN et al. 1991; TIMM and ERDIN 1992) demonstrate that effective inhibition of COMT markedly reduces the peripheral formation of 3-*O*-methoxy dopa, increases the bioavailability of L-dopa, and more effectively presents the straitum with dopamine. These early studies suggest that the new COMT inhibitors may be promising as adjuncts to dopamine replacement therapy in the treatment of Parkinson's disease.

4. Molecular and Structural Biology

In the last 3–5 years, there has been a spectacular increase in our knowledge of the structure of COMT. It has been known for some time that COMT is present in tissues in two forms: the larger fraction, present as a cytoplasmic, soluble form (S-COMT) and a quantitatively smaller membrane-bound fraction (M-COMT) which exhibits a significantly higher affinity for catecholamines. For a recent discussion of the role of M-COMT, see ROTH (1992). Two research teams, one Finnish (Orion Corporation and Laboratory of Molecular Genetics, Institute of Biotechnology, University of Helsinki) and one Swiss (Pharma Research and Central Research Units, Hoffmann-La Roche Ltd., Basel), have reported the molecular cloning and characterization of the two forms of COMT. These studies include rodent (SALMINEN et al. 1990), porcine (BERTOCCI et al. 1991a), and human (LUNDSTROM et al. 1991; BERTOCCI et al. 1991b) COMT. The initial sequencing of S-COMT was accomplished by purification of the native protein, isolation and sequencing several COMT-specific peptides, followed by the preparation and use of oligonucleotides as DNA probes. The soluble form of COMT, S-COMT, was purified from rat (KORKOLAINEN and NISSINEN 1989; TILGMANN and KALKINEN 1991) and porcine (BERTOCCI et al. 1990, 1991a,b) liver, and human placenta (TILGMANN and KALKKINEN 1991; NORIN and TIPTON 1991). The final purification was accomplished by high-performance anion exchange, reversed-phase (see VESER and MAY 1986) and immunoaffinity chromatography (BERTOCCI et al. 1991b).

Analysis of the resultant cDNAs has essentially solved the primary peptide structure of both S- and M-COMT and revealed a great similarity in the amino acid sequences of the two forms. For example, peptide sequence of rat S-COMT is virtually identical to the core peptide of M-COMT (SALMINEN et al. 1990). Furthermore, the amino acid sequences of COMT from different species, while not identical, are highly homologous. Comparisons between the sequence deduced from porcine cDNA (amino acids 1–186) and the deduced human sequence (amino acids 86–271) showed a homology of 83%–93% (BERTOCCI et al. 1991b). Seven cysteines are present in the porcine and human COMT, of which two are present in identical 71-residue sequences – amino acids 79–150 and 164–235, respectively. BERTOCCI et al. (1991b) have suggested that these cysteines may be part of the catalytic center. This is in agreement with the previous studies with partially pure COMT which implicated the presence of two cysteines in the catalytic site (MORRIS et al. 1973; BORCHARDT and THAKKER 1977).

With the tools available in molecular biology, several aspects of the structure and control of COMT have been elucidated, including the chromosomal site, an initial crystal structure, the presence of a hydrophobic signal anchor at the N-terminal, and regulation of the formation of the S- and M-COMT. Analysis of genomic DNA by Southern blotting, cell hybrids, and in situ hybridization indicates that in mammalian genomes, there is a single gene for COMT. The site for human (placental) COMT is on chromosome 22 at q11.1 to 11.2 (GROSSMAN et al. 1992a; WINDQUVIST et al. 1992 in agreement with findings of TILGMANN et al. 1992; LUNDSTROM et al. 1991). The single gene locus for COMT may provide insight into the genetic control and implied structural differences between the low- and high-activity forms of human red blood cell (RBC) COMT (WEINSHILBOUM 1988a, 1989; GROSSMAN et al. 1992b).

The protein-coding capacities of these COMT cDNAs have been used to express recombinant forms of both S- and M-COMT. The cDNAs for S-COMT from rat liver and human placenta were transfected into *Escherichia coli* with the successful expression of large amounts (10% of the bacterial protein) of COMT-specific rat (24.7 kDa) and human (24.4 kDa) polypeptides (LUNDSTROM et al. 1991). The COMT-specific rat polypeptide was purified and crystalized (in the presence of AdoMet and the COMT inhibitor 1,5-dinitrocatechol) by vapor diffusion hanging drop techniques to yield asymmetric trigonal crystals. An initial X-ray analysis has been reported (VIDGREN et al. 1991).

Hydropathy plots of the sequences of S-COMT from rat and human failed to reveal the presence of membrane-spanning domains (LUNDSTROM et al. 1991). However, upstream from the initiator ATG of S-COMT is an open reading frame with another initiation codon (ATG) region which contains a stretch of hydrophobic amino acids. This structure resembles a signal peptide, suggesting that translation from the first ATG could be responsible for synthesis of M-COMT. Accordingly, the sequence of M-COMT from rat carries an extention of 43 amino acid residues at the N-terminal, while the human M-COMT has a 50-residue extension. These apparent hydrophobic signal anchors could subserve insertion of M-COMT into the cytoplasmic side of membranes (ULMANEN and LUNDSTROM et al. 1991; LUNDSTROM et al. 1991). These N-terminal extentions may also be related to the increased affinity of M-COMT towards dopamine and other catechols as well as the marked preference for *meta O*-methylation exhibited by M-COMT (NISSINEN 1984).

Enzymatically active recombinant S-COMT (25 kDa) and M-COMT (30 kDa) were expressed in insect cells infected with baculovirus expression constructs (TILGMANN et al. 1992). The resultant M-COMT (30 kDa) cosedimented with plasma membrane markers. However, pulse-chase experiments with ^{35}S-methionine labeled cells infected with M-COMT baculovirus suggested that M-COMT is not processed from S-COMT (25 kDa). BERTOCCI et al. (1990, 1991a) in studies with human kidney 293 cells transfected with a plasmid containing human COMT clone showed a membrane fraction with a 29-kDa COMT peptide and a 25.5-kDa cytosolic COMT peptide, suggesting that the 25.5-kDa peptide arises from the 29-kDa M-COMT peptide. The nature and site of the control mechanism(s) determining the amount and fraction of COMT as S- and M-COMT remain to be clarified. This question is of particular interest at tissue sites such as the luminal epithelium of the uterus and collecting ducts of breast, where induction of COMT is under progesterone dominance (INOUE and CREVELING 1991).

III. Hydroxyindole *O*-Methyltransferase

1. Enzymology

HIOMT, first described in 1960 (AXELROD and WEISSBACH 1960) and latter purified to homogeneity (JACKSON and LOVENBERG 1971), is found almost exclusively in the pineal gland of vertebrates and catalyzes the *O*-methylation of *N*-acetyserotonin to form the hormone melationin. HIOMT, unlike the initial enzyme in the melatonin pathway, serotonin-*N*-acetyltransferase, does not display large circadian variations. The changes in HIOMT activity occur gradually over several days when the animal is continuously exposed to light (see SUGDEN et al. 1987).

While HIOMT is fairly specific for *N*-acetylserontonin, it does catalyze *O*-methylation of other hydroxyindoles such as 5-hydroxytryptamine and 5-hydroxyindoleacetic acid (AXELROD and WEISSBACH 1961). The kinetic mechanism of the reaction catalyzed by HIOMT appears to be of the ordered bi–bi type that involves binding of AdoMet first, followed by addition of the methyl acceptor substrates (SATAKE and MORTON 1979). The purification, assay, and biochemical properties of HIOMT have been reviewed (SUGDEN et al. 1987). Like many other methyltransferases, HIOMT is inhibited very effectively by AdoHcy. HIOMT tolerates less structural modifications in AdoHcy than many other methyltransferases when the analogs of AdoHcy are evaluated as inhibitors of these enzymes (BORCHARDT et al. 1978). The selective and tight binding of AdoHcy to HIOMT may play an important role in modulating the in vivo activity of this enzyme. Interestingly, bovine HIOMT purified to homogeneity was found to contain AdoHcy (KUWANO and TAKAHASHI 1980). It was later reported that the enzyme–AdoHcy complex could be dissociated by excess of AdoMet or by AdoHcy hydrolase (KUWANO and TAKAHASHI 1984).

2. Molecular and Structural Biology

The molecular cloning and nucleotide sequencing of cDNA encoding pineal HIOMT have been reported for cow (ISHIDA et al. 1987; DONOHUE et al.

1992), chicken (VOISIN et al. 1992), and human (DONOHUE et al. 1992). Polyadenylated RNA isolated from pineal tissues was used to prepare cDNA libraries in λgt11, followed by antibody screening and selection of cDNA clones. ISHIDA et al. (1987) reported a primary 250 amino acid sequence for a 37.8-kDa HIOMT deduced from a 1050-nucleotide region of bovine cDNA. More recently, DONOHUE et al. (1992), resequenced this cDNA to yield a 1430-bp oligonucleotide which included the entire 5′- and 3′-coding regions. Translation of the revised sequence gave a primary sequence of 315 residues for a 38-kDa HIOMT, in good agreement with estimates of the native protein (KUWANO et al. 1978; JACKSON and LOVENBERG 1971). VOISIN et al. (1992), using a similar approach, isolated a cDNA clone from chicken pineal gland to yield a 1038-nucleotide sequence coding for a 346-amino acid 38-kDa HIOMT. VOISIN et al. (1992) were able to demonstrate the presence of HIOMT mRNA transcripts in the retina and brain. DONOHUE et al. (1992) isolated a cDNA clone from human pineal glands and reported a 1122-bp sequence coding for a slightly larger (41.6-kDa) HIOMT protein. The human nucleotide sequence is unusual in that it contains a 84-bp fragment of the LINE I sequence, which is a repetitive sequence present in the human, primate, and some rodent genomes. The function of this inclusion is unknown. Exclusive of this LINE I sequence, the human HIOMT is 75% and 63% homologous to both bovine and avian HIOMT clones, respectively. Sites predictive of post-translational modifications for casein kinase II phosporylation, protein kinase C, tyrosine kinase phosphorylation, and myristolation are present in these sequences as well as conservation sites for seven cysteine residues. The deduced amino acid sequences of bovine and avian HIOMT are 81% and 73% similar to human HIOMT, respectively.

It is of interest that a 26-residue stretch (Lys 262-Leu 287) in chicken HIOMT showed a much closer homology with similar sequences in bovine HIOMT (69%), neurosprene *O*-methyltransferase (42%), PNMT (50%), and COMT (31%), suggesting the presence of a conserved sequence and perhaps indicating a common site for *S*-adenosyl-L-methionine binding.

E. *N*-Methylation

I. Overview

Since the first demonstration of *N*-methylation of pyridine by HIS (1887) over a century ago, this reaction has been shown to be an important metabolic step in the transformation of many endogenous and xenobiotic molecules containing primary, secondary, or tertiary amino groups, including important endogenous molecules such as histamine and epinephrine. As is the case with *O*-methylation, *N*-methylation also occurs by transfer of a methyl group from AdoMet to the nucleophilic amino groups. The resultant produts are *N*-methylated metabolites and AdoHcy. Amine *N*-

methyltransferase catalyzes the *N*-methylation of amines with a wide variety of structures and thus exhibits very broad substrate specificity. The enzyme, despite its broad selectivity, does not catalyze the *N*-methylation of such important molecules as histamine and norepinephrine. Interestingly, the highly specific enzymes HMT and PNMT catalyze the methylation of histamine and norepinephrine, respectively (see ANSHER and JAKOBY 1990 for a recent review of *N*-methyltransferases).

The product of *N*-methylation of norepinephrine is epinephrine, a neurotransmitter in the CNS that modulates such important physiological processes as temperature regulation, reproduction, cardiovascular function, and food intake. Hence, PNMT plays a crucial role in several metabolic and physiological functions by participating in the biosynthesis of epinephrine. Because of this, PNMT activity is regulated by several factors, including product inhibition and hormonal modulation (see ANSHER and JAKOBY 1990).

Histamine, a putative neurotransmitter or neuromodulator in the CNS (WADA et al. 1985), is synthesized from histidine by histidine decarboxylase. It has been localized immunocytochemically in a widespread fiber system dispersed throughout the CNS which appears to originate from a small group of cell bodies located in the posterior hypothalamus (WATANABE et al. 1984). More recently, the anatomical localization of histamine-containing neurons has been confirmed using histidine decarboxylase mRNA derived from the cloning of a cDNA-encoding fetal rat liver. Histaminergic perikarya were found exclusively in the tubermammillary nucleus (BAYLISS et al. 1990). HMT plays a key role in the termination of the histamine action by catalyzing methylation of one of the imidazole nitrogens. In addition to brain, HMT is also distributed in skin and gastric mucosa (see ANSHER and JAKOBY 1990), suggesting its role in histamine inactivation also in those tissues. The *N*-methylation reaction must play a very important role in metabolic inactivation of drugs, because a large number of drug molecules contain amino functionality. However, in a selected cases, *N*-methylation may result in the formation of active metabolites. This is best illustrated by conversion of apomorphine to pharmacologically active morphine by *N*-methylation. In a few cases, the metabolic activation of some xenobiotics by amine *N*-methyltransferases may lead to the formation of highly toxic or carcinogenic products. The most notable example of metabolic activation by amine *N*-methyltransferases to toxic products is provided by *N*-methylation of 4-phenyl-1,2,3,6-tetrahydropyridine to 1-methyl-4-phenyltetrahydropyridine (MPTP) by liver and brain amine *N*-methyltransferases (ANSHER et al. 1986). This metabolite is oxidatively converted to a highly toxic metabolite 1-methyl-4-phenylpyridinium ion (MPP^+), which is implicated in the destruction of dopamine neurons in substantia nigra and development of Parkinson-like syndrome (CALNE et al. 1985; also see ANSHER and JAKOBY 1990). *N*-Methylation and subsequent oxidation of 4-aminoazobenzene by flavin monooxygenases results in the formation of *N*-hydroxyarylamine, which is a proximate carcinogen. Further metabolic transformation of this

N-hydroxyarylamine results in the formation of the ultimate hepatocarcinogen (ZIEGLER et al. 1988). These examples show that the amine *N*-methyltransferases can collaborate with other oxidative enzymes to produce highly toxic and/or carcinogenic metabolites.

II. Phenethanolamine *N*-Methyltransferase

1. Enzymology

PNMT is the terminal enzyme in the catecholamine pathway and catalyzes the *N*-methylation of norepinephrine to yield epinephrine. The enzyme is present in the adrenal medulla, SIF cells of sympathetic ganglia, and sensory nuclei of the vagus nerve. Periperally located PNMT is regulated by glucocorticoids. PNMT is also found in the CNS, including cell groups in the medulla oblongata, hypothalamus, amygdala, and in retinal and amacrine cells of the retina. Centrally located PNMT does not appear to be under the regulation of glucocorticoids.

Unlike the amine *N*-methyltransferases, PNMT is highly specific for its methyl acceptor substrates. The enzyme requires the presence of a phenethanolamine moiety and does not accept phenethylamines as substrates. The endogenous substrates of PNMT include norepinephrine and epinephrine. Thus, with very few exceptions (RAFFERTY and GRUNEWALD 1982), the β-hydroxyl group on the ethylamine side chain is essential for the enzyme activity. It is of interest to note that the compounds in which the aromatic ring is replaced by a cyclohex-3-enyl, cyclohexyl, or cyclooctyl rings are good substrates for PNMT (GRUNEWALD et al. 1975). FULLER (1987) showed that the apparent K_m of the various ring-substituted phenethanolamine substrates varied over a wide range (1–680 mM), whereas the V_{max} values remained essentially unchanged.

2. Molecular and Structural Biology

In a pioneering study, JOH et al. (1983) and BAETGE et al. (1986) reported the complete nucleotide sequence and deduced amino acid sequence of bovine PNMT. A full-length clone was isolated using PNMT mRNA from bovine adrenal medulla. The PNMT cDNA was capable of directing the synthesis in a hamster kidney cell line of enzymatically active PNMT with a relative molecular mass of 21 kDa. Subsequently, the complete PNMT-coding sequences have been characterized and the primary amino acid sequences determined for bovine (BATTER et al. 1988), human (KANADA et al. 1988; SASAOKA et al. 1989), and rat (MEZEY 1989). The cDNA and amino acid sequences for PNMT are remarkably similar. Thus, the cDNA from rat adrenal medulla shows 83% and 84% homology to the coding region of bovine and human cDNAs, respectively. The amino acid sequence of rat PNMT has an 83%–85% correspondence to the sequence for bovine and

92% homology to human PNMT. The human enzyme consists of 282 amino acid residues with a predicted mass of 30.9 kDa (KANADA et al. 1988). Using mouse–human somatic cell hybrids, the gene for human PNMT was assigned to a single gene on chromosome 17. More recently, SASAOKA et al. (1989) observed a minor PNMT mRNA (type B) in addition to the major mRNA (type A) and suggested that the single PNMT gene is capable of producing multiple forms of mRNAs under the control of alternate promoters. MEZEY (1989) reported the presence of two types of PNMT-specific mRNAs in young rat brain; however, only one form is expressed in the adult brain. These observations suggest that the selection of the transcription site for PNMT may be developmentally regulated. Of importance is the presence of at least three sequences for the glucocorticoid regulatory element, one in the first intron and two or more upstream from the cap site of the major type A mRNA (SASAOKA et al. 1989; BAETGE et al. 1988). EVINGER and JOH (1989) compared the transcriptional rate of PNMT mRNA in the adrenal medulla of rat strains which possess distinctive levels of epinephrine and PNMT. It is apparent that the rate of PNMT gene transcription is a major factor responsible for strain-specific levels of PNMT mRNA among the rat strains examined. Thus, intrinsic genetic components as well as neural and steroid elements determine the levels of PNMT gene expression.

III. Histamine *N*-Methyltransferase

1. Enzymology

Histamine appears to be metabolized in the brain exclusively by transfer of the methyl group from AdoMet, catalyzed by HMT to form *N*-methylhistamine, followed by oxidative deamination by monoamine oxidase B. HMT is a highly specific *N*-methyltransferase and accepts only those histamine derivatives as substrates in which positions 1, 2, and 3 are unsubstituted (see ANSHER and JAKOBY 1990). The enzyme also requires a positive charge on the side chain and does not accept compounds with a negative charge on the side chain as substrates. Methylation of the primary amino group of histamine reduces its K_m by almost one order of magnitude (HOUGH et al. 1981). The enzyme is inhibited by histamine at concentrations that are tenfold higher than the K_m; however, the transferase purified to homogeneity from ox brain is not inhibited by histamine. While this enzyme exhibits kinetic behavior that is consistent with the formation of a ternary complex without the requirement of any order for the binding of the two substrates (GITOMER and TIPTON 1986), partially purified enzyme from human skin exhibits kinetics suggestive of ordered steady state mechanism involving ternary complexes (FRANCIS et al. 1980). As indicated in Sect. B, the methyl transfer from AdoMet to histamine occurs via direct transfer to the histamine nitrogen and is accompanied by inversion of the configuration when a chiral methyl group containing hydrogen, deuterium, and tritium (CH^2H^3H) is used (ASANO et al. 1984).

2. Molecular and Structural Biology

Recently a cDNA clone of 1.3 kb was derived from a rat kidney cDNA library consisting of an eight-nucleotide 5′-noncoding region, a coding region of 885 nucleotides, and 369 nucleotide 3′-noncoding region. The encoded HMT protein has an amino acid sequence of 295 residues with a calculated mass of 33 940. Expression of the cDNA in *E. coli* yielded a catalytically active HMT identical with native HMT (TAKEMURA et al. 1992).

F. *S*-Methylation

I. Overview

Unlike *O*- and *N*-methylation reactions, which play crucial roles in both metabolic detoxication of xenobiotics as well as biosynthesis of physiologically important hormones and neurotransmitters, AdoMet-dependent *S*-methylation appears to be associated almost exclusively with the metabolic detoxication function (WEISIGER and JAKOBY 1980). A study of the distribution of thiol methyltransferase activity in rat tissues showed the highest specific activity in cecal and colonic mucosa (WEISIGER and JAKOBY 1980), suggesting its role in the detoxification of hydrogen sulfide formed by anaerobic bacteria in the intestinal tract. Thiol methyltransferases, like many metabolic enzymes, have broad substrate specificity toward thiol-containing compounds (see STEVENS and BAKKE 1990, and references therein). Many therapeutic agents are metabolized by thiol methyltransferases – these include captopril (DRUMMER et al. 1983), thiopurines (WEINSHILBOUM 1986), cephalosporins (secondary metabolism; KERREMANS et al. 1985), penicillamine (KEITH et al. 1985), and many others (see STEVENS and BAKKE 1990). It is noteworthy that many substrates for thiol methylation are generated by initial conjugation of the xenobiotics with glutathione, followed by enzymatic degradation to the cysteine conjugates, and finally cleavage of the cysteine conjugates by the enzymes known as β-lyases (see STEVENS and BAKKE 1990). *S*-Methylation of the thiol metabolites generated by β-lyases is known as the thiomethyl shunt, as this reaction diverts the cysteine conjugates from their normal metabolic course, leading to the formation and excretion of mercapturic acids (JAKOBY et al. 1984).

II. *S*-Methyltransferases

The presence of thiol methyltransferases was first suspected when sulfhydryl compounds were found to inhibit choline biosynthesis, presumably by serving as alternate methyl acceptors (BREMER and GREENBERG 1961a). The *S*-methylation activity was detected in rat liver microsomes (BREMER and GREENBERG 1961b). Later, a soluble enzyme was described that catalyzed the methylation of thiopurine and thiouracil (REMY 1963). To date, three thiol methyltransferases have been described, i.e., the microsomal enzyme thiol methyltransferase (TMT, EC 2.1.1.9; BORCHARDT and CHENG 1978), the soluble enzyme thiopurine methyltransferase (TPMT, EC 2.1.1.67; WEINSHILBOUM 1991), and a cytosolic thioether *S*-methyltransferase (TEMT; WARNER 1992). Whether the microsomal and soluble enzymes are uniquely different enzymes is uncertain (WEISIGER and JAKOBY 1980; STEVENS and BAKKE 1990). TPMT catalyzes methyl transfer to the sulfur of aromatic and heterocyclic sulfhydryl compounds, TMT catalyzes the transfer to aliphatic sulfhydryl compounds, and TEMT catalyzes the methylation to molecules with a thio-, seleno-, or telluroether bond. Substrates for TEMT include sulfhydryl compounds such as 2-mercaptoethanol, 2,3-dimercaptopropanol, methylmercaptan, and hydrogen sulfide as well as dimethylsulfide, telluride, and selenide (STEEL and BENEVENGA 1979; MOZIER et al. 1988). Many of the products of TMT are substrates for TEMT and provide a pathway for the detoxification and excretion of selenite (WARNER 1992).

TEMT has been purified to homogeneity and the cDNA sequence determined (WARNER 1992). TEMT, with a molecular mass 29460, has a K_m value of $1\,\mu M$ for both AdoMet and telluro-, seleno-, or thioethers. Cloning and sequencing of the cDNA for TEMT yielded a coding region of 792 nucleotides to give a peptide of 264 amino acid residues. The sequence of the 3′-untranslated region was also reported. Sequence analysis indicated that both the nucleotide and amino acid sequences for TEMT have significant homology with PNMT. Both transferases have two areas of highly conserved sequences which may relate to an AdoMet-binding site.

G. Pharmacogenetics of Methyltransferases

While methylation of endogenous and xenobiotic compounds has been studied for a long time, the interindividual variations in the activities of these important metabolic enzymes and the factors responsible for these variations have been investigated only recently. WEINSHILBOUM (1989, 1991) and his colleagues have shown in a series of studies that inheritance is a significant factor responsible for the inter-individual variations of at least four methyltransferases in humans affecting *O*-, *N*-, and *S*-methylation of endogenous and xenobiotic compounds. These studies were performed by measuring the methyltransferase activities in easily accessible human cell, i.e., RBC (GROSSMAN et al. 1992b; see references in WEINSHILBOUM 1989). While the methyltransferase activities in RBC do not play a significant role in the biosynthesis and/or metabolism of endogenous compounds or drug molecules, it has been postulated that the biochemical properties and regulation of methyltransferases in the RBC might reflect those of the methyltransferases in the target tissues. This hypothesis has been proven correct for the four methyltransferases by showing that the variations in the enzyme activities are related to the variations among individuals in the metabolism, therapeutic effects, and toxicity of drugs. The four methyltransferases that have been studied by WEINSHILBOUM and his colleagues (see WEINSHILBOUM 1989) are COMT, HMT, TPMT, and TMT. An excellent example of the impact of the genetic variation of a methyltransfer activity on drug toxicity has been provided by the studies involving the 6-mercaptopurine therapy (LENNARD et al. 1987). It is believed that thioguanine nucleotides cause myelosuppression in patients who are being treated with thiopurines. A significant correlation was found between myelosuppression in these patients and low TPMT activity in their RBC (LENNARD et al. 1987). Thus, it appears that inherited variations in various methyltransferase activities play a significant role in the interindividual variations in the metabolism of thiopurine and catechol drugs, with a consequent potential for variations in susceptibility to toxicity due to these drugs.

H. Conclusion

It must become evident from the discussions in the previous sections that methyltransferases play a pivotal role in numerous physiological and metabolic functions in humans and other mammalian species. Insufficient activity of many of the methyltransferases may severely compromise normal physiological functions and may also result in numerous adverse toxic reactions to many pharmacological agents.

The study of methyltransferases has entered a new state of the art, resulting from the successes of molecular biology in the cloning and derivation of cDNA, mRNA, and amino acid sequences of a growing multitude of methyltransferases. The successful expression of enzymatically competent methyltransferase proteins through a variety of vectors and in a number of cell types has virtually eliminated the need for the isolation of such proteins from tissue sources except as reference materials. The enzymologist can design experiments where the quantity of available enzyme is no longer the limiting factor. The avenue is now open for site-mutational studies whereby the structure of the active site can be systematically altered and information obtained on the specific amino acid residues for binding of substrates, cofactors, activators, and inhibitors. Establishment of the structure of active sites should permit the rational synthesis of new medicinal agents with high affinity for methyltransferases. The ability to measure specific mRNAs for various methyltransferases allows studies at the molecular level to not only determine the regional and cellular localization of methyltransferase proteins, but also to gain insight into their rates of formation and degradation, as well as operative hormonal and genetic control mechanisms in both normal and pathological states.

References

Acquas E, Carboni E, de Ree RHA, Da Prada M, Di Chiara G (1992) Extracellular concentrations of dopamine and metabolites in the rat caudate after oral administration of a novel catechol-*O*-methyltransferase inhibitor Ro 40-7592. J Neurochem 59:326–330

Amin AM, Creveling CR, Lowe MC (1983) Immunocytochemical localization of catechol *O*-methyltransferase in normal and cancerous breast tissues of mouse and rat. JNCI 70:337–342

Ansher SS, Jakoby WB (1990) *N*-methylation. In: Mulder GJ (ed) Conjugation reactions in drug metabolism. Taylor and Francis, London, p 233

Ansher SS, Cadet JL, Jakoby WB, Baker JK (1986) Role of *N*-methyltransferases in the neurotoxicity associated with the metabolites of 1-methyl-4-phenyl-1,2,3,4-tetrahydropyridine (MPTP) and other 4-substituted pyridines present in the environment. Biochm Pharmacol 35:3359–3363

Asano Y, Woodward WB, Houck DR, Floss HG (1984) Stereochemical course of the tranmethylation catalyzed by histamine *N*-methyltransferase. Arch Biochem Biophys 231:253–256

Assicot M, Contesso G, Bohuon C (1977) Catechol-*O*-methyltransferase in human breast cancers. Eur J Cancer 13:961–966

Axelrod J, Tomchick R (1958) Enzymatic *O*-methylation of epinephrine and other catechols. J Biol Chem 233:702–705

Axelrod J, Weissbach H (1960) Enzymatic *O*-methylation of *N*-acetylserotonin to melatonin. Science 131:1312

Axelrod J, Weissbach H (1961) Purification and properties of hydroxyindol *O*-methyltransferase. J Biol Chem 236:211–213

Backstrom R, Honkanen E, Pippuri A, Kairisalo P, Pystynen J, Heinola K, Nissinen E, Linden I-B, Mannisto PT, Kaakkloa S, Pohto P (1989) Synthesis of some novel potent and selective catechol-*O*-methyltransferase inhibitors. J Med Chem 32:841–846

Baetge EE, Suh YH, Joh TH (1986) Complete nucleotide and deduced amino acid sequence of bovine phenylethanolamine *N*-methyltransferase: partial amino acid homology with rat tyrosine hydroxylase. Proc Natl Acad Sci USA 83:5454–5458

Baetge EE, Behringer RR, Messing A, Brinster RL, Palmiter RD (1988) Transgenic mice express the human phenylethanolamine *N*-methyltranferase gene in adrenal medulla and retina. Proc Natl Acad Sci USA 85:3648–3652

Batter DK, D'Mello SR, Turzai LM, Hughes HB III, Gioio AE, Kaplan BB (1988) The complete nucleotide sequence and structure of the gene encoding bovine phenylethanolamine *N*-methyltransferase. J Neurosci Res 19:367–376

Bayliss DA, Wang Y-M, Zahnow CA, Joseph DR, Millhorn DE (1990) Localization of histidine decarboxylase mRNA in rat brain. Mol Cell Neurosci 1:3–9

Bertocci B, Garotta G, Zurcher G, Miggiano V, Da Prada M (1990) Monoclonal antibodies recognizing both soluble and membrane bound catechol-*O*-methyltransferase. J Neural Transm Suppl 32:369–374

Bertocci B, Garotta G, Da Prada M, Lahm H-W, Zurcher G, Virgallita G, Miggiano V (1991a) Immunoaffinity purification and partial amino acid sequence analysis of catechol-*O*-methyltranferase from pig liver. Biochim Biophys Acta 1080: 103–109

Bertocci B, Miggiano V, Da Prada M, Dembic Z, Lahm H-W, Malherbe P (1991b) Human catechol-*O*-methyltransferase: cloning and expression of the membrane-associated form. Proc Natl Acad Sci USA 88:1416–1420

Blaschko E, Hertting G (1971) Enzymatic methylation of L-ascorbic acid by catechol *O*-methyltransferase. Biochem Pharmacol 20:1363–1370

Borchardt RT, Cheng CF (1978) Purification and characterization of rat liver microsomal thiol methyltransferase. Biochim Biophys Acta 522:340–353

Borchardt RT, Thakker DR (1977) Evidence for sulfhydryl groups at the active site of catechol-*O*-methyltransferase. In: Usdin E, Weiner N, Youdim MBH (eds) Structure and function of monoamine enzymes. Dekker, New York, p 707

Borchardt RT, Wu YS (1974) Potential inhibitors of *S*-adenosylmethionine-dependent methyltransferases. I. Modification of the amino acid portion of *S*-adenosylhomocysteine. J Med Chem 17:862–867

Borchardt RT, Wu YS (1975) Potential inhibitors of *S*-adenosylmethionine-dependent methyltransferases. III. Modifications of the sugar portion of *S*-adenosylhomocysteine. J Med Chem 18:300–304

Borchardt RT, Huber JA, Wu YS (1974) Potential inhibitors of *S*-adenosylmethionine-dependent methyltransferases. II. Modification of the base portion of *S*-adenosylhomocysteine. J Med Chem 17:868–873

Borchardt RT, Huber JA, Wu YS (1976a) Potential inhibitors of *S*-adenosylmethionine dependent methyltransferases. IV. Futher modification of the amino acid and base portions of *S*-adenosylmethionine. J Med Chem 19:1094–1099

Borchardt RT, Wu YS, Huber JA, Wycpalek AF (1976b) Potential inhibitors of *S*-adenosylmethionine-dependent methyltransferases. V. The role of the asymmetric sulfonium pole in the enzymatic binding of *S*-adenosyl-L-methonine. J Med Chem 19:1104–1110

Borchardt RT, Wu YS, Wu BS (1978) Potential inhibitors of *S*-adenosylmethionine-dependent methyltransferases. VII. Role of the ribosyl moiety in enzymatic binding of *S*-adenosyl-L-homocysteine and *S*-adenosyl-L-methionine. J Med Chem 21:1307–1310

Borchardt RT, Creveling CR, Ueland PM (eds) (1986) Biological methylation and drug design: experimental and clinical roles of *S*-adenosylmethionine. Humana, Clifton

Borgulya J, Bruderer H, Bernauer K, Zurcher G, Da Prada M (1989) Catechol-*O*-methyltransferase-inhibiting pyrocatechol derivatives: synthesis and structure-activity studies. Helv Chim Acta 72:952–968

Boudikova B, Szumlanski C, Maidak B, Weinshilboum R (1990) Human liver catechol-*O*-methyltransferase pharmacogenetics. Clin Pharmacol Ther 48:381–389

Brannan T, Martinez T, Yahr MD (1992) Catechol-*O*-methyltransferase inhibition increases striatal L-dopa and dopamine: an in vivo study in rats. Neurology 42:683–685

Bremer J, Greenberg DM (1961a) Methyltransferring enzyme system of microsome in the biosynthesis of lecithin (phosphatidylcholine). Biochim Biophys Acta 46:205–216

Bremer J, Greenberg DM (1961b) Enzymic methylation of foreign compounds. Biochim Biophys Acta 46:217–224

Calne DB, Langstrom JE, Martin WRW, Stoessl AJ, Ruth TJ, Adam MJ, Pate BD, Schulzer M (1985) Positron emission tomography after MPTP, observations relating to the cause of Parkinson's disease. Nature 317:246–248

Cantoni GL (1953) *S*-Adenosylmethionine; a new intermediate formed enzymatically from L-methionine and ATP. J Biol Chem 204:403–416

Cedarbaum J, Leger G, Reches A, Guttman M (1990) Effect of nitecapone (OR-462) on the pharmacokinetics of levodopa and 3-*O*-methyldopa formation in cynomolgus monkeys. Clin Neuropharmacol 13:544–52

Cedarbaum JM, Leger G, Guttman M (1991) Reduction of circulating 3-*O*-methyldopa by inhibition of catechol-*O*-methyltransferase with OR-611 and OR-462 in Cynomolgus monkeys: implications for the treatment of Parkinson's disease. Clin Neuropharmacol 14:330–342

Chakraborty C, Davis DL, Dey SK (1990) The *O*-methylation of catechol oestrogrens by pig conceptuses and endometrium during the peri-implantation period. J Endocrinol 127:77–84

Cornforth JW, Reichard SA, Talalay P, Correll HL, Glusker JP (1977) Determination of the absolute configuration at the sulfonium center of *S*-adenosylmethionine. Correlation with the absolute configuration of the diastereomeric *S*-carboxymethyl-(S)-methionine salts. J Am Chem Soc 99:7292–7300

Coward JK, Slisz EP (1973) Analogs of *S*-adenosylhomocysteine as potential inhibitors of biological transmethylation. Specificity of the *S*-adenosylhomocysteine binding site. J Med Chem 16:460–463

Coward JK, Sweet WD (1972) Analogs of *S*-adenosylhomocysteine as potential inhibitors of biological transmethylation. Synthesis and biological activity of homocysteine derivatives bridged to adenine. J Med Chem 15:381–384
Coward JK, D'Urso-Scott M, Sweet WD (1972) Inhibition of catechol-*O*-methyltransferase by *S*-adenosylhomocysteine and by *S*-adenosylhomocysteine sulfoxide, a potential transition-state analog. Biochem Pharmacol 21:1200–1203
Coward JK, Bussolloti DL, Cheng CD (1974) Analogs of *S*-adenosylhomocysteine as potential inhibitors of biological transmethylation: inhibition of several methylases by *S*-Tubercidinylhomocysteine. J Med Chem 17:1286–1289
Creveling CR (1993) Catechol-*O*-methyltransferase. In: Nagatsu T, Parvez SN, Parvez S (eds) Methods in neurotransmitter research. Elsevier, Amsterdam, pp 375–406
Creveling CR, Hartman BK (1982) Relationships between the cellular localization and the physiological function of catechol-*O*-methyl transferase. In: Usdin E, Borchardt RT, Creveling CR (eds) Biochemistry of *S*-adenosylmethionine and related compounds. Macmillan, London, p 479
Da Prada M (1990) Catechol-*O*-methyltransferase inhibitors: their role in the therapy of Parkinson's disease. Eur J Pharmacol 183:4–5
Da Prada M (1991) New approaches to the treatment of age-related brain disorders. Can J Neurol Sci 18:384–386
De La Haba G, Jamieson GA, Mudd SH, Richards HH (1959) *S*-adenosylmethionine: the relation of configuration at the sulfonium center to enzymatic activity. J Am Chem Soc 81:3975–3980
Donohue SJ, Roseboom PH, Klein DC (1992) Bovine hydroxyindole *O*-methyltransferase: significant sequence revision. J Biol Chem 267:5184–5185
Drummer OH, Miach P, Jarrott B (1983) *S*-methylation of captopril: demonstration of captopril thiol methyltransferase activity in human eruthrocytes and enzyme distribution in rat tissues. Biochem Pharmacol 32:1557–1562
Eloranta TO (1977) Tissue distribution of *S*-adenosylmethionine and *S*-adenosylhomocysteine in the rat. Biochem J 166:521–529
Evered D, Clark C (eds) (1985) Photoperiodism, melatonin and the pineal. Ciba Found Symp 117
Evinger MJ, Joh TH (1989) Strain-specific differences in transcription of the gene for the epinephrine-synthesizing enzyme phenylethanolamine *N*-methyltransferase. Mol Brain Res 5:141–147
Falany CN, Vazquez ME, Heroux JA, Roth JA (1990) Purification and characterization of human liver phenol-sulfating phenolsulfotransferase. Arch Biochem Biophys 278:312–318
Feldman JM, Reintgen DS, Seigler HF (1979) Monoamine oxidase and catechol *O*-methyltransferase activity in hamster and rat insulinomas. Diabetologia 17: 249–256
Floss G, Woodward R (1982) Further stereochemical studies on methyl transfer reactions. In: Usdin E, Borchardt RT, Creveling CR (eds) Biochemistry of *S*-adenosylmethionine and related compounds. Macmillan, London, p 539
Francis DM, Thomson MF, Greaves MW (1980) The kinetic properties and reaction mechanism of histamine methyltransferase from human skin. Biochem J 187: 819–828
Friedgen B, Halbrugge T, Graefe K-H (1993) The part played by catechol-*O*-methyltransferase in the plasma kinetics of 3,4-dihydroxyphenylglycol and 3,4-dihydroxyphenylalanine in the anesthetized rabbit. Naunyn Schmiedebergs Arch Pharmacol 347:155–161
Fuller RW (1987) Norepinephrine *N*-methyltransferase from rabbit adrenal glands. Methods Enzymol 142:655–660
Fuller RW, Perry KW, Hemrick-Luecke SK (1983) Tropolone antagonism of the L-dopa-induced elevation of *S*-adenosylhomocysteine: *S*-adenosylmethionine ratio but not depletion of adrenaline in rat hypothalamus. J Pharm Pharmacol 36:419–429

Gitomer WL, Tipton KF (1986) Purification and kinetic properties of ox brain histamine *N*-methyltransferase. Biochem J 233:669–676

Goldstein DS, Grossman E, Tamrat M, Chang PC, Eisenhofer G, Bacher J, Kirk KL, Bacharach S, Kopin IJ (1991) Positron emission imaging of cardiac sympathetic innervation and function using ^{18}F-6-fluorodopamine: effects of chemical sympathectomy by 6-hydroxydopamine. J Hypertens 9:417–423

Griffith OW, Anderson ME, Meister A (1979) Inhibition of glutathione biosynthesis by protamine sulfoxime (*S*-n-propylhomocysteine sulfoxime), a selective inhibitor of γ-glutamylcysteine synthetase. J Biol Chem 254:1205–1210

Grossman MH, Creveling CR, Rybcznski R, Braverman M, Isersky C, Breakfield XO (1985) Soluble and particulate forms of rat cetechol-*O*-methyltransferase distinguished by gel electrophoresis and immune fixation. J Neurochem 44: 421–432

Grossman MH, Creveling CR, Breakfield XO (1989) Isolation of the mRNA encoding rat liver catechol-*O*-methyltransferase. Biochem Biophys Res Commun 158:776–782

Grossman MH, Emanuel BS, Budarf ML (1992a) Chromosomal mapping of the human catechol-*O*-methyltransferase gene to 22q11.1 to q11.2. Genomics 12: 822–825

Grossman MH, Szumlanski C, Littrell JB, Weinstein R, Weinshiboum RM (1992b) Electrophoretic analysis of low and high activity forms of catechol-*O*-methyltransferase in human erythrocytes. Life Sci 50:473–480

Grunewald GL, Grindel JM, Vincek WC, Borchardt RT (1975) Importance of aromatic ring in adrenergic amines. Nonaromatic analogues of phenethanolamine as substrates for phenethanolamine *N*-methyltransferase. Mol Pharmacol 11:694–699

Guldberg HC, Marsden CA (1975) Catechol-*O*-methyltransferase: pharmacological aspects and physiological role. Pharmacol Rev 27:135–206

Halbrugge T, Friedgen B, Ludwig J, Graefe K-H (1993) Effects of catechol-*O*-methyltransferase inhibition on the plasma clearance of noradrenaline and the formation of 3,4-dihydroxyphenylglycol in the rabbit. Naunyn Schmiedebergs Arch Pharmacol (in press)

Higazi MF, Borchardt RT, Schowen RL (1976) SN_2-like transition state for methyltransfer catelyzed by catechol-*O*-methyltransferase. J Am Chem Soc 98:3048–3049

His W (1887) Über das Stoffwechselproduct des Pyridine. Arch Exp Pathol Pharmakol 22:253–260

Hoffman AR, Paul SM, Axelrod J (1979) Catecholestrogens: synthesis and metabolism by human breast tumors in vitro. Cancer Res 39:4584–4587

Hoffman JL (1979) Inhibition of *S*-adenosyl sulfur amino acid metabolism: periodate-oxidized nucleosides as potent inhibitors of *S*-adenosylhomocysteine hydrolase. In: Usdin E, Borchardt RT, Creveling CR (eds) Transmethylation. Elsevier North Holland, New York, p 181

Hoffman JL (1993) Xenobiotic activation by *S*-adenosylation and *N*- and *S*-methylation. In: Anders MV (ed) Conjugation-dependent bioactivation. University of Rochester Press, Rochester

Horn AS, Dijkstra D, Mulder TBA, Rollema H, Westerink BHC (1981) Eur J Med Chem 16:469–472

Hough LB, Khandelwal JK, Mittag TW (1981) Alpha-methylhistamine methylation by histamine methyltransferase. Agents Action 11:425–428

Inoue K, Creveling CR (1991) Induction of catechol-*O*-methyltransferase in the luminal epithelium of rat uterus by progesterone. J Histochem Cytochem 39: 823–828

Ishida I, Obinata M, Deguchi T (1987) Molecular cloning and nucleotide sequence of cDNA encoding hydroxyindole *O*-methyltransferase of bovine pineal glands. J Biol Chem 262:2895–2899

Jackson RL, Lovenberg W (1971) Isolation and characterization of multiple forms of hydroxyindole-*O*-methyltransferase. J Biol Chem 246:4280–4285
Jakoby WB, Stevens J, Duffel MW, Weisiger RA (1984) The terminal enzymes of mercapturate formation and the thiomethyl shunt. Rev Biochem Toxicol 6:158–169
Joh TH, Baetge EE, Ross ME, Feis DJ (1983) Evidence for the exsistence of homologous gene coding regions for the catecholamine biosynthetic enzymes. Cold Spring Harbor Symp Quant Biol 48:327–335
Joh TH, Baetge EE, Ross ME, Lai C-Y, Docherty M, Bradford H, Reis DJ (1985) Genes for neurotransmitter synthesis, storage and uptake. Fed Proc 44:2723–2779
Kaakkola S, Gordin A, Jarvinen M, Wikberg T, Schultz E, Nissinen E, Pentikainen PJ, Rita H (1990) Effect of a novel catechol-*O*-methyltransferase inhibitor, nitecapone, on the metabolism of L-DOPA in healthy volunteers. Clin Neuropharmacol 13:436–447
Kaneda N, Ichinose H, Kobayashi K, Oka K, Kishi F, Nakazawa Y, Fujita K, Nagatsu T (1988) Molecular cloning of cDNA and chromosomal assignment of the gene for human phenylethanolamine *N*-methyltransferase, the enzyme for epinephrine biosynthesis. J Biol Chem 263:7672–7677
Karsch FJ, Woodfill CJI, Malpaus B, Robinson JE, Wayne NL (1991) Melatonin and mammalian photoperiodism; synchronization and annual reproductive cycles. In: Klein DC, Moore RY, Repert S (eds) Suprachiasmatic nucleus. The mind's clock. Oxford University Press, New York, p 217
Keith RA, Otterness DM, Kerremans AL, Weinshilboum RM (1985) *S*-methylation of D- and L-penicillamine by human erythrocyte membrane thiol methyltransferase. Drug Metab Dispos 13:669–676
Keller BT, Borchardt RT (1986) Metabolism and mechanism of action of nepanocin A – a potent inhibitor of *S*-adenosylhomocysteine hydrolase. In: Borchardt RT, Creveling CR, Ueland PM (eds) Biological methylation and drug design. Experimental and clinical roles of *S*-adenosylmethionine. Humana, New York, p 385
Kerremans AL, Lipsky JJ, van Loon J, Gallego MO, Weishilboum RM (1985) Cephalosporin-induced hypothrombinemia: possible role for thiol methylation of 1-methyltetrazole-5-thiol and 2-methyl-1,2,3-thiadiazole-5-thiol. J Pharmacol Exp Ther 235:382–388
Klein DC, Roseboom PH, Donohue SJ, Marrs BL (1992) Evolution of melatonin as a night signal: contribution from a primitive photosynthetic organism. Mol Cell Neurosci 3:181–183
Korkolainen T, Nissinen E (1989) Purification of rat liver soluble catechol-*O*-methyltransferase by high performance liquid chromatography. Biomed Chromatogr 3:127–130
Kredich NM, Hershfield MS (1980) Perturbations in *S*-adenosylhomocysteine and *S*-adenosylmethionine metabolism. Adv Enzyme Regul 18:181–191
Kuwano R, Takahashi Y (1980) *S*-adenosylhomocysteine is bound to pineal hydroxyindole *O*-methyltransferase. Life Sci 27:1321–1326
Kuwano R, Takahashi Y (1984) Binding of *S*-adenosylhomocysteine to hydroxyindole *O*-methyltransferase. Biochim Biophys Acta 787:1–7
Kuwano R, Yoshida Y, Takahashi Y (1978) Purification of bovine pineal hydroxylindole-*O*-methyltransferase by immunoadsorption chromatography. J Neurochem 31:815–824
Lennard L, van Loon JA, Lilleyman JS, Weinshilboum RM (1987) Thiopurine pharmacogenetics in leukemia: correlation of erythocyte thiopurine methyltransferase activity and 6-thioguanine nucleotide concentrations. Clin Pharmacol 41:18–25
Li SA, Purdy RH, Li JJ (1989) Variation in catechol *O*-methyltransferase activity in rodent tissues: possible role in estrogen carcinogenicity. Carcinogenesis 10: 63–67

Linden I-B, Nissinen E, Etemadzadeh E, Kaakola S, Mannisto R, Pohto P (1988) Favorable effects of catechol-*O*-methyltransferase inhibition by OR-462 in experimental models of Parkinson's disease. J Pharmacol Exp Ther 247:289–293
Longcope C (1983) Assay and metabolism of catechol estrogens. In: Merriam GR, Lipsett MB (eds) Catechol estrogens. Raven, New York, p 144
Lotta T, Takinen J, Backstrom R, Nissinen E (1992) PLS modelling of structure–activity relationships of catechol-*O*-methyltranferase inhibitors. J Comput Aided Mol Des 6:253–257
Lundstrom K, Salminen M, Jalanko A, Savolainen R, Ulmanen I (1991) Cloning and characterization of hyman placental catechol-*O*-methyltransferase cDNA. DNA Cell Biol 10:181–189
Lundstrom K, Tilgmann C, Peranen J, Kalkkinen N, Ulmanen I (1992) Expression of enzymatically active rat liver and human placental catechol-*O*-methyltransferase in *Escherichia coli*; purification and partial characterization of the enzyme. Biochim Biophys Acta 1129:149–154
Luwano R, Takahashi Y (1984) Binding of *S*-adenosylhomocysteine to hydroxyindole *O*-methyltransferase. Biochim Biophys Acta 787:1–7
Maj J, Rogoz Z, Sowinska H, Superata J (1992) Behavioural and neurochemical effects of R0 40-7592, a new COMT inhibitor with a potential therapeutic activity in Parkinson's disease. J Neural Transm Park Dis Dement Sect 2:101–112
Mannisto PT, Kaakkola S (1990) Rationale for selective COMT inhibitors as adjuncts in the drug treatment of Parkinson's disease. Pharmacol Toxicol 66:317–323
Mannisto PT, Kaakkola S, Nissinen E, Linden I-B, Pohto P (1988) Properties of novel effective and highly selective inhibitors of catechol-*O*-methyltransferase. Life Sci 43:1465–1471
Mannisto PT, Tuomainen P, Tuomainen RK (1992) Different in vivo properties of three new inhibitors of catechol-*O*-methyltransferase in the rat. Br J Pharmacol 105:569–574
Mezey E (1989) Cloning of the rat medullary phenylethanolamine *N*-methyltransferase. Nucleic Acids Res 17:2125
Morris ND, McNeal ET, Creveling CR (1973) On the role of sulfhydryl groups in the active site of catechol-*O*-methyltransferase (Abst F19). ACS Middle Atlantic Regional Meeting, Jan 14–17, Washington
Mozier NM, McConnell KP, Hoffman JL (1988) *S*-adenosyl-L-methionine:thioether *S*-methyltransferase, a new enzyme in sulfur and selenium metabolism. J Biol Chem 263:4527–4531
Mulder GJ, Krijgsheld KR (1984) In: Roe DA, Campbell TC (eds) Drugs and nutrients. Dekker, New York, p 119
Nic a'Bhaird N, Goldberg R, Tipton KF (1990) Catechol-*O*-methyltransferase and its role in catecholamine metabolism. Adv Neurol 53:489
Nikodejevic B, Senoh S, Daly JW, Creveling CR (1970) Catechol-*O*-methyltransferase II: a new class of inhibitors of catechol-*O*-methyltransferase; 3,5-dihydroxy-4-methylbenzoic acid and related compounds. J Pharmacol Exp Ther 174:83–93
Nissinen E (1984) The site of *O*-methylation by membrane-bound catechol-*O*-methyltransferase. Biochem Pharmacol 33:3105–3108
Nissinen E, Linden I-B, Schultz E, Kaakkola S (1988a) Catechol-*O*-methyltransferase activity in human and rat small intestine. Life Sci 42:2609–2614
Nissinen E, Linden I-B, Schultz E, Kaakkola S, Mannisto PT, Pohto P (1988b) Inhibition of catechol-*O*-methyltransferase by two novel disubstituted catechols in the rat. Eur J Pharmacol 153:263–269
Norin NAB, Tipton KF (1991) Catechol-*O*-methyltransferase from human placenta: purification and some properties. Biochem Soc Trans 19:20S
Nosenko ND (1990) Neuroendocrine effects of neonatal action of catechol-*O*-methyltransferase and sex steroids inhibitor. Neurosci Behav Physiol 20:462–465

Ozawa S, Nagata K, Gong D, Yamazoe Y, Kato R (1990) Nucleotide sequence of a full-length cDNA (PST-1) for aryl sulfotransferase from rat liver. Nucleic Acids Res 18:4001
Piedrafita FJ, Elorriaga C, Fernadez-Alvarez E, Nieto O (1990) Inhibition of catechol-*O*-methyltransferase by *N*-(3,4-dihyroxyphenyl)maleimide. J Enzym Inhib 4:43–50
Rafferty MF, Grunewald GL (1982) The remarkable substrate activity for phenethanolamine *N*-methyltransferase of some configurationally defined phenethylamines lacking a side chain hydroxyl group: conformationally defined adrenergic agents 6. Mol Pharmacol 22:127–132
Remy CN (1963) Metabolism of thiopyrimidines and thiopurines. J Biol Chem 238:1078–1084
Roth JA (1992) Membrane-bound catechol-*O*-methyltransferase: a reevaluation of its role in the *O*-methylation of the catecholamine neurotransmitters. Rev Physiol Biochem Pharmacol 120:2–29
Roth JA, Grossman MH, Adolf M (1990) Variation in hepatic membrane-bound catechol-*O*-methyltransferase activity in Fischer and Wistar-Furth strain of rat. Biochem Pharmacol 40:1151–1153
Roy D, Weisz J, Liehr JG (1990) The *O*-methylation of 4-hydroxyestradiol is inhibited by 2-hydroxyestradiol: implications for estrogen-induced carcinogenesis. Carcinogenesis 11:459–462
Salminen M, Lundstrom K, Tilgmann C, Savolainen R, Kalkkinen N, Ulmanen I (1990) Molecular cloning and characterization of rat liver catechol-*O*-methyltransferase. Gene 93:241–247
Sasaoka T, Kanada N, Kurosawa Y, Fujita K, Nagatsu T (1989) Structure of human phenylethanolamine *N*-methyltransferase gene: existence of two types of mRNA with different transcription initiation site. Neurochem Int 15:555–565
Satake N, Morton B (1979) Pineal hydroxyindol *O*-methyltransferase: mechanism, and inhibition by scotophobin A. Pharmacol Biochem Behav 10:457–462
Schultz E (1991) Catechol-*O*-methyltransferase and aromatic L-amino acid decarboxylase activies in human gastrointesinal tissues. Life Sci 49:721–725
Schultz E, Tapila S, Bachstrom A-C, Gordin A, Nissinen E, Pohto P (1991) Inhibition of human erythrocyte and gastroduodenal catechol-*O*-methyltransferase activity by nitecapone. Eur J Clin Pharmacol 40:577–580
Shinagawa Y (1992) Molecular orbital studies on the structure–activity relationships of catechol *O*-methyltransferase inhibitors. Jpn J Pharmacol 58:95–106
Shull KH, McConomy J, Vogt M, Castillo A, Farber E (1966) On the mechanism of induction of hepatic adenosine triphosphate deficiency by ethionine. J Biol Chem 241:5060–5070
Steel RD, Benevenga NJ (1979) The metabolism of 3-methylthiopropionate in rat liver homogenates. J Biol Chem 254:8885–8890
Stevens JL, Bakke JE (1990) *S*-methylation. In: Mulder GJ (ed) Conjugation reactions in drug metabolism. Taylor and Francis, London, p 251
Sugden D, Cena V, Klein DC (1987) Hydroxyindole *O*-methyltransferase. Methods Enzymol 142:590–596
Takemura M, Tanaka T, Taguchi Y, Imamura I, Mizuguchi H, Kuroda M, Fukui H, Yamatodani A, Wada H (1992) Histamine *N*-methyltransferase from rat kidney: cloning, nucleotide sequence, and expression in E. coli cells. J Biol Chem 267:15687–15691
Taskinen J, Vidgren J, Ovaska M, Backstrom R, Pippuri A, Nissinen E (1989) QSAR and binding model for inhibition of rat liver catechol-*O*-methyltransferase by 1,5-substituted-3,4-dihydroxybenzenes. Quant Struct Act Relat 8:210–213
Taskinen J, Wikberg T, Ottoila P, Kanner L, Lotta T, Pippuri A, Backstrom R (1991) Identification of major metabolites of the catechol-*O*-methyltransferase-inhibitor nitecapone in human urine. Drug Metab Dispos 19:178–183
Thakker DR, Creveling CR (1990) *O*-Methylation. In: Mulder GJ (ed) Conjugation reactions in drug metabolism. Taylor and Francis, London, p 193

Thakker DR, Boehlert C, Kirk KL, Antkowiak R, Creveling CR (1986) Regioselectivity of catechol-*O*-methyltransferase. J Biol Chem 261:178–184

Thithapandha A, Cohn VH (1978) Brain histimine *N*-methyltransferase purification, mechanism of action, and inhibition by drugs. Biochem Pharmacol 27:263–271

Tilgmann C, Kalkkinen N (1991) Purification and partial sequence analysis of the soluble catechol-*O*-methyltransferase from human placenta: comparison to the rat liver enzyme. Biochem Biophys Res Commun 174:995–1002

Tilgmann C, Melen K, Lundstrom K, Jalanko A, Julkunen I, Kalkkinen N, Ulmanen I (1992) Expression of recombinant soluble and membrane-bound catechol *O*-methyltranferase in eukaryotic cells and identification of the respective enzymes in rat brain. Eur J Biochem 207:813–821

Timm U, Erdin R (1992) Determination of the catechol-*O*-methyltransferase inhibitor Ro 40-7592 in human plasma by high performance liquid chromatography with coulometric detection. J Chromatogr 593:63–68

Tisdale MJ (1980) The effect of the methionine antagonist L-2-amino-4-methoxy-trans-3-butenoic acid on the growth and metabolism of Walker carcinoma in vitro. Biochem Pharmacol 29:501–508

Tornwall M, Mannisto PT (1991) Acute toxicity of three new selective COMT inhibitors in mice with special emphasis on interactions with drugs increasing catecholaminergic neurotransmission. Pharmacol Toxicol 69:64–70

Tsukuda K, Yamano S, Abe T, Okada G (1980) Ethionine-induced changes in the activities of *S*-adenosylmethionine synthetase isozymes form rat liver. Biochem Biophys Res Commun 95:1160–1167

Ulmanen I, Lundstrom K (1991) Cell-free synthesis of rat and human catechol *O*-methyltransferase; insertion of the membrane-bound from into microsomal membranes in vitro. Eur J Biochem 202:1013–1020

Usdin E, Borchardt RT, Creveling CR (eds) (1982) Biochemistry of *S*-adenosylmethionine and related compounds. Macmillan, London

Veser J, May W (1986) A rapid purification procedure for *S*-adenosyl-L-methionine: catechol-*O*-methyltransferase by high-performance ion exchange chromatography and subsequent affinity chromatography. Chromatographia 22:7–12

Vidgren J, Tilgmann C, Lunstrom K, Lijas A (1991) Crystallization and preliminary X-ray investigation of a recombinant form of rat catechol *O*-methyltransferase. Proteins Struct Funct Genet 11:233–236

Villa-Trevino S, Shull KH, Farber E (1966) The inhibition of liver ribonucleic acid synthesis by ethionine. J Biol Chem 241:4670–4676

Voisin P, Guerlotte J, Bernard M, Collin JP, Cogne M (1992) Molecular cloning and nucleotide sequence of a cDNA encoding hyroxyindole-*O*-methyltransferase from chicken pineal gland. Biochem J 282:571–576

Wada H, Watanabe T, Yamatodani A, Maeyama K, Itoi N, Cacabelos R, Seo M, Kiyono S, Nagai K, Nagagawa H (1985) Physiological function of histamine in the brain. Adv Biosci 51:225

Wade L, Katzman R (1975) 3-*O*-Methyldopa inhibition of L-dopa at the blood-brain barrier. Life Sci 17:131–136

Waldmeier PC, Baumann PA, Feldtrauer J-J, Hauser K, Bittiger H, Bischoff S, von Sprecher G (1990) CGP 28014, a new inhibitor of catechol-*O*-methylation with a non-catechol structure. Naunyn Schmiedebergs Arch Pharmacol 342:305–311

Warner DR (1992) Cloning and active site labelling of thioether methyltransferase. PhD dissertation, University of Louisville

Watanabe R, Taguche Y, Shiosaka S, Tanaka J, Kubota H, Terano Y, Tohyama M, Wada H (1984) Distribution of the histaminergic neuron system in the central nervous system of rats: a fluorescent immunohistochemical analysis with histidine decarboxylase as a marker. Brain Res 295:13–25

Weinshilboum R (1986) Sulfate conjugation of neurotransmitters and drugs. Fed Proc 45:2220–2222

Weinshilboum R (1988a) Phenol sulfotransferase inheritance. Cell Mol Neurobiol 8:27–34

Weinshilboum R (1988b) Pharmacogenetics of methylation: relationship to drug metabolism. Clin Biochem 21:201–210

Weinshilboum R (1989) Methyltransferase pharmacogenetics. Pharmacol Ther 43: 77–90

Weinshilboum R (1991) In: Damani LA (ed) Sulfur drugs and related organic chemicals: chemistry, biochemistry, and toxicology. Horwood, Chichester

Weisiger RA, Jakoby WB (1979) Thiol *S*-methyltransferase from rat liver. Arch Biochem Biophys 196:631–637

Weisiger RA, Jakoby WB (1980) *S*-Methylation: thiol *S*-methyltransferases. In: Jakoby WB (ed) Enzymatic basis of detoxification, vol 2. Academic, New York, p 131

Windquist R, Lundstrom K, Salminen M, Laatikainen M, Ulmanen I (1992) The human catechol-*O*-methyltransferase (COMT) gene maps to band q11.2 of chromosome 22 and shows a frequest RFLP with Bg/I. Cytogenet Cell Genet 59:253–257

Woodward RW, Tsai MD, Floss HG, Gooks PA, Coward JK (1980) Stereochemical course of the transmethylation catalyzed by catechol-*O*-methyltransferase. J Biol Chem 255:9124–9127

Youde IR, Raxworthy MJ, Gulliver PA, Dijkstra D, Horn AS (1984) The metabolism of dopamine, *N,N*-dialkylated dopamines and derivatives of dopamine agonist 2-amino-dihydroxy-1,2,3,4-tetrahydronaphthaliene (ADTN) by catechol *O*-methyltransferase. J Pharm Pharmacol 36:309–313

Zapia V, Zydeck-Cwich CR, Schlenk F (1969) The specificiy of *S*-adenosylmethionine derivatives in methyltransfer reactions. J Biol Chem 214:4499–1509

Ziegler DM (1985) Molecular basis for N-oxygenation of *sec*- and *tert*-amines. In: Gorrod J, Damani LA (eds) Biological oxidation of nitrogen in organic molecules. Horwood, Chichester, p 43

Ziegler DM, Ansher SS, Nagata T, Kadluber FF, Jakoby WB (1988) *N*-Methylation: potential mechanism for metabolic activation of carcinogenic primary arylamines. Proc Natl Acad Sci USA 85:2514–2517

Zimmerman TP, Wolberg G, Duncan GS, Elion GB (1980) Adenosine analogues as substrates and inhibitors of *S*-adenosylhomocysteine hydrolase in intact lymphocytes. Biochemistry 19:2252–2259

Zurcher G, Colzi A, Da Prada M (1990) Ro 40-7592: inhibition of COMT in rat brain and extracerebral tissues. J Neural Transm Suppl 32:375–380

Section II
Regulation of Phase II Conjugation: Deconjugation Reactions in Intact Cells and Tissues

CHAPTER 8

Cofactor Supply as a Rate-Limiting Determinant of Hepatic Conjugation Reactions

L.A. REINKE, F.C. KAUFFMANN, and R.G. THURMAN

A. Introduction

The metabolism of drugs, other xenobiotics, and endogenous compounds by conjugation is usually catalyzed by specific transferases; the notable exceptions are the non-enzymatic conjugation of highly reactive intermediates with glutathione (GSH) and the formation of acyl-linked glucuronides (reviewed in Chaps. 13 and 16 of this volume). Because of the important role of transferases in catalyzing conjugation reactions, these enzymes have been studied extensively, and the properties of the important conjugating enzymes are described in Chaps. 1–7.

Conjugation of drugs and xenobiotics is dependent on the biosynthesis of the required cofactors by the body. Although there are many differences in cofactor requirements among various pathways, two properties are common to all conjugation reactions: a requirement for energy and enhanced excretion of metabolic intermediates generated via conjugation.

I. Energy Requirements for Conjugation

The energy required for conjugation reactions is used primarily in the biosynthesis of cofactors needed for conjugation reactions. The exception is conjugation of simple acids with glycine or glutamate, where the acidic drug is converted into a drug coenzyme A (CoA) derivative in a step requiring adenosine triphosphate (ATP), followed by addition of the amino acid. Uridine triphosphate (UTP) is used for the formation of uridine diphosphate (UDP)-glucose and UDP-glucuronic acid (UDP-GA), while ATP is required for the biosynthesis of the other cofactors. A good example of the relationship between conjugation and cellular energy status is inhibition of sulfation and glucuronidation in hepatocytes incubated under hypoxic conditions (AW and JONES 1982). Under normal metabolic conditions, cells have no difficulty in meeting the energy requirements for conjugation; however, production of high-energy phosphate intermediates are increased during high rates of conjugation, so that other energy-requiring processes are not compromised.

II. Metabolic Burden of Conjugation

In addition to the expenditure of energy, a naturally occurring metabolic intermediate is added to the chemical being metabolized, and the resulting conjugate is exported from the cell. Thus, conjugation invariably leads to the loss of key cellular intermediates, such as carbohydrate (glucuronidation), amino acids (conjugation with GSH and amino acids), and acetate (acetylation). Abnormally low concentrations of many of these building blocks and other closely related intermediates have been documented to occur as a result of rapid rates of drug conjugation. In the case of GSH, excessive loss of the tripeptide may have toxicological significance (discussed in Sect. E.II).

III. Drug Substrate Concentration as a Rate-Determining Factor for Conjugation Reactions

In general, the metabolism and clearance of most drugs follow first-order kinetics, i.e., the rate of metabolism is directly dependent on the concentration of the drug. This principle is also true of most conjugation pathways. Substrate concentration is a particularly important rate-determining factor in the case of drugs which may be conjugated with either glucuronic acid or sulfate.

Numerous studies have demonstrated that sulfate conjugates are formed primarily when drug concentrations are low and that glucuronides predominate when drug concentrations are high (e.g., MINCK et al. 1973; SCHWARZ 1980; KOSTER et al. 1981; REINKE et al. 1981). This phenomenon is easily understandable from the typical K_m values of the respective transferase enzymes for substrate; in general, sulfotransferase enzymes have a much lower K_m for substrates than glucuronosyltransferases. The result is that sulfate conjugates readily form at low substrate concentrations, but increasing concentrations of drug saturate this conjugation pathway (REINKE et al. 1981; KOSTER and MULDER 1982). In contrast, glucuronidation has a high capacity for substrate and is difficult to saturate. The relevance of these observations is that conjugates are often formed from metabolites of cytochrome P-450 and other pathways of oxidative metabolism, so that the type of conjugate which predominates is influenced primarily by the rate of the oxidative metabolism.

The same principles apply to rates of conjugation after exposure of animals to agents which induce drug-metabolizing enzymes. Phenobarbital, aromatic hydrocarbons, and many other compounds increase several forms of both cytochrome P-450 and glucuronosyltransferase in the liver. Thus, higher rates of glucuronide formation after induction of drug metabolism might be explained by increased glucuronosyltransferase activity, but cofactor supply must also be taken into consideration. For example, *p*-nitroanisole *O*-demethylation and the subsequent conjugation of the product, *p*-nitrophenol, were elevated in perfused livers from phenobarbital-treated rats compared to controls (REINKE et al. 1981); however, livers from well-fed control rats had the same capacity to glucuronidate *p*-nitrophenol as livers from well-fed phenobarbital-treated rats at all but the highest substrate concentrations tested (Fig. 1). Maximal rates of *p*-nitrophenol conjugation in the three dietary groups (fasted, fed, and fasted–refed) correlated closely with glycogen content of those livers, suggesting that the supply of UDP-GA was rate limiting. Increased *p*-nitrophenol glucuronidation after phenobarbital treatment is better explained by the greater rate of *p*-nitroanisole metabolism and therefore higher concentration of the substrate *p*-nitrophenol, rather than by the induction of glucuronosyltransferase by phenobarbital (REINKE et al. 1981).

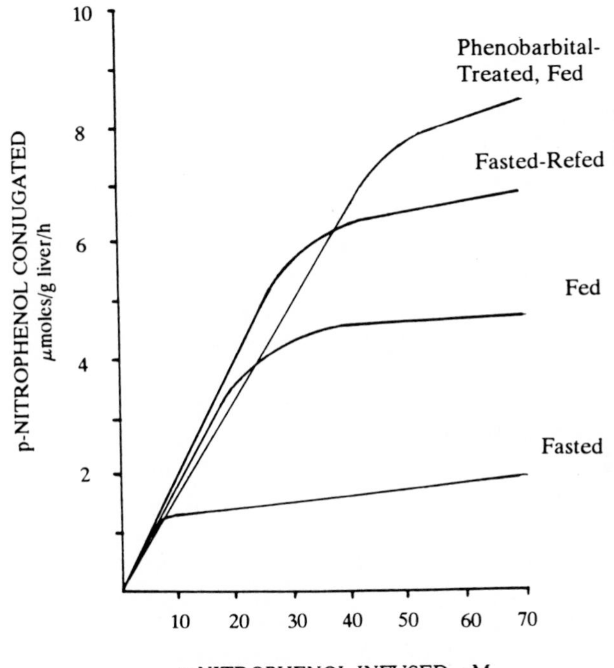

Fig. 1. Effect of the nutritional state on *p*-nitrophenol conjugation in perfused rat livers. Rates of *p*-nitrophenol conjugation were measured in perfused livers from rats which had been allowed free access to lab chow (*fed*), fasted for 24 h (*fasted*), or fasted for 48 h and then allowed free access to chow for an additional 24 h (*fasted–refed*). Similar experiments were performed with rats allowed free access to lab chow, but which also received phenobarbital (1 mg/ml) in their drinking water (*phenobarbital-treated, fed*). The *curves* represent average conjugation rates in at least five rats per treatment group. Other experiments showed that rates of *p*-nitrophenol sulfation were unaffected by the nutritional state and that differences in conjugation rates were due to changes in glucuronidation

The concentration of substrate chosen for studies of regulation of conjugation may make comparison of results obtained in different laboratories difficult. For example, UDP-GA in the liver of a fasted rat may be adequate to glucuronidate aglycones at low concentrations, but not at higher concentrations (REINKE et al. 1981). Thus, some of the conflicting data in the literature regarding the role of cofactor supply to limit conjugation may be due to the fact that the concentration of substrates employed in the various studies often varies between laboratories.

B. Models Used to Study Regulation of Conjugation

The enzymology of the transferase enzymes is most appropriately studied in vitro, in purified or semipurified preparations. However, whole cell preparations are required for studies in which rate limitation by cofactor supply is being tested, because the metabolic pathways which form the cofactor in intact cells must be operational. Studies in intact, living animals, which probably have the most biological relevance, suggest that events regulating the availability of cofactor may be limiting. Pharmacokinetic methods (e.g., PRICE et al. 1987) and measurement of tissue concentrations of cofactors following a drug challenge (e.g., HJELLE et al. 1985) have been performed. In studies involving whole animals, the concentrations of the drug under study and any required precursors (such as inorganic sulfate, glucose, and sulfur-containing amino acids) are supplied by the circulation. Manipulation of these determinants of conjugation in vivo is difficult. Consequently, two in vitro models, the perfused liver and isolated hepatocytes, have been used extensively to study the regulation of drug conjugation.

Isolated perfused livers have the advantage that normal liver structure is maintained, and venous perfusate and biliary efflux may be sampled separately. Both of these properties are lost when hepatocytes are used, but isolated cells offer the advantage of efficiency. Both freshly isolated hepatocytes and hepatocyte cultures have been employed in conjugation studies, but the usefulness of cultured cells is hampered by loss of cytochrome P-450 activity and changes in some conjugating transferases after a few days of culture. Additional comparisons among hepatocytes, liver slices, perfused livers, and intact animals have been made elsewhere (THURMAN et al. 1989). In general, comparable results have been obtained with perfused livers and freshly isolated hepatocytes, and studies with these models have been very useful in extending and interpreting results obtained with laboratory animals.

C. Glucuronidation

I. Uridine Diphosphate Glucuronic Acid Metabolism

A simplified schematic of UDP-GA metabolism is shown in Fig. 2. UDP-GA is biosynthesized from glucose-1-phosphate (G-1-P), which is derived either from glycogenolysis or from glucose-6-phosphate (G-6-P) by the phosphoglucomutase reaction. UDP-Glucose (UDP-G) is formed from UTP and G-1-P by the action of UDP-glucose pyrophosphorylase, and the rapid catabolism of pyrophosphate (PP_i) in the cell makes the reaction essentially irreversible. UDP-G normally provides the glucosyl units for glycogen biosynthesis; however, UDP-G may be oxidized by the cytosolic enzyme UDP-glucose dehydrogenase to form UDP-GA. The dehydrogenase step requires NAD^+ as a cofactor and is essentially irreversible.

The degradation of UDP-GA is catalyzed primarily by UDP-glucuronate pyrophosphatase to form glucuronate-1-P (Fig. 2). This intermediate is sub-

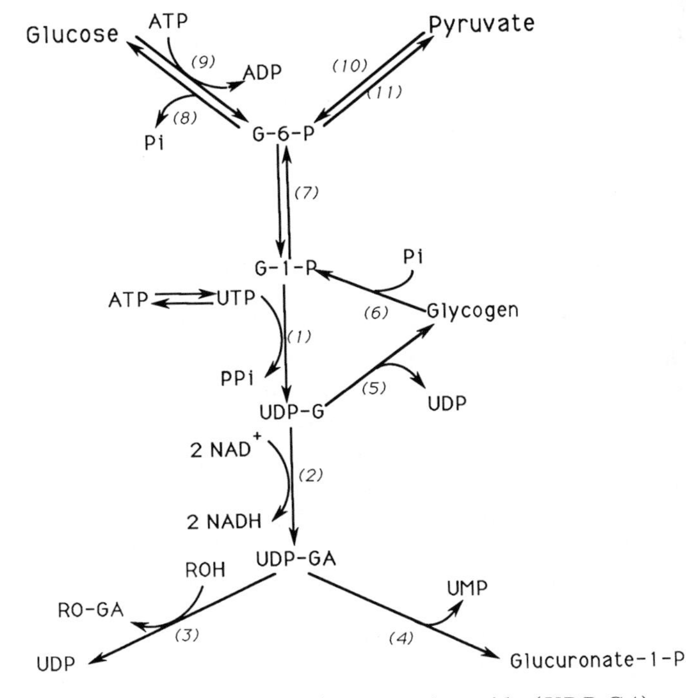

Fig. 2. Uridine diphosphate (*UDP*)-glucuronic acid (*UDP-GA*) metabolism. Enzymes: (*1*) UDP-glucose pyrophosphorylase; (*2*) UDP-glucose dehydrogenase; (*3*) UDP-glucuronosyltransferase(s): (*4*) UDP-glucuronate pyrophosphatase; (*5*) glycogen synthase; (*6*) glycogen phosphorylase; (*7*) phosphoglucomutase; (*8*) glucose-6-phosphatase; (*9*) hexokinase and glucokinase; (*10*) gluconeogenic pathway; (*11*) glycolytic pathway. See text for abbreviations

sequently dephosphorylated to form GA, which may then be metabolized to ascorbate, pentose cycle intermediates, and other metabolic products (AARTS 1966).

The K_m values of glucuronosyltransferases for UDP-GA are usually reported to be in the range of 0.1–0.4 mM (e.g., BOCK et al. 1973), which approximates the concentration of UDP-GA in the liver. For this reason, it should be expected that changes in cellular metabolism which increase or decrease the availability of UDP-GA will cause corresponding changes in the rates of glucuronidation. In fact, several laboratories have shown direct correlations between the rates of glucuronidation and the intracellular concentrations of UDP-GA (SINGH and SCHWARZ 1981; AW and JONES 1984; REINKE et al. 1981). A variety of biochemical and physiological factors have been shown to alter rates of glucuronidation via availability of UDP-GA and are discussed in the following sections.

II. Carbohydrate Supplies

1. Glycogen Levels

Glycogen was shown to be the probable source of UDP-GA many years ago (DZIEWIATKOWSKI and LEWIS 1944), and the close relationship which exists between glycogen metabolism and UDP-GA biosynthesis is illustrated in Fig. 2. Not only do glycogen and UDP-GA both arise from a common precursor (UDP-G), glycogen breakdown also serves as a major source of glucosyl units for UDP-GA biosynthesis.

Experiments using perfused rat livers emphasize the importance of glycogen stores in determining the rate of glucuronidation (REINKE et al. 1981). Rats were divided into three nutritional groups (fed ad libitum, fasted for 24 h, or fasted for 48 h and then refed for 24 h) and rates of *p*-nitrophenol conjugation were measured in perfused livers from these animals (Fig. 1). Rates of *p*-nitrophenol glucuronidation and hepatic levels of glycogen were both lowest in livers from fasted rats, and highest in livers of fasted–refed rats. The lowest hepatic concentrations of UDP-G and UDP-GA were also measured in the livers of fasted rats, while the glycogen-rich livers from fasted–refed rats generally had the highest concentrations of these intermediates (REINKE et al. 1981). Other examples of decreased drug glucuronidation following a period of fasting include studies of acetaminophen conjugation in rat hepatocytes (AW and JONES 1984) and intact rats (PRICE and JOLLOW 1988), 7-hydroxycoumarin conjugation in both periportal and pericentral regions of the rat liver lobule (CONWAY et al. 1985), and glucuronidation of *p*-nitrophenol in hepatocytes from mice (BANHEGYI et al. 1988). Fasting may also exaggerate decreases in glucuronidation observed with other metabolic stresses, such as hypoxia (ANGUS et al. 1988).

Because of the well-known decreases in rates of glucuronidation associated with fasting, addition of glucose or gluconeogenic precursors to intact cells predictably provides a carbohydrate source for UDP-GA biosynthesis and increase rates of glucuronidation. In support of this hypothesis, modest increases in rates of glucuronidation have been reported when glucose was provided to perfused livers or isolated hepatocytes (REINKE et al. 1981; EACHO et al. 1981a; AW and JONES 1984; CONWAY et al. 1985). However, in other studies, glucose addition has had a negligible effect (BANHEGYI et al. 1988). For example, administration of glucose or gluconeogenic precursors to fasted rats that also received a hepatotoxic dose of acetaminophen failed to increase hepatic concentrations of UDP-G or UDP-GA, did not increase rates of acetaminophen glucuronidation, and did not protect against acetaminophen-induced liver damage (PRICE and JOLLOW 1989).

2. Endocrine Disorders and Glucuronidation

Streptozotocin-induced diabetes increases the glucuronidation of *p*-nitrophenol in freshly isolated hepatocytes from male rats without affecting the activity of the glucuronosyltransferase enzymes (EACHO et al. 1981). Similarly, diabetic male Long-Evans rats were more resistant to acetaminophen hepatotoxicity and glucuronidated the drug at higher rates than nondiabetic controls (PRICE and JOLLOW 1982). In both studies, the effects of diabetes were reversed by insulin treatment. A subsequent study showed that UDP-GA levels in the diabetic Long-Evans rats were not different from those of control rats in the absence of a drug substrate, but that the biosynthesis of UDP-GA during acetaminophen metabolism was increased in the diabetic state (PRICE and JOLLOW 1986). In contrast, there have been occasional reports of decreased glucuronidation in experimental diabetes (see DUTTON 1980). These conflicting data could possibly be explained by sex-dependent (EACHO et al. 1981a,b) and strain-dependent (PRICE and JOLLOW 1986) effects of diabetes on glucuronidation. Further studies of the influence of diabetic states on glucuronidation of drug substrates are needed because of the importance of this disease to human pathology.

Although hepatic glucose metabolism is influenced by a number of hormones, there have been relatively few studies on the effects of altered endocrine function on hepatic glucuronidation. Some effects of hormones and pregnancy on glucuronidation, and especially effects on glucuronosyltransferase activity, have been reviewed by DUTTON (1980). In more recent studies, decreased rates of *p*-nitrophenol glucuronidation in perfused livers from hypophysectomized rats were attributed to low hepatic carbohydrate stores (AL-TURK and REINKE 1983).

III. Cellular Energetics and Glucuronidation

UTP is required for the biosynthesis of UDP-G and UDP-GA from G-1-P (Fig. 2). When glycogen serves as the source of carbohydrate, only UTP is required for UDP-GA biosynthesis. However, additional energy in the form of ATP is required if the G-1-P is derived from gluconeogenesis or in the form of exogenously added glucose (Fig. 2). Hepatic concentrations of UTP are also most likely in equilibrium with ATP. Thus, it is not surprising that physiological conditions which impair normal cellular energetics tend to lower hepatic concentrations of UDP-GA and decrease rates of glucuronidation.

1. Hypoxia

Because mitochondrial oxidative phosphorylation is of primary importance in generation of ATP, cellular energetics are readily influenced by changes in the availability of oxygen. The liver, which receives most of its blood supply from the portal circulation, may be especially sensitive to cellular oxygen deficiency. In addition, an oxygen gradient exists in the liver lobule, with cells in the periportal area exposed to higher oxygen concentrations than cells in the pericentral region. When 7-hydroxycoumarin glucuronidation was measured in periportal and pericentral areas of the liver lobule, changes in the availability of UDP-GA over relatively short time periods caused corresponding changes in conjugation in both sublobular regions (Conway et al. 1985).

Low concentrations of oxygen resulted in diminished rates of *p*-nitroanisole oxidation, as well as *p*-nitrophenol conjugation, in perfused rat livers (Wu et al. 1990). Because similar effects of hypoxia were not observed in isolated microsomes, the effects of oxygen in perfused livers were attributed to changes in hepatic concentrations of reduced nicotinamide adenine dinucleotide phosphate (NADPH) required for mixed-function oxidation and UDP-GA needed for glucuronidation. Decreased conjugation of harmol in perfused livers has also been observed during periods of hypoxia (Angus et al. 1987, 1988).

Effects of hypoxia on hepatic conjugation have been studied extensively in freshly isolated hepatocytes (Aw and Jones 1982, 1984). In these studies, rates of glucuronidation were proportional not only to UDP-GA, but also to UDP-G, G-1-P, and UTP. The authors concluded that rates of glucuronidation during hypoxia were controlled by the UDP-glucose pyrophosphorylase reaction, which requires a steady supply of UTP (Fig. 2).

2. Metabolic Inhibitors

In order to define further the relationship which exists between cellular energetics and conjugation, a variety of known metabolic inhibitors have been evaluated. Freshly isolated hepatocytes or perfused livers were used in most of these studies in order to avoid the complication of the toxicity of these compounds to the animal. Inhibitors of mitochondrial oxidative phosphorylation, such as cyanide (Reinke et al. 1981), rotenone (Wiebkin et al. 1979), and antimycin-A (Reinke et al. 1987), all decrease rates of conjugation in intact cells. Agents which decrease hepatic concentrations of ATP by uncoupling oxidative phosphorylation, such as dinitrophenol (WIEBKIN et al. 1979; REINKE et al. 1981), also have similar inhibitory effects. Although fructose might be expected to increase the availability of carbohydrate for UDP-GA biosynthesis, inhibition of *p*-nitrophenol conjugation occurs both in isolated hepatocytes (EACHO et al. 1981) and perfused livers (REINKE et al. 1981) due, most likely, to depletion of ATP. Fructose lowers hepatic concentrations of ATP because it is rapidly phosphorylated to generate fructose-1-phosphate.

DILLS and KLAASSEN (1986a) attempted to determine whether mitochondrial inhibitors decrease hepatic concentrations of UDP-GA, 3′-phosphoadenosine-5′-phosphosulfate (PAPS), and GSH when administered in vivo. Although the agents tested all decreased hepatic concentrations of ATP, the expected decreases in cofactor supply were not observed. However, in these studies, no substrate for conjugation was administered, and the toxicity of the inhibitors may have complicated the results. When studies of this type were repeated with the less toxic agents fructose and ethionine, hepatic concentrations of UDP-GA were decreased by 40%–50%, and rates of acetaminophen conjugation with glucuronic acid and sulfate were both diminished (DILLS and KLAASSEN 1986b).

Galactosamine is a well-characterized inhibitor of hepatic glucuronidation. In the liver, galactosamine reacts rapidly with UTP to form UDP-galactosamine. Under these conditions, hepatic concentrations of UTP and UDP-GA are rapidly depleted, resulting in decreased rates of glucuronidation both in vitro and in vivo (MOLDEUS et al. 1979; SINGH and SCHWARZ 1981; GREGUS et al. 1988b).

IV. The Cellular Oxidation–Reduction State and Glucuronidation

UDP-glucose dehydrogenase is an enzyme that requires NAD^+ (Fig. 2), and its activity is inhibited when cellular concentrations of reduced nicotinamide adenine dinucleotide (NADH) are elevated. The occurrence of this phenomenon in intact cells was proven by MOLDEUS et al. (1978), who showed that ethanol inhibited the glucuronidation of harmol in isolated hepatocytes. The inhibition is explained by metabolism of ethanol by alcohol dehydrogenase, which increased cellular levels of NADH and inhibited the biosynthesis of UDP-GA. Inhibitors of mitochondrial respiration such as cyanide, which also increase cellular levels of NADH, may likewise inhibit glucuronidation through this mechanism (REINKE et al. 1981). Cellular concentrations of NADH would also be expected to increase during hypoxia, but experiments with hepatocytes indicate that the UDP-glucose pyrophosphorylase step of UDP-GA synthesis, which requires UTP, is more sensitive to low concentrations of oxygen than the UDP-glucose dehydrogenase step (AW and JONES 1984).

V. Other Factors Influencing Glucuronidation

1. Volatile Anesthetics

Diethyl ether rapidly depletes hepatic concentrations of UDP-GA and causes corresponding decreases in the glucuronidation of acetaminophen (WATKINS et al. 1984) and bilirubin (DILLS and KLAASSEN 1984). These observations could not be explained by ether-induced changes in glucuronosyltransferase activity or in any of the precursors to UDP-GA. More recently, volatile anesthetics have been shown to increase the activity of hepatic nucleotide pyrophosphatase activity (WATKINS et al. 1990). Thus, enhanced catabolism of UDP-GA (Fig. 2) provides the most plausible explanation for the effects of volatile anesthetics on hepatic glucuronidation.

2. Effects of Drugs and Other Chemicals

a) Increased Glucuronidation

A number of drugs which are capable of inducing hepatic monooxygenase and glucuronosyltransferase enzymes, such as aromatic hydrocarbons, phenobarbital, and butylated hydroxyanisole, also increase hepatic concentrations of UDP-GA (WATKINS and KLAASSEN 1983; GOON and KLAASSEN 1992). However, the mechanisms and biological significance of these effects are largely unknown. Addition of ascorbic acid to suspensions of hepatocytes increases glucuronidation of 4-hydroxybiphenyl, possibly because of increased cellular concentrations of UDP-GA (PATERSON and FRY 1983).

b) Impaired Glucuronidation

Hepatic concentrations of UDP-GA are decreased by a number of drugs which are rapidly glucuronidated, such as acetaminophen (HJELLE et al. 1985; PRICE and JOLLOW 1986), salicylamide (KAMISAKO et al. 1990), clofibric acid, valproic acid, and chloramphenicol (HOWELL et al. 1986). Thus, rates of glucuronidation could become limited by cofactor supply when the demand is high, even though the available experimental evidence suggests that the liver has a high capacity for UDP-GA biosynthesis.

Hepatic concentrations of UDP-GA are also decreased by a number of hepatotoxic compounds (WATKINS and KLAASSEN 1983). These observations are not surprising, given the close relationship between UDP-GA and other pathways of carbohydrate and energy metabolism. Similarly, various forms of liver disease influence glucuronidation through effects on transferase activity, cofactor supply, or activation of glucuronidase activity (DUTTON 1980). Chronic alcohol administration to rats decreases both rates of 7-hydroxycoumarin glucuronidation and UDP-GA levels in perfused livers, without causing overt liver damage (REINKE et al. 1986). Hind limb ischemia has also been shown to decrease chloramphenicol glucuronidation and hepatic concentrations of UDP-GA (GRIFFETH et al. 1985). Although the mechanism for impaired glucuronidation during trauma is unknown, this observation raises the interesting possibility that chemical mediators in the blood influence hepatic metabolism and decrease glucuronidation. In this regard, it should be noted that both adenosine and dibutyryl cyclic adenosine monophosphate (AMP) decrease UDP-GA biosynthesis in isolated hepatocytes (SHIPLEY et al. 1986; SHIPLEY and WEINER 1987). Alternatively, hormonal disturbances in microcirculation could indirectly impair glucuronidation by producing local hypoxia.

In a recent review of drug glucuronidation in humans (MINERS and MACKENZIE 1991), probenecid and several other drugs were reported to inhibit glucuronidation when administered concomitantly. Diet, disease states, and various hormonal changes were also shown to affect glucuronidation in human patients in this review. The authors presumed that all of these changes resulted from alterations in glucuronosyltransferase activity; however, direct measurements of the enzyme were not made. The data reviewed in the preceding sections, which were obtained with experimental animals, indicate that all of these effects may also be explained, at least in part, by changes in UDP-GA levels.

VI. Intracellular Transport of Uridine Diphosphate Glucuronic Acid

The activities of all glucuronosyltransferases in microsomes can be increased by the addition of detergents, UDP-*N*-acetylglucosamine, or various forms of mechanical disruption (DUTTON 1980). Experiments using perfused livers indicate that this "latency" of glucuronosyltransferases also exists in the intact liver (BOCK et al. 1977). Data indicating enzyme latency have generally been explained by either a conformational restriction on the enzymes or by the possibility that the active site of the enzyme is located in the lumen of the endoplasmic reticulum (reviewed by ZAKIM and DANNENBERG 1992). In either case, cytoplasmic UDP-GA may not be freely accessible to binding sites on the transferase, and some type of transport mechanism may be required to deliver the cofactor to the active site (HAUSER et al. 1988a,b). While this topic is controversial and poorly understood, intracellular UDP-GA transport could provide another way in which glucuronidation is regulated by cofactor supply.

D. Sulfate Conjugation

I. 3′-Phosphoadenosine-5′-Phosphosulfate Metabolism

The biosynthesis of PAPS (also referred to as adenosine 3′-phosphate 5′-sulfatophosphate) is illustrated in Fig. 3. The reaction of inorganic sulfate with ATP to form adenosine-5′phosphosulfate (APS) is catalyzed by ATP sulfurylase. Although the equilibrium of this reaction favors the formation

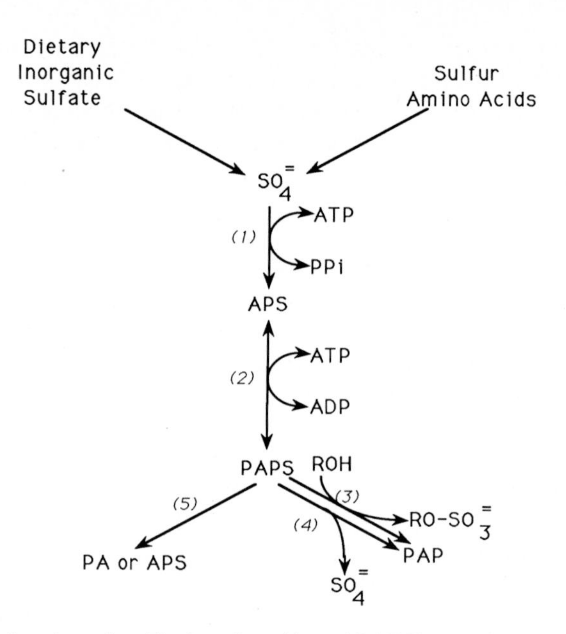

Fig. 3. 3′-Phosphoadenosine-5′-phosphosulfate (*PAPS*) metabolism. Enzymes: (*1*) ATP sulfurylase; (*2*) APS kinase; (*3*) sulfotransferase(s); (*4*) sulfohydrolase; (*5*) 3′- and 5′-nucleotidases. See text for abbreviations

of ATP and sulfate, the reaction is completed by the rapid metabolism of PP_i and APS. The ATP sulfurylase reaction has been studied extensively, and additional information on the enzyme and its reaction mechanism has been reviewed elsewhere (MULDER 1981). APS is phosphorylated by ATP in a reaction catalyzed by APS kinase. The APS kinase reaction is essentially irreversible and provides "active sulfate" required for sulfate conjugation. PAPS is a chemically labile intermediate, and reliable methods to measure its cellular concentrations have only recently been devised (e.g., HJELLE et al. 1985; SWEENY and REINKE 1988). PAPS is also catabolized by hydrolysis of the sulfate ester by sulfohydrolase enzymes or by cleavage of the phosphate groups by various tissue nucleotidases (Fig. 3).

The reported K_m values of partially purified phenol sulfotransferases for PAPS are usually in the range of 10–40 μM (ROY 1981). Steady state concentrations of PAPS in the liver are known to be highly dependent on the availability of inorganic sulfate, but normally range from 30 to 70 μM in the rat liver (BRZEZNICKA et al. 1987). Because hepatic concentrations of PAPS are approximately the same range as the K_m of the sulfotransferases, it is likely that rates of hepatic sulfation are regulated, at least in part, by cofactor supply.

The PAPS biosynthetic enzymes and the sulfotransferases are widely distributed throughout the body. The regulation of sulfate conjugation has been studied extensively in the liver, and the reactions catalyzed by the phenol sulfotransferase enzymes have received the most attention (see Chap. 2 for review). However, it is not known whether the sulfation of endogenous compounds such as steroids and neurotransmitters, or the extrahepatic conjugation of drugs, are regulated in same way as hepatic sulfation.

II. Availability of Inorganic Sulfate and Rates of Hepatic Sulfation

Rates of hepatic sulfate conjugation are highly dependent on the availability of inorganic sulfate in blood or incubation medium. For example, if hepatocytes are incubated in sulfate-free medium, rates of sulfate conjugation are essentially zero (MOLDEUS et al. 1979; SCHWARZ 1980, 1984; SUNDHEIMER and BRENDEL 1984). In experiments of this type, rates of sulfation increased as the concentration of sulfate in the medium was increased up to about 5 m*M*, after which higher concentrations of sulfate had little effect. Similarly, when sulfate was removed from the perfusion buffer, rates of *p*-nitrophenol sulfation in perfused rat livers decreased rapidly and were restored quickly when sulfate was reintroduced (REINKE et al. 1981). As was observed with hepatocytes, excess sulfate did not increase rates of sulfation in perfused rat livers. Sulfite serves as an excellent source of sulfate required for sulfate conjugation in isolated hepatocytes (SUN et al. 1989).

When a drug which is a good substrate for sulfate conjugation (e.g., acetaminophen) is administered, concentrations of inorganic sulfate in the blood often decline dramatically (KRIJGSHELD et al. 1981a; HJELLE et al. 1985; KIM et al. 1992). In accord with the concept that circulating inorganic sulfate is an important determinant of drug sulfation, administration of inorganic sulfate to acetaminophen-treated rats increased rates of acetaminophen sulfation (GALINSKY and LEVY 1981; LIN and LEVY 1986). Thus, sulfation of drugs in vivo as well as in vitro appears limited by extracellular inorganic sulfate. Conditions which decrease the availability of sulfate in vivo include administration of large amounts of sodium chloride and the feeding of diets low in sulfur-containing amino acids (KRIJGSHELD et al. 1981).

A number of cellular and exogenous compounds have been evaluated as sources of sulfate for drug conjugation. In the absence of inorganic sulfate, cysteine partially restores rates of sulfate conjugation in isolated hepatocytes (MOLDEUS et al. 1979; SCHWARZ 1980). Although both L- and D-cysteine can be oxidized rapidly and serve as a source of inorganic sulfate, D-cysteine is a more efficient sulfur donor, because it is not used in other metabolic pathways (KRIJGSHELD et al. 1981). *N*-Acetylcysteine also increases rates of sulfate conjugation in the rat (GALINSKY and LEVY 1981). GSH is a potential source of cysteine, and GSH depletion with phorone or diethylmaleate decreases rates of acetaminophen and harmol sulfation (GALINSKY 1986; GREGUS et al. 1988a). Although methionine is also metabolized to cysteine, it does not increase rates of sulfation in isolated hepatocytes (MOLDEUS et al. 1979).

Relationships between rates of sulfation and the availability of inorganic sulfate illustrate that concentrations of PAPS in hepatocytes must be quite small and are depleted rapidly by sulfate conjugation, particularly in the absence of inorganic sulfate. Indeed, concentrations of PAPS in liver range from 16 to 80 nmol/g in several animal species (BRZEZNICKA et al. 1987). Although hepatocytes contain sulfur amino acids in proteins and GSH, these reserves are not readily available to generate PAPS and support sulfate conjugation when inorganic sulfate concentrations are low. In addition, rapid restoration of rates of sulfation upon addition of a source of sulfate suggests that PAPS biosynthesis can occur rapidly despite the unfavorable equilibrium of the ATP-sulfurylase reaction (Fig. 3).

III. Rate-Limiting Factors for Sulfate Conjugation

As noted earlier, conjugation of drugs with sulfate is a low-capacity pathway for drug metabolism, due to low sulfotransferase activity, limited cofactor supply, or high arylsulfatase activity (see Chap. 9). Decreased rates of sulfation when inorganic sulfate is not available are best explained by lack of the cofactor PAPS. However, when sulfate is present in excess, corresponding increases in sulfate conjugation are not observed (REINKE et al. 1981), suggesting that sulfotransferase activity is the limiting factor in the presence of saturating amounts of sulfate. An alternative explanation is that cellular concentrations of PAPS may remain low even at high sulfate concentrations, because of the lability of the cofactor, its enzymatic degradation, or unfavorable conditions for its biosynthesis. Experiments designed to test directly the relationship between PAPS concentrations and rates of acetaminophen sulfation were performed using freshly isolated hepatocytes (SWEENY and REINKE 1988). Addition of acetaminophen caused an initial decrease in cellular levels of PAPS, but concentrations of PAPS in the presence of acetaminophen were linearly dependent on the concentration of sulfate in the medium, even at supraphysiological concentrations (e.g., 4 m*M* sulfate). When rates of acetaminophen sulfation were compared to steady state levels of PAPS in the same cells, maximal rates of conjugation occurred with 50 pmol of PAPS per 10^6 cells. Although cellular PAPS levels could be increased by three- to fourfold, rates of acetaminophen sulfation were not increased. These data directly demonstrate that the sulfotransferase enzymes are rate limiting for acetaminophen conjugation when sulfate (and therefore PAPS) concentrations are high. However, with normal sulfate concentrations in the blood (approximately 0.9 m*M* in rats), intracellular levels of PAPS most likely determine the rate of acetaminophen sulfation (SWEENY and REINKE 1988). An excellent correlation between serum sulfate concentrations and hepatic PAPS levels has also been reported in vivo in normal and acetaminophen-treated rats (HJELLE et al. 1985).

IV. Cellular Energetics and Sulfation

Because 2 mol ATP is required to synthesize 1 mol PAPS (Fig. 3) and because PAPS turnover is rapid, sulfate conjugation would be expected to be impaired when energy metabolism is depressed. This hypothesis was tested experimentally by Aw and Jones (1982), who showed a close relationship between the rate of acetaminophen sulfation in isolated hepatocytes and ATP to ADP ratios. In these studies, conditions used to lower ATP levels of the cells included hypoxia, the ATP translocase inhibitor atractyloside, the uncoupling agent FCCP (carbonyl cyanide-*p*-trifluoromethoxyphenylhydrazone), and the ATP-trapping agent ethionine. Similar results to those of Aw and Jones (1982) were noted after administration of ethionine or fructose to acetaminophen-treated rats, i.e., hepatic ATP to ADP ratios, PAPS concentrations, and rates of acetaminophen sulfation were decreased (Dills and Klaassen 1986a,b).

V. Other Metabolic Factors Affecting 3′-Phosphoadenosine-5′-Phosphosulfate Levels

Because the biosynthesis of PAPS requires only sulfate and ATP (Fig. 3), sulfate conjugation is relatively insensitive to changes in other metabolic intermediates. Unlike glucuronidation, sulfation is not affected by fasting (Reinke et al. 1981) or increases in cellular concentrations of NADH (Moldeus et al. 1978). A number of inhibitors of the ATP sulfurylase reaction (Fig. 2) have been reported; however, it is not known whether these agents have physiological significance in regulating rates of sulfate conjugation in intact cells.

Although changes in drug sulfation are correlated with corresponding alterations in hepatic levels of PAPS, changes can occur without measurable changes in energetics or sulfate concentrations. For example, addition of lithium to hepatocytes inhibits harmol sulfation, possibly due to inhibition of sodium-dependent transport of sulfate across the cell membrane (Sundheimer and Brendel 1984). When buthionine sulfoximine, a GSH synthesis inhibitor, is used to deplete hepatic GSH, rates of sulfation of acetaminophen increase (Galinsky 1986). This effect of buthionine sulfoximine is best explained by diversion of cysteine from GSH synthesis toward production of sulfate for PAPS synthesis. Perfused livers from ethanol-treated rats were unable to maintain 7-hydroxycoumarin sulfation for prolonged periods (Reinke et al. 1986). The decreasing rates of sulfation correlated with declining concentrations of PAPS in livers from ethanol-fed rats, but the mechanism for depletion of PAPS after ethanol administration has not been established. Paradoxically, when the uncoupling agent, dinitrophenol, was administered to rats to lower hepatic energetics (Dills and Klaassen 1986), PAPS levels were actually increased. A possible explanation is that dinitrophenol inhibited phenol sulfotransferase activity, which may block the use of hepatic PAPS for sulfation of endogenous compounds.

VI. Futile Cycling of Sulfate Conjugates

The previous discussion has focused on the limitation of sulfate conjugation by hepatic levels of PAPS. However, hydrolysis of the conjugates also limits the efficiency of this pathway and places additional demands on the liver for PAPS synthesis. Futile cycling of sulfate conjugates is reviewed in Chap. 9.

E. Glutathione

GSH is widely distributed throughout the body and is present at especially high concentrations (e.g., 5–10 m*M*) in liver. In addition to conjugation with reactive metabolites, GSH functions in the metabolism of hydroperoxides and aldehydes, transport of amino acids, calcium homeostasis, and regulation of cellular thiols. A detailed discussion of the importance of GSH in renal toxicity is presented in Chap. 16. Other important aspects of GSH are presented in a number of excellent reviews on this topic (e.g., see Sies and Wendel 1978; Larsson et al. 1983; Ross 1988).

I. Glutathione Synthesis and Metabolism

The pathways of GSH biosynthesis and catabolism are illustrated in Fig. 4. Regulation of GSH synthesis and degradation are covered in two recent reviews by Meister (1988, 1991). GSH biosynthesis involves the formation of two peptide bonds, first between γ-glutamic acid (GLU) and cysteine (CYS), which is catalyzed by γ-glutamyl-cysteine synthetase. In the subsequent step, GSH synthetase adds glycine (GLY). Both of these synthetic steps require energy in the form of ATP. The catabolism of GSH to its constituent amino acids is also illustrated in Fig. 4. γ-Glutamyltranspeptidase (GGT) transfers glutamate to another amino acid, producing the dipeptides CYS–GLY and GLU–amino acid. GGT is localized in the hepatic cell membrane and functions to transfer amino acids into the cell. The CYS–GLY bond is cleaved by peptidases, while the GLU–amino acid bond is hydrolyzed by γ-glutamyl cyclotransferase to form 5-oxoproline (OxoPro). This cyclic compound is subsequently hydrolyzed at the expense of ATP to regenerate glutamate. Conjugation of GSH with electrophilic, reactive compounds occurs either spontaneously or via catalysis by one of a family of GSH *S*-transferases (Fig. 4).

GSH is released from the liver in both its reduced and oxidized forms. Both the sinusoidal and canalicular transport of GSH may involve passive carrier systems, whereas the transport of oxidized GSH (GSH disulfide,

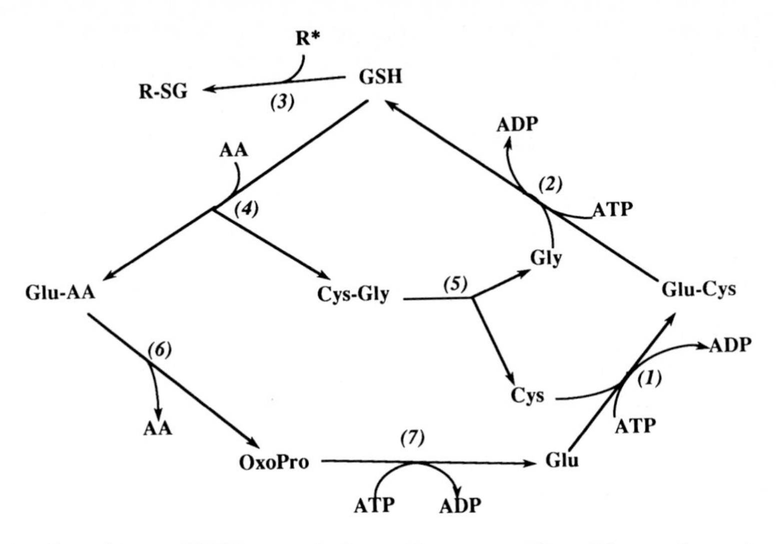

Fig. 4. Glutathione (GSH) metabolism. Enzymes: (*1*) γ-Glutamyl-cysteine synthetase; (*2*) glutathione synthetase; (*3*) glutathione *S*-transferase(s); (*4*) γ-glutamyl transpeptidase; (*5*) nonspecific peptidases; (*6*) γ-glutamyl cyclotransferase; (*7*) 5-oxoprolinase. See text for abbreviations

GSSG) into the bile depends on active transport against a concentration gradient (reviewed in KAPLOWITZ et al. 1985). Sinusoidal plus biliary efflux of GSH accounts quantitatively for nearly all of the turnover of hepatic GSH (LAUTERBURG et al. 1984).

Very few studies have explored the relationship between hepatic GSH concentrations and rates of GSH conjugation. In one study of this type, rates of 2-bromoisovalerylurea conjugation were reduced only when GSH levels were markedly decreased (POLHUIJS et al. 1992).

II. Mechanisms of Depletion of Hepatic Glutathione

Factors affecting cellular concentrations of GSH have been studied extensively, because GSH protects cells from the toxic effects of many exogenous chemicals that are converted to reactive electrophiles. Emphasis has most often been on the toxicological significance of GSH depletion, rather than the relationship between GSH levels and rates of conjugation. For this reason, the following discussion focuses on experimental conditions which decrease hepatic GSH concentrations, rather than on a rigorous discussion of the involvement of GSH in conjugation. The demand for hepatic GSH associated with the metabolism of many chemicals exceeds the capacity of the liver to regenerate this tripeptide. As a result, all GSH-requiring processes may be compromised to varying extents during rapid conjugation with GSH.

1. Conjugation of Electrophilic Compounds

One of the most widely studied and best-known examples of GSH conjugation involves the metabolism of acetaminophen. Acetaminophen is metabolized by cytochrome P-450 to a reactive metabolite (thought to be *N*-acetyl-*p*-benzoquinone imine), which is subsequently detoxified by reaction with GSH. Most covalent binding of acetaminophen to hepatic proteins occurs after depletion of GSH, and the severity of hepatic necrosis is related to the degree of covalent binding (JOLLOW et al. 1973; MITCHELL et al. 1973). When sulfhydryl compounds such as *N*-acetylcysteine are provided, the covalent binding, loss of cellular thiols, and toxicity of acetaminophen are antagonized (BUCKPITT et al. 1979; MASSEY and RACZ 1981). Administration of *N*-acetylcysteine is currently recommended as an antidote to acetaminophen poisoning in humans. Studies with acetaminophen have clearly demonstrated that GSH conjugation can be limited by GSH availability. Thus, modulating hepatic levels of GSH has important clinical relevance.

GSH antagonizes the toxicity of many chemicals other than acetaminophen which are activated by oxidative metabolism. GSH depletion associated with such chemicals could be caused by covalent binding or by the initiation of other oxidative processes (reviewed by COMPORTI 1987). GSH depletion alone does not appear to injure cells, but inadequate levels of GSH allow other cytotoxic processes to progress.

A number of agents have been used experimentally to deplete hepatic GSH. These chemicals are conjugated with GSH by GSH *S*-transferases, and the conjugates are transported from cells. Agents of this type are usually α,β-unsaturated carbonyl compounds (PLUMMER et al. 1981), with diethylmaleate and phorone representing two of the most common examples.

2. Oxidative Stress

GSH levels are perturbed markedly under a number of oxidative conditions (reviewed by ROSS 1988). Although changes in GSH that occur with oxidative stress do not involve conjugation per se, they constitute physiologically important mechanisms of GSH depletion, which decrease the ability of the liver to form GSH conjugates.

The role of GSH in the metabolism of peroxides is illustrated in Fig. 5. A peroxide (ROOH) is reduced by GSH peroxidase to yield the corresponding alcohol and water. GSSG formed in this reaction is reduced by GSH reductase at the expense of NADPH, which in turn is regenerated by other pathways of intermediary metabolism. Because one form of GSH peroxidase is a selenium-containing enzyme, selenium deficiency may increase the sensitivity of tissue to oxidative challenges (SIES et al. 1983). Increased rates of hepatic GSH synthesis and efflux have also been reported in selenium-deficient animals (HILL and BURK 1982). The GSH reductase inhibitor BCNU (BABSON and REED 1978), which prevents reduction of

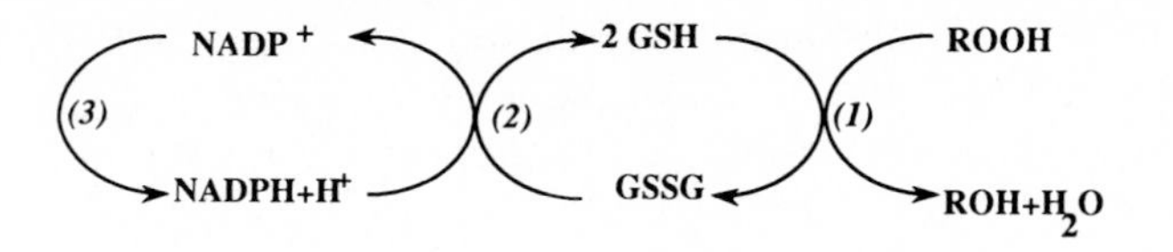

Fig. 5. Glutathione oxidation–reduction reactions. Enzymes: (*1*) glutathione peroxidase; (*2*) glutathione reductase; (*3*) enzymes catalyzing the reduction of $NADP^+$ to NADPH, such as glucose-6-phosphate dehydrogenase, $NADP^+$-specific isocitrate dehydrogenase, etc. See text for abbreviations

GSSG, has been used in many experimental applications to study GSH homeostasis. NADPH is a cofactor for GSH reductase, and its concentration may become rate limiting for GSSG reduction under certain conditions, such as hypoxia (Tribble and Jones 1990).

GSH is critically involved in the maintenance of cellular thiols, as indicated in Eqs. 1 and 2 below, where RSSR and RSH depict protein disulfides and thiols, respectively, and RSSG represents mixed GSH–protein disulfides.

$$\mathrm{RSSR + GSH \leftrightarrow RSH + RSSG} \tag{1}$$

$$\mathrm{RSSG + GSH \leftrightarrow RSH + GSSG} \tag{2}$$

GSH may add to free radical intermediates to form GSH conjugates (Ross 1988; Connor et al. 1990), as indicated in Fig. 4. Alternatively, a free radical (R·) can abstract a hydrogen atom from GSH to form a sulfur-centered glutathionyl radical (GS·), as shown in Eq. 3. The GS· radical is then reduced by a variety of cellular antioxidants such as ascorbate, or may react to form GSSG as shown in Eq. 4.

$$\mathrm{R\cdot + GSH \rightarrow RH + GS\cdot} \tag{3}$$

$$\mathrm{GS\cdot + GS\cdot \rightarrow GSSG} \tag{4}$$

Under conditions of oxidative stress, GSH can be depleted by at least five distinct, but related, pathways: (1) formation of conjugates with free radicals and the export of the conjugates from the cells; (2) formation of GSH mixed thiols; (3) GSSG formation during peroxide metabolism; (4) GSSG formation during free radical reactions; and (5) export of GSSG from the hepatocyte into the bile (Sies 1985).

3. Inhibition of Glutathione Synthesis

Inhibitors have been identified for each of the enzymes involved in GSH biosynthesis and catabolism shown in Fig. 4 (Meister 1988, 1991). Most of these inhibitors are structural analogs of the peptide substrates for the respective reactions. The inhibitor used most effectively in experimental situations is buthionine sulfoximine, an irreversible inhibitor of γ-glutamyl-cysteine synthetase. Inhibitors of other steps of GSH synthesis tend to be poorly tolerated and may result in metabolic acidosis (Meister 1991). An interesting potential therapeutic application of the inhibition of GSH synthesis is to increase the sensitivity of tumor cells to chemotherapeutic agents that act by electrophilic mechanisms (Meister 1991).

4. Fasting and Nutritional Influences

Modest decreases in hepatic levels of GSH occur in fasted animals in many laboratories. In addition, diurnal variations in hepatic GSH levels occur which are related closely to feeding schedules (Meister 1991), because amino acids which comprise GSH can be obtained from proteins and amino acids in the diet. Experiments designed to measure the rate of hepatic GSH turnover also indicate that fasting increases both the rate of GSH biosynthesis and its efflux from the liver (Lauterburg and Mitchell 1980; Lauterburg et al. 1984). The concentration of cysteine appears to be particularly important in determining rates of glutathione, sulfate, and taurine production in hepatocytes (Stipanuk et al. 1992). Hepatic GSH concentrations were depleted by feeding diets deficient in sulfur amino acids to rats and were not restored by addition of inorganic sulfate to drinking water (Rozman et al. 1992).

5. Hepatic Energetics

Because ATP is required for GSH synthesis, GSH would be expected to decrease when hepatic ATP concentrations are lowered; however, when low doses of mitochondrial inhibitors were administered to rats, no decreases in hepatic GSH levels were observed (Dills and Klaassen 1986a). In contrast, administration of large doses of ethionine or fructose lowers hepatic GSH and ATP levels and decreases the rate of formation of GSH conjugates of acetaminophen (Dills and Klaassen 1986b).

6. Other Factors Which Decrease Glutathione

A variety of stresses (shock, cold, exercise) deplete hepatic concentrations of GSH (Beck and Linkenheimer 1952; Pyke et al. 1986). Although the mechanism(s) for these effects remain uncertain, increased circulating levels of epinephrine are possibly involved. Hepatic GSH levels are decreased by α_2-adrenergic activation (James et al. 1983), which may be explained by stimulation of GSH turnover resulting from elevated levels of calcium and cyclic AMP (Lauterburg and Mitchell 1980).

GSH metabolism is also compromised by aging. Hepatic levels of GSH are significantly lower in old (30 months of age) mice, and recovery of GSH following a challenge with acetaminophen is markedly impaired compared to that noted in younger animals (Chen et al. 1990). However, the explanations for these age-dependent effects in GSH metabolism are not known.

III. Methods of Increasing Hepatic Concentrations of Glutathione

Because of the important role of GSH in protecting cells against reactive metabolites and oxidants, development of strategies to increase hepatic levels of GSH is of considerable interest. Unfortunately, GSH administration is ineffective, because very little of the tripeptide enters hepatocytes. A number of alternate approaches have been developed (MEISTER 1991). In general, these methods are based on increasing the availability of cysteine for GSH biosynthesis. Toxicity of cysteine requires the use of other agents which are cysteine precursors. The use of *N*-acetylcysteine in the treatment of an acetaminophen overdose is the most common example of a therapeutic application for stimulation of GSH biosynthesis.

F. Other Pathways of Hepatic Conjugation

Little information is available regarding the possible role of cofactor supply in determining rates of methylation, amino acid conjugation, or acetylation of drugs. Conjugation of benzoic acid with glycine in hepatocytes is sensitive to hypoxia, possibly due to decreased ATP availability for benzoyl-CoA formation (JONES 1984). *S*-Adenosylmethionine administration may be of value in some forms of liver disease (FRIEDEL et al. 1989), but the effects of this treatment on the methylation of drug substrates are unknown.

Acetylation, an important pathway of conjugation for drugs containing arylamine or hydrazine groups, requires acetyl-CoA as a cofactor. Most of the studies of acetylation have focused on the phenotypic expression and other properties of the acetyltransferases (see Chap. 4 of this volume). Apparently the effects of altered acetyl-CoA levels in drug acetylation have not been vigorously studied, but several facts suggest that further studies of acetyl-CoA as a rate-limiting factor for drug conjugation would be an interesting area for research. First, acetyl-CoA is an important intermediate for several metabolic pathways and its steady state hepatic concentrations only range from 20 to 50 nmol/g (GREENBAUM et al. 1971), about the same as PAPS. Secondly, sulfamethoxazole is rapidly acetylated in hepatocytes and can be used as a probe to sample the hepatic acetyl-CoA pool (HELLERSTEIN et al. 1991). Taken together, these data suggest that high rates of acetylation and lipogenesis could compete for a limited pool of acetyl-CoA.

References

Aarts EM (1966) Differentiation of the barbiturate stimulation of the glucuronic acid pathway from de novo enzyme synthesis. Biochem Pharmacol 15:1469–1477

Al-Turk W, Reinke LA (1983) Diminished conjugation of products of mixed-function oxidation in perfused livers from hypophysectomized rats. Pharmacology 27: 74–84

Angus PW, Mihaly GW, Morgan DJ, Smallwood RA (1987) Hypoxia impairs conjugation and elimination of harmol in the isolated perfused rat liver. J Pharmacol Exp Ther 240:931–936

Angus PW, Mihaly GW, Morgan DJ, Smallwood RA (1988) Synergistic effects of hypoxia and fasting on harmol elimination in the isolated perfused rat liver. Biochem Pharmacol 37:1207–1212

Aw TY, Jones DP (1982) Secondary bioenergetic hypoxia: inhibition of sulfation and glucuronidation reactions in isolated hepatocytes at low O_2 concentration. J Biol Chem 257:8997–9004

Aw TY, Jones DP (1984) Control of glucuronidation during hypoxia: limitation by UDP-glucose pyrophosphorylase. Biochem J 219:707–712

Babson JR, Reed DJ (1978) Inactivation of glutathione reductase by 2-chloroethyl nitrosourea-derived isocyanates. Biochem Biophys Res Commun 83:754–762

Bànhegyi G, Garzò T, Antoni F, Mandl J (1988) Glycogenolysis – and not gluconeogenesis – is the source of UDP-glucuronic acid for glucuronidation. Biochim Biophys Acta 967:429–435

Bànhegyi G, Puskàs R, Garzò T, Antoni F, Mandl J (1991) High amounts of glucose and insulin inhibit *p*-nitrophenol conjugation in mouse hepatocytes. Biochem Pharmacol 42:1299–1302

Beck LV, Linkenheimer W (1952) Effects of shock and cold on mouse liver sulfhydryls. Proc Soc Exp Biol Med 81:291–294

Bock KW, Fröhling W, Remmer H, Rexer B (1973) Effects of phenobarbital and 3-methylcholanthrene on substrate specificity of rat liver microsomal UDP-glucuronyltransferase. Biochim Biophys Acta 327:46–56

Bock KW, Huber E, Schlote W (1977) UDP-glucuronyltransferase in perfused rat liver and in microsomes. Effects of CCl_4 injury. Naunyn Schmiedebergs Arch Pharmacol 296:199–203

Brzeznicka EA, Hazelton GA, Klaassen CD (1987) Comparison of adenosine 3′-phosphate 5′-phosphosulfate concentrations in tissues from different laboratory animals. Drug Metab Dispos 15:133–135

Buckpitt AR, Rollins DE, Mitchell JR (1979) Varying effects of sulfhydryl nucleophiles on acetaminophen oxidation and sulfhydryl adduct formation. Biochem Pharmacol 28:2941–2946

Chen T, Richie JP, Lang CA (1990) Life span profiles of glutathione and acetaminophen detoxification. Drug Metab Dispos 18:882–887

Comporti M (1987) Glutathione depleting agents and lipid peroxidation. Chem Phys Lipids 45:143–169

Connor HD, LaCagnin LB, Knecht KT, Thurman RG, Mason RP (1990) Reaction of glutathione with a free radical metabolite of carbon tetrachloride. Mol Pharmacol 37:443–451

Conway JG, Kauffman FC, Thurman RG (1985) Effect of glucose on 7-hydroxycoumarin glucuronide production in periportal and pericentral regions of the liver lobule. Biochem J 226:749–756

Dills RL, Klaassen CD (1984) Decreased glucuronidation of bilirubin by diethyl ether anesthesia. Biochem Pharmacol 33:2813–2814

Dills RL, Klaassen CD (1986a) The effect of inhibitors of mitochondrial energy production on hepatic glutathione, UDP-glucuronic acid, and adenosine 3′-phosphate-5′-phosphosulfate concentrations. Drug Metab Dispos 14:190–196

Dills RL, Klaassen CD (1986b) Effect of reduced hepatic energy state on acetaminophen conjugation in rats. J Pharmacol Exp Ther 238:463–472

Dutton GJ (ed) (1980) Glucuronidation of drugs and other compounds. CRC, Boca Raton

Dziewiatkowski DD, Lewis HB (1944) Glucuronic acid synthesis and the glycogen content of the liver of the rat. J Biol Chem 153:49–52

Eacho PI, Sweeny D, Weiner M (1981a) Effects of glucose and fructose on conjugation of *p*-nitrophenol in hepatocytes of normal and streptozotocin-diabetic rats. Biochem Pharmacol 30:2616–2619

Eacho PI, Sweeny D, Weiner M (1981b) Conjugation of *p*-nitroanisole and *p*-nitrophenol in hepatocytes isolated from streptozotocin diabetic rats. J Pharmacol Exp Ther 218:34–40

Friedel HA, Goa KL, Benfield P (1989) *S*-Adenosyl-L-methionine: a review of its pharmacological properties and therapeutic potential in liver dysfunction and affective disorders in relation to its physiological role in cell metabolism. Drugs 38:389–416

Galinsky RE (1986) Role of glutathione turnover in drug sulfation: differential effects of diethylmaleate and buthionine sulfoximine on the pharmacokinetics of acetaminophen in the rat. J Pharmacol Exp Ther 236:133–139

Galinsky RE, Levy G (1981) Dose- and time-dependent elimination of acetaminophen in rats: pharmacokinetic implications of cosubstrate depletion. J Pharmacol Exp Ther 219:14–20

Goon D, Klaassen CD (1992) Effects of microsomal enzyme inducers upon UDP-glucuronic acid concentration and UDP-glucuronosyltransferase activity in the rat intestine and liver. Toxicol Appl Pharmacol 115:254–260

Greenbaum AL, Gumaa KA, McLean P (1971) The distribution of hepatic metabolites and the control of the pathways of carbohydrate metabolism in animals of different dietary and hormonal status. Arch Biochem Biophys 143: 617–663

Gregus Z, White C, Howell S, Klaassen CD (1988a) Effect of glutathione depletion on sulfate activation and sulfate ester formation in rats. Biochem Pharmacol 37:4307–4312

Gregus Z, Madhu C, Goon D, Klaassen CD (1988b) Effect of galactosamine-induced hepatic UDP-glucuronic acid depletion on acetaminophen elimination in rats: dispositional differences between hepatically and extrahepatically formed glucuronides of acetaminophen and other chemicals. Drug Metab Dispos 16: 527–533

Griffeth LK, Rosen GM, Rauckman EJ (1985) Effects of model traumatic injury on hepatic drug metabolism in the rat. IV. Glucuronidation. Drug Metab Dispos 13:391–397

Hauser SC, Ransil BJ, Ziurys JC, Gollan JL (1988a) Interaction of uridine 5′-diphosphoglucuronic acid with microsomal UDP-glucuronosyltransferase in primate liver: the facilitating role of uridine 5′-diphospho-N-acetylglucosamine. Biochim Biophys Acta 967:141–148

Hauser SC, Ziurys JC, Gollan JL (1988b) A membrane transporter mediates access of uridine 5′-diphosphoglucuronic acid from the cytosol into the endoplasmic reticulum of rat hepatocytes: implications for glucuronidation reactions. Biochim Biophys Acta 967:149–157

Hellerstein MK, Wu K, Kaempfer S, Kletke C, Shackleton CHL (1991) Sampling the lipogenic hepatic acetyl-CoA pool in vivo in the rat: comparison of xenobiotic probe to values predicted from isotopomeric distribution in circulating lipids and measurement of lipogenesis and acetyl-CoA dilution. J Biol Chem 266:10912–10919

Hill KE, Burk RF (1982) Effect of selenium deficiency and vitamin E deficiency on glutathione metabolism in isolated rat hepatocytes. J Biol Chem 257:10668–10672

Hjelle JJ, Hazelton GA, Klaassen CD (1985) Acetaminophen decreases adenosine 3′-phosphate 5′-phosphosulfate and uridine diphosphoglucuronic acid in rat liver. Drug Metab Dispos 13:35–41

Howell SR, Hazelton GA, Klaassen CD (1986) Depletion of hepatic UDP-glucuronic acid by drugs that are glucuronidated. J Pharmacol Exp Ther 236:610–614

James RC, Roberts SM, Harbison RD (1983) The perturbation of hepatic glutathione by α_2-adrenergic agonists. Fundam Appl Toxicol 3:303–308

Jollow DJ, Mitchell JR, Potter WZ, Davis DC, Gillette JR, Brodie BB (1973) Acetaminophen-induced hepatic necrosis. II. Role of covalent binding in vivo. J Pharmacol Exp Ther 187:195–202

Jones DP (1984) Benzylamine metabolism at low O_2 concentrations: relative sensitivities of monoamine oxidase, aldehyde dehydrogenase and hippurate synthesis to hypoxia. Biochem Pharmacol 33:413–417

Kamisako T, Adachi Y, Yamamoto T (1990) Effect of UDP-glucuronic acid depletion by salicylamide on biliary bilirubin excretion in the rat. J Pharmacol Exp Ther 254:380–382

Kaplowitz N, Aw TY, Ookhtens M (1985) The regulation of hepatic glutathione. Annu Rev Pharmacol Toxicol 25:715–744

Kim HJ, Rozman P, Madhu C, Klaassen CD (1992) Homeostasis of sulfate and 3′-phosphoadenosine 5′-phosphosulfate in rats after acetaminophen administration. J Pharmacol Exp Ther 261:1015–1021

Koster H, Halsema I, Scholtens E, Knippers M, Mulder GJ (1981) Dose-dependent shifts in the sulfation and glucuronidation of phenolic compounds in the rat in vivo and in isolated hepatocytes: the role of saturation of phenolsulfotransferase. Biochem Pharmacol 18:2569–2575

Koster H, Mulder GJ (1982) Apparent aberrancy in the kinetics of intracellular metabolism of a single substrate by two enzymes: an alternative explanation for anomalies in the kinetics of sulfation and glucuronidation. Drug Metab Dispos 10:330–335

Krijgsheld KR, Scholtens E, Mulder GJ (1981a) An evaluation of methods to decrease the availability of inorganic sulphate for sulphate conjugation in the rat in vivo. Biochem Pharmacol 30:1973–1979

Krijgsheld KR, Glazenburg EJ, Scholtens E, Mulder GJ (1981b) The oxidation of L- and D-cysteine to inorganic sulfate and taurine in the rat. Biochim Biophys Acta 677:7–12

Larsson A, Orrenius S, Holmgren A, Mannervik B (eds) (1983) Functions of glutathione: biochemical, physiological, toxicological, and clinical aspects. Raven, New York

Lauterburg BH, Mitchell JR (1980) In vivo regulation of hepatic glutathione synthesis: effects of food deprivation or glutathione depletion by electrophilic compounds. In: Snyder R, Parke DV, Kocsis JJ, Jollow DJ, Bogson CG, Witmer CM (eds) Biological reactive intermediates – II: chemical mechanisms and biological effects. Adv Exp Med Biol 136A: 453

Lauterburg BH, Adams JD, Mitchell JR (1984) Hepatic glutathione homeostasis in the rat: efflux accounts for glutathione turnover. Hepatology 4:586–590

Lin JH, Levy G (1986) Effect of prevention of inorganic sulfate depletion on the pharmacokinetics of acetaminophen in rats. J Pharmacol Exp Ther 239:94–98

Massey TE, Racz WJ (1981) Effects of N-acetylcysteine on metabolism, covalent binding, and toxicity of acetaminophen in isolated mouse hepatocytes. Toxicol Appl Pharmacol 60:220–228

Meister A (1988) Glutathione metabolism and its selective modification. J Biol Chem 263:17205–17208

Meister A (1991) Glutathione deficiency produced by inhibition of its synthesis, and its reversal; applications in research and therapy. Pharmacol Ther 51:155–194

Minck K, Schupp RR, Illing PA, Kahl GF, Netter KJ (1973) Interrelationship between demethylation of p-nitroanisole and conjugation of p-nitrophenol in rat liver. Naunyn Schmiedebergs Arch Pharmacol 279:347–360

Miners JO, Mackenzie PI (1991) Drug glucuronidation in humans. Pharmacol Ther 51:347–369

Mitchell JR, Jollow DJ, Gillette JR, Brodie BB (1973) Drug metabolism as a cause of drug toxicity. Drug Metab Dispos 1:418–423

Moldeus P, Andersson B, Norling A (1978) Interaction of ethanol oxidation with glucuronidation in isolated hepatocytes. Biochem Pharmacol 27:2583–2588

Moldeus P, Andersson B, Gergely V (1979) Regulation of glucuronidation and sulfate conjugation in isolated hepatocytes. Drug Metab Dispos 7:416–419

Mulder GJ (1981) Sulfate activation. In: Mulder GJ (ed) Sulfation of drugs and related compounds. CRC, Boca Raton, p 53

Paterson P, Fry JR (1983) The effect of ascorbic acid on the conjugation of 4-hydroxybiphenyl in rat isolated hepatocytes. Xenobiotica 13:607–610

Plummer JL, Smith BR, Sies H, Bend JR (1981) Chemical depletion of glutathione in vivo. In: Jacoby WB (ed) Detoxication and drug metabolism: conjugation and related systems. Methods Enzymol 77:50

Polhuijs M, Lankhaar G, Mulder GJ (1992) Relationship between glutathione content in liver and glutathione conjugation rate in the rat in vivo. Effect of buthionine sulphoximine pretreatment on conjugation of the two 2-bromoisovalerylurea enantiomers during intravenous infusion. Biochem J 285: 401–404

Price VF, Jollow DJ (1982) Increased resistance of diabetic rats to acetaminophen-induced hepatotoxicity. J Pharmacol Exp Ther 220:504–513

Price VF, Jollow DJ (1986) Strain differences in susceptibility of normal and diabetic rats to acetaminophen hepatotoxicity. Biochem Pharmacol 35:687–695

Price VF, Miller MG, Jollow DJ (1987) Mechanisms of fasting-induced potentiation of acetaminophen hepatotoxicity in the rat. Biochem Pharmacol 36:427–433

Price VF, Jollow DJ (1988) Mechanism of decreased acetaminophen glucuronidation in the fasted rat. Biochem Pharmacol 37:1067–1075

Price VF, Jollow DJ (1989) Effect of glucose and gluconeogenic substrates on fasting-induced suppression of acetaminophen glucuronidation in the rat. Biochem Pharmacol 38:289–297

Pyke S, Lew H, Quintanilha A (1986) Severe depletion in liver glutathione during physical exercise. Biochem Biophys Res Commun 139:926–931

Reinke LA, Belinsky SA, Evans RK, Kauffman FC, Thurman RG (1981) Conjugation of *p*-nitrophenol in the perfused rat liver: the effect of substrate concentration and carbohydrate reserves. J Pharmacol Exp Ther 217:863–870

Reinke LA, Moyer MJ, Notley KA (1986) Diminished rates of glucuronidation and sulfation in perfused rat liver after chronic ethanol administration. Biochem Pharmacol 35:439–447

Reinke LA, Tupper JS, Sweeny DJ (1987) 7-Ethoxycoumarin O-deethylation in perfused livers from ethanol-fed rats: evidence for an important role of mitochondrial reducing equivalents. Pharmacology 34:167–175

Ross D (1988) Glutathione, free radicals and chemotherapeutic agents: mechanisms of free-radical induced toxicity and glutathione-dependent protection. Pharmacol Ther 37:231–249

Roy AB (1981) Sulfotransferases. In: Mulder GJ (ed) Sulfation of drugs and related compounds. CRC, Boca Raton, p 83

Rozman P, Kim HJ, Madhu C, Gregus A, Klaassen CD (1992) Homeostasis of sulfate and 3′-phosphoadenosine 5′-phosphosulfate in rats with deficient dietary intake of sulfur. Drug Metab Dispos 20:374–378

Schwarz LR (1980) Modulation of sulfation and glucuronidation of 1-naphthol in isolated rat liver cells. Arch Toxicol 44:137–145

Schwarz LR (1984) Sulfation of 1-naphthol in isolated rat hepatocytes: dependence on inorganic sulfate. Hoppe Seylers Z Physiol Chem 365:43–48

Shipley LA, Weiner M (1987) Effects of adenosine on glucuronidation and uridine diphosphate glucuronic acid (UDPGA) synthesis in isolated hepatocytes. Biochem Pharmacol 36:2993–3000

Shipley LA, Eacho PI, Sweeny DJ, Weiner M (1986) Inhibition of glucuronidation and sulfation by dibutyryl cyclic AMP in isolated rat hepatocytes. Drug Metab Dispos 14:526–531

Sies H (1985) Hydroperoxides and thiol oxidants in the study of oxidative stress in intact cells and organs. In: Sies H (ed) Oxidative stress. Academic, London, p 73

Sies H, Wendel A (eds) (1978) Functions of glutathione in liver and kidney. Springer, Berlin Heidelberg New York

Sies H, Brigelius R, Wefers H, Muller A, Cadenas E (1983) Cellular redox changes and response to drugs and toxic agents. Fundam Appl Toxicol 3: 200–208

Singh J, Schwarz LR (1981) Dependence of glucuronidation rate on UDP-glucuronic acid levels in isolated hepatocytes. Biochem Pharmacol 30:3252–3254

Stipanuk MH, Coloso RM, Garcia RAG, Banks MF (1992) Cysteine concentration regulates cysteine metabolism to glutathione, sulfate and taurine in rat hepatocytes. J Nutr 122:420–427

Sun Y, Cotgreave I, Lindeke B, Moldeus P (1989) The metabolism of sulfite in liver: stimulation of sulfate conjugation and effects on paracetamol and allyl alcohol toxicity. Biochem Pharmacol 38:4299–4305

Sundheimer DW, Brendel K (1984) Factors influencing sulfation in isolated rat hepatocytes. Life Sci 34:23–29

Sweeny DJ, Reinke LA (1988) Sulfation of acetaminophen in isolated rat hepatocytes: relationship to sulfate ion concentrations and intracellular levels of 3′-phosphoadenosine-5′-phosphosulfate. Drug Metab Dispos 16:712–715

Thurman RG, Ganey PE, Belinsky SA, Conway JG, Badr MZ, Kauffman FC (1989) Advantages of the perfused liver as a model to study hepatotoxicity in periportal and pericentral regions of the liver lobule. In: McQueen CA (ed) In vitro toxicology: model systems and methods. Telford, London, p 69

Tribble DL, Jones DP (1990) Oxygen dependence of oxidative stress: rate of NADPH supply for maintaining the GSH pool during hypoxia. Biochem Pharmacol 39:729–736

Watkins JB, Klaassen CD (1983) Chemically-induced alteration of UDP-glucuronic acid concentration in rat liver. Drug Metab Dispos 11:37–40

Watkins JB, Siegers C-P, Klaassen CD (1984) Effect of diethyl ether on the biliary excretion of acetaminophen. Proc Soc Exp Biol Med 177:168–175

Watkins JB, Engles DR, Beck LV (1990) Effect of volatile anesthetics on the hepatic UDP-glucuronic acid pathway in mice. Biochem Pharmacol 40:731–735

Wiebkin P, Parker GL, Fry JR, Bridges JW (1979) Effect of various metabolic inhibitors on biphenyl metabolism in isolated rat hepatocytes. Biochem Pharmacol 28:3315–3321

Wu I-R, Kauffman FC, Qu W, Ganey P, Thurman RG (1990) Unique role of oxygen in regulation of hepatic monooxygenation and glucuronidation. Mol Pharmacol 38:128–133

Zakim D, Dannenberg AJ (1992) How does the microsomal membrane regulate UDP-glucuronosyltransferases? Biochem Pharmacol 43:1385–1393

CHAPTER 9

Regulation of Drug Conjugate Production by Futile Cycling in Intact Cells

F.C. KAUFFMAN

A. Introduction

Conjugation of drugs and xenobiotics in liver and extrahepatic tissues is a complex process involving the availability of activated substrates such as uridine diphosphate (UDE)-glucuronic acid (REINKE et al. 1986) and adenosine 3′-phosphate-5′-phosphosulfate (PAPS) (GLAZENBURG et al. 1984), the uptake of substrates across various cellular membranes, and the formation and release of conjugated products (DEVRIES et al. 1985) as well as the activities of transferases and hydrolases (DEVRIES et al. 1985; EL MOUELHI and KAUFFMAN 1986; SCHOLLHAMMER et al. 1975).

Often overlooked in discussion of the regulation of drug conjugate formation in intact cells is the involvement of futile cycling via specific transferases and hydrolases localized in the same or adjacent subcellular compartments. The term futile cycling is used because conjugated metabolites of drugs, endogenous substrates, and toxic chemicals may undergo successive cycles of synthesis to the conjugate and hydrolysis back to the free metabolite. Futile cycling of conjugates is potentially an important site of regulation, because factors that affect either the activity of a transferase or an associated hydrolase will alter rates of cycling and, thus, net conjugate production or utilization in intact cells. Theoretically, futile cycling of a wide array of phase II metabolites such as glucuronide, sulfate, methoxy, and acetyl conjugates may occur. Recent studies (DWIVEDI et al. 1987; EL MOUELHI and KAUFFMAN 1986; KAUFFMAN et al. 1991) indicate that futile cycling of sulfate and glucuronide conjugates and deconjugated free metabolites in liver as well as extrahepatic tissues is an important determinant for the net production of drug conjugates. This chapter reviews recent studies illustrating the involvement of futile cycling in regulating net sulfate and glucuronide conjugate production. Although futile cycling is possible with other types of conjugates, e.g., methoxy and acetyl, there is little information on this possibility.

B. Properties of Hydrolases and Transferases Related to Futile Cycling of Conjugates

Studies in laboratory animals and isolate cells indicate that glucuronide and sulfate conjugates of various substrates undergo futile cycling in the liver because of the relatively high activities of β-glucuronidase and arylsulfatase in this tissue. Enzymes involved in futile cycling are localized in the same or adjacent subcellular compartments and have relatively high affinities for conjugates and deconjugated substrates. The pH optimum of β-glucuronidase is 4–5, while that of sulfatase is approximately 7.3. Similarities in the pH optima of related sulfotransferases and sulfatases, as well as high affinities of these enzymes for their respective substrates, favors futile cycling of sulfate conjugates compared to glucuronide conjugates. Activities of arylsulfatase and sulfotransferase are essentially the same at neutral pH, while the activity of β-glucuronidase is nearly 30-fold less at pH 7.3 compared to its activity at 4.7 (EL MOUELHI and KAUFFMAN 1986). If an enzyme and substrate are localized within the same cellular compartment and the concentration of substrate(s) is low compared to the K_m, flux through this enzyme will generally follow a first-order rate determined by the expression: rate = (S) (V_{max}/K_m) (LOWRY and PASSONNEAU 1964). Thus, substrate concentration, as well as the K_m of the transferase or hydrolase for their respective substrates in addition to maximum activities measured in vitro, are important determinants of futile cycling in intact cells. pH optima sensitivities to various intracellular inhibitors and activators need to be considered as determinants of futile cycling.

Significant activities of arylsulfatase and β-glucuronidase are localized in the hepatic endoplasmic reticulum, and these enzymes share common sites with associated transferases. Approximately one third of the ubiquitous enzyme β-glucuronidase is localized in the endoplasmic reticulum of hepatocytes, with the remainder of this enzyme activity confined to lysosomes (SWANK et al. 1986). Futile cycling involving synthesis via UDP-glucuronosyltransferase and hydrolysis via β-glucuronidase located in the hepatic endoplasmic reticulum is clearly possible, because β-glucuronidase is compartmentalized within the lumen of the endoplasmic reticulum (PAIGEN 1979), as is the active site of glucuronosyl transferases (BERRY et al. 1975). Thus, glucuronide conjugates produced via glucuronosyltransferase are exposed to β-glucuronidase localized on the luminal side of the endoplasmic reticulum.

Arylsulfatase is located on the cytosolic surface of the endoplasmic reticulum (ROY 1976) and may have ready access to sulfate conjugates formed via sulfotransferases in the cytosolic compartment. The affinities of enzymes involved in the formation and hydrolysis of sulfate conjugates tend to be greater than those associated with futile cycling of glucuronide conjugates. For example, the K_m of sulfotransferase(s) for 4-methylumbelliferone is about $1\,\mu M$ (KAUFFMAN et al. 1991) while that of glucuronosyltransferase for the same substrate is approximately, $250\,\mu M$ (CONWAY et al. 1988). Affinities of the two hydrolytic enzymes β-glucuronidase and arylsulfatase for methylumbelliferyl-glucuronide and sulfate are about $100\,\mu M$. The higher affinity of sulfotransferase compared to glucuronosyltransferase facilitates reconjugation of the hydrolyzed sulfate conjugate.

In line with the idea that futile cycling may more readily apply to sulfate conjugates than to glucuronide conjugates, futile cycling of the former, but not the latter, is readily demonstrated using the highly fluorescent substrate 4-methylumbelliferone as substrate in liver homogenates (EL MOUELHI and KAUFFMAN 1986) and a reconstituted system of liver microsomes and cytoplasm (KAUFFMAN et al. 1991). Sulfate conjugate production in liver homogenates is also stimulated following addition of 250 μM sodium sulfite, an inhibitor of sulfatase (half-maximal inhibition with 20 μM), to this system. In contrast, addition of 1 mM saccharolactone, which completely inhibits β-glucuronidase activity, does not enhance methylumbelliferone glucuronide formation in liver homogenates incubated with the aglycone and UDP-glucuronic acid (EL MOUELHI and KAUFFMAN 1986).

Futile cycling of the sulfate, but not the glucuronide, conjugate of methylumbelliferone is also easily demonstrated in a reconstituted system consisting of liver microsomes, cytosol, and PAPS (KAUFFMAN et al. 1991). Rates of hydrolysis of 4-methylumbelliferone sulfate in this system remain constant until PAPS is added and then decrease dramatically until the cofactor is consumed (Fig. 1). Subsequent repeated additions of PAPS decrease formation of the sulfate conjugate during periods of futile cycling. Finally, addition of sodium sulfite followed by PAPS markedly stimulated

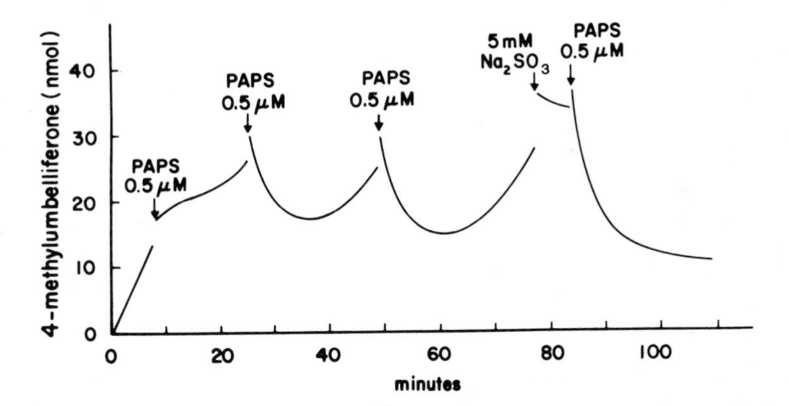

Fig. 1. Futile cycling of *4-methylumbelliferone* and 4-methylumbelliferone sulfate in a reconstituted system. A mixture of rat liver microsomes and cytosol were incubated with buffer containing 5 μM 4-methylumbelliferyl sulfate. At various intervals indicated by *arrows* 0.5 μM adenosine 3′-phosphate-5′-phosphosulfate (*PAPS*) was added to the system. Production of 4-methylumbelliferone was monitored by the appearance of fluorescence (366–450 nm). Na_2SO_3 (5 mM) was added at 60 min to inhibit arylsulfatase. Note greater and prolonged loss of fluoresence reflecting formation of the sulfate conjugate after inhibition of arylsulfatase with Na_2SO_3. (From KAUFFMAN et al. 1991)

the formation of methylumbelliferone sulfate, as reflected by a marked loss of fluorescence (Fig. 1). Similar experiments employing methylumbelliferyl glucuronide and additions of UDP-glucuronic acid to the reconstituted system failed to demonstrate futile cycling of the glucuronide conjugate. Although such experiments demonstrate that futile cycling of the sulfate conjugate is more likely to occur than that of the glucuronide conjugate in this particular cell-free system, evidence reviewed below indicates that futile cycling may be involved in the regulation of net glucuronide conjugation production in vivo. There is also at least one report (SCHOLLHAMMER et al. 1975) of futile cycling involving glucuronosyltransferase and β-glucuronidase in liver homogenates. Approximately 20% of β-glucuronidase activity is retained at pH 7.5 compared to activity measured at its pH optimum of 4.5, and addition of glucaro-1,4-lactone increases the production of glucuronide conjugates in microsomes isolated from rat liver (SCHOLLHAMMER et al. 1975).

β-Glucuronidase is localized mainly in periportal hepatocytes (POSO et al. 1991) or evenly distributed across the liver lobule (EL MOUELHI and KAUFFMAN 1986), yet glucuronidation of at least one substrate, 7-hydroxycoumarin, is highest in pericentral hepatocytes (CONWAY et al. 1985). Glucuronosyltransferases are localized mainly in pericentral hepatocytes (EL MOUELHI and KAUFFMAN 1986). Thus, the amount of synthetic enzyme relative to the hydrolytic enzyme is likely an important determinant of net glucuronide formation in sublobular zones of the liver.

In addition to activities of the intracellular hydrolases and transferases, transport of conjugated and free substrates across cellular membranes and protein binding influence rates of futile cycling. In studies of futile cycling of methylumbelliferyl conjugates in isolated hepatocytes (KAUFFMAN et al. 1991) and perfused rat livers (RATNA et al. 1993), the glucuronide conjugate underwent futile cycling to a much lesser extent than the sulfate conjugate due, in part, to a marked reduction in the transport of the glucuronide conjugate compared to the sulfate. Binding of substrate to extracellular protein has also clearly been shown to be an important determinant of futile cycling of low concentrations of methylumbelliferyl sulfate (CHIBA and PANG 1993).

C. Futile Cycling of Glucuronide Conjugates

A study describing the net glucuronidation of bilirubin in inbred and outbred strains of rats that differ markedly in hepatic β-glucuronidase, but not in glucuronosyltransferase, showed that glucuronidation of bilirubin varies inversely with activities of the former enzyme (DWIVEDI et al. 1987). Subpopulations of Sprague-Dawley and Wistar rats having an approximately twofold variation in hepatic β-glucuronidase with essentially the same activities of UDP-glucuronosyltransferase have been identified (DWIVEDI et al. 1987). Subpopulations that have high ratios of hepatic hydrolase related to transferase activity have low amounts of circulating bilirubin glucuronide. Studies using D-glucaro-1,4-lactone or calcium glucurate to inhibit microsomal β-glucuronidase (DWIVEDI et al. 1987) indicated that agents inhibiting this enzyme increase circulating glucuronide conjugates. Both glucaro-1,4-lactone and calcium glucurate selectively inhibit the microsomal form of the enzyme because they are excluded from lysosomes (LLOYD and FORSTER 1986). Treatment of either Fisher 344 or Wistar rats with the lactone increased the level of glucuronidated bilirubin and decreased free bilirubin in serum of the two rat strains. Although this result may be explained, in part, by an action of the inhibitors on serum β-glucuronidase, inhibition of hepatic microsomal β-glucuronidase is the more likely site of action of the inhibitor.

The intriguing possibility that some procarcinogens circulate as glucuronide conjugates is raised by the finding that inhibitors of β-glucuronidase reduce the incidence of several types of chemically induced tumors in laboratory animals. For example, the frequency of dimethylbenzanthracene-induced mammary tumors in rats (WALASZEK et al. 1984, 1986a) and mice (WALASZEK et al. 1986b) is reduced by treating animals exposed to the carcinogen with inhibitors of β-glucuronidase. It has been known for some years that β-glucuronidase catalyzes the hydrolysis of benzo(a)pyrene-3-glucuronide to a derivative that binds to DNA to a far greater extent than 3-hydroxy-benzo(a)pyrene (KINOSHITA and GELBOIN 1978). A reactive species, possibly a quinone, may be formed prior to the ultimate phenol. Further work in this area is clearly warranted, because glucuronide conjugates of polycyclic aromatic hydrocarbon metabolites are formed and released from the liver in relatively large amounts after oxidative metabolism (ZALESKI et al. 1991).

Evidence that microsomal β-glucuronidase in liver is involved in futile cycling has also been obtained in experiments employing perfused rat livers (BELINSKY et al. 1984; CHIBA and PANG 1993). Futile cycling between 4-methylumbelliferone and its sulfate and glucuronide conjugates was examined recently in a single pass perfused rat liver (CHIBA and PANG 1993). Hydrolysis of the glucuronide conjugate and resynthesis was demonstrated in this preparation; however, the rate of futile cycling was at least 20-fold lower than that noted with the sulfate conjugate.

Additional support for the idea that microsomal β-glucuronidase is involved in regulating net glucuronide conjugate production is also derived from studies of p-nitrophenol metabolism in isolated perfused rat livers. Production of p-nitrophenyl glucuronide by isolated perfused rat livers was decreased by infusion of epinephrine in a dose-dependent manner (half-maximal inhibition at $5\,\mu M$; BELINSKY et al. 1984). The effect of epinephrine is best explained by its action on α-adrenergic receptors and subsequent increases in intracellular Ca^{2+}. The α-antagonist phentolamine, but not the β-antagonist propranolol, inhibited glucuronidation (Fig. 2). Inhibition of glucuronidation by epinepherine was calcium dependent, because epinephrine failed to inhibit glucuronidation when livers were perfused with

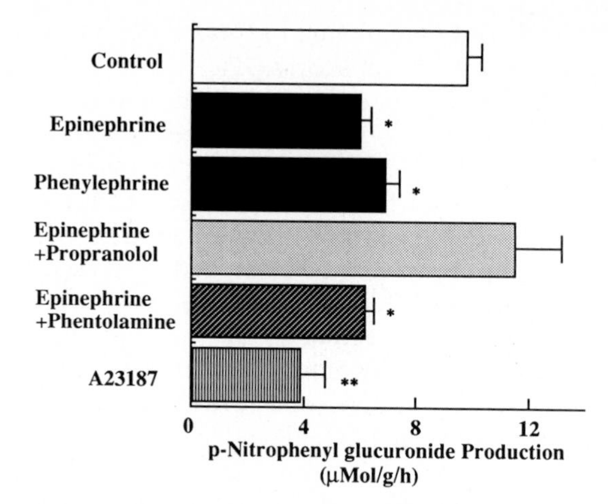

Fig. 2. Actions of adrenergic agonists and antagonists and *A23187* on *p-nitrophenyl glucuronide production* by isolated perfused rat livers. Isolated livers from phenobarbital-treated rats were perfused with 0.1 m*M* *p*-nitrophenol in Krebs Hensileit bicarbonate buffer in a nonrecirculating system and the production of *p*-nitrophenyl glucuronide measured in samples of effluent perfusate incubated with β-glucuronidase. The concentration of all agents added was 100 μM with the exception of A23187, which was 5 μM. Length of *bars* are averages of at least four livers $\pm$ S.E.M. (Figure is adopted from data presented in BELINSKY et al. 1984)

calcium-free medium. Further, the calcium ionophore A23187 markedly inhibited glucuronidation (Fig. 2; BELINSKY et al. 1984).

Involvement of futile cycling in regulating net *p*-nitrophenylglucuronide production was suggested by the finding that ionized calcium comparable to physiological intracellular concentrations (0.1–2 μM) increased microsomal β-glucuronidase in a dose-dependent manner, but had no effect on microsomal glucuronosyltransferases (BELINSKY et al. 1984). In further support of the idea that the action of epinephrine is mediated via activation of microsomal β-glucuronidase and not secondary to actions on hepatic microvasculature or glucose metabolism, epinephrine failed to inhibit glucuronide production in perfused livers from β-glucuronidase-deficient C3H/HeJ mice (Fig. 3).

Regulation of microsomal β-glucuronidase by ionized calcium in the physiological range has been implicated in the glucuronidation of at least two other substrates, 3-hydroxybenzo(a)pyrene (WHITTAKER et al. 1985) and 3-methylumbelliferone (SOKOLOVE et al. 1984). Hydrolysis of 3-benzo(a)-pyrenyl glucuronide and 3-methylumbelliferyl glucuronide via β-glucuronidase is stimulated by micromolar concentrations of Ca^{2+} (half-maximal stimulation with approximately 0.3 μM Ca^{2+}). Dissociation of the enzyme from microsomal membranes by various treatments such as exposure to detergents or mellitin increased basal β-glucuronidase and markedly decreased the sensitivity of the enzyme to ionized calcium

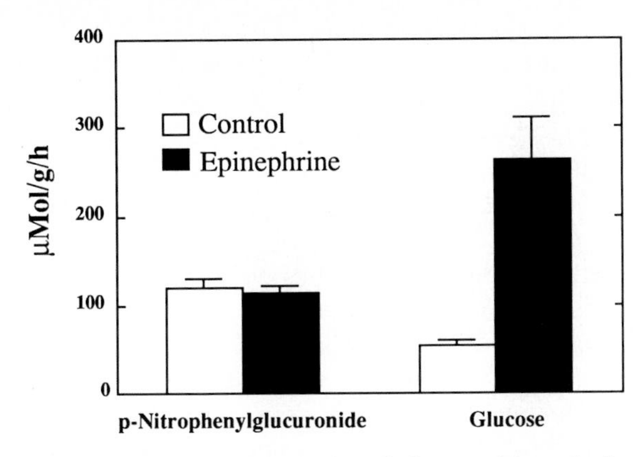

Fig. 3. Actions of *epinephrine* on *p-nitrophenyl-glucuronide* and *glucose* production in perfused livers from β-glucuronidase-deficient C3H/HeJ mice. Livers from C3H/HeJ mice were perfused with or without *p*-nitrophenol (0.1 m*M*) or epinephrine, as described in Fig. 2. Values are means ± S.E. from four livers. (Data adopted from BELINSKY et al. 1984)

(SOKOLOVE et al. 1984). Thus, interaction of cytosolic Ca^{2+} with membrane-bound β-glucuronidase modulates glucuronidation of various hydroxylated substrates in intact hepatocytes. Stimulation of microsomal β-glucuronidase by Ca^{2+} does not involve calmodulin, since addition of either calmodulin inhibitors or exogenous calmodulin failed to alter Ca^{2+} stimulation of the enzyme (SOKOLOVE et al. 1984).

D. Futile Cycling of Sulfate Conjugates

Studies of the hydrolysis and resynthesis of 4-methylumbelliferyl sulfate and 4-methylumbelliferyl glucuronide using isolated rat hepatocytes (KAUFFMAN et al. 1991) and perfused livers (RATNA et al. 1993) as experimental systems suggest that futile cycling may be more important to the regulation of net sulfate conjugate production than net glucuronide formation. The sulfate conjugate was taken up and hydrolyzed considerably more rapidly than the glucuronide in both preparations. This may be explained by the higher lipophilicity of the sulfate anion (MIYAUCHI et al. 1987) as well as by the presence of a marked permeability barrier to methylumbelliferyl glucuronide (RATNA et al. 1993). Using intact hepatocytes or homogenates of hepatocytes, compounds have been identified that inhibit either the uptake of sulfate conjugates or their hydrolysis via arylsulfatase (KAUFFMAN et al. 1991). For example, sodium sulfate inhibits hydrolysis of 4-methylumbelliferyl sulfate by intact hepatocytes (half-maximal inhibition, 0.1 m*M*), but not by homogenates, suggesting a selective action on the uptake of organic sulfate at the plasma membrane. Compounds that inhibit hydrolysis of sulfate conjugates in both intact hepatocytes and homogenates include sodium sulfite (half-maximal inhibition, 0.1 m*M*), pregnenolone sulfate (half-maximal inhibition, 1 μM), and estrone sulfate (half-maximal inhibition, 10 μM). Cholesterol sulfate, which does not readily enter hepatocytes, inhibits 4-methylumbelliferyl sulfate hydrolysis in homogenates, but not in intact cells, suggesting that cholesterol sulfate does not compete at anion transport sites on the plasma membrane.

To test whether agents that inhibit arylsulfatase modify production of sulfate conjugates in intact cells, the actions of pregnenolone sulfate on the formation of 4-methylumbelliferyl sulfate from free 4-methylumbelliferone was studied in isolated hepatocytes (KAUFFMAN et al. 1991). Addition of pregnenolone sulfate (100 μM) to intact cells increased the rate of 4-methylumbelliferyl sulfate production and decreased the fraction of 4-methylumbelliferyl converted into the glucuronide conjugate (Fig. 4). Although the rate of utilization of free 4-methylumbelliferyl was unchanged by the addition of pregnenolone sulfate, glucuronide production decreased about 27% in the presence of the competitive inhibitor of arylsulfatase. Simultaneously, sulfate conjugate production increased and essentially balanced the decrease in glucuronide production. Although these results argue strongly that sulfate conjugate production within hepatocytes is regulated by futile cycling, further research employing other substrates is needed.

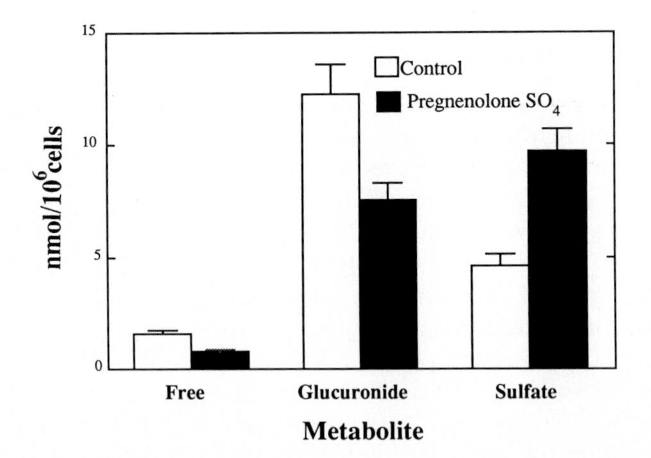

Fig. 4. Effect of *pregnenolone* SO_4 on conjugation of 4-methylumbelliferone by isolated hepatocytes. Hepatocytes (1×10^6 cells/ml were incubated with 20 μM 4-methylumbelliferone in the absence (*open bars*) or presence of 0.1 m*M* pregnenolone SO_4 in Krebs Henseliet bicarbonate buffer at 37°C for 30 min. Samples were assayed for free 4-methylumbelliferone glucuronide and sulfate conjugates (BETHUNE 1974)

E. Conclusion

Results indicating that futile cycling of both glucuronide and sulfate conjugates occurs in hepatocytes suggest that drugs and endogenous substrates that affect microsomal arylsulfatase and β-glucuronidase modulate the net production of sulfate and glucuronide conjugates by the liver. The involvement of futile cycling in regulating the net production of acetyl and methoxy conjugates in intact cells has not been evaluated. Available evidence indicates that net sulfate conjugate production is regulated to a greater extent by futile cycling than is the net production of glucuronide conjugates. Additional studies employing various inhibitors of the hydrolytic enzymes need to consider the actions of such compounds on transmembrane anion carriers and protein binding, which also are important determinants of futile cycling. Finally, futile cycling, which involves more than one enzyme, must be distinguished from reversible metabolism which occurs via a single enzyme.

Since many hormones, including estrogen (Tseng et al. 1983), catecholamines (Gaudin et al. 1985), and thyroxin (Kung et al. 1988), circulate mainly as sulfate conjugates in vivo, it is worthwhile to consider whether sulfate conjugation of a variety of drugs and toxic chemicals in the liver is altered by changes in circulating levels of sulfated hormones or by agents used to inhibit sulfatase in extrahepatic tissues. This consideration is particularly pertinent in view of recent work to develop inhibitors of estrone sulfatase in mammary tissue as an approach to reducing the availability of estrogen in estrogen-dependent breast tumors (Duncan et al. 1993). Future research directed at evaluating the role of futile cycling of drug conjugates in extrahepatic tissues is also warranted in view of the wide tissue distribution of various hydrolases localized in close proximity to related transferases.

Acknowledgement. Studies on futile cycling of glucuronide and sulfate conjugates carried out in our laboratory were supported, in part, by grants CA-20807 and ES from the U.S. Public Health Service. The author is grateful to Marybeth Sarsfield for her expert assistance in assembling the manuscript.

References

Belinsky SA, Kauffman FC, Sokolove PM, Tsukuda T, Thurman RG (1984) Calcium-mediated inhibition of glucuronide production by epinephrine in the perfused rat liver. J Biol Chem 259(12):7705–7711

Berry C, Stellon A, Hallinan T (1975) Guinea pig liver microsomal UDP-glucuronosyltransferase: compartmented or phospholipid-constrained. Biochim Biophys Acta 403:335–344

Bethune JE (1974) The adrenal cortex. UpJohn, Kalamazoo

Chiba M, Pang KS (1993) Effect of protein binding on 4-methylumbelliferyl sulfate desulfation kinetics in perfused rat liver. J Pharmacol Exp Ther (in press)

Conway JG, Kauffman FC, Thurman RG (1985) Effect of glucose on 7-hydroxycoumarin glucuronide production in periportal and pericentral regions of the liver lobule. Biochem J 226:749–756

Conway JG, Kauffman FC, Tsukuda T, Thurman RG (1988) Glucuronidation of 7-hydroxycoumarin in periportal and pericentral regions of the lobule in livers from untreated and 3-methylcholanthrene-treated rats. Mol Pharmacol 33: 111–119

DeVries MH, Groothuis GMM, Mulder GJ, Nguyen H, Meijer DKF (1985) Secretion of the organic anion harmol sulfate from liver into blood. Biochem Pharmacol 34:2129–2135

Duncan L, Purohit A, Howarth NM, Potter VL, Reed J (1993) Inhibition of estrone sulfatase activity by estrone-3-methylthiophosphonate: a potential therapeutic agent in breast cancer. Cancer Res 53:298–303

Dwivedi C, Downie A, Webb T (1987) Net glucuronidation in different rat strains: importance of microsomal β-glucuronidase. FASEB J 1:303–307

El Mouelhi M, Kauffman FC (1986) Sublobular distribution of transferases and hydrolases associated with glucuronide, sulfate and glutathione conjugation in human liver. Hepatology 6:450–456

Gaudin C, Ruget G, Selz F, Cuche JL (1985) Free and conjugated catecholamines in digestive tissues of rats. Life Sci 37:1469–1474

Glazenburg EJ, Jekel-Halsema IMC, Baranczyk-Kuzma A, Krijgscheld KR, Mulder GJ (1984) D-Cysteine as a selective precursor for inorganic sulfate in the rat in vivo: effect of D-cysteine on the sulfation of hormol. Biochem Pharmacol 33: 625–628

Kauffman FC, Whittaker M, Anundi I, Thurman RG (1991) Futile cycling of a sulfate conjugate by isolated hepatocytes. Mol Pharmacol 39:414–420

Kinoshita N, Gelboin HV (1978) β-Glucuronidase catalyzed hydrolysis of benzo(a)pyrene-3-glucuronide and binding to DNA. Science 199:307–309

Kung MP, Spaulding SW, Roth JA (1988) Desulfation of 3,5,3′-triiodothronine sulfate by microsomes from human and rat tissues. Endocrinology 122:1195–1200

Lloyd JB, Forster S (1986) The lysosome membrane. Trends Biochem Sci 11: 365–368

Lowry OH, Passonneau JV (1964) The relationships between substrates and enzymes of glycolysis in brain. J Biol Chem 239:31–42

Miyauchi S, Sugiyama Y, Sawada Y, Iga T, Hanano M (1987) Conjugative metabolism of 4-methylumbelliferone in the rat liver: verification of the sequestration process in multiple indicator dilution experiments. Chem Pharm Bull (Tokyo) 35:4241–4248

Paigen J (1979) Acid hydrolases as models of genetic control. Annu Rev Genet 13:417–466

Poso AR, Penttila KE, Lindros KO (1991) Heterogenous zonal distribution of lysosomal enzymes in rat liver. Enzyme 145:174–179

Ratna S, Chiba M, Bandyopadhyay L, Pang KS (1993) Futile cycling between 4-methylumbelliferone and its conjugates in perfused rat liver. Hepatology (in press)

Reinke LA, Moyer MJ, Notley KA (1986) Diminished rates of glucuronidation and sulfation in perfused rat liver after chronic ethanol administration. Biochem Pharmacol 35:439–447

Roy AB (1976) Sulfatase, lysosomes and disease. Aust J Exp Biol Med Sci 54: 111–135

Schollhammer I, Poll DS, Bickel MH (1975) Liver microsomal β-glucuronidase and UDP-glucuronyltransferase. Enzyme 20:269–276

Sokolove PM, Wilcox MA, Thurman RG, Kauffman FC (1984) Stimulation of hepatic microsomal β-glucuronidase by calcium. Biochem Biophys Res Commun 121:987–993

Swank RT, Pfister K, Miller D, Chapman V (1986) The egasin gene affects the processing of oligosaccharides of lysosomal β-glucuronidase in liver. Biochem J 240:445–454

Tseng L, Mazella J, Lee LY, Stone ML (1983) Estrogen sulfatase and estrogen sulfotransferase in human primary mammary carcinoma. J Steroid Biochem 19:1413–1417

Walaszek Z, Hanausek-Walaszek M, Webb TE (1984) Inhibition of 7,12-dimethylbenz(a)anthracene-induced rat mammary tumorigenesis by 2,5-di-*O*-acetyl-D-glucaro-1-4:6,3-dilactone, and in vivo *β*-glucuronidase inhibitor. Carcinogenesis 5:767–772

Walaszek Z, Hanausek-Walaszek M, Minton JP, Webb TE (1986a) Dietary glucarate as an anti-promoter of 7,12-dimethylbenz(a)anthracene-induced mammary tumorigenesis. Carcinogenesis 7:1463–1466

Walaszek Z, Hanausek-Walaszek M, Webb TE (1986b) Dietary glucurate-mediated reduction of sensitivity of murine strains to chemical carcinogenesis. Cancer Lett 33:25–32

Whittaker M, Sokolove PM, Thurman RG, Kauffman FC (1985) Stimulation of 3-benzo(a)pyrenyl glucuronide hydrolysis by calcium activation of microsomal *β*-glucuronidase. Cancer Lett 26:145–152

Zaleski J, Kwei GY, Thurman RG, Kauffman FC (1991) Suppression of benzo(a)pyrene metabolism by accumulation of triacylglycerols in rat hepatocytes: effect of high-fat and food restricted diets. Carcinogenesis 12:2073–2079

CHAPTER 10

Pharmacokinetic Modeling of Drug Conjugates

K.S. PANG and M. CHIBA

A. Introduction

The liver is the most important drug-eliminating organ that is capable of both conjugation and biliary excretion. Much has been reported on the liver's role as a highly specialized and heterogeneous organ (NOVIKOFF 1959; MILLER et al. 1979; DE LEEUE and KNOOK 1984; GOODING et al. 1978; JUNGERMAN and KATZ 1982), and an accurate physiological description of hepatic drug conjugation and conjugate processing by the liver necessitates consideration of the structure of the liver and its microcirculation (PANG and STILLWELL 1983; GORESKY and GROOM 1984; PANG 1990; PANG et al. 1991, 1992). The attendant heterogeneities – in enzymic zonation (BARON et al. 1982; ULLRICH et al. 1984; KNAPP et al. 1988; THURMAN et al. 1987; PANG et al. 1983; PANG and TERRELL 1981a), biliary excretion (GUMUCIO et al. 1978; BOYER et al. 1979), capillary transit times (GORESKY 1963; GORESKY and GROOM 1984), cosubstrate abundance (ASGHER et al. 1975; SMITH et al. 1979; MURRAY et al. 1986), intracellular binding (BRAAKMAN et al. 1987, 1989; BASS et al. 1989) and transport (BURGER et al. 1989; MCFARLANE et al. 1990), together with clearance modifiers, such as organ blood flow, drug and conjugate binding to vascular proteins, transmembrane clearance, and the K_m and V_{max} of the saturable eliminatory pathways (for reviews, see GORESKY and GROOM 1984; PANG and XU 1988; PANG 1990; PANG et al. 1991, 1992; GORESKY et al. 1993a,b) – must be viewed as a whole in order to accurately relate the occurrences involved during drug and conjugate processing within the liver. The rate-limiting step in the overall removal process is highly dependent on these variables as well as on the concentration of drug at the inlet of the liver.

Within the intact liver, drug (an already existing chemical entity) disappearance is a result of uptake by the organ and occurs as a distributed-in-space phenomenon, directed by flow along the sinusoids and described according to its position along the sinusoidal flow path (GORESKY et al. 1973; WINKLER et al. 1973; PANG and STILLWELL 1983). This leads to the observed concentration gradient between the inlet and outlet of the liver (JONES et al. 1980; GUMUCIO et al. 1981, 1984; WEISIGER et al. 1986). Drug uptake is governed by time-related events, including drug transport into and out of hepatocytes, binding to red cells, plasma, and tissue proteins, and conjugation by enzymes or excretion into bile, events which occur as a function of the unbound concentration. The events on substrate influx for recruitment of metabolic–excretory activities and efflux are linked to the delivery by flow (Fig. 1A) and are modulated by substrate binding to red blood cells

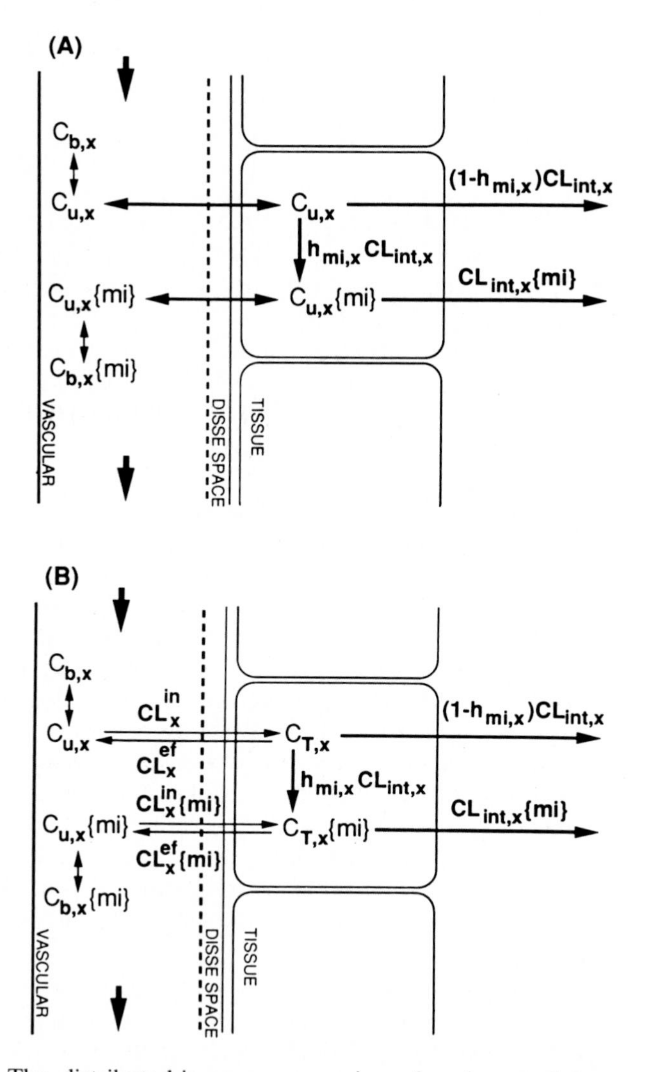

Fig. 1A,B. The distributed-in-space processing of a drug and its conjugate, *mi*, whose distributions are flow-limited **A** or barrier-limited **B**, at any point x. The liver is viewed as three compartments: expanded vascular (sinusoidal space + *Disse space*), *tissue*, and bile (not shown) compartments, receiving unidirectional flow (*bold arrow* in vascular compartment). The bound ($C_{b,x}$) and unbound ($C_{u,x}$) species in the vascular compartment are in equilibrium. See text for details

(GORESKY et al. 1975, 1988; PANG et al. 1988a), and plasma (WOLKOFF et al. 1979; GILLETTE 1973; XU et al. 1993) and tissue (FLEISCHNER et al. 1975; GORESKY et al. 1978; GÄRTNER et al. 1982; THEILMANN et al. 1985) proteins; the generally accepted view is that the unbound substrate is the species that is transported across membranes and becomes eliminated (LEVY and YACOBI 1974; GRAUSZ and SCHMID 1971; BARNHART and CLARENBURG 1973; SORRENTINO et al. 1989a). The rates at which the conjugation and excretory processes proceed, however, are dependent on the amounts and localization of enzymatic activity for conjugate formation and the activities towards biliary excretion.

Similar consideration must then be given to conjugate formation and excretion within hepatocytes (Fig. 1A). After formation, each conjugate is potentially immediately excreted or acted on by hydrolases, events which lead to a sequential first-pass effect of the formed conjugate (PANG and GILLETTE 1979). The conjugate will, in parallel fashion, efflux into the sinusoid and become exposed to hepatocytes downstream from its site of formation; the metabolite re-enters the liver cell and is prone to elimination. These processes are repeated before the conjugate eventually re-enters the general circulation (for reviews, see PANG and XU 1988; ST-PIERRE et al. 1992; GORESKY et al. 1993a,b). Thus, metabolic processing is also a distributed-in-space phenomenon, and a conjugate formed within the liver is expected to undergo different extents of metabolism–excretion in comparison to a preformed conjugate entering the liver from the circulation. The disparity is due to different points of conjugate introduction in the organ, even though the events underlying the elimination and transport are interrelated, because of involvement of the same enzymic–excretory processes (for reviews, see PANG and XU 1988; PANG 1990; PANG et al. 1991, 1992; GORESKY et al. 1993a). The whole must thus be viewed within the context of the microcirculatory events and the functional heterogeneities in the liver.

This chapter focuses on the functional microcirculatory unit of the liver, the acinus (RAPPAPORT et al. 1954; RAPPAPORT 1958, 1980), in its relation to enzyme zonation and clearance modifiers on the modeling of substrate removal and conjugate formation. Special attention is given to the binding and transport characteristics of the conjugate. As will be emphasized in this chapter, major discrepancies between the fates of preformed and generated conjugates after administration of the precursor and conjugate have been found to exist in the liver (GORESKY et al. 1992; PANG and TERRELL 1981b; RATNA et al. 1993). Cellular membranes acting as barriers for permeation for polar conjugates have unequivocally rendered higher extents of intrahepatic conjugate elimination, usually via biliary excretion, than those from preformed conjugate administration; otherwise, the converse will be true (GORESKY et al. 1992; RATNA et al. 1993). The effect of zonal distribution of the cosubstrate, glutathione (GSH), on conjugation is being addressed in a distributed-in-space fashion for the first time.

B. Hepatic Modeling: Tubular Flow Model

In view of the fact that heterogeneity exists for capillary transit times, tissue binding, enzyme zonation, and transport, a general strategy has been evolved in our laboratory to interrelate these determinants and to effectively encompass structural heterogeneities in order to describe drug conjugation under steady state conditions. In this approach, the liver is viewed as an organ receiving a series of nonsegregated, parallel flows surrounded by identical, single sheets of hepatocytes of uniform ("parallel tube" model; WINKLER et al. 1973, 1974) or nonuniform ("enzyme-distributed") enzymatic activities (PANG et al. 1983; PANG and STILLWELL 1983). Since the liver outflow concentration and extraction ratio depend not only on the abundance and distribution of the activity of the enzyme, represented by V_{max}, but also on the distribution of sinusoidal transit times (GORESKY et al. 1973; PANG et al. 1988c), the assumption that all sinusoids have the same transit time and the same V_{max} in the tubular flow model will result in a slight underestimation of the true V_{max} (GONZALES-FERNANDEZ and ATTA 1973; BASS 1983, 1985; BASS and ROBINSON 1981).

The simplified, steady state approach has been utilized to interrelate liver blood flow (Q), the influx (CL^{in}) and efflux (CL^{ef}) clearances, and the total eliminatory capacity (CL_{int} or intrinsic clearance) with drug conjugation reactions. The condition is further simplified when the distribution of the parent compound is perfusion rate limited, i.e., there is rapid equilibration of drug between the perfusing blood and the intracellular enzyme sites (CL^{in} or CL^{ef} for drug and metabolite $\gg Q$) and the concentrations of unbound drug and metabolite in the sinusoidal blood at any locale (x) equal those within the hepatic tissue at x and reflect events occurring at the cellular level. As will soon become evident in the ensuing mass–balance relationships, the influx and efflux transmembrane clearances, the intrinsic clearance, and the unbound fraction for both drug and conjugate may be varied from x to (x + dx) to encompass aspects of heterogeneity in transport and zonation, as well as induced changes in protein binding (Fig. 1A). The shape of the concentration gradient that develops along the length of the sinusoid due to irreversible drug removal becomes highly dependent on the interrelations of these factors.

When the distribution of a substrate is flow limited (transmembrance clearance $\gg Q$), the mass–balance equation that describes drug removal at x by a sun of nth metabolic and excretory pathways is given by the sum of the Michaelis-Menten reactions at x.

For the rate of disappearance of drug,

$$\frac{Q\mathrm{d}C_x}{\mathrm{d}x} = -\frac{1}{L}\sum_{i=1}^{n}\frac{V_{maxi,x}C_{u,x}}{K_{mi} + C_{u,x}} \tag{1}$$

For the rate of conjugate formation (when sequential removal of conjugate is absent),

$$\frac{Q\mathrm{d}C_{\mathrm{x}}\{\mathrm{mi}\}}{\mathrm{d}x} = \frac{1}{L}\left\{\frac{V_{\mathrm{maxi,x}}C_{\mathrm{u,x}}}{K_{\mathrm{mi}} + C_{\mathrm{u,x}}}\right\} \tag{2}$$

where C_{x} and $C_{\mathrm{u,x}}$ are the total and unbound concentrations of drug in sinusoidal blood at point x, respectively; $C_{\mathrm{x}}\{\mathrm{mi}\}$ is the metabolite concentration in the sinusoid at x; $V_{\mathrm{maxi,x}}$ is the maximum velocity for each ith pathway at x, which may vary along the length of the sinusoid (see Sect. B.II on enzyme zonation), whereas K_{mi}, the corresponding Michaelis-Menten constant for the pathway, is considered to be identical for all x. As shown with Eq. 2, the rate of formation of the conjugate at x relies on the local unbound concentration of its parent compound and the V_{max} and K_{m} for the formation pathway and is independent of the modes of disposal of the conjugate. However, most conjugates, instead of complete efflux into the sinusoidal space, usually undergo biliary excretion and, in some cases, even endure metabolism. Consequently, what is observed in sinusoidal blood becomes the difference between its rate of formation and rate of removal.

For the rate of appearance of conjugate in hepatic venous blood,

$$\frac{Q\mathrm{d}C_{\mathrm{x}}\{\mathrm{mi}\}}{\mathrm{d}x} = \frac{1}{L}\Bigg\{\underbrace{\frac{V_{\mathrm{maxi,x}}C_{\mathrm{u,x}}}{K_{\mathrm{mi}} + C_{\mathrm{u,x}}}}_{\text{rate of conjugate formation}} - \underbrace{\sum_{i=1}^{\mathrm{m}}\frac{V_{\mathrm{maxi,x}}\{\mathrm{mi}\}C_{\mathrm{u,x}}\{\mathrm{mi}\}}{K_{\mathrm{mi}}\{\mathrm{mi}\} + C_{\mathrm{u,x}}\{\mathrm{mi}\}}}_{\text{rate of conjugate removal}}\Bigg\} \tag{3}$$

Alternately, the term $\mathrm{CL}_{\mathrm{int,x}}$, or the intrinsic clearance at x, is the sum of all of the ith excretory and metabolic intrinsic clearances at x:

$$\mathrm{CL}_{\mathrm{int,x}} = \sum_{i=1}^{n}\frac{V_{\mathrm{maxi,x}}}{K_{\mathrm{mi}} + C_{\mathrm{u,x}}} \tag{4}$$

$\mathrm{CL}_{\mathrm{int,x}}$ is also viewed as the volume of hepatocyte water which is cleared of drug per unit time at x by the liver (WILKINSON and SHAND 1975). By summing the individual $\mathrm{CL}_{\mathrm{int,x}}$, then averaging this over the length, L, the length-averaged intrinsic clearance ($\mathrm{CL}_{\mathrm{int}}$) or $\int_0^L \mathrm{CL}_{\mathrm{int,x}}\mathrm{d}x/L$ may be obtained (PANG and STILLWELL 1983).

At $x = L$, C_{x} in Eq. 1 becomes the hepatic venous drug concentration, C_{Out}, at steady state. For a single removal scheme wherein binding is constant, the output concentration at steady state under apparent first-order conditions may be expressed as (WINKLER et al. 1974)

$$C_{\mathrm{Out}} = C_{\mathrm{In}}e^{-f_{\mathrm{B}}\mathrm{CL}_{\mathrm{int}}/Q} \tag{5}$$

where C_{In} and C_{Out} denote the steady state input and output concentrations across the organ, respectively; f_{B} is the unbound fraction in blood. On rearrangement of Eq. 5, the steady state extraction ratio of drug, estimated as the arterio-venous concentration difference divided by the arterial concentration, is:

$$E = (1 - e^{-f_{\mathrm{B}}\mathrm{CL}_{\mathrm{int}}/Q}) \tag{6}$$

The simplest form of expressing the velocity (v^{mi}) of formation of the conjugate, mi, within this steady state system is given by integration of Eq. 2:

$$v^{mi} = \frac{1}{L}\int_0^L \left\{\frac{V_{maxi}C_{u,x}}{K_{mi} + C_{u,x}}\right\}dx \tag{7}$$

Upon additional integration of the conjugate removal rate for all x along L (right term on the right side of Eq. 3), the overall conjugate removal rate, $v\{mi\}$, which for most conjugates is the biliary excretion rate, and the apparent extraction ratio of the formed conjugate $E\{mi,P\}$ are obtained as:

$$E\{mi,P\} = \frac{v^{mi} - v\{mi\}}{v^{mi}} \tag{8}$$

and its complement fraction, the apparent availability of the formed conjugate, $F\{mi,P\}$, is given by (ST-PIERRE et al. 1992)

$$F\{mi,P\} = \frac{[F\{mi\} - F\{P\}]\ln(F\{P\})}{E\{P\}\ln[F\{P\}/F\{mi\}]} \tag{9}$$

which relates to the availability of the preformed conjugate $F\{mi\}$ and for the parent drug $F\{P\}$. The estimation of $F\{mi,P\}$ exceeds $F\{mi\}$ in all cases and is independent of the value of h_{mi} (or fractional elimination), whether competing pathways are absent ($h_{mi} = 1$) or present ($h_{mi} < 1$) (ST-PIERRE et al. 1992). Conversely, the model predicts that the extent of sequential metabolism of endogenously formed mi is less than that of its preformed counterpart ($E\{mi,P\} < E\{mi\}$).

Often unknown are the V_{max}s and K_ms of the enzymic systems for conjugate formation. These estimates, as shown in comparative studies on hepatic clearance models, are strongly dependent on the type of assumptions made for the liver with regard to its flow behavior (LEVENSPIEL 1972) and what is viewed as the average (unbound) substrate concentration in the liver (ST-PIERRE et al. 1992). For an unbound substrate, the average substrate concentration in liver is approximated by the logarithmic average of the inlet and outlet concentrations ($\hat{C}$) (WINKLER et al. 1974)

$$\hat{C} = \frac{C_{In} - C_{Out}}{\ln(C_{In}/C_{Out})} \tag{10}$$

whereas when protein binding occurs, the substrate concentration should be approximated by the unbound logarithmic average of the unbound inlet and outlet concentrations, $\hat{C}_u$ (XU et al. 1993)

$$\hat{C} = \frac{C_{In,u} - C_{Out,u}}{\ln(C_{In,u}/C_{Out,u})} \tag{11}$$

where $C_{In,u}$ and $C_{Out,u}$ are the unbound concentrations at the inlet and outlet, respectively. With this definition of the substrate concentration, the formation of conjugate (v^{mi}) may be estimated with respect to the following Michaelis-Menten equation:

$$v^{mi} = \frac{V_{maxi}\hat{C}_u}{K_{mi} + \hat{C}_u} \tag{12}$$

where the intrinsic clearance, CL_{int}, as conceived by GILLETTE (1971) and introduced by WILKINSON and SHAND (1975), is re-expressed as

$$CL_{int} = \sum_{i=1}^{n} \frac{V_{maxi}}{K_{mi} + \hat{C}_u} \tag{13}$$

which dwindles to a constant, $\Sigma(V_{maxi}/K_{mi})$, at low substrate concentration ($\ll K_{mi}$) or first-order conditions. With metabolic data on v^{mi} and the input and output concentrations or their unbound counterparts, Eq. 12 may be applied to obtain estimates of the V_{maxi} and K_{mi} of individual conjugation processes (PANG et al. 1983; MORRIS et al. 1988; XU et al. 1990, 1993).

I. Transmembrane Barrier

The plasma membrane of hepatocytes imposes a substantial barrier for the entry of substrates. Transmembrane transport is a process which can constitute the rate-determining factor. For lipophilic substrates, the mode of entry via passive diffusion is rapid, and the flux across the membrane is sufficiently high such that the membrane is seldom rate limiting. Many conjugates which are organic anions are expected to encounter the membrane as an austere barrier unless specific transport carriers exist (for reviews, see MEIJER 1987; NATHANSON and BOYER 1991). Carrier-mediated influx has been reported for the sulfate conjugates of harmol (SUNDHEIMER and BRENDEL 1983) and 4-methylumbelliferone (4MU; CHIBA et al. 1993) and the GSH conjugate of bromosulfophthalein (SORRENTINO et al. 1988, 1989b; GENG et al. 1993). In the absence of facilitated transport, hydrophilic compounds will be barred from entry (DE LANNOY and PANG 1987; MIYAUCHI et al. 1987a–c; GORESKY et al. 1992) and their uptake is often retarded. Conceptual frameworks for a membrane barrier for polar compounds, which may be applied to preformed polar conjugates, have been presented (GILLETTE and PANG 1977; SATO et al. 1986; MIYAUCHI et al. 1987a, 1989). Instantaneous equilibration at any point x would not occur in this instance, i.e., the unbound bood concentration at point x would not reflect that in the liver tissue at the same locale.

The following section highlights the effect of such a barrier on the difference in the apparent handling between a preformed (administered) conjugate and a conjugate generated within cells (derived from precursor). The equations described by DE LANNOY and PANG (1986, 1987) for enalaprilat as a formed metabolite from enalapril versus preformed enalaprilat may be readily used to illustrate the importance of a transmembrane barrier for polar conjugates. For the modeling of such barrier-limited events, discrete compartments for the vascular space (expanded plasma volume or plasma plus interstitial space), liver tissue, and bile are used to describe fluxes across the sinusoidal and canalicular membranes (Fig. 1B). Accordingly, the mass–balance steady state relationships for the change of drug concentrations in the vascular compartment and tissue with respect to their position, x, in liver, are:

For drug in vascular compartment,

$$\frac{Q\mathrm{d}C_x}{\mathrm{d}x} = \frac{f_{T,x}C_{T,x}\mathrm{CL}_x^{ef} - f_{B,x}C_x\mathrm{CL}_x^{in}}{L} \tag{13}$$

and for drug in tissue,

$$\frac{Q\mathrm{d}C_{T,x}}{\mathrm{d}x} = 0 = \frac{1}{L}\{f_{B,x}C_x\mathrm{CL}_x^{in} - f_{T,x}C_{T,x}[\mathrm{CL}_x^{ef} + \mathrm{CL}_{int,x}]\} \tag{14}$$

where C_x and $C_{T,x}$ are the concentrations of drug in the vascular and tissue compartments at x, respectively, and $f_{B,x}$ and $f_{T,x}$ denote the corresponding unbound fractions of drug in the vascular and tissue compartments; CL_x^{in}, CL_x^{ef}, and $\mathrm{CL}_{int,x}$ are the influx and efflux transmembrane and intrinsic clearances, respectively, at x. These acinar clearances may be comprised of more than one component consisting of saturable and nonsaturable processes. The equation describing the generated metabolite in blood and tissue following input of drug to liver are:

For the generated conjugate in the vascular compartment,

$$\frac{Q\mathrm{d}C_x\{mi\}}{\mathrm{d}x} = \left\{\frac{f_{T,x}\{mi\}C_{T,x}\{mi\}\mathrm{CL}_x^{ef}\{mi\} - f_{B,x}\{mi\}C_x\{mi\}\mathrm{CL}_x^{in}\{mi\}}{L}\right\} \tag{15}$$

and for the generated conjugate in tissue,

$$\frac{Q\mathrm{d}C_{T,x}\{mi\}}{\mathrm{d}x} = 0 = \frac{1}{L}(f_{B,x}\{mi\}C_x\{mi\}\mathrm{CL}_x^{in}\{mi\} + f_{T,x}C_{T,x}h_{mi,x}\mathrm{CL}_{int,x} - f_{T,x}\{mi\}C_{T,x}\{mi\}[\mathrm{CL}_x^{ef}\{mi\} + \mathrm{CL}_{int,x}\{mi\}]) \tag{16}$$

where $C_x\{mi\}$ and $C_{T,x}\{mi\}$ are the concentrations of the formed conjugate in the vascular and tissue compartments at point x, respectively, and $f_{B,x}\{mi\}$ and $f_{T,x}\{mi\}$ correspond to the unbound fractions of the conjugate in the vascular compartment and in liver tissue; $h_{mi,x}$ is the fraction of total drug intrinsic clearance which forms the primary metabolite at x; $\mathrm{CL}_x^{in}\{mi\}$, $\mathrm{CL}_x^{ef}\{mi\}$, and $\mathrm{CL}_{int,x}\{mi\}$ denote the influx and efflux transmembrane clearances and intrinsic clearance for elimination of the metabolite, respectively, at point x. Other pathway(s) for removal of drug, denoted by the intrinsic clearance $(1 - h_{mi,x})\mathrm{CL}_{int,x}$, represent metabolic or excretory pathways other than formation of the particular conjugate of interest, whereas $CL_{int}\{mi\}$ mostly represent the biliary excretion intrinsic clearance of the conjugate (Fig. 1B). The biliary excretion rates of the drug and metabolite are:

For the parent drug,

$$\frac{dB_x}{dx} = f_{T,x}C_{T,x}CL_x^b \tag{17}$$

and for the formed conjugate,

$$\frac{dB_x\{mi\}}{dx} = f_{T,x}\{mi\}C_{T,x}\{mi\}CL_{int,x}\{mi\} \tag{18}$$

where B_x and $B_x\{mi\}$ are the amounts of drug and conjugate excreted into bile, and CL_x^b and $CL_{int,x}\{mi\}$ are the biliary intrinsic clearances for drug and conjugate excretion. These biliary excretion rates are modulated by the corresponding efflux clearances for the drug and conjugate, since efflux poses as a competing process for the intracellular substrate.

Analytical solutions exist when CL_x^{in}, CL_x^{ef}, $CL_{int,x}$, $h_{mi,x}$, $CL_x^{in}\{mi\}$, $CL_x^{ef}\{mi\}$, $CL_{int,x}\{mi\}$, and the unbound fractions are invariant with x. The steady state extraction ratios are (PANG and CHIBA 1994):

For the drug,

$$E = 1 - e^{-\left\{\frac{f_B CL_{int} CL^{in}}{Q(CL_{int} + CL^{ef})}\right\}} \tag{19}$$

and for the formed conjugate, $E\{mi,P\}$,

$$E\{mi,P\} = 1 - \left\{\frac{f_B CL_{int} CL^{in}}{f_B CL_{int} CL^{in}[CL_{int}\{mi\} + CL^{ef}\{mi\}] - f_B\{mi\}CL_{int}\{mi\}CL^{in}\{mi\}[CL_{int} + CL^{ef}]}\right\} \times \left\{\frac{e^{-\frac{f_B\{mi\}CL_{int}\{mi\}CL^{in}\{mi\}}{Q(CL_{int}\{mi\} + CL^{ef}\{mi\})}} - e^{-\frac{f_B CL_{int} CL^{in}}{Q(CL_{int} + CL^{ef})}}}{\left(1 - e^{-\frac{f_B CL_{int} CL^{in}}{Q(CL_{int} + CL^{ef})}}\right)}\right\} \tag{20}$$

Note that $E\{mi,P\}$ is independent of the fraction of total intrinsic clearance for the formation of the metabolite, but is dependent on other parameters (binding, transmembrane clearances, and intrinsic clearance) pertaining to the parent compound.

One of the uses of the model equations, as shown below and elsewhere, is to provide simulations for an improved understanding of the system. Simulations of the vascular and tissue concentrations are readily obtained, as shown by DE LANNOY and PANG (1987). The hepatocyte membrane barrier will render differences in handling between a preformed (administered) conjugate and a conjugate generated within hepatocytes (derived from precursor). A general trend emerges: the hepatic extraction ratio of the preformed metabolite, $E\{\text{mi}\}$, and the apparent extraction ratio of a formed conjugate, ($E\{\text{mi,P}\}$), are influenced by the transmembrane clearance, ($CL^{in}\{\text{mi}\} = CL^{ef}\{\text{mi}\} = CL^{d}\{\text{mi}\}$), for a given finite $CL_{int}\{\text{mi}\}$ in opposite directions. When $CL^{d}\{\text{mi}\}/Q \gg CL_{int}\{\text{mi}\}/Q$, the rate-limiting step (RLS) is biliary excretion for both the preformed and formed conjugate. However, at $CL^{d}\{\text{mi}\}/Q \ll CL_{int}\{\text{mi}\}/Q$, the RLS for preformed metabolite is the transmembrane transport for influx; the same transmembrane transport (for efflux) entraps the formed metabolite and steers it towards excretion (Fig. 2). There will be an apparent enhancement in removal of the generated, polar conjugate via biliary excretion, in relation to that for preformed conjugate. This trend was indeed observed for several sulfate (GORESKY et al. 1992), glucuronide (MIYAUCHI et al. 1989; RATNA et al. 1993), and GSH (VAN ANDA et al. 1979; STEELE et al. 1981; SMITH et al. 1983; POLHOUIJS et al. 1991, 1993) conjugates suspected of barrier-limited entry (Table 1).

II. Zonation of Enzymic Activities

Much acinar distribution of enzymes exists in the liver with regard to conjugation reactions (Table 2). The role of enzyme zonation on formation of conjugates has been illustrated both theoretically and experimentally. Enzymic localization at any point x along the sinusoid of length L can be conceptualized as a distribution of enzyme content or $V_{max,x}$ along L. Two such enzymic systems are depicted schematically in Fig. 3, one for sulfation and one for glucuronidation. For these conjugation systems, the relative location of each system may be described with respect to its median (or center) of enzymic distribution, the plane which divides total enzymatic activity (total V_{max} or $\int_0^L V_{max,x}dx/L$) into halves. The median or the "median distance" serves to interrelate the distance between inlet of the liver and the bulk of the enzyme. System I (sulfation activity) is viewed as an anterior pathway in relation to system II (glucuronidation), since its median (or center) of distribution precedes that for system II.

Sulfation and glucuronidation are common competing conjugation pathways of most phenolic substrates. Sulfation is often a higher-affinity, lower-capacity pathway than glucuronidation. According to the scheme, the substrate first accesses the anteriorly located enzyme system (system I, sulfotransferases) to generate the corresponding sulfate conjugate; glucuronidation by system II, the posteriorly located competitive system, occurs when residual substrate arrives downstream for recruitment of such activities. Hence, the concentration of substrate at x is related to its removal at points preceding x and at x. In this instance, individual conjugation rates may be readily predicted by Eq. 2.

From theoretical simulations (PANG et al. 1987; MORRIS and PANG 1987), it is shown that for highly cleared (high E) compounds for which outflow concentrations are much lower than the corresponding input concentrations, a steep intrahepatic gradient exists during the steady state flow of substrate into the liver; the converse is true for poorly extracted compounds. Thus, the

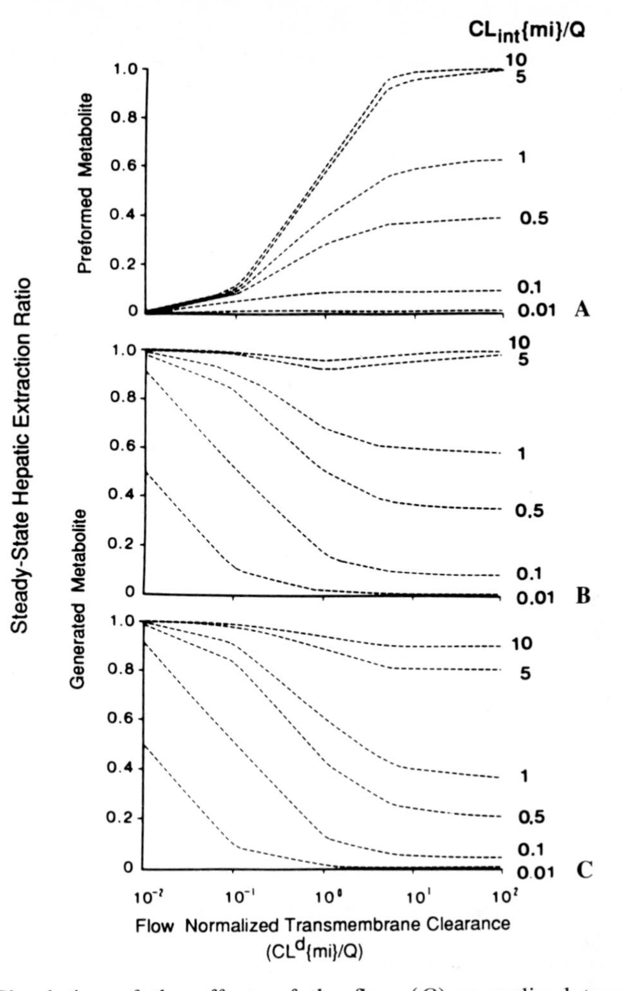

Fig. 2A–C. Simulation of the effects of the flow (Q)-normalized transmembrane clearances of drug (CL^d/Q) and conjugate ($CL^d\{mi\}/Q$), and the flow-normalized intrinsic clearances of drug (CL_{int}/Q) and conjugate ($CL_{int}\{mi\}/Q$) on the extraction ratio of a preformed ($E\{mi\}$) **A** and generated conjugate ($E\{mi,P\}$) **B**, **C**. In this simulation, the liver was viewed as three compartments (see DE LANNOY and PANG 1987); all transmembrane (CL^d) and intrinsic clearances (CL_{int}) are assumed to be evenly distributed at any point x along the length of the sinusoid (L). Values of drug intrinsic clearance and transmembrane clearance were varied: CL_{int}/Q values were 10, 5, 1, 0.5, 0.1, 0.01, of which half (h_{mi}, 0.5) was involved in conjugate formation; CL^d/Q were 10^2, 10^1, 10^0, 10^{-1}, and 10^{-2} (not all simulations were shown). **A** The steady state hepatic extraction ratio of conjugate, $E\{mi\}$, is independent of clearance parameters of drug, but increases with $CL_d\{mi\}/Q$, especially when the metabolite is reasonably highly cleared ($CL_{int}\{mi\}/Q \gg 1$). In contrast, $E\{mi,P\}$ decreases with increasing $CL^d\{mi\}/Q$ due to rapid efflux into sinusoids and is altered only slightly by drug parameters CL_{int} and CL^d; similar trends are seen for $CL_{int}/Q = 10$, when $CL^d/Q = 100$ or 10 **B**, and for $CL_{int}/Q = 0.01$ and $CL^d/Q = 10^{-2}$ **C**. The fractional elimination, h_{mi}, had no effect on the shapes of the graphs **B**, **C**. The *numbers* next to each graph denote the flow-normalized intrinsic clearance of the metabolite, $CL_{int}\{mi\}/Q$

Table 1. Effect of transmembrane barrier on the extents of elimination of preformed versus formed conjugates

Metabolite	Preformed conjugate	Generated conjugate		References
	E{mi}[a]	E{mi,P}	Precursor	
Acetaminophen sulfate	0.003			GORESKY et al. (1992)
		0.03[b]	Acetaminophen	PANG and TERRELL (1981b)
4-Methylumbelliferyl glucuronide	0.073			RATNA et al. (1993)
		0.479[b]	4-Methylumbelliferone	ibid.
		0.647[b]	4-Methylumbellifereryl sulfate	ibid.
α-Bromoisovalerylurea (S) glutathione conjugate	0.0003			POLHUIJS et al. (1991)
		0.79[c]	(R)-α-Bromoisovalerylurea	POLHUIJS et al. (1993)
α-Bromoisovalerylurea (R) glutathione conjugate	0.0003			POLHUIJS et al. (1991)
		1.00[c]	(S)-α-Bromoisovalerylurea	POLHUIJS et al. (1993)

[a] Extraction ratio of the preformed, adminstered conjugate.

[b] These conjugates are primarly biliarily excreted; E{mi,P} was estimated as $\left[\frac{\text{biliary excretion rate of conjugate}}{\text{formation rate of conjugate}}\right]$.

[c] The glutathione conjugate is of opposite configuration to its precursor and undergoes cleavage; E{mi,P} was estimated as $\left[1 - \frac{\text{rate out of conjugate in venous perfusate}}{\text{formation rate of conjugate}}\right]$.

Table 2. Zonation of conjugation and deconjugation activities found by immunohistochemical and staining techniques, microdissection, and by prograde and retrograde, and HAPV (hepatic artery-portal vein) and HAHV (hepatic artery-hepatic vein) perfusion of the rat liver

Noted metabolic heterogeneities			Drug examples	References
Anterior	Even	Posterior		
		UDP-glucuronyltransferase		Ullrich et al. (1984), Knapp et al. (1988)
		Glutathione *S*-transferase		Redick et al. (1982)
	Arylsulfatase			Anundi et al. (1986), El Mouelhi and Kauffman (1986)
	β-Glucuronidase			ibid.
Sulfation			Acetaminophen	Pang and Gillette (1979); Pang and Terrell (1981a); Pang et al. (1988b)
Sulfation			*N*-OH-2-Acetylaminofluorene	de Baun et al. (1971); Meerman and Mulder (1981)
Sulfation	Glucuronidation		Gentisamide	Morris et al. (1988)
Sulfation	Glucuronidation		Harmol	Dawson et al. (1985)
Sulfation	Glucuronidation		7-Hydroxycoumarin	Conway et al. (1987)
Sulfation		Glucuronidation	7-Hydroxycoumarin	Conway et al. (1984)
Sulfation	Glucuronidation		Salicylamide	Xu and Pang (1989)
		Glycine conjugation	Benzoic acid	Chiba et al. (1994)
		Glutathione conjugation	Bromosulfophthalein	Zhao et al. (1993)

UDP, uridine diphosphate.

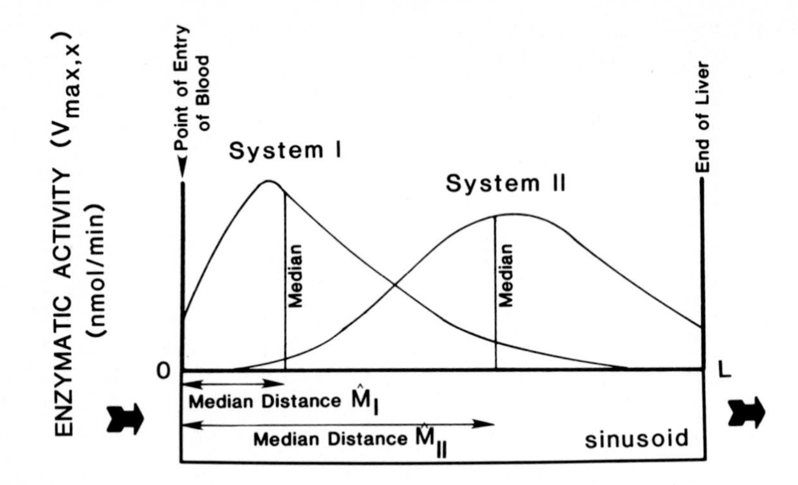

Fig. 3. The distributed-in-space phenomenon in drug processing. A schematic representation of uneven distribution of drug-metabolizing enzymes in the liver, *systems I and II*, which are either involved in parallel, competing, or sequential metabolic pathways. Drug processing occurs along the direction of flow of substrate, from *left* to *right*, in a distributed-in-space fashion. The enzymic distributions of systems I and II are described by the *median distances*, the distance from the inlet of the liver to the *median* (plane which divides the amount of enzyme into equal halves). As shown, system I is anteriorly localized relative to system II along the direction of flow of substrate

anterior pathways exert an effect on formation of metabolites downstream, especially for highly cleared compounds. This occurs at low concentration, wherein the anterior pathway is operating linearly and maximally such that not all downstream hepatocytes are metabolically recruited due to substrate depletion. At intermediate concentrations that are saturating for the anterior sulfation system, a proportionally higher substrate flux reaches the downstream region to recruit glucuronidation activities, rendering disproportionately higher glucuronidation rates; at higher concentration ($\gg K_m$), all enzymic systems (anterior and posterior) will be recruited by substrate, and the role of enzymic heterogeneity in metabolite formation becomes attenuated and unimportant (MORRIS and PANG 1987).

Another question which arises is the accuracy of the K_m and V_{max} estimates for the anterior and posterior conjugation pathways. Since the posterior pathway is under modulation of the anterior pathway capable of depletion of substrate, the metabolic data for glucuronidation with increasing concentration usually display a "S" curve instead of a rectangular hyperbola described for Michaelis-Menten behavior. The premise was tested by MORRIS and PANG (1987), who employed a variety of K_m and V_{max} values for various intermediately (E, 0.5) or highly (E, approximately 1) cleared phenolic substrates to simulate sulfation and glucuronidation rates to refit to the Michaelis-Menten equation (Eq. 12). Among the examples, good estimates were obtained for the anterior sulfation pathway and for the K_m and V_{max} for the posterior glucuronidation pathway when the K_m values for sulfation and glucuronidation were similar; however, overestimates of these constants for glucuronidation resulted when the K_m for glucuronidation exceeded that for sulfation. The error was obliterated upon suppression of the anterior sulfation pathway (MORRIS and PANG 1987).

These metabolic reactions have been modeled, using knowledge of binding characteristics to blood and albumin and the enzymatic parameters for the conjugation pathways (obtained with Eq. 12), for highly cleared phenolic substrates such as harmol, gentisamide, and salicylamide in single-pass perfused rat liver studies. For these highly cleared phenolic substrates, compensatory increases in glucuronidation with input concentration were observed (Fig. 4). Inferences about zonation of conjugation of enzymes were obtained from studies with retrograde liver perfusion, which effectively reversed the order of recruitment of enzymatic activities, namely, that more glucuronide and less sulfate conjugate was formed (PANG et al. 1981, 1983; MORRIS et al. 1987, 1988; XU and PANG 1989; XU et al. 1990). The derived enzymatic constants (Table 3) and variations in the $V_{max,x}$ were employed with Eqs. 1 and 2 to simulate data for drug disappearance and conjugate formation. The criterion for selection of the optimized distribution was based on the weighted sum of squares of residuals (WSSR) between predictions and observations among different enzyme-distributed models. Among the models examined (from 5 to 150), the optimized enzymic model – a descending gradient of sulfation activities (from high to zero), an evenly distributed glucuronidation activities, and an ascending gradient for hydroxylation activities (from zero to maximum value, for salicylamide) – was highly consistent with observations for the progradely and retrogradely perfused liver. Moreover, upon suppression of the anterior sulfation pathway with a specific inhibitor, 2,6-dichloro-4-nitrophenol (DCNP), the compensatory glucuronidation of harmol and salicylamide disappeared (KOSTER et al. 1982; XU et al. 1990); Michaelis-Menten-like kinetics were observed and predicted for the glucuronidation of harmol and salicylamide in the presence of DCNP (Fig. 5).

III. Nonlinear Protein Binding

The influence of drug–protein binding on drug disposition has been both well recognized and intensively studied (WOLKOFF et al. 1979; GILLETTE 1973; WEISIGER 1985; SCHARY and ROWLAND 1983; SORRENTINO et al. 1989b; JUSKO and GRETCH 1976; ROWLAND 1984; ØIE 1986; HUANG and ØIE 1984; JANSEN 1981; SMALLWOOD et al. 1988; RUBIN and TOZER 1986). The generally accepted view is that that the physiological, biochemical, and pharmacological processes are related to the unbound species. Changes in the unbound concentration, often expressed as changes in the unbound fraction, may elicit toxic or subtherapeutic outcomes. This is especially true for highly

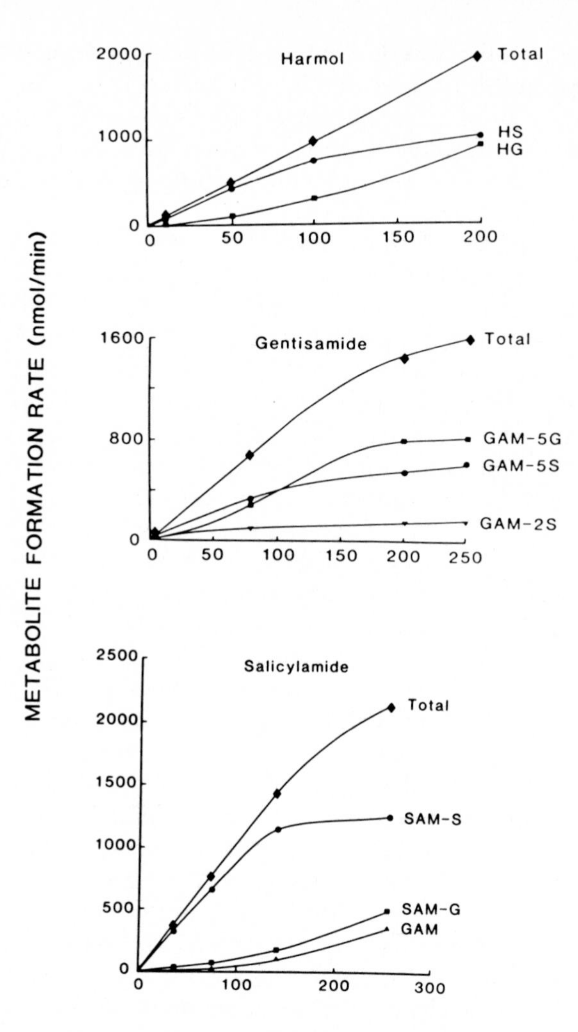

Fig. 4. Concentration-dependent elimination of *harmol* (H), *gentisamide* (GSM), and *salicylamide* (SAM) in the single-pass perfused rat liver preparation (10 ml/min). At increasing substrate concentration to the liver, sulfation (*S*) was apparently becoming saturated for all three substrates, whereas glucuronidation (*G*) and hydroxylation (to form *GAM*, for salicylamide only) rates increased disproportionately with *input concentration*. (Data from PANG et al. 1981; MORRIS et al. 1988; XU and PANG 1989)

bound drugs such as warfarin, bilirubin, dicumarol, and valproic acid (WOSILAIT and GARTEN 1972; ØIE and LEVY 1975; GUGLER and MUELLER 1978).

Due to irreversibile drug loss, the concentration gradient along the liver sinusoid leads to an outlet concentration that is much lower than the inlet

Table 3. Kinetic constants for harmol, gentisamide, salicylamide, and 4-methylumbelliferone metabolism

Drug	Metabolite	Estimated Km^{a} (μM)	Estimated $V_{max}{}^{a}$ (nmol/min/liver)	References
Harmol	Sulfate	9	35	Mulder and Hagedoorn (1974)
	Glucuronide	144	65	
Gentisamide	2-Sulfate	22 ± 14	24 ± 9.7	Morris et al. (1988)
	5-Sulfate	26 ± 12	81 ± 15	
	5-Glucuronide	71 ± 22	88 ± 38	
Salicylamide	Sulfate	15 ± 3.5	155 ± 30	Xu et al. (1990)
	Glucurnonide[b]	151 ± 41	200 ± 44	
	Gentisamide[b]	281 ± 24	89 ± 28	Xu and Pang (1989)
4-Methylumbelliferone	Sulfate[c]	6 ± 3[c]	361 ± 110	Ratna et al. (1993)
	Glucuronide[c]	15 ± 5[c]	1250 ± 320	

[a] Estimated with Eq. 12.
[b] Estimated in the presence of 2,6-dichloro-4-nitrophenol (40–50 μM).
[c] Values denote net conjugation.

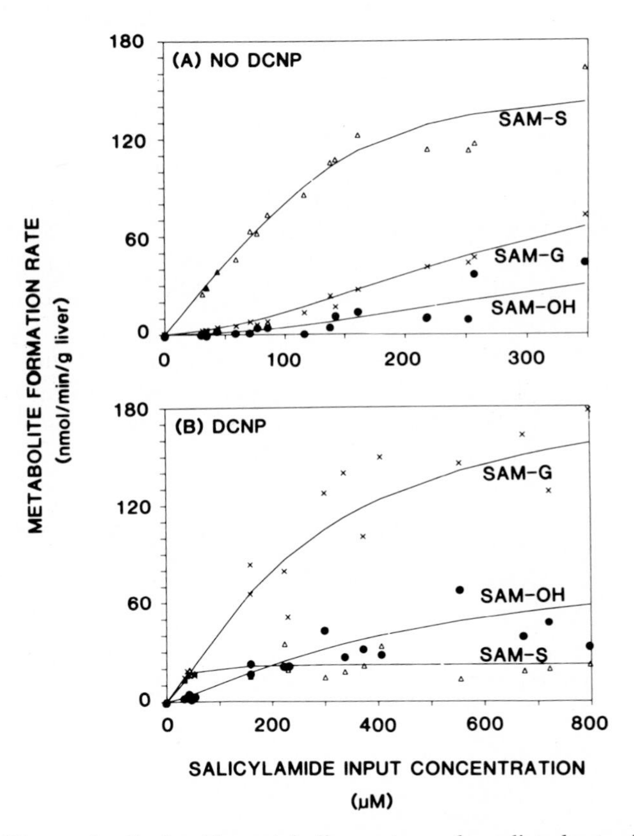

Fig. 5A,B. Observed salicylamide metabolism rates and predicted rates based on the enzymatic parameters (Table 3) and enzymic distributions for the perfused rat liver preparations in an absence **A** and presence **B** of 2,6-dichloro-4-nitrophenol (*DCNP*), the sulfation inhibitor. Good match was obtained for observations versus predictions (____) from the enzyme-distributed model. (From Xu and Pang 1989)

concentration. The reduced substrate to protein ratio at the outlet is expected to result in decreases of the unbound fraction, and this is more apt to occur for drugs which are highly cleared, since the concentration gradient along the sinusoid is the steepest (HUANG and ØIE 1984; XU et al. 1993). The dynamics of substrate removal and the induced changes in the unbound fraction along the flow path at varing inlet concentrations in the presence of heterogeneously distributed enzymic systems have been examined in concert for substrate removal under varying input substrate concentrations (XU et al. 1993).

Conventionally, protein binding is viewed as a reversible process that can be described by the Langmuir isotherm; the unbound plasma concentration for a single class of N equivalent binding sites of identical affinity constant, K_A, can be solved analytically and described with respect to the total plasma concentration, C_P, in the following fashion (XU et al. 1993):

$$C_{P,u} = \frac{-(1 + NK_A[P_t] - K_A C_P) + \{(1 + NK_A[P_t] - K_A C_P)^2 + 4K_A C_P\}^{\frac{1}{2}}}{2K_A} \tag{21}$$

and equals the unbound blood concentration in absence of red cell concentrative mechanisms. The characteristic dependence of the unbound fraction on the K_A and protein concentration for the binding isotherms is depicted in Fig. 6. At low K_A, the binding isotherm changes only slightly and gradually with concentration; at high K_A ($>10^5\,M^{-1}$) where binding is considerably tighter, the unbound fractions are reduced, especially at low concentrations. However, there are sharp and precipitous increases in unbound fraction upon small increments of the drug concentration at various regions of the binding isotherms which appear to be dependent on K_A and the protein concentration; the latter represents the capacity of binding sites (Fig. 6A,B). These marked changes in binding occur when binding is near its saturation capacity such that further small increments in concentration will cause a sharp rise in the unbound fraction.

Often, the unbound concentration is expressed relative to the total plasma concentration, C_P, as an unbound fraction, f_P:

$$f_P = \frac{C_{P,u}}{C_P} \tag{22}$$

The unbound fraction in blood, f_B, is related to the unbound fraction in plasma as:

$$f_B = \frac{C_{B,u}}{C_B} = \frac{f_P}{(C_B/C_P)} \tag{23}$$

where C_B/C_P is the blood to plasma concentration ratio.

The manner in which heterogeneous enzymic systems (one, two, and three parallel enzymic systems) modify the unbound fraction along the

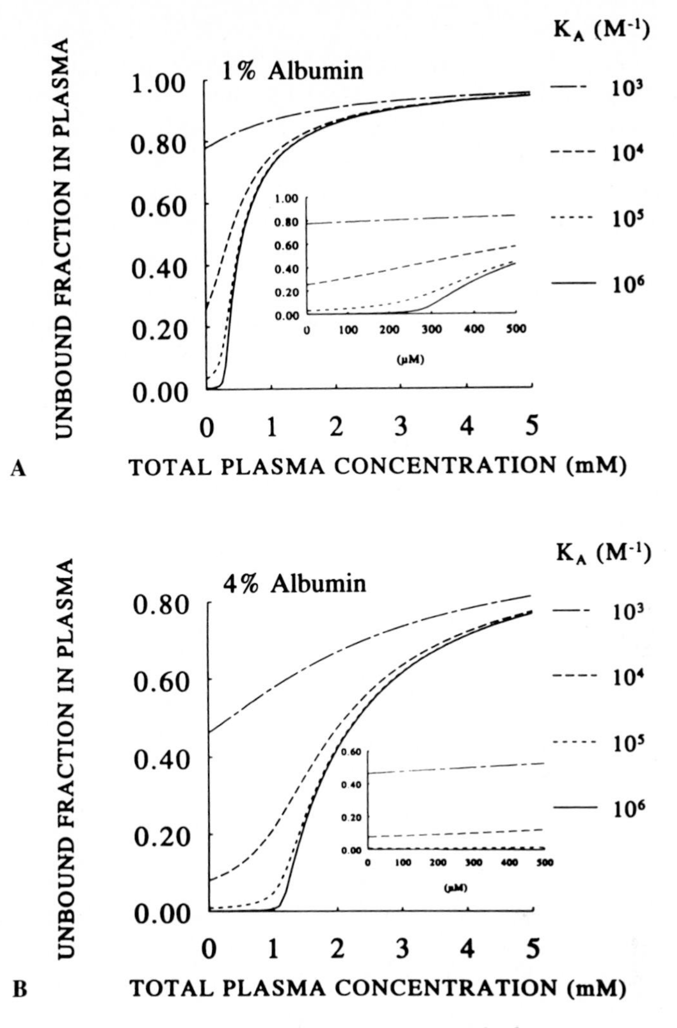

Fig. 6A,B. *Unbound fraction in plasma* versus *total plasma concentration* for the binding of a drug to a single class of two equivalent binding sites. The K_A values vary from 10^3 to $10^6 M^{-1}$ at albumin concentrations of 1% **A** and 4% **B**. Note that the *inflexion points* of the binding isotherms are displaced to the right at the higher protein concentration (1% versus 4% albumin)

length of the sinusoid ($f_{B,x}$) was studied recently (Xu et al. 1993). The mass–balance consideration for the change of the concentration (dC_x/dx) of a flow-limited substrate (Fig. 1A) over a small increment of length, dx, across the single-pass liver preparation at steady state has been described previously (Eq. 1), and the unbound fraction at x is given by the ratio of unbound concentration to the total (unbound and bound) concentration, or $C_{u,x}/(C_{u,x} + C_{b,x})$. Due to removal, changes in $C_{u,x}$ results, thus invoking changes in $f_{B,x}$. For substrates which are metabolized by enzymic systems with appreciable V_{max} and low K_m, large changes in $C_{u,x}$ and $f_{B,x}$ are expected to result along the length of the sinusoid.

In a series of simulations based on Eq. 1 at constant protein concentration (1% albumin), XU et al. (1993) showed that the binding association constant, K_A, strongly influence E and $f_{B,x}$ along the sinusoidal length. They described this overall change in f_B, or the percentage change in f_B (defined as $(f_{B,In} - f_{B,Out})/f_{B,In} \times 100\%$ where subscripts "In" and "Out" denote the inlet and outlet of the liver sinusoid, respectively), for correlation with changes in E at x. Given an enzymic system of appreciable affinity (low K_m, $10\,\mu M$) and capacity (V_{max}, 1000 nmol/min), E was found to display the characteristic decreasing trend with concentration due to saturation of the enzymic system for drugs which were poorly bound ($K_A < 10^3\,M^{-1}$); the effect of protein binding on metabolism was minimal, and the percentage change in f_B was insignificant (Fig. 7, left panel). For tightly bound drugs ($K_A = 10^6\,M^{-1}$), $f_{B,In}$ was close to zero at low input concentration. With increasing concentration, values of E showed an uncharacteristic rise, then became attenuated with concentration. The upward trend of E was explained by the saturation of binding sites for tightly bound and highly cleared drugs, causing disproportionately greater increments in unbound drug (shown in

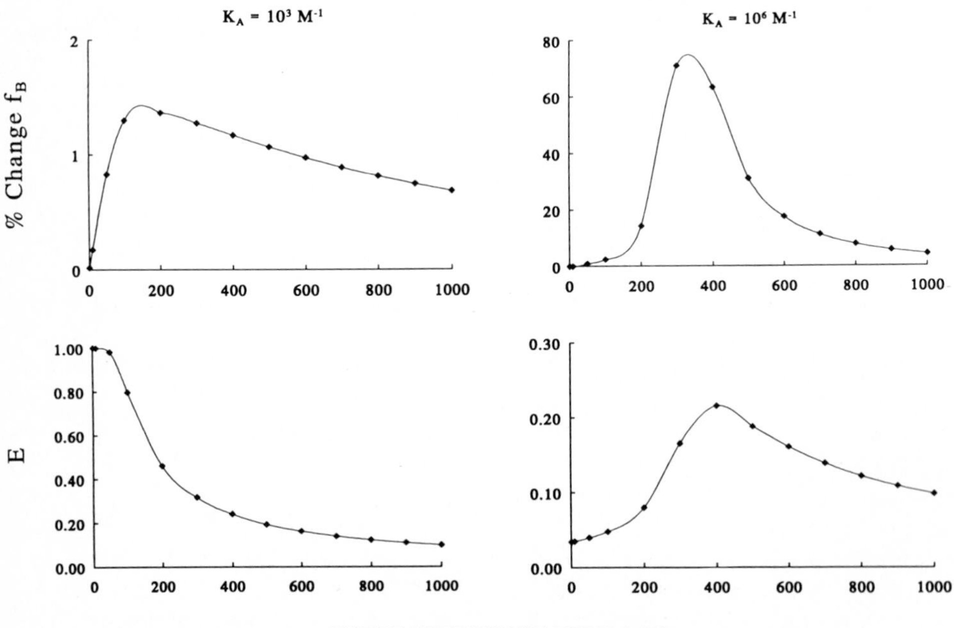

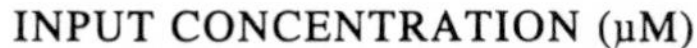

Fig. 7. Changes in percent change in f_B and E with C_{In} for an unienzyme system. Simulations were done based on a hypothetical single enzymic system ($K_m = 10\,\mu M$, $V_{max} = 1000$ nmol/min) for $K_A = 10^3$ (*left*) and 10^6 (*right*) M^{-1}. The profiles were identical for all enzymic distribution patterns, but greatly differed for the different K_A.

Fig. 6), which tends to promote elimination; the percentage change in f_B was significant and paralleled the changes in E (Fig. 7, right panel). With increasing concentration, saturation of enzymes ensued. A comparison of the changes in protein binding revealed that the percentage change in f_B between the inlet and outlet of the liver was considerably greater (>100 fold) at high K_A than at low K_A (10^6 and $10^3 M^{-1}$; Fig. 7). For drugs of high K_A, the RLS will switch from the saturation of protein binding sites to saturation of the enzymic system (K_D or $1/K_A < K_m$, where K_D is the dissociation constant) with increasing concentration. A variation in enzyme distribution for unienzyme systems altered only the profile of $f_{B,x}$ (Fig. 8), but was without an overall effect on $f_{B,Out}$ and percentage change in f_B. Further exploration with multiple enzymic systems and K_A showed exceedingly similar trends, although small differences of E and percentage change f_B were observed with a variation in enzymic distribution (Xu et al. 1993).

These simulations have clearly aided the interpretation of the mechanism underlying the unusual profile (e.g., ascending–descending profile) of E for 4MU sulfate (4MUS) observed in the single-pass perfused liver preparation with 1% albumin in the perfusate, for which nonlinear protein binding due to a single class of binding site (K_A, $1.08 \times 10^4 M^{-1}$; N, 2.5) was found (Ratna et al. 1993). The unusual profile for E was found to disappear when a perfusate without albumin was substituted for 1% albumin in the preparation (Fig. 9; Chiba and Pang 1993a). The model (Fig. 10) is slightly more complicated than previously described due to futile cycling, and the encompassing equations are described in detail in Sect. B.IV. When numerical calculations were performed, the simulated data for E at the K_A of $10^4 M^{-1}$ mimicked the observed values of E for 4MUS (Fig. 9B); the corresponding simulated data for the percentage change in f_B with concentration (Fig. 9A) implied that, for 4MUS, protein binding became saturated prior to desulfation with concentration (K_D, $90 \mu M$; K_m, $267 \mu M$). The early saturation of protein binding would liberate unbound 4MUS to enter the liver cell for desulfation, thus raising the E; upon further increases in concentration, saturation of desulfation followed. The alternating limiting conditions are responsible for the parabolic behavior of E with concentration.

Upon using the same strategy of Morris and Pang (1987), Xu et al. (1993) assessed the use of the logarithmic average concentration in Eq. 12 on parameter estimates of kinetic constants. With nonlinear protein binding, overestimates of these constants for glucuronidation were obtained when the K_m for glucuronidation greatly exceeded that for sulfation. The error was circumvented upon suppression of the anterior sulfation pathway (Xu et al. 1993).

IV. Futile Cycling

The interconversion between a drug and its conjugate(s) involving conjugating enzymes and hydrolases has been reported for clofibric acid and its

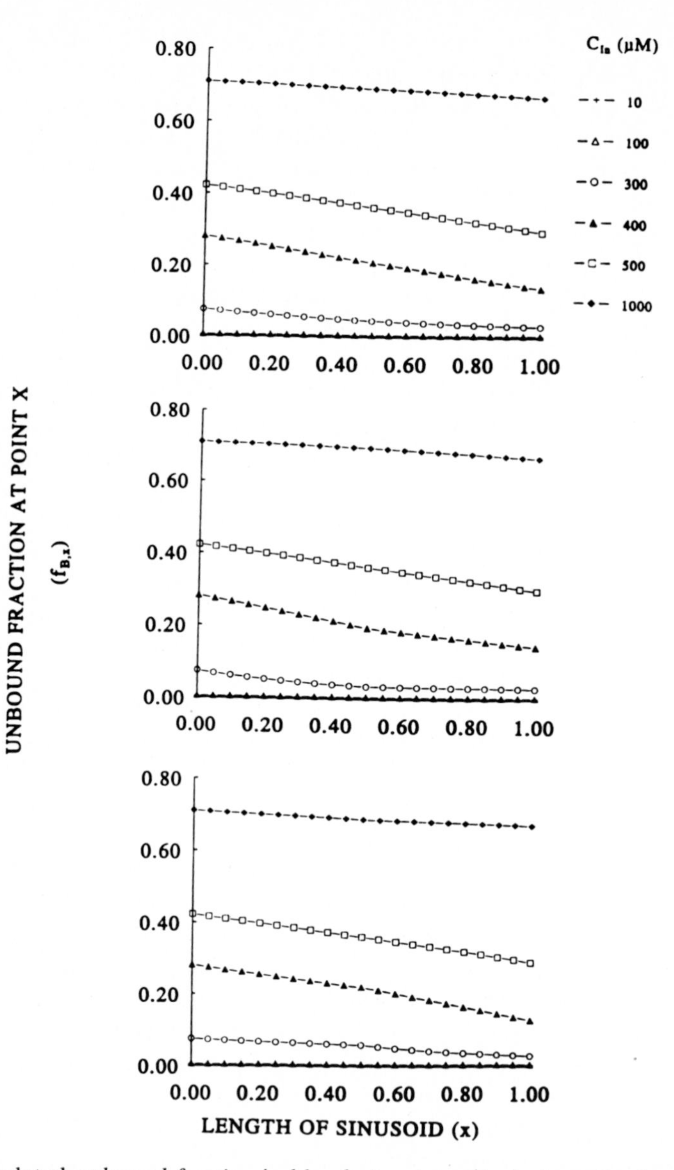

Fig. 8. Simulated *unbound fraction* in blood at *point x* ($f_{B,x}$) along the *length of the sinusoid* for a drug which is metabolized by an unienzyme enzyme system at various input concentrations. The K_m ($10\,\mu M$) and total enzymatic activity (V_{max} or 1000 nmol/min) were held constant, while the enzymatic activity at differents point of x, $V_{max,x}$, is allowed to vary along the sinusoidal flow path (from $x = 0$ to $x = L$). The change in unbound fraction, $f_{B,x}$ for the K_A of $10^6 M^{-1}$ is shown for the following distributions: enzyme is evenly distributed (*top*); enzymic concentration gradient is descending linearly, from a high value at $x = 0$ to zero at $x = L$ (middle); enzymic concentration gradient is ascending linearly, from zero at $x = 0$ to a high value at $x = L$ (*bottom*). Data for the K_A of $10^3 M^{-1}$ showed little or no change in $f_{B,x}$. (From XU et al. 1993)

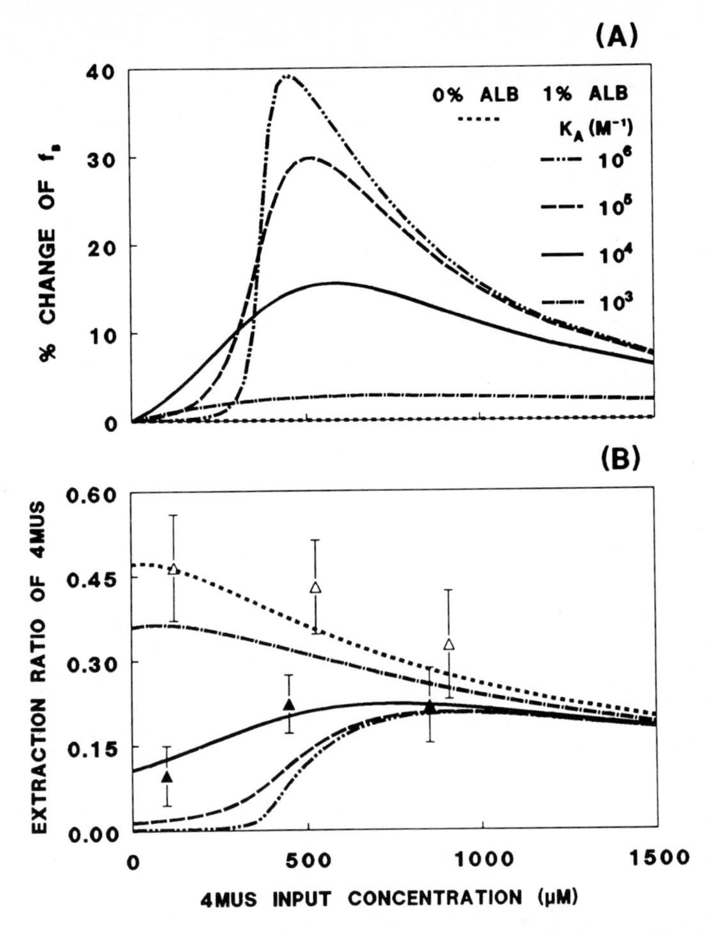

Fig. 9A,B. Predicted changes in **A** unbound fraction of 4-methylumbelliferone sulfate (*4MUS*) in blood between the inlet and outlet of the liver (% change in f_B) and **B** the corresponding steady state *extraction ratio of 4MUS* for various K_As versus *4MUS input concentration*. Predictions were carried out at K_A values at 0 (----), 10^3 (—·—·—), 10^4 (—), 10^5 (———), and 10^6 (—··—··) M^{-1}, with other parameters shown in Table 4. Predictions were matched against the mean ± SD of the observed steady state extraction ratios for liver studies conducted in absence (△) and presence (▲) of albumin. (Data from CHIBA and PANG 1993a)

glucuronide (MEFFIN et al. 1983), 4MU, 4MUS, and 4MU glucuronide (4MUG) conjugates (EL-MOUELHI and KAUFFMAN 1986; ANUNDI et al. 1986; MIYAUCHI et al. 1987b,c, 1989; KAUFFMAN et al. 1991; RATNA et al. 1993; CHIBA and PANG 1993a; Fig. 11). The topic of interconversion has been the subject of several theoretical communications (LEVENSPIEL 1972; FROMENT and BISHOFF 1976; HWANG et al. 1981; WAGNER et al. 1981; EBLING and JUSKO 1986; FERRY and WAGNER 1986). The consequence of futile cycling is that total drug removal and net formation of the metabolite undergoing interconversion are apparently reduced. By inference, the interconversion

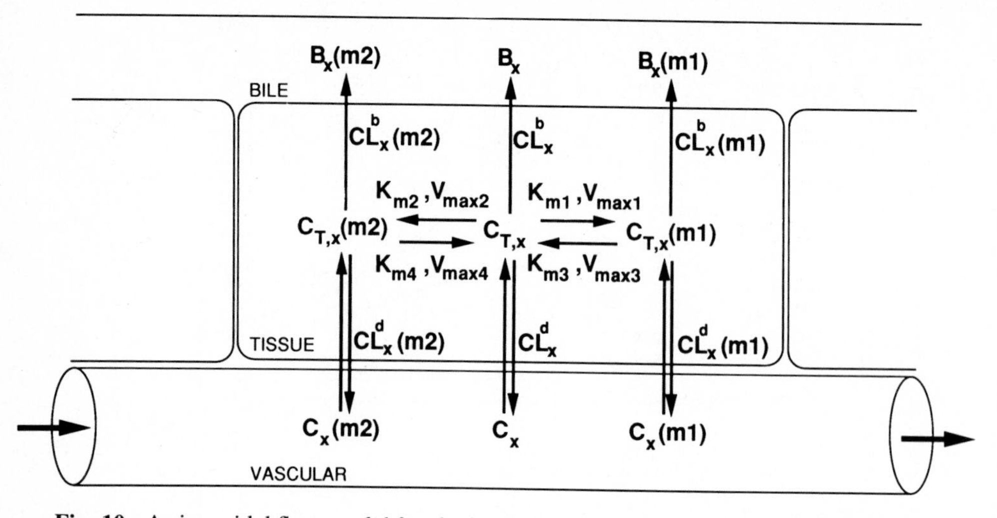

Fig. 10. A sinusoidal flow model for the hepatic elimination of 4-methylumbelliferone (4MU), its sulfate (4MUS), and its glucuronide (4MUG). The figure presents an enlarged view at point x along the length of the sinusoid (L) and the direction of flow (*bold arrow* in the vascular compartment). The liver is viewed as three compartments: expanded *vascular* (sinusoidal space + Disse space), *tissue*, and *bile*. 4MU in tissue ($C_{T,x}$) undergoes futile cycling with 4MUS [$C_{T,x}$(m1)] and 4MUG [$C_{T,x}$(m2)]. See text for details

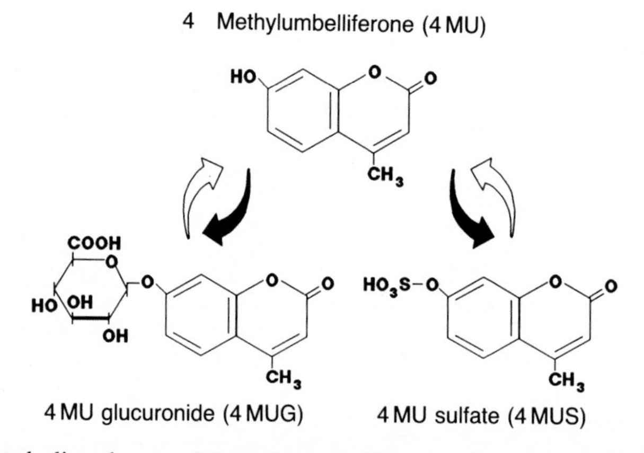

Fig. 11. Metabolic scheme of 4-methylumbelliferone (7-hydroxy-4-methylcoumarin, 4MU) in rat liver. Facile futile cycling exists between 4MU and its sulfate conjugate, 4MUS, whereas deglucuronidation of *4MUG* was low. (From CHIBA and PANG 1993a)

between a drug and its conjugate reduces the sequential first-pass metabolism (PANG and GILLETTE 1979) of that formed conjugate. It is further expected that the extent of metabolite removal–interconversion is strongly modulated by the transmembrane (described above) and protein-binding characteristics of both the precursor and the usually more polar metabolite.

The quantitative prediction about the futile cycling of 4MU as a model compound was developed with the tubular flow model that was modified to encompass futile cycling (Fig. 10) for the single-pass rat liver experiments. The following mass–balance equations, incorporating the binding properties of each species, are based on the assumption that $CL_x^{in} = CL_x^{ef} = CL_x^d$ and f_T are constant along L for all species.

For 4MU in the vascular compartment,

$$\frac{Q\mathrm{d}C_x}{\mathrm{d}x} = \frac{1}{L}[f_T C_{T,x} - f_{B,x} C_x]CL_x^d \tag{24}$$

For 4MUS (metabolite, m1) in the vascular compartment:

$$\frac{Q\mathrm{d}C_x\{m1\}}{\mathrm{d}x} = \frac{1}{L}[f_T\{m1\}C_{T,x}\{m1\} - f_{B,x}\{m1\}C_x\{m1\}]CL_x^d\{m1\} \tag{25}$$

For 4MUG (metabolite, m2) in the vascular compartment:

$$\frac{Q\mathrm{d}C_x\{m2\}}{\mathrm{d}x} = \frac{1}{L}[f_T\{m2\}C_{T,x}\{m2\} - f_{B,x}\{m2\}C_x\{m2\}]CL_x^d\{m2\} \tag{26}$$

At steady state, the rates of change of 4MU and 4MU conjugates in tissue at any point x are described by the following equations:

For 4MU in tissue,

$$0 = \frac{1}{L}\left[f_{B,x}CL_x^d C_x + \frac{V_{max3} f_T\{m1\}C_{T,x}\{m1\}}{K_{m3} + f_T\{m1\}C_{T,x}\{m1\}} + \frac{V_{max4} f_T\{m2\}C_{T,x}\{m2\}}{K_{m4} + f_T\{m2\}C_{T,x}\{m2\}} - \left(\frac{V_{max1}}{K_{m1} + f_T C_{T,x}} + \frac{V_{max2}}{K_{m2} + f_T C_{T,x}}\right) f_T C_{T,x} - (CL_x^b + CL_x^d) f_T C_{T,x}\right] \tag{27}$$

For 4MUS in tissue,

$$0 = \frac{1}{L}\left(f_{B,x}\{m1\}CL_x^d\{m1\}C_x\{m1\} + \frac{V_{max1} f_T C_{T,x}}{K_{m1} + f_T C_{T,x}} - \frac{V_{max3} f_T\{m1\}C_{T,x}\{m1\}}{K_{m3} + f_T\{m1\}C_{T,x}\{m1\}} - [CL_x^b\{m1\} + CL_x^d\{m1\}] f_T\{m1\}C_{T,x}\{m1\}\right) \tag{28}$$

and for 4MUG in tissue,

$$0 = \frac{1}{L}\left(f_{B,x}\{m2\}CL_x^d\{m2\}C_x\{m2\} + \frac{V_{max2} f_T C_{T,x}}{K_{m2} + f_T C_{T,x}}\right.$$

$$- \frac{V_{max4} f_T\{m2\} C_{T,x}\{m2\}}{K_{m4} + f_T\{m2\} C_{T,x}\{m2\}} - [CL_x^b\{m2\} + CL_x^d\{m2\}] f_T\{m2\} C_{T,x}\{m2\} \Bigg) \quad (29)$$

where C_x, $C_x\{m1\}$, and $C_x\{m2\}$ are the concentrations of 4MU, 4MUS, and 4MUG, respectively, in blood and $C_{T,x}$, $C_{T,x}\{m1\}$, and $C_{T,x}\{m2\}$ are their corresponding concentrations in tissue at any point x; $f_{B,x}$, $f_{B,x}\{m1\}$, and $f_{B,x}\{m2\}$, respectively, denote the unbound fractions of 4MU, 4MUS, and 4MUG in blood at x, and f_T, $f_T\{m1\}$, and $f_T\{m2\}$ are the unbound fractions of 4MU, 4MUS, and 4MUG in tissue. CL_x^d, $CL_x^d\{m1\}$, and $CL_x^d\{m2\}$, respectively, denote the transmembrane clearances ($CL^{in} = CL^{ef} = CL^d$) for 4MU, 4MUS, and 4MUG at any point x. CL_x^b, $CL_x^b\{m1\}$, and $CL_x^b\{m2\}$ are the biliary intrinsic clearances for 4MU, 4MUS, and 4MUG, respectively. Metabolic parameters (Michaelis-Menten constant, K_{mi}, and maximum velocity, V_{maxi}, subscript i = 1, 2, 3, and 4) representing parameters for sulfation and glucuronidation of 4MU, desulfation of 4MUS, and deglucuronidation of 4MUG, respectively, were assigned values obtained experimentally with Eq. 12 (Table 4).

The rates of 4MU (dB_x/dx), 4MUS ($dB_x\{m1\}/dx$), and 4MUG ($dB_x\{m2\}/dx$) excretion into the bile at any point x are proportional to their tissue concentrations.

Table 4. Kinetic parameters used for simulation of 4-methylumbelliferone (4MU), its sulfate (4MUS), and its glucuronide (4MUG)

	Parameters 4MU	4MUS (ml)	4MUG (m2)
C_B/C_P [a]	1.18	0.839	0.849
f_P [a]	0.436	–	–
K_A ($\times 10^4 M^{-1}$)[a,b]	–	1.08	0.122
N [a,b]	–	2.5	1.18
CL^d (ml/min per g liver)[c]	50	5	0.5
CL^b (ml/min per g liver)[c]	0.015	0.015	0.15
Q (ml/min per g liver)[d]	1.0		
K_{m1} (μM)[a]	6		
V_{max1} (nmol/min per g liver)[a]	36		
K_{m2} (μM)[a]	14.6		
V_{max2} (nmol/min per g liver)[a]	125		
K_{m3} (μM)[e]	382		
V_{max3} (nmol/min per g liver)[e]	370		
K_{m4} (μM)[a]	114		
V_{max4} (nmol/min per g liver)[a]	5.5		

[a] Kinetic parameters were obtained from RATNA et al. (1993).
[b] Concentration-dependent plasma protein binding was observed.
[c] Appropriate values were assigned, after optimization by trial simulations.
[d] A 10 g liver and a flow rate of 10 ml/min per g liver were used.
[e] Averaged parameters for net desulfation, with and without albumin.

For 4MU excretion into bile,

$$\frac{dB_x}{dx} = \frac{1}{L}[f_T CL_x^b C_{T,x}] \tag{30}$$

For 4MUS excretion into bile,

$$\frac{dB_x\{m1\}}{dx} = \frac{1}{L}[f_T\{m1\}CL_x^b\{m1\}C_{T,x}\{m1\}] \tag{31}$$

For 4MUG excretion into bile,

$$\frac{dB_x\{m2\}}{dx} = \frac{1}{L}[f_T\{m2\}CL_x^b\{m2\}C_{T,x}\{m2\}] \tag{32}$$

In order to solve Eqs. 27–29 simultaneously for $C_{T,x}$, $C_{T,x}\{m1\}$, and $C_{T,x}\{m2\}$ at given concentrations in the sinusoid, C_x, $C_x\{m1\}$, and $C_x\{m2\}$ (Eqs. 24–26), an iterative procedure similar to that described by MAIS et al. (1974) was utilized for a program written in FORTRAN on a PC computer. By incorporating the obtained $C_{T,x}$, $C_{T,x}\{m1\}$, and $C_{T,x}\{m2\}$ into Eqs. 27–29, the changes in concentration of 4MU, 4MUS, and 4MUG for any x along the sinusoidal flow path were estimated. Similarly, the changes in biliary excretion rate with distance at steady state for 4MU, 4MUS, and 4MUG were numerically obtained by incorporating $C_{T,x}$, $C_{T,x}\{m1\}$, and $C_{T,x}\{m2\}$ into Eqs. 30–32. Since plasma protein binding of 4MUS and 4MUG showed concentration dependence, the unbound concentrations (C_x) and the unbound fraction in perfusate ($f_{B,x}$) at any point x are estimated with Eq. 21.

A protocol encompassing the simultaneous delivery of tracer [^{3}H]4MU, which is predominantly sulfated, and the unlabeled 4MU conjugate was employed to delineate deconjugation in single-pass rat liver perfusion studies (RATNA et al. 1993). By virtue of deconjugation, the rise in intracellular concentration of 4MU would shift tracer [^{3}H]4MU metabolism from sulfation to glucuronidation (Fig. 12). The marked desulfation contrasted strongly the meager deglucuronidation in these studies: 4MUS, and not 4MUG, had shifted the net formation of [^{3}H]4MUS to [^{3}H]4MUG in a concentration-dependent fashion (Fig. 13).

Protein-binding parameters, together with enzymatic constants for net conjugation and deconjugation reactions obtained experimentally for single-pass 4MU, 4MUS, and 4MUG liver perfusion experiments (Table 4), were used to simulate the disposition of 4MU and its conjugates in the presence or absence of albumin (only for 4MUS). Model predictions (lines), when matched against observations on E and the net rates of metabolism for 4MU, 4MUG, and 4MUS at the various input concentrations, were similar, although the predictions slightly underscored the net deglucuronidation of 4MUG and net sulfation of 4MUS (Fig. 14). The model was further used to examine the absence of desulfation (Fig. 15A) or deglucuronidation (Fig.

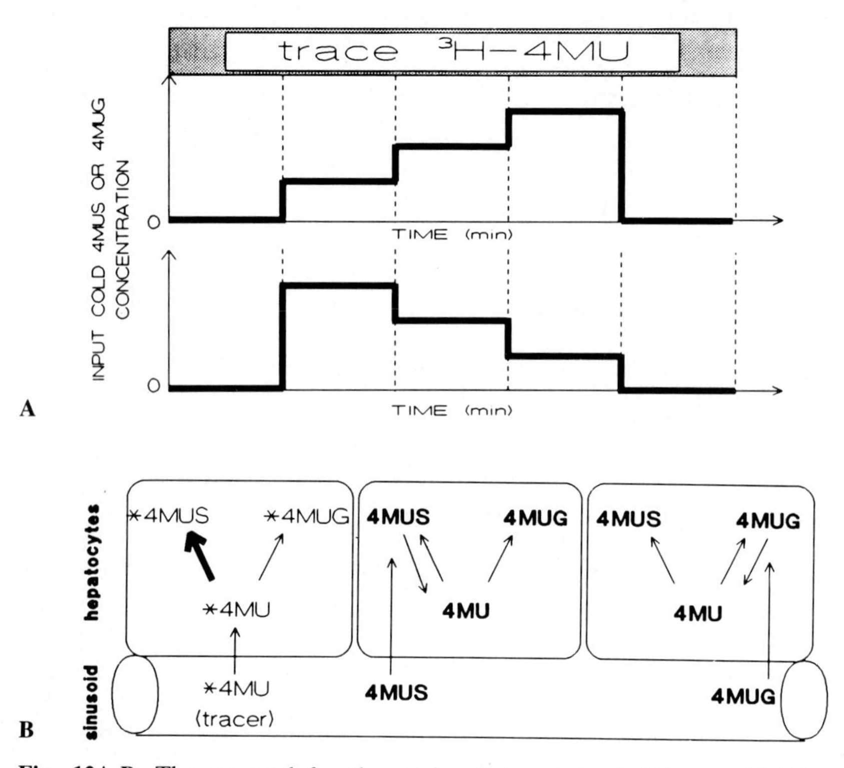

Fig. 12A,B. The protocol for the study of 4-methylumbelliferone (*4MU*) sulfate (*4MUS*) and glucuronide (*4MUG*) deconjugation **A** and intracellular metabolic events upon entry of the unlabeled conjugate and tracer [^{3}H]4MU into hepatocytes **B**. **A** Input tracer [^{3}H]4MU concentration was maintained constant during the entire experiment. In most studies, 4MUS or 4MUG input concentrations were increased stepwise from the second to the fourth periods of perfusion (each of 40 min duration); in some studies, 4MUS and 4MUG concentrations were decreased stepwise. The first (40 min) and last (40–60 min) periods (without 4MUS and 4MUG) were rendered identical for viability check of the liver preparation. **B** Metabolism of tracer [^{3}H]4MU (*left cell*) when 4MUS and 4MUG was present. Net conjugation for tracer [^{3}H]4MU formed predominantly [^{3}H]4MUS; deconjugation of 4MUS (*middle cell*) and 4MUG (*right cell*) would raise the intracellular concentration of 4MU and perturb tracer [^{3}H]4MU conjugation. (From RATNA et al. 1993)

15B) on the overall disposition of 4MU. When desulfation parameters were set as zero (backward resulfation process was absent), an appreciable increase in sulfation rate (15%) and an unaltered net glucuronidation rate were observed; the overall *E* for 4MU was increased slightly, since the pathway of 4MU sulfation is an unimportant pathway due to its low capacity (Fig. 15A). When deglucuronidation was absent, a similar pattern, albeit attenuated, was observed: total glucuronidation rate was increased very slightly (3%), but there was little change in the net sulfation rate (Fig. 15B); the overal *E* for 4MU was slightly increased. These small changes were due

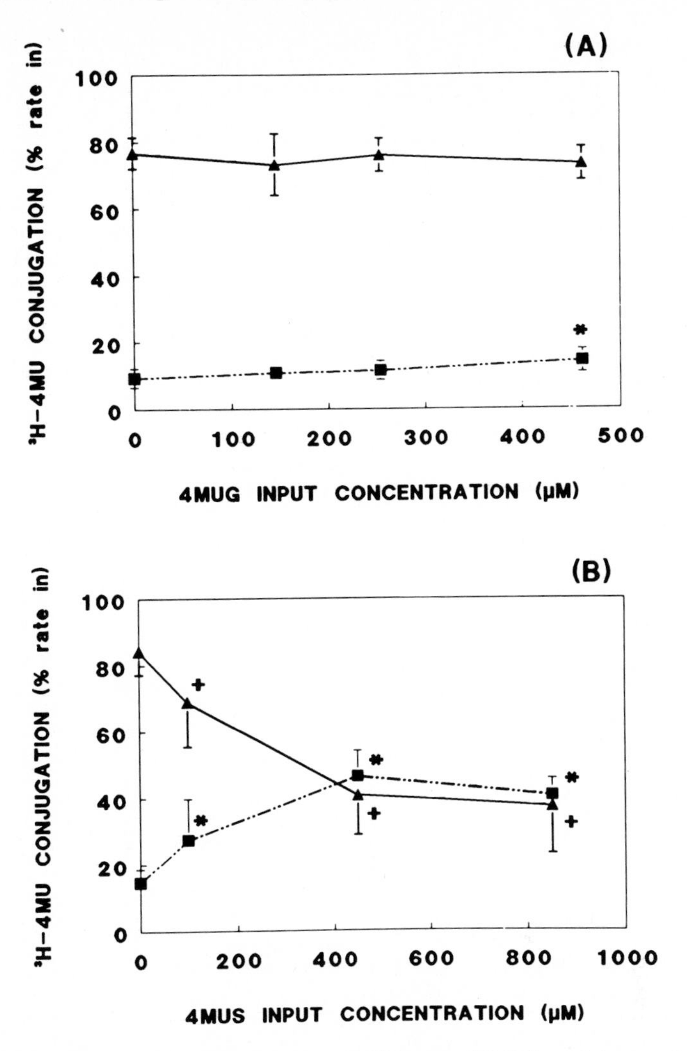

Fig. 13A,B. Futile cycling of 4-methylumbelliferone (*4MU*) and its conjugates. A shift of net sulfation (▲) and glucuronidation (■) of tracer [^{3}H]4MU, which ordinarily formed mainly [^{3}H]4MUS and little [^{3}H]4MUG (see 0 μM on x-axis), was used to detect futile cycling of unlabeled 4MU glucuronide (*4MUG*) and sulfate (*4MUS*) given to the perfused rat liver. **A** A lack of deglucuronidation of 4MUG was evidenced by its inability to perturb tracer [^{3}H]4MU metabolism. **B** Evidence for desulfation of 4MUS was inferred, since tracer metabolism of [^{3}H]4MU (depicted at 0 μM 4MUS) was perturbed in the presence of unlabeled 4MUS, which underwent desulfation and raised the intrahepatic concentration of 4MU. The latter shifted [^{3}H]4MU metabolism from [^{3}H]4MUS to [^{3}H]4MUG formation. The symbols (+) and (*), respectively, denote differences between net sulfation and glucuronidation rates of tracer [^{3}H]4MU compared to those for the controls (at 0 μM 4MUS or 4MUG). (From RATNA et al. 1993)

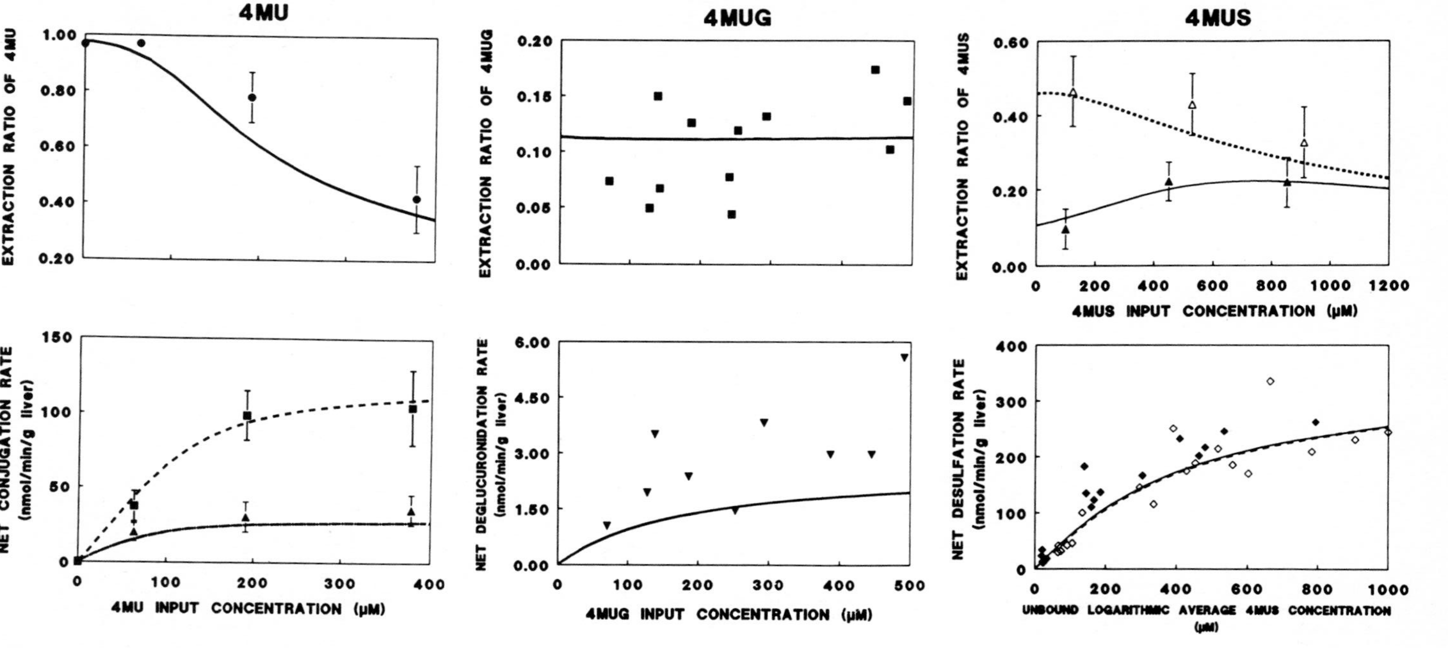

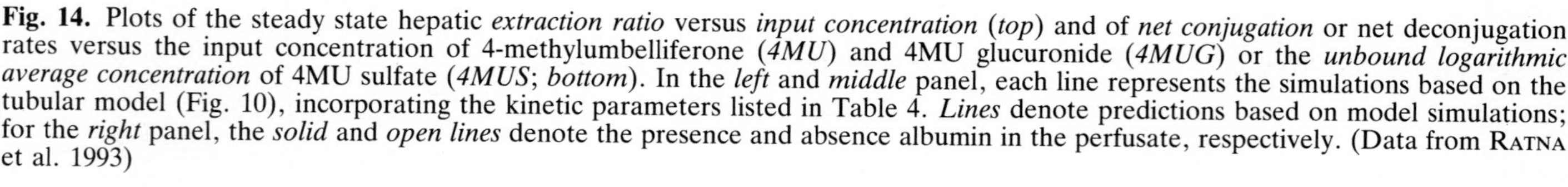

Fig. 14. Plots of the steady state hepatic *extraction ratio* versus *input concentration* (*top*) and of *net conjugation* or net deconjugation rates versus the input concentration of 4-methylumbelliferone (*4MU*) and 4MU glucuronide (*4MUG*) or the *unbound logarithmic average concentration* of 4MU sulfate (*4MUS*; *bottom*). In the *left* and *middle* panel, each line represents the simulations based on the tubular model (Fig. 10), incorporating the kinetic parameters listed in Table 4. *Lines* denote predictions based on model simulations; for the *right* panel, the *solid* and *open lines* denote the presence and absence albumin in the perfusate, respectively. (Data from RATNA et al. 1993)

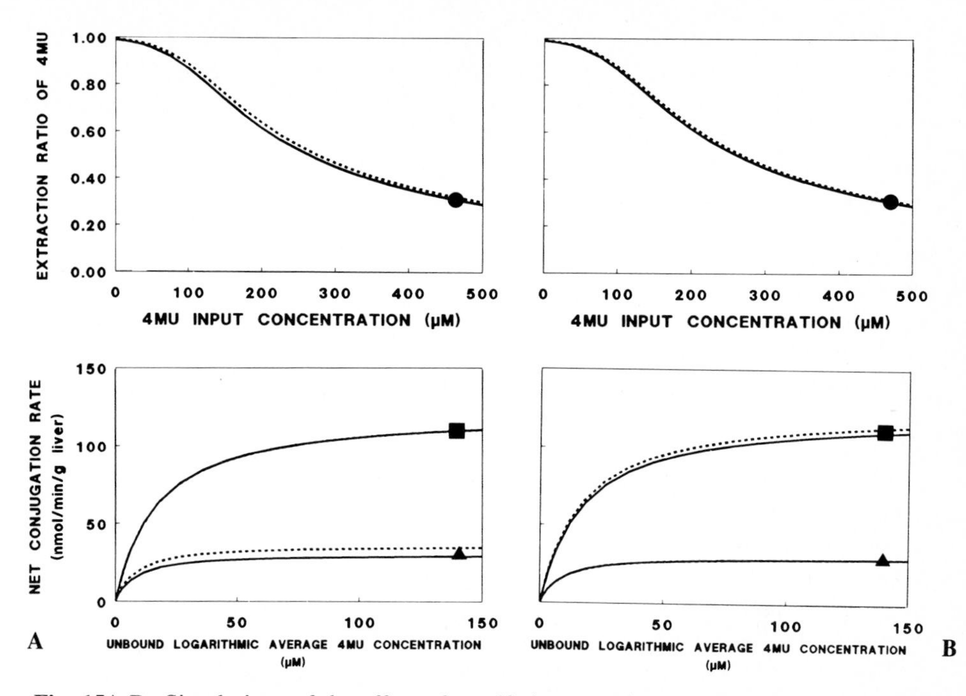

Fig. 15A,B. Simulations of the effect of resulfation **A** and reglucuronidation **B** on the net *extraction ratio* of 4-methylumbelliferone (*4MU; top*) and the total or net formation rates of 4MU conjugates (*bottom*) versus *input concentration* of 4MU. Absence of desulfation (---) **A** and deglucuronidation (---) on E and total/net conjugation rates were compared to those when conjugation and deconjugation pathways were intact (____). The symbols (●), (■), and (▲) denote the net extraction ratio and net glucuronidation and sulfation of 4MU, respectively. (From RATNA et al. 1993)

in this case to the unimportance of the deglucuronidation pathway (very low V_{max}). For other examples of drug and its conjugate(s) undergoing futile cycling with K_m values for conjugation and deconjugation being more comparable, an absence or the suppression of futile cycling will induce a greater conjugation rate of that pathway and an attenuation of formation of other metabolites when its backward deconjugation is suppressed; the increase in E will also be greater.

V. Flow

The role of hepatic blood flow on drug removal has been well studied (PANG and ROWLAND 1977b; PANG et al. 1988b,c; BRAUER et al. 1956; WHITSETT et al. 1971; KEIDING and CHIARANTINI 1978; SHAND et al. 1975; AHMAD et al. 1983), but is seldom extended to describe conjugate formation. When substrates are categorized as highly ($E \cong 1$), intermediately, or poorly ($E \cong 0.1$) extracted compounds, a systematic variation in behavior is found. A highly cleared compound is almost completely removed due to the underlying high liver metabolic–excretory activities, and hence the clearance of these compounds becomes rate limited by organ blood flow rate; for poorly cleared compounds, clearance is restricted by the intrinsically poor removal ability of the organ for the substrate (ROWLAND et al. 1973; PANG and ROWLAND 1977a; WINKLER et al. 1973; WILKINSON 1987).

The manner in which sulfation and glucuronidation pathways compete in drug removal under varying flow rates was examined for harmol in perfused liver studies (DAWSON et al. 1985) and explained by PANG and MULDER (1990). Since harmol is fairly highly cleared, a faster flow rate brought about only a slight reduction in E; changes in sulfation, the anterior, higher-affinity pathway, paralleled those for E due to a reduction in transit time at faster flow rates. For glucuronidation, no change was observed with flow (Fig. 16). When the enzymatic parameters for conjugation of harmol and the enzymic zonation for conjugation (periportal for sulfation and even distribution for glucuronidation) were used in model equations (Eqs. 1, 2) to simulate conjugation events, the data were well predicted. Glucuronidation is subjected to the dual influence of substrate supply and drug transit time, two diametrically opposed factors induced by flow, which appeared to counterbalance each other (PANG and MULDER 1990). The condition prevailed at low input concentrations ($\ll K_m$), where substrate availability and not enzyme is rate limiting. When the simulations were repeated with other K_ms for conjugation, glucuronidation, the posterior pathway, was found to vary. Its rate could potentially increase with flow, when the flow effects on

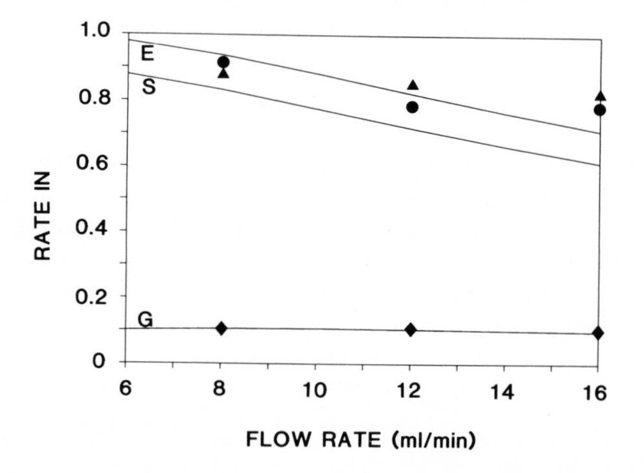

Fig. 16. Influence of organ blood flow on the extraction ratio of harmol (10 μM) and formation of harmol sulfate and harmol glucuronide conjugates. The flow-induced changes of harmol sulfation (S,▲) parallel those for harmol extraction ratio (E,●). No apparent change is observed for harmol glucuronidation (G,◆) due to the counter effects of reduced sojourn time for drug, and higher availability of substrate downstream at increased flow rates. (Data from PANG and MULDER 1990)

substrate sparing from upstream sulfation surpassed that for the reduction in drug transit time (PANG and MULDER 1990).

VI. Cosubstrate

Conjugation reactions require the presence of cosubstrates, such as 3′-phosphoadenosine-5′-phosphosulfate (PAPS), uridine disphosphoglucuronic acid (UDPGA) and glutathione (GSH) for conjugation reactions. In rat livers, levels as high as 77 nmol PAPS/g liver have been reported (BREZNICKA et al. 1987). UDPGA levels in liver vary from 0.41 μmol/g wet weight in guinea pig to 0.02 μmol/g in carp (DUTTON 1980). The hepatic synthesis rates of uridine diphosphate (UDP)-glucose (UDPG) and UDPGA have been determined in rats to be both 100 nmol/g liver (DILLS and KLAASSEN 1987). The liver GSH concentration is higher than that of PAPS and UDPGA and is present at around 4.5–6 μmol/g rat liver (LAUTERBURG and MITCHEL 1981). Much work has been done on GSH due to its abundance and importance. The synthesis and efflux of GSH into the sinusoid (GRIFFITH and MEISTER 1979; KAPLOWITZ et al. 1980; BALLATORI and CLARKSON 1983; AW et al. 1986; OOHKTENS et al. 1985; SIES and GRAF 1985; FERNANDES-CHECA and KAPLOWITZ 1990), degradation (MEISTER and ANDERSON 1983; ELING et al. 1986), and biliary excretion by carrier-mediated system(s) (KITAMURA et al. 1990), followed by intrabiliary degradation (BALLATORI et al. 1986), maintain the intrahepatic GSH pool at a fairly constant level. GSH is synthesized readily from cysteine, glutamine, and glycine, with the rate of incorporation of cysteine being rate limiting (LAUTERBURG et al. 1980). Methionine also serves as an alternate precursor amino acid to cysteine (FINKELSTEIN and MUDD 1967; REED and ORRENIUS 1977; TATEISHI et al. 1981; MEISTER and ANDERSON 1983). The GSH turnover rate is also prone to feedback inhibition (LAUTERBURG and MITCHEL 1981; LAUTERBURG et al. 1982). An enriched periportal distribution in GSH was suggested mostly from reports on what was the labeling of liver thiol groups (ASGHER et al. 1975; SMITH et al. 1979; MURRAY et al. 1986). The acinar difference in GSH, however, is expected to be somewhat attenuated, especially in guinea pig liver, since the abundance of the ectoactivity of the γ-glutamyltransferases in the sinusoidal pole will diminish the heterogeneous distribution of GSH: as much as 60% of the effluxed GSH in the periportal region can be cleaved to its cysteinyl–glycine dipeptide metabolite, which upon reuptake, may be used for synthesis of GSH downstream (SPEISKY et al. 1990; LANÇA and ISRAEL 1991).

In the depleted state, however, the supply of cosubstrates may limit the rate of conjugation (HJELLE et al. 1985; DILLS and KLAASSEN 1986, 1987; GALINSKY and LEVY 1981). The dependency of the rate of conjugation on cosubstrate supply becomes apparent when faster rates of conjugation are obtained upon repletion of precursors of cosubstrates, e.g., inorganic sulfate for PAPS (MULDER and KEULEMANS 1978; KRIJGSHELD et al. 1979, 1982; GALINSKY and LEVY 1981; LIN and LEVY 1986; HJELLE et al. 1985; SCHWARZ and SCHWENK 1984; SWEENY and REINKE 1988) and glucose for UDPGA (CONWAY et al. 1985). The limiting role of inorganic sulfate in controlling periportal necrosis from the highly reactive sulfate conjugate of *N*-hydroxy-2-acetylaminofluorene (MEERMAN and MULDER 1981) has revealed indirectly the importance of PAPS precursor. There are also indications that cellular UDPGA may be a determinant of glucuronidation in vivo (WATKINS and KLAASSEN 1983; SINGH and SCHWARZ 1981; HOWELL et al. 1986; HJELLE et al. 1985). The amount of UDPGA required for glucuronidation of acetaminophen after a therapeutic dose was nearly equal to the total content of UDPGA in the liver; after a toxic dose, the UDPGA demand was over 100-fold greater than the normal basal level (PRICE and JOLLOW 1984). Like PAPS and UDPGA, GSH is rapidly depleted with loading of acceptor substrates (TATEISHI et al. 1981; ORRENIUS et al. 1983; MEISTER and ANDERSON 1983; KAPLOWITZ et al. 1985) such as acetaminophen (JOLLOW et al. 1974; LAUTERBURG et al. 1980; LAUTERBURG and MITCHEL 1981; LAUTERBURG et al. 1982) and styrene oxide (SMITH et al. 1983). The depletion is associated with reduced rates of GSH adduct formation. All of these effectively reduce the intrahepatic GSH concentrations or alter intrahepatic energy supply, which influences GSH synthesis (DILLS and KLAASSEN 1986).

Modeling of conjugation reactions with respect to levels of the cosubstrate has rarely been explored. CHEN and GILLETTE (1988) provided the first quantitative description of the kinetics of GSH depletion by acetaminophen via the electrophilic attack of a reactive intermediate (JOLLOW et al. 1974). Detoxifcation pathways such as glucurondiation and sulfation, normally operating under first-order conditions, also exist for acetaminophen. The account was able to predict the time dependence of GSH depletion in the liver. Subsequently, CHIBA and PANG (1993b) presented a similar set of equations to describe the acinar distribution of GSH in the liver (Fig. 17A) and the depletion of GSH by acetaminphen (Fig. 17B), both viewed as a distributed-in-space phenomenon. As a starting point for modeling, the GSH cycle was simplified. The intrasinusoidal and intrabiliary degradation of GSH, denoting either GSH oxidation, cleavage, and/or biliary excretion, was represented by intrinsic clearance ($CL_{int,x}\{GSH\}$), whereas $k_{o,x}\{GSH\}$ was the rate of synthesis in the liver. The influx transmembrane clearance ($CL_x^{in}\{GSH\}$) was assumed to be first order, and the efflux of GSH was described as a saturable process of $V_{max,x}^{ef}\{GSH\}$ and $K_m^{ef}\{GSH\}$ in a Hill's equation (AW et al. 1986). In the absence of any added GSH acceptor substrate, the rate equations for GSH were given by CHIBA and PANG (1993b):

For the rate of change of GSH in the vascular compartment,

$$\frac{Q dC_x\{GSH\}}{dx} = \frac{1}{L}\left[\frac{V_{max,x}^{ef}\{GSH\}(C_{T,x}\{GSH\})^n}{K_m^{ef}\{GSH\} + (C_{T,x}\{GSH\})^n} - C_x\{GSH\}CL_x^{in}\{GSH\}\right] \quad (33)$$

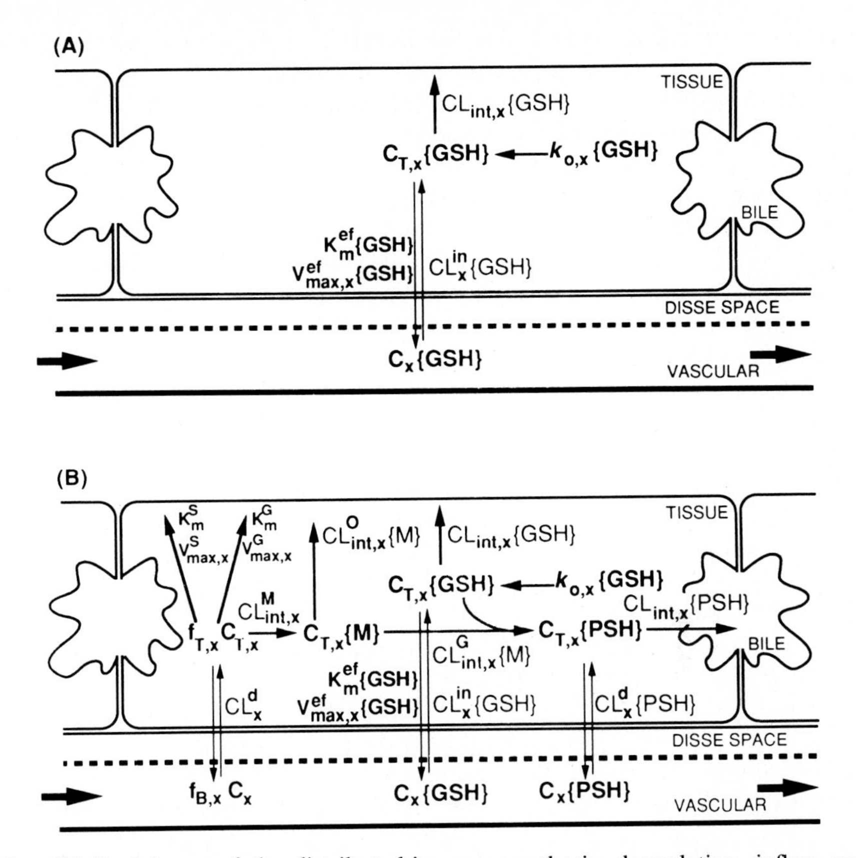

Fig. 17A,B. Schema of the distributed-in-space synthesis, degradation, influx, and efflux of glutathione (*GSH*) at any point *x* along the direction of flow (*bold arrow* in *vascular* compartment) in absence **A** and presence **B** of an acceptor substrate, the reactive metabolite of acetaminophen, *M*, which either undergoes electrophilic attack onto GSH or to other macromolecules. Two other saturable metabolic pathways, sulfation and glucuronidation, also exist for acetaminophen. The formed glutathione adduct, *PSH*, either undergoes biliary excretion or effluxes into sinusoidal blood. See text for details

and for the rate of change of GSH in liver,

$$0 = \frac{1}{L}\Bigg[k_{o,x}\{\mathrm{GSH}\} + \mathrm{CL}_x^{in}\{\mathrm{GSH}\}C_x\{\mathrm{GSH}\} - \frac{V_{max,x}^{ef}\{\mathrm{GSH}\}(C_{T,x}\{\mathrm{GSH}\})^n}{K_m^{ef}\{\mathrm{GSH}\} + (C_{T,x}\{\mathrm{GSH}\})^n} - C_{T,x}\{\mathrm{GSH}\}\mathrm{CL}_{int,x}\{\mathrm{GSH}\}\Bigg] \quad (34)$$

To simulate the effect of acetaminophen depletion of GSH, three possible pathways for acetaminophen removal were described: one was for the formation of the reactive intermediate M of intrinsic clearance, $\mathrm{CL}_{int,x}^{M}$;

the remainder two alternate saturable detoxication pathways were by sulfation and glucuronidation of enzymatic parameters, $V^{S}_{max,x}$, K^{S}_{m}, $V^{G}_{max,x}$, and K^{G}_{m}. The short-lived intermediate M, which never left the cell, underwent conjugation with GSH (represented by $CL^{G}_{int,x}\{M\}$ at x) or with thiol groups of macromolecules (represented by $CL^{O}_{int,x}\{M\}$ at x). Upon formation, the GSH adduct PSH was either excreted (with intrinsic clearance at x, $CL_{int,x}\{PSH\}$; passive bidirectional transmembrane clearances for drug (CL^{d}_{x}) and for the GSH adduct ($CL^{d}_{x}\{PSH\}$) were assumed (Fig. 17B)), or effluxes into sinusoidal blood.

Acknowledging that formation of the GSH adduct is bimolecular in nature, the presence of a known depletor such as the reactive intermediate of acetaminophen is expected to consume GSH. The mass balance equations are:

For the rate of change of acetaminophen in the vascular compartment,

$$\frac{Q\mathrm{d}C_x}{\mathrm{d}x} = \frac{1}{L}[CL^{d}_{x}(f_{T,x}C_{T,x} - f_{B,x}C_x)] \tag{35}$$

For the rate of change of GSH in the vascular compartment,

$$\frac{Q\mathrm{d}C_x\{GSH\}}{\mathrm{d}x} = \frac{1}{L}\left[\frac{V^{ef}_{max,x}\{GSH\}(C_{T,x}\{GSH\})^n}{K^{ef}_{m}\{GSH\} + (C_{T,x}\{GSH\})^n} - C_x\{GSH\}CL^{in}_{x}\{GSH\}\right] \tag{36}$$

For the rate of change of the GSH adduct, PSH, in the vascular compartment,

$$\frac{Q\mathrm{d}C_x\{PSH\}}{\mathrm{d}x} = \frac{1}{L}[CL^{d}_{x}\{PSH\}(C_{T,x}\{PSH\} - C_x\{PSH\})] \tag{37}$$

For the rate of change of acetaminophen in tissue,

$$0 = \frac{1}{L}\left[CL^{d}_{x}(f_{B,x}C_x - f_{T,x}C_{T,x}) - f_{T,x}C_{T,x}\left(CL^{M}_{int,x} + \frac{V^{G}_{max,x}}{K^{G}_{m} + f_{T,x}C_{T,x}} + \frac{V^{S}_{max,x}}{K^{S}_{m} + f_{T,x}C_{T,x}}\right)\right] \tag{38}$$

For the rate of change of the short-lived reactive metabolite M in tissue,

$$0 = \frac{1}{L}[f_{T,x}C_{T,x}CL^{M}_{int,x} - C_{T,x}\{M\}(CL^{G}_{int,x}\{M\}C_{T,x}\{GSH\} + CL^{O}_{int,x}\{M\})] \tag{39}$$

For the rate of change of GSH in the tissue,

$$0 = \frac{1}{L}\Big[k_{o,x}\{GSH\} + CL^{in}_{x}\{GSH\}C_x\{GSH\}$$

$$- \left(\frac{V_{max,x}^{ef}\{GSH\}(C_{T,x}\{GSH\})^n}{K_m^{ef}\{GSH\} + (C_{T,x}\{GSH\})^n}\right)$$

$$\left. - C_{T,x}\{GSH\}(CL_{int,x}\{GSH\} + C_{T,x}\{M\}CL_{int,x}^{G}\{M\})\right] \quad (40)$$

For the rate of change of PSH in tissue, and

$$0 = \frac{1}{L}[CL_x^d\{PSH\}(C_x\{PSH\} - C_{T,x}\{PSH\}) + C_{T,x}\{GSH\}C_{T,x}\{M\}CL_{int,x}^{G}\{M\} - C_{T,x}\{PSH\}CL_{int,x}\{PSH\}] \quad (41)$$

For the rate of biliary excretion of PSH,

$$\frac{dB_x\{PSH\}}{dx} = \frac{1}{L}C_{T,x}\{PSH\}CL_{int,x}\{PSH\} \quad (42)$$

where C_x and $C_{T,x}$ denote the concentrations, and $f_{B,x}$ and $f_{T,x}$ the unbound fractions, in the vascular compartment and tissue, respectively, at x for the parent compound and for the other species, when classified: {M} for reactive intermediate, {GSH} for glutathione, {PSH} for the glutathione adduct.

To understand the effect of acinar distribution of GSH on GSH conjugation, the GSH synthesis rate at x, or $k_{o,x}\{GSH\}$, was altered from a decreasing (model A) to an increasing (model B) distribution, or kept constant (model C), whereas $CL_{int,x}\{GSH\}$, the intrinsic clearance for GSH removal, was maintained constant at all x (Fig. 18). Model A was most consistent with the known acinar distribution of GSH. A low influx transmembrane clearance and literature values for the saturable efflux system of GSH (Aw et al. 1986) and for GSH synthesis rate, taken as the average of those during normal (undepleted GSH) and GSH-depleted conditions (Fernandes-Checa and Kaplowitz 1990), were used for the simulations; the acinar variation in the intrinsic clearances (or $V_{max,x}$) and transmembrane clearance was avoided in the modeling (same for all x). Sulfation and glucuronidation enzymatic parameters were taken from Watari et al. (1983); values for the formation of the reactive intermediate and for the bimolecular GSH conjugation reaction were taken from Chen and Gillette (1988). Parameters which are not available were assigned values, based on known physicochemical characteristics of the species. These parameters are summarized in Table 5.

With the varying distributions (models A–C), acinar distributions of intrahepatic GSH ($C_{T,x}\{GSH\}$) were found accordingly and paralleled the various distribution for the synthesis rates (Fig. 19A); the length-averaged intrahepatic GSH (or $\int_0^L C_{T,x}\{GSH\}dx/L$) were around 5.8, 5.7, and 5.8 μmol/g liver, respectively, for models A, B, and C, and were not different from experimentally observed concentrations of intrahepatic GSH. The efflux

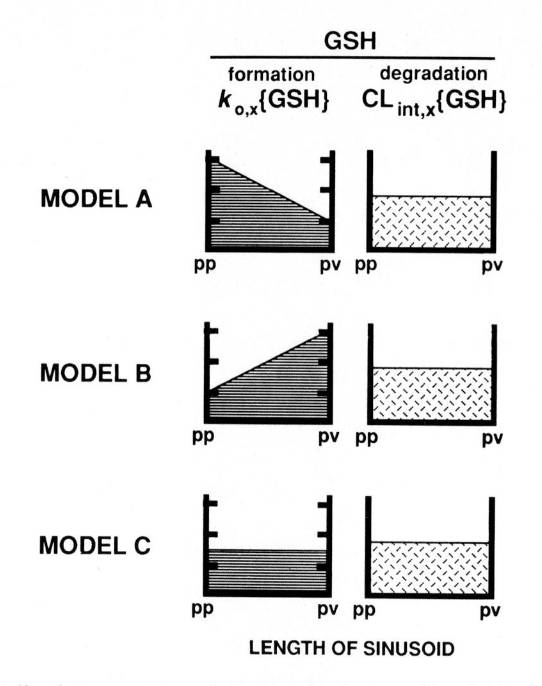

Fig. 18. The distribution patterns of the synthesis rate ($k_{o,x}\{GSH\}$) and the degradation intrinsic clearance ($CL_{int,x}\{GSH\}$) of glutathione (*GSH*) from the periportal region (*pp*) to the perihepatic venous (*pv*) region

patterns of GSH in the plasma, $C_x\{GSH\}$, were similar and converged to exceedingly similar outflow concentrations (C_x at $L = C_{Out}$) of around $15\,\mu M$ (Fig. 19B), a value observed by ADAMS et al. (1983) for the GSH in plasma. When a low (0.01 mM) versus a high (10 mM) acetaminophen input concentration was used for simulation, tissue GSH was unaltered at 0.01 mM, but became readily depleted, in a manner which paralleled the formation of the reactive intermediate in tissue (Fig. 20A,B). The higher the concentration of the reactive intermediate in tissue, the greater the GSH depletion at x. Despite the fact that these changes at x were dependent on the acinar distribution for GSH (Fig. 20A,B; models A, B, and C), the length-averaged intrahepatic GSH concentrations were depleted to similar levels (3 µmol/g liver) for all models. Moreover, identical formation and efflux rates of the acetaminophen GSH adduct were observed among the models (Fig. 20C,D).

Since the acinar distribution of GSH was devoid of influence on the formation and efflux rates of the acetaminophen GSH adduct, simulation with model A was used to examine the effect of input concentration on the depletion kinetics of intrahepatic GSH. Upon increasing the acetaminophen input concentration from 0.01 to 10 mM, increased formation of the reactive intermediate was observed and paralleled the decrease in intracellular GSH

Table 5. Parameters for simulation of glutathione synthesis and depletion in the presence of depletors

Parameter	Definition	Assigned value
Glutathione parameters		
$k_o\{GSH\}$ (nmol/min)	Length-averaged glutathione synthesis rate	730[a]
$CL_{int}\{GSH\}$ (ml/min)	Length-averaged intrinsic clearance of GSH degradation	0.1[b]
$CL_x^{in}\{GSH\}$ (ml/min)	First-order influx clearance at x	1[b]
$V_{max}^{ef}\{GSH\}$ (nmol/min)	Length-averaged capacity for carrier mediated efflux	200[c]
$K_m^{ef}\{GSH\}$ (μM)	Michaelis-Menten constant for the efflux process	3200[c]
n	Hill's coefficient for the efflux process	2.9[c]
Parent drug parameters		
$f_{B,x}$	Unbound fraction in blood at x	unity
$f_{T,x}$	Unbound fraction in tissue at x	unity
CL_x^d (ml/min)	Bidirectional transmembrane clearance at x	100[b]
V_{max}^S (nmol/min)	Length-averaged maximum velocity for sulfation	1230[d]
K_m^S (μM)	Michaelis-Menten constant for sulfation	109[d]
V_{max}^G (nmol/min)	Length-averaged maximum velocity for glucuronidation	690[d]
K_m^G (μM)	Michaelis-Menten constant for glucuronidation	915[d]
CL_{int}^M (ml/min)	Length-averaged intrinsic clearance for formation of M	0.035[e]
Reactive intermediate (M) parameters		
$CL_{int}^G\{M\}$ (ml/min)	Length-averaged intrinsic clearance for formation of acetaminophen glutathione adduct	50[b]
$CL_{int}^O\{M\}$ (ml/min)	Length-averaged intrinsic clearance for formation of other adducts	0[b]
Glutathione adduct {PSH} parameters		
$CL_{int}\{PSH\}$ (ml/min)	Length-averaged intrinsic clearance for biliary excretion	5.0[b]
$CL_x^d\{PSH\}$ (ml/min)	Bidrectional transmembrane clearance at x	1.0[b]

[a] Taken from FERNANDES-CHECA and KAPLOWITZ (1990), average of depleted and repleted glutathione conditions.
[b] Assigned.
[c] Taken from AW et al. (1986).
[d] Taken from WATARI et al. (1983).
[e] Taken from CHEN and GILLETTE (1988).

concentration (Fig. 21A,B); the length-averaged intrahepatic GSH concentration was reduced from 5.8 to 4.4 and 3 μmol/g liver at 1, 5, and 10 m*M* acetaminophen, respectively. Although the formation and efflux rates of the GSH adduct were found to increase with input acetaminophen concentration, formation of the GSH adduct, when expressed as a percentage of

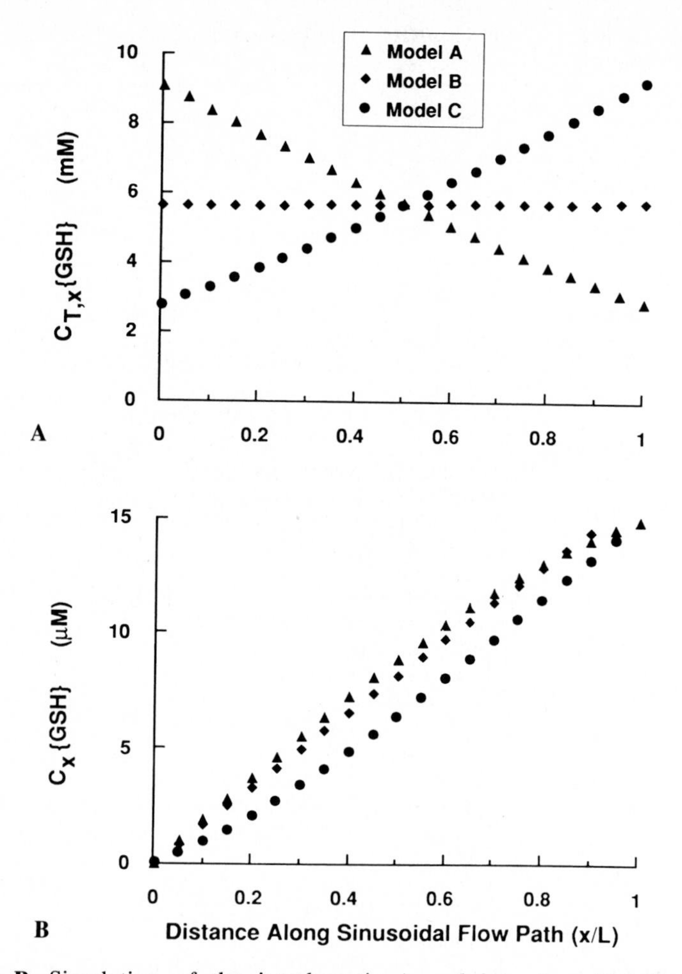

Fig. 19A,B. Simulation of the intrahepatic **A** and intrasinusoidal **B** glutathione (GSH) levels without depletor for models A, B, and C (Fig. 18). The length averaged GSH content was around 5.7–5.8 μmol/g liver, and the outflow GSH concentration (C_{Out}) was around 15 μM

the total input rate of acetaminophen, was decreased due to GSH as a rate-limiting factor (Fig. 21C,D).

The final application of the rate equations (Eqs. 35–42) was found in the remarkable resemblance of simulated data versus the observed sulfation,

---

Fig. 20A–D. Effect of acinar distribution (models A, B, and C) on the liver concentrations of the reactive intermediate of acetaminophen, M **A**, and GSH **B**, and on the formation rate **C** and total efflux rate (venous blood and bile) **D** of the acetaminophen glutathione conjugate. The acinar GSH was without effect on PSH formation and efflux

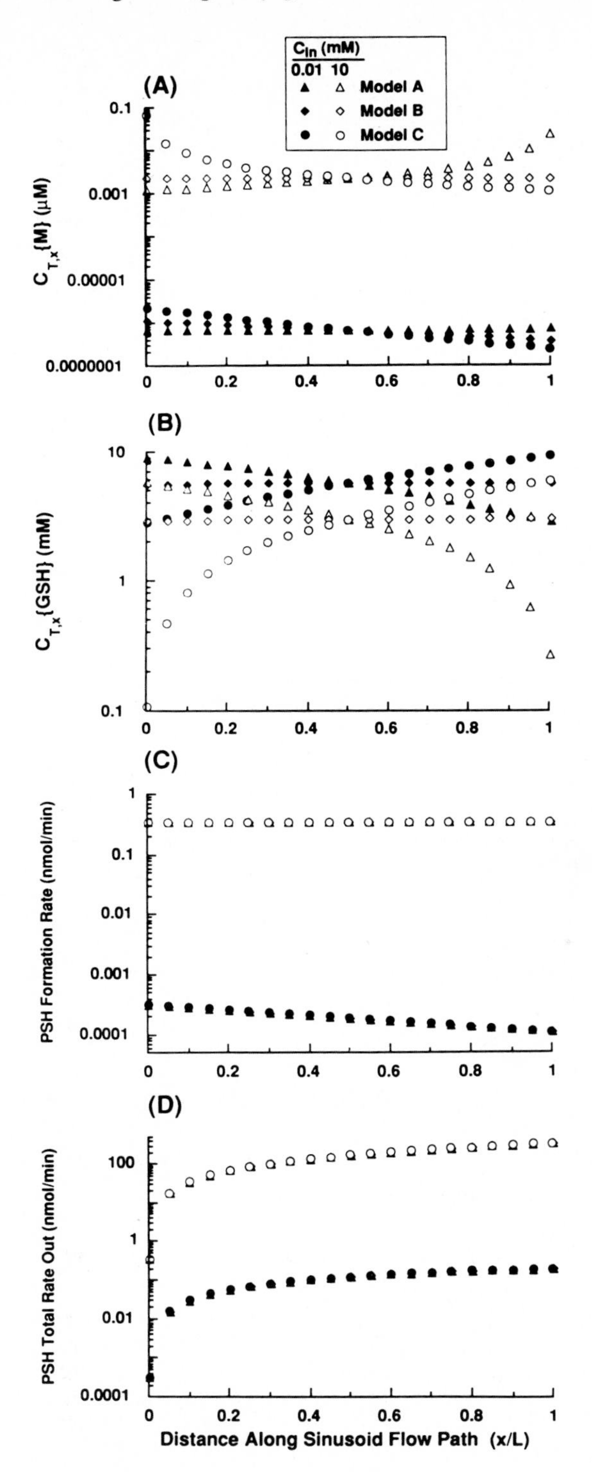

C_{in} (mM)
0.01 10
Model A
Model B
Model C
(A)
$C_{T,x}${M} (μM)
0.1
0.001
0.00001
0.0000001
0
0.2
0.4
0.6
0.8
1
(B)
$C_{T,x}${GSH} (mM)
10
1
0.1
(C)
PSH Formation Rate (nmol/min)
1
0.1
0.01
0.001
0.0001
(D)
PSH Total Rate Out (nmol/min)
100
1
0.01
0.0001
Distance Along Sinusoid Flow Path (x/L)

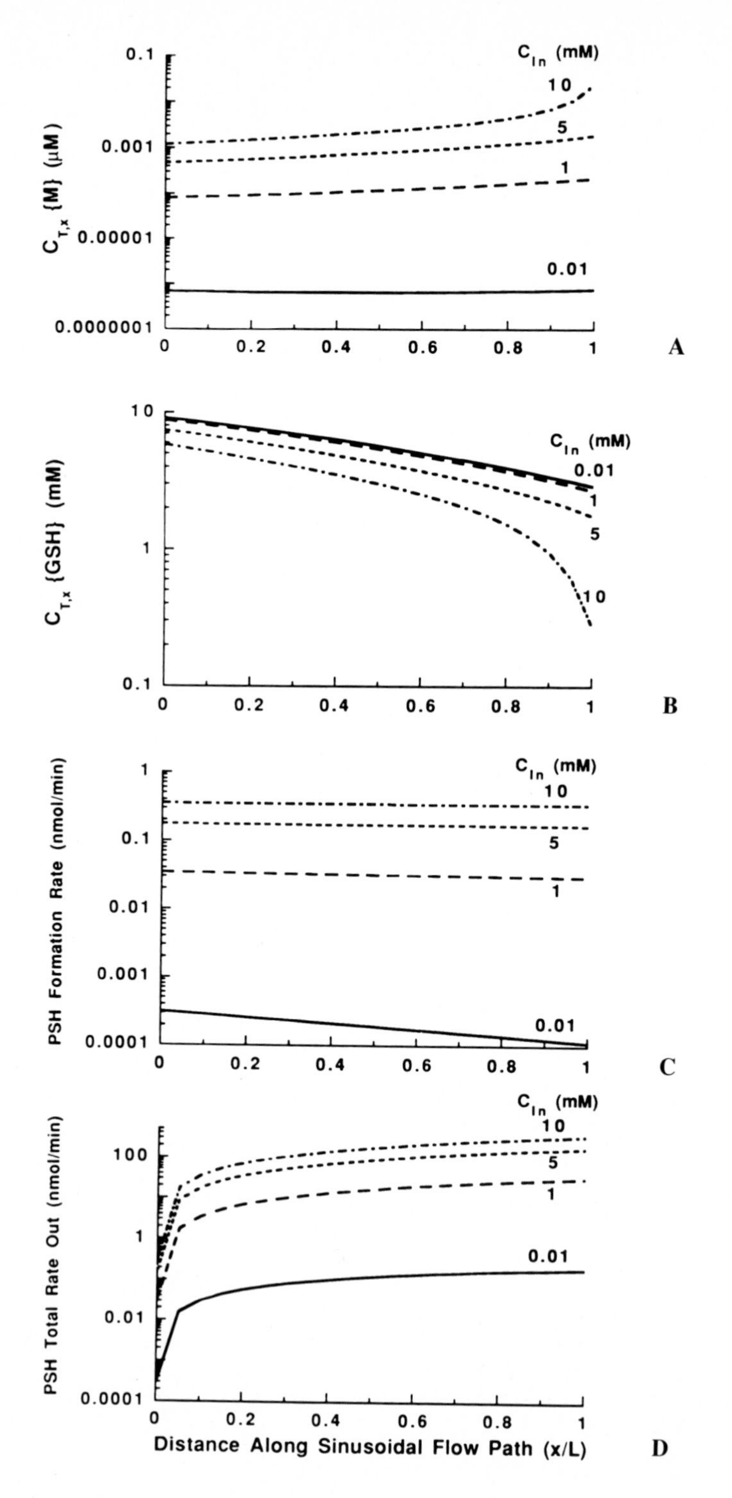

0.1
0.001
0.00001
0.0000001
C_T,x {M} (μM)
C_In (mM)
10
5
1
0.01
0
0.2
0.4
0.6
0.8
1
A
10
1
0.1
C_T,x {GSH} (mM)
C_In (mM)
0.01
1
5
10
B
1
0.1
0.01
0.001
0.0001
PSH Formation Rate (nmol/min)
C_In (mM)
10
5
1
0.01
C
100
1
0.01
0.0001
PSH Total Rate Out (nmol/min)
C_In (mM)
10
5
1
0.01
Distance Along Sinusoidal Flow Path (x/L)
D

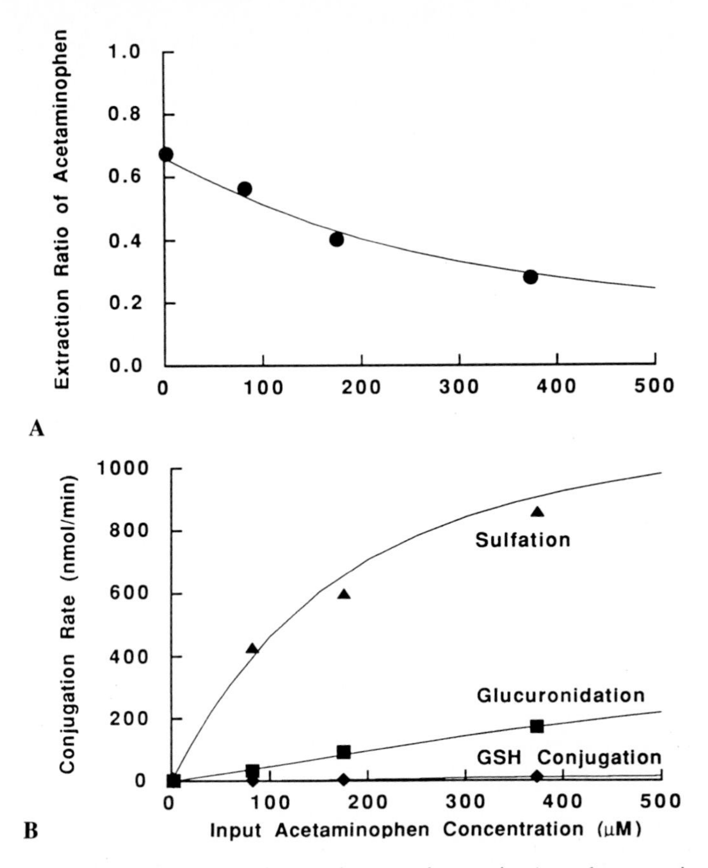

Fig. 22A,B. Simulated versus observed extraction ratio **A** and acetaminophen sulfation, glucuronidation, and glutathione conjugation rates **B** in the single-pass perfused rat liver (from FAYZ et al. 1984). Simulations were performed with the model equations (Eqs. 35–42) and parameters shown in Table 5

glucuronidation, and GSH conjugation rates (summed efflux rates in venous perfusate and bile) of acetaminophen in single-pass perfused rat liver studies (FAYZ et al. 1984). The close match for this data (Fig. 22) and between the simulated length-averaged GSH levels in liver tissue (5–6 μmol/g liver) and for the plasma GSH concentration (15 μM) attests to the success of this type of approach.

←

Fig. 21A–D. Effect of acetaminophen concentration on the liver concentrations of the reactive metabolite, M **A**, and GSH **B**, and on the formation rate **C** and total efflux rate **D** of the acetaminophen glutathione conjugate according to model A (Fig. 18)

C. Concluding Remarks

This chapter summarized the steady state rate equations for the simulation of conjugation and deconjugation reactions; tissue binding need not be considered. The parameters for vascular binding, transport, and removal in the rate equations are allowed to vary at any point x to incorporate heterogeneity. In order to approximate the experimental condition, data on plasma protein binding, red cell partitioning, and metabolic data with concentration (conjugate formation rates) are needed for simulation. Transmembrane clearances are usually unavailable in steady state approaches, but these can be acquired with the multiple indicator dilution technique as proposed by GORESKY et al. (1973, 1992) or with isolated hepatocyte studies (SUNDHEIMER and BRENDEL 1983; MIYAUCHI et al. 1989; FERNANDES-CHECA and KAPLOWITZ 1990). Otherwise, assignment of the values on a trial and error basis for optimization becomes necessary (DE LANNOY and PANG 1987; RATNA et al. 1993). Simulation with these simple mass–balance equations have proven useful in the understanding of membrane-limited processes, zonation of enzymes, the effect of protein binding and futile cycling, and the role of the cosubstrate GSH on conjugation and deconjugation processes. Through these endeavors, a more quantitative interpretation of metabolic data on conjugation reactions is provided.

Acknowledgement. This work was supported by the Medical Research Council of Canada (MA9104, MA9765) and the National Institutes of Health (GM-38250).

References

Adams JD Jr, Lauterburg BH, Mitchell JR (1983) Plasma glutathione and glutathione disulfide in the rat: regulation and response to oxidative stress. J Pharmacol Exp Ther 227:749–754

Ahmad AB, Bennett PN, Rowland M (1983) Models of hepatic drug clearance: discrimination between the "well-stirred" and "parallel-tube" models. J Pharm Pharmacol 35:219–224

Anundi IM, Kauffman FC, EL-Mouelhi M, Thurman RG (1986) Hydrolysis of organic sulfates in periportal and pericentral regions of the liver lobule: studies with 4-methylumbelliferyl sulfate in the perfused rat liver. Mol Pharmacol 29:599–605

Asghar K, Reddy BK, Krishna G (1975) Histochemical localization of glutathione in tissues. J Histochem Cytochem 23:774–779

Aw TY, Ookhtens RC, Kaplowitz N (1986) Kinetics of glutathione efflux from isolated rat hepatocytes. Am J Physiol 250:G236–G243

Ballatori N, Clarkson TW (1983) Biliary transport of glutathione and methylmercury. Am J Physiol 244:G435–G441

Ballatori N, Jacob R, Boyer JL (1986) Intrabiliary glutathione hydrolysis: a source of glutamate in bile. J Biol Chem 261:7860–7865

Barnhart JR, Clarenburg R (1973) Factors determining the clearance of bilirubin in perfused rat liver. Am J Physiol 225:497–508

Baron J, Redick RA, Guengerich FP (1982) Effect of 3-methyl-cholanthrene, β-naphthoflavone, and phenobarbital on the 3-methyl-cholanthrene inducible isozyme of cytochrome P-450 within centrilobular, midzonal, and periportal hepatocytes. J Biol Chem 257:953–957

Bass L (1983) Saturation kinetics in hepatic drug removal: a statistical approach to functional heterogeneity. Am J Physiol 244:G583–G589

Bass L (1985) Heterogeneity within observed regions: physiologic basis and effects on estimation of rates of biodynamic processes. Circulation 72 Suppl 4:47–52

Bass L, Robinson PJ (1981) Effects of capillary heterogeneity on rates of steady state uptake of substances by the intact liver. Microvas Res 22:43–57

Bass NM, Barker ME, Manning JA, Jones AL, Ockner RK (1989) Acinar heterogeneity of fatty acid binding protein expression in livers of male, female, and clofibrate-treated rats. Hepatology 9:12–21

Boyer JL, Elias E, Layden TJ (1979) The paracellular pathway and bile formation. Yale J Biol Med 52:61–67

Braakman I, Groothuis GMM, Meijer DKF (1987) Acinar heterogeneity in hepatic transport of the organic cation rhodamine B in rat liver. Hepatology 7:849–855

Braakman I, Groothuis GMM, Meijer DKF (1989) Zonal compartmentation of perfused rat liver: plasma reapparance of rhodamine B explained. J Pharmacol Ther 239:869–873

Brauer RW, Leong GF, McElroy RF, Holloway RJ (1956) Circulatory pathways in the rat liver as revealed by P^{32} chromic phosphate colloid uptake in the perfused rat liver. Am J Physiol 184:593–598

Breznicka EA, Hazelton GA, Klaassen CD (1987) Comparison of adenosine 3′-phosphate 5′-phosphosulfate concentrations in tissues from different laboratory animals. Drug Metab Dispos 15:133–135

Burger HJ, Gebhardt R, Mayer C, Mecke D (1989) Different capacities for amino acid transport in periportal and perivenous hepatocytes isolated by digitonin/collagenase perfusion. Hepatology 9:22–28

Chen R, Gillette JR (1988) Pharmacokinetic procedures for the estimation of organ clearances for the formation of short-lived metabolites. Acetaminophen induced glutathione depletion in hamster. Drug Metab Dispos 16:373–385

Chiba M, Hollands, Pang KS (1993) Hepatic uptake of 4-methylumbelliferyl sulfate: a multiple indicator dilution study in perfused rat liver (Abstr). FASEB J 7:A481

Chiba M, Pang KS (1993a) Effect of protein binding on 4-metylumbelliferyl sulfate desulfation kinetics in perfused rat liver. J Pharmacol Exp Ther 266:492–499

Chiba M, Pang KS (1993b) The acinar distribution of glutathione (GSH) on its depletion kinetics: a simulation study. ASPET, abstract, San Francisco

Chiba M, Poon K, Hollands J, Pang KS (1994) Glycine conjugation of benzoic acid and its acinar localization in liver. J Pharmacol Exp Ther 268:409–416

Conway JG, Kauffman FC, Tsukada T, Thurman RG (1984) Glucuronidation of 7-hydroxycoumarin in periportal and pericentral regions of the liver lobule. Mol Pharmacol 25:487–493

Conway JG, Kauffman FC, Thurman RG (1985) Effect of glucose on 7-hydroxycoumarin glucuronide production in periportal and pericentral regions of the liver lobule. Biochem J 226:749–756

Conway JG, Kauffman FC, Tsukuda T, Thurman RG (1987) Glucuronidation of 7-hydroxycoumarin in periportal and pericentral regions of the lobule in livers from untreated and 3-methyl-cholanthrene-treated rats. Mol Pharmacol 33: 111–119

Dawson JR, Weitering JG, Mulder GJ, Stillwell RN, Pang KS (1985) Alteration of transit time and direction of flow to probe the heterogeneous distribution of conjugation activities for harmol in the perfused rat liver preparation. J Pharmacol Exp Ther 234:691–697

DeBaun JR, Smith JYR, Miller EC, Miller JA (1971) Reactivity in vivo of the carcinogen N-hydroxy-2-acetylaminoflourene: increase by sulfate ion. Science 167:184–186

De Lannoy IAM, Pang KS (1986) A commentary. The presence of diffusional barriers on drug and metabolite kinetics. Enalaprilat as a generated versus preformed metabolite. Drug Metab Dispos 14:513–520

De Lannoy IAM, Pang KS (1987) Diffusional barriers on drug and metabolite kinetics. Drug Metab Dispos 15:51–58
De Leeue AM, Knook DL (1984) The ultrastructure of sinusoidal liver cells in the intact rat at various ages. In: van Bezooijen CFA (ed) Pharmacological, morphological and physiological aspects of aging. Eurage, Rijswik, pp 91–96
Dills RL, Klaassen CD (1986) The effect of inhibitors of mitochondrial energy production on hepatic glutathione, UDP-glucuronic acid, and adenosine 3′-phosphate-5′-phosphosulfate concentrations. Drug Metab Dispos 14:190–196
Dills RL, Klaassen CD (1987) Hepatic UDP-glucose and UDP-glucuronic acid sysnthesis rates in rats during a reduced energy state. Drug Metab Dispos 15:281–288
Dutton GJ (1980) Glucuronidation of drugs and other compounds. CRC, Boca Raton
Ebling WF, Jusko WJ (1986) The determination of essential clearance, volume, and residence time parameters of recirculating metabolic systems: the reversible metabolism of methylprednisolone and methylprednisone in rabbits. J Pharmacokinet Biopharm 14:557–599
El Mouelhi M, Kauffman FC (1986) Sublobular distribution of transferases and hydrolases associated with glucuronide, sulfate, and glutathione conjugation in human liver. Hepatology 6:450–456
Eling TE, Curtis JF, Harman LS, Mason RP (1986) Oxidation of glutathione to its thiyl free radical metabolite by prostaglandin H synthase. J Biol Chem 261: 5023–5028
Fayz S, Cherry WF, Dawson JR, Mulder GJ, Pang KS (1984) Inhibition of acetaminophen sulfation by 2,6-dichloro-4-nitrophenol in the perfused rat liver preparation. Lack of a compensatory increase in glucuronidation. Drug Metab Dispos 12:323–329
Fernandes-Checa JC, Kaplowitz N (1990) The use of monochlorobimane to determine hepatic GSH levels and synthesis. Anal Biochem 190:212–219
Ferry JJ Jr, Wagner JG (1986) The non-linear pharmacokinetics of prednisone and prednisolone. I. Theoretical. Biopharm Drug Dispos 7:91–101
Finkelstein TD, Mudd SH (1967) Trans-sulfuration in mammals: the methione-sparing effect of cysteine. J Biol Chem 242:873–880
Fleischner G, Meijer DKF, Levine WG, Gatmaitan Z, Gluck R, Arias IM (1975) Effect of hypolipidemic drugs, nafenopin and clofibrate, on the concentration of ligandin and Z protein in rat liver. Biochem Biophys Res Commun 67:1401–1407
Froment GF, Bischoff KB (1976) In: Chemical reactor analysis and design. Wiley, New York, p 10
Galinsky RE, Levy G (1981) Dose- and time-dependent elimination of acetaminophen in rats: pharmacokinetic implications of cosubstrate depletion. J Pharmacol Exp Ther 210:14–20
Gärtner U, Stockert RJ, Levine WG, Wolkoff AW (1982) Effect of nafenopin on the uptake of bilirubin and sulfobromophthalein by the isolated perfused rat liver. Gastroenterology 83:1163–1169
Geng WP, Barker F, Schwab AJ, Goresky CA, Pang KS (1993) Hepatic uptake of bromosulfophthalein-glutathione conjugate in perfused rat liver. A multiple indicator dilution study (Abstr). FASEB J 7:A481
Gillette JR (1971) Factors affecting drug metabolism. Ann NY Acad Sci 179: 43–46
Gillette JR (1973) Overview of drug-protein binding. NY Acad Sci 226:6–17
Gillette JR, Pang KS (1977) Theoretical aspects of pharmacokinetic drug interactions. Clin Pharmacol Ther 22:623–639
Gonzalez-Fernandez JM, Atta SE (1973) Maximal substrate transport in capillary networks. Microvasc Res 5:180–198
Gooding PE, Chayen J, Sawyer B, Slater TF (1978) Cytochrome P-450 distribution in rat liver and the effect of sodium phenobarbitone administration. Chem Biol Interact 20:299–310

Goresky CA (1963) A linear method for determining liver sinusoidal and extravascular volumes. Am J Physiol 204:626–640
Goresky CA, Groom AC (1984) Microcirculatory events in the liver and the spleen. In: Renkin EM, Michel CC (eds) The cardiovascular system IV. American Physiological Society, Washington, pp 689–780 (Handbook of Physiology)
Goresky CA, Bach GG, Nadeau E (1973) On the uptake of materials by the intact liver: the transport and net removal of galactose. J Clin Invest 52:991–1009
Goresky CA, Bach GG, Nadeau E (1975) Red cell carriage of label. Its limiting effect on the exchange of materials in the liver. Circ Res 36:328–351
Goresky CA, Daly DS, Mishkin D, Arias IM (1978) Uptake of labeled palmitate by the intact liver: role of intracellular binding sites. Am J Physiol 234:E542–E553
Goresky CA, Schwab AJ, Rose CP (1988) Xenon handling in the liver: red cell capacity effect. Circ Res 63:767–778
Goresky CA, Pang KS, Schwab AJ, Barker F III, Cherry WF, Bach GG (1992) Uptake of a protein bound polar compound, acetaminophen sulfate, by perfused rat liver. Hepatology 16:173–190
Goresky CA, Bach GG, Schwab AJ (1993a) Distributed-in-space product formation in vivo: linear kinetics. Am J Physiol 264:H2007–H2028
Goresky CA, Bach GG, Schwab AJ (1993b) Distributed-in-space product formation in vivo: enzyme kinetics. Am J Physiol 264:H2029–H2050
Grausz H, Schmid R (1971) Reciprocal relation between plasma albumin level and hepatic sulfobromophthalein removal. N Engl J Med 284:1403–1404
Griffith OW, Meister A (1979) Translocation of intracellular glutathione to membrane-bound gamma-glutamyltranspeptidase as a discrete step in the gamma-glutamyl cycle: glutathionuria after inhibition of transpeptidase. Proc Natl Acad Sci USA 76:268–272
Gugler R, Mueller G (1978) Plasma protein binding of valproic acid in healthy subjects and in patients with renal disease. Br J Clin Pharmacol 5:441–446
Gumucio DL, Gumucio JJ, Wilson JAP, Cutter C, Krauss M, Caldwell R, Chen E (1984) Albumin influences sulfobromophthalein transport by hepatocytes of each acinar zone. Am J Physiol 246:G86–G95
Gumucio JJ, Balabaud C, Miller DL, Demason LF, Appleman HD, Stoecker TJ, Franzblau DR (1978) Bile secretion and liver cell heterogeneity in the rat. J Lab Clin Med 91:350–362
Gumucio JJ, Miller DL, Krauss MD, Zanolli CC (1981) Transport of fluorescent compounds into hepatocytes and the resultant zonal labeling of the hepatic acinus in the rat. Gastroenterology 80:639–646
Hjelle JJ, Hazelton GA, Klaassen CD (1985) Acetaminophen decreases adenosine 3′-phosphate 5′-phosphosulfate and uridine diphosphoglucuronic acid in rat liver. Drug Metab Dispos 13:35–41
Howell SR, Hazelton GA, Klaassen CD (1986) Depletion of hepatic UDP-glucuronic acid by drugs that are glucuronidated. J Pharmacol Exp Ther 236:610–614
Huang JD, Øie S (1984) Hepatic elimination of drugs with concentration-dependent serum protein binding. J Pharmacokinet Biopharm 12:67–81
Hwang S, Kwan KC, Albert KS (1981) A linear model of reversible metabolism and its bioavailability assessment. J Pharmacokinet Biopharm 9:693–709
Jansen JA (1981) Influence of plasma protein binding kinetics on hepatic clearance assessed from a "tube" model and a "well-stirred" model. J Pharmacokinet Biopharm 19:15–26
Jollow DJ, Thorgeirsson SS, Potter WZ, Hashimoto M, Mitchell JR (1974) Acetaminophen-induced hepatic necrosis. VI. Metabolic disposition of toxic and nontoxic doses of acetaminophen. Pharmacology 12:251–271
Jones AL, Hreadek GT, Renston RH, Wong KY, Karlagnais G, Paumgartner G (1980) Autoradiographic evidence for hepatic lobular concentration gradient of bile acid derivative. Am J Physiol 238:G233–G237
Jungerman K, Katz N (1982) Functional hepatocellular heterogeneity. Hepatology 2:385–395

Jusko WJ, Gretch M (1976) Plasma and tissue protein binding of drugs in pharmacokinetics. Drug Metab Rev 5:43–140
Kaplowitz N, Kuhlenkamp J, Goldstein L, Reeve J (1980) Effect of salicylates and phenobarbital on hepatic glutathione in the rat. J Pharmacol Exp Ther 212: 240–245
Kaplowitz N, Aw TK, Ookhtens M (1985) The regulation of hepatic glutathione. Annu Rev Pharmacol Toxicol 25:715–744
Kauffman FC, Whittaker M, Anundi I, Thurman RG (1991) Futile cycling of a sulfate conjugate by isolated hepatocytes. Mol Pharmacol 39:414–420
Keiding E, Chiarantini E (1978) Effect of sinusoidal perfusion on galactose elimination kinetics in perfused rat liver. J Pharmacol Exp Ther 205:465–470
Kitamura T, Jansen P, Hardenbrook C, Kamimoto Y, Gatmaitan Z, Arias IM (1990) Defective ATP-dependent bile canalicular transport of organic anions in mutant (TR^{-1}) rats with conjugated hyperbilirubinemia. Proc Natl Acad Sci USA 87:3557–3561
Knapp SA, Green MD, Tephly TR, Baron J (1988) Immuno-histochemical demonstration of isozyme- and strain- specific differences in the intralobular localizations and distributions of UDP-glucuronosyltransferases in livers of untreated rats. Mol Pharmacol 33:14–21
Kosower NS, Kosower EM (1978) The glutathione status of cells. Int Rev Cytol 54:109–160
Koster H, Halsema I, Pang KS, Scholtens E, Mulder GJ (1982) Kinetics of sulfation and glucuronidation of harmol in the perfused rat liver preparation. Disappearance of aberrancies in glucuronidation kinetics by inhibition of sulfation. Biochem Pharmacol 31:3023–3038
Krijgsheld KR, Frankena H, Scholtens E, Zweens J, Mulder GJ (1979) Absorption, serum levels and urinary excretion of inorganic sulfate after oral administration of sodium sulfate in the conscious rat. Biochim Biophys Acta 586:492–500
Krijgsheld KR, Scholtens E, Mulder GJ (1982) The dependence of the rate of sulphate conjugation on the plasma concentration of inorganic sulphate in the rat in vivo. Biochem Pharmacol 31:3997–4000
Lança AJ, Israel Y (1991) Histochemical demonstration of sinusoidal gamma-glutamyltransferase activity by substrate protection fixation: comparative studies in rat and guinea pig liver. Hepatology 14:857–863
Lauterburg BH, Vaishnav Y, Stillwell WG, Mitchell JR (1980) The effect of age and glutathione depletion on hepatic glutathione turnover in vivo determined by acetaminophen probe analysis. J Pharmacol Exp Ther 213:54–58
Lauterburg BH, Mitchel JR (1981) Regulation of hepatic glutathione turnover in rats in vivo and evidence for kinetic homogeneity of the hepatic glutathione pool. J Clin Invest 67:1415–1424
Lauterburg BH, Smith CV, Hughes H, Mitchell JR (1982) Determinants of hepatic glutathione turnover: toxicolgical significance. Trends Pharmacol Sci 3:245–248
Levenspiel O (1972) In: Chemical reaction engineering, 2nd edn. Wiley, New York, pp 182–185
Levy G, Yacobi A (1974) Effect of protein binding on elimination of warfarin. J Pharm Sci 63:805–806
Lin JH, Levy G (1986) Effect of prevention of inorganic sulfate depletion on the pharmacokinetics of acetaminophen in rats. J Pharmacol Exp Ther 239:94–98
Mais RF, Kereszies-Nagy S, Zaroslinski JF, Oester YT (1974) Interpretation of protein–drug interaction through fraction unbound and relative contribution of secondary sites. J Pharm Sci 63:1423–1427
McFarlane BM, Spios J, Gove CD, McFarlane IG, Williams R (1990) Antibodies against the hepatic asialoglycoprotein receptor perfused in situ preferentially attach to periportal liver cells in the rat. Hepatology 11:408–415
Meerman JHN, Mulder GJ (1981) Prevention of the hepatotoxic action of N-hydroxy-2-acetylaminofluorene in the rat by inhibition of N-O-sulfation by pentachlorophenol. Life Sci 21:2361–2365

Meffin PJ, Zilm DM, Veenendaal JR (1983) Reduced clofibric acid clearance in renal dysfunction is due to a futile cycle. J Pharmacol Exp Ther 227:732–738
Meijer DKF (1987) Current concepts on hepatic transport of drugs. J Hepatol 4:259–268
Meister A, Anderson ME (1983) Glutathione. Annu Rev Biochem 52:711–760
Miller DL, Zanolli CS, Gumucio JJ (1979) Quantitative morphology of the sinusoids in the hepatic acinus. Gastroenterology 76:965–969
Miyauchi S, Sugiyama Y, Sato H, Sawada Y, Iga I, Hanano M (1987a) Effect of a diffusional barrier to a metabolite across hepatocytes on its kinetics in "enzyme-distributed" models: a computer-aided simulation study. J Pharmacokinet Biopharm 15:399–421
Miyauchi S, Sugiyama Y, Sawada Y, Iga T, Hanano M (1987b) Conjugative metabolism of 4-methylumbelliferone in the rat liver: verification of the sequestration process in multiple indicator dilution experiments. Chem Pharm Bull (Tokyo) 35:4241–4248
Miyauchi S, Sugiyama Y, Sawada Y, Morita K, Iga T, Hanano M (1987c) Kinetics of transport of 4-methylumbelliferone in rats. Analysis by multiple indicator dilution method. J Pharmacokinet Biopharm 15:25–38
Miyauchi S, Sugiyama Y, Iga T, Hanano M (1989) The conjugative metabolism of 4-methylumbelliferone and deconjugation to the parent drug examined by isolated perfused liver and in vitro homogenate of rats. Chem Pharm Bull (Tokyo) 37:475–480
Morris ME, Pang KS (1987) Competition between two enzymes for substrate removal in liver: modulating effects of competitive pathways. J Pharmacokinet Biopharm 15:473–496
Morris ME, Yuen V, Pang KS (1987) Competing pathways in drug metabolism. II. Competing pathways in drug metabolism. Enzymic systems for 2- and 5-sulfoconjugation are distributed anterior to 5-glucuronidation in the metabolism of gentisamide by the perfused rat liver. J Pharmacokinet Biopharm 16:633–656
Morris ME, Yuen V, Tang BK, Pang KS (1988) Competing pathways in drug metabolism. I. Effect of varying input concentrations on gentisamide conjugation in the once-through in situ perfused rat liver preparation. J Pharmacol Exp Ther 245:614–652
Mulder GJ, Hadgedoorn AH (1974) UDP-glucuronyltransferase and phenolsulfotransferase in vivo and in vitro. Conjugation of harmol and harmolol. Biochem Pharmacol 23:2101–2109
Mulder GJ, Keulemans K (1978) Metabolism of inorganic sulfate in the isolated perfused rat liver. Biochem J 176:959–965
Murray GI, Burke MD, Even SWB (1986) Glutathione lozalization by a novel *o*-phthalaldehyde histofluorescence method. Histochem J 18:434–440
Nathanson MH, Boyer JL (1991) Special article. Mechanisms and regulation of bile secretion. Hepatology 14:551–566
Novikoff AB (1959) Cell heterogeneity within the hepatic lobule of the rat (staining reactions). J Histochem Cytochem 7:240–244
Øie S (1986) Drug distribution and binding. J Clin Pharmacol 26:583–586
Øie S, Levy G (1975) Effect of plasma protein binding on elimination of bilirubin. J Pharm Sci 64:1433–1434
Ookhtens M, Hobdy K, Corvasce MC, Aw TY, Kaplowitz N (1985) Sinusoidal efflux of glutathione in the perfused rat liver. Evidence for a carrier-mediated process. J Clin Invest 75:258–265
Orrenius S, Ormstad K, Thor H, Jewell SA (1983) Turnover and functions of glutathione studies with isolated hepatic and renal cells. Fed Proc 42:3177–3188
Pang KS (1990) Kinetics of conjugation reactions in eliminating organs. In: Mulder GJ (ed) Conjugation reactions in drug metabolism: an integrated approach. Taylor and Francis, London, pp 5–39

Pang KS, Barker F III, Schwab AJ, Goresky CA (1988a) Red cell carriage of acetaminophen as studied by the technique of multiple indicator dilution in perfused rat liver. Hepatology 8:1384 (abstract No 667)

Pang KS, Cherry WF, Accaputo J, Schwab AJ, Goresky CA (1988b) Combined hepatic arterial-portal venous or hepatic venous flows once-through the in situ perfused rat liver to probe the abundance of drug metabolizing activities. Perihepatic venous O-deethylation activity for phenacetin and periportal sulfation activity for acetaminophen. J Pharmacol Exp Ther 247:690–700

Pang KS, Chiba M (1994) Metabolism: scaling up from in vitro to organ and whole body. In: Welling PG, Balant LP (eds) Handbook of Experimental Pharmacology. Springer, Berlin Heidelberg New York 101–187

Pang KS, Gillette JR (1979) Sequential first-pass elimination of a metabolite derived from its precursor. J Pharmacokinet Biopharm 7:275–290

Pang KS, Goresky CA, Schwab AJ (1991) Deterministic factors underlying drug and metabolite clearances in rat liver perfusion studies. In: Ballet F, Thurman RG (eds) Research in perfused liver: clinical and basic applications. INSERM, Paris; Libbey, London, pp 259–302

Pang KS, Koster H, Halsema ICM, Scholtens E, Mulder GJ (1981) Aberrant pharmacokinetics of harmol in the perfused rat liver preparation: sulfate and glucuronide conjugations. J Pharmacol Exp Ther 219:134–140

Pang KS, Koster H, Halsema ICM, Scholtens E, Mulder GJ, Stillwell RN (1983) Normal and retrograde perfusion to probe the zonal distribution of sulfation and glucuronidation activities of harmol in the perfused rat liver preparation. J Pharmacol Exp Ther 224:647–653

Pang KS, Lee WF, Cherry WF, Yuen V, Accaputo J, Schwab AJ, Goresky CA (1988c) Effects of perfusate flow rate on measured blood volume, Disse space, intracellular water spaces, and drug extraction in the perfused rat liver preparation: characterization by the technique of multiple indicator dilution. J Pharmacokinet Biopharm 16:595–605

Pang KS, Mulder GJ (1990) A commentary: effect of flow on formation of metabolites. Drug Metab Dispos 18:270–275

Pang KS, Rowland M (1977a) Hepatic clearance of drugs. I. Theoretical consideration of a "well-stirred" model and a "parallel tube" model. Influence of hepatic blood flow, plasma and blood cells binding, and the hepatocellular activity on hepatic drug clearance. J Pharmacokinet Biopharm 5:625–653

Pang KS, Rowland M (1977b) Hepatic clearance of drugs. II. Experimental evidence for acceptance of the "well-stirred" model over the "parallel tube" model using lidocaine in the perfused rat liver in situ preparation. J Pharmacokinet Biopharm 5:655–680

Pang KS, Stillwell RN (1983) An understanding of the role of enzymic localization of the liver on metabolite kinetics: a computer simulation. J Pharmacokinet Biopharm 11:451–468

Pang KS, Terrell JA (1981a) Retrograde perfusion to probe the heterogeneous distribution of hepatic drug metabolizing enzymes in rats. J Pharmacol Exp Ther 216:339–346

Pang KS, Terrell JA (1981b) Conjugation kinetics of acetaminophen by the perfused liver preparation. Biochem Pharmacol 38:1959–1965

Pang KS, Xu X (1988) Drug metabolism factors in drug discovery and design. In: Welling PG, Tse FL-S (eds) Pharmacokinetics: regulatory–industrial–academic perspectives. Dekker, New York, pp 383–447

Pang KS, Xu X, St-Pierre MV (1992) Determinants of metabolite disposition. Annu Rev Pharmacol 32:623–669

Pang KS, Xu X, Morris ME, Yuen V (1987) Kinetic modeling of conjugations in liver. Fed Proc 46:2439–2441

Polhuijs M, Meijer DKF, Mulder GJ (1991) The fate of diastereomeric glutathione conjugates of alpha-bromoisovalerylurea in blood in the rat in vivo and in the perfused liver. Stereoselectivity in biliary and urinary excretion. J Pharmacol Exp Ther 256:458–461

Polhuijs M, Cherry WF, Gasinska I, Mulder GJ, Pang KS (1993) Stereoselective glutathione conjugation and amidolysis of R-(+)- and S-(−)-α-bromoisovalerylurea in the perfused rat liver preparation. J Pharmacol Exp Ther 265:1402–1412

Price VF, Jollow DJ (1984) Role of UDPGA flux in acetaminophen clearance and hepatotoxicity. Xenobiotica 7:553–559

Rappaport AM (1958) The structural and functional unit in the human liver (liver acinus). Anat Rec 130:673–689

Rappaport AM (1980) Hepatic blood flow: Morphologic aspects and physiologic regulation. Int Rev Physiol 21:1–63

Rappaport AM, Borowy ZJ, Lougheed WM, Lotto WN (1954) Subdivision of hexagonal liver lobules into a structural and functional unit: role in hepatic physiology and pathology. Anat Rec 119:11–34

Ratna S, Chiba M, Bandyophdhyay L, Pang KS (1993) Futile cycling between 4-methylumbelliferone and its conjugates in perfused rat liver. Hepatology 17: 838–853

Redick JA, Jakoby WB, Baron J (1982) Immunohistochemical localization of glutathione-S-transferase in livers of untreated rats. J Biol Chem 257:15200–15203

Reed RG, Orrenius S (1977) The role of methionine in glutathione biosynthesis by isolated hepatocytes. Biochem Biophys Res Commun 77:1257–1264

Rowland M (1984) Protein binding and drug clearance. Clin Pharmacokinet 9 Suppl 1:10–17

Rowland M, Benet LZ, Graham GG (1973) Clearance concepts in pharmacokinetics. J Pharmacokinet Biopharm 1:123–136

Rubin GM, Tozer TN (1986) Hepatic binding and Michaelis-Menten metabolism of drugs. J Pharm Sci 75:660–663

Sato H, Sugiyama Y, Miyauchi S, Sawada Y, Iga T, Hanano M (1986) A simulation study on the effect of a uniform diffusional barrier across hepatocytes on drug metabolism by evenly or unevenly distributed uni-enzyme in the liver. J Pharm Sci 75:3–8

Schary WL, Rowland M (1983) Protein binding and hepatic clearance: studies with tolbutamide, a drug of low intrinsic clearance, in the isolated perfused rat liver preparation. J Pharmacokinet Biopharm 11:225–243

Schwarz LR, Schwenk M (1984) Sulfation in isolated enterocytes of guinea-pig: dependence on inorganic sulfate. Biochem Pharmacol 33:3353–3356

Shand DG, Kornhauser DM, Wilkinson GR (1975) Effects of route of administration and blood flow on hepatic elimination. J Pharmacol Exp Ther 195:424–432

Sies H, Graf P (1985) Hepatic thiol and glutathione efflux under the influence of vasopressin, phenylephrine and adrenaline. Biochem J 226:545–549

Singh J, Schwarz LR (1981) Dependence of glucuronidation rate on UDP-glucuronic acid levels in isolated hepatocytes. Biochem Pharmacol 30:3252–3254

Smallwood RH, Mihaly GW, Smallwood RA, Morgan DJ (1988) Effect of a protein binding change on unbound and total plasma concentrations for drugs of intermediate hepatic extraction. J Pharmacokinet Biopharm 16:529–542

Smith BR, van Anda J, Fouts JR, Bend JR (1983) Estimation of the styrene 7,8-oxide-detoxifying potential of epoxide hydrolase in glutathione-depleted, perfused rat liver. J Pharmacol Exp Ther 227:491–498

Smith MT, Loveridege N, Wills ED, Chayen J (1979) The distribution of glutathione content in the rat liver lobule. Biochem J 182:103–108

Sorrentino D, Licko V, Weisiger RA (1988) Sex difference in sulfobromophthalein glutathione transport by perfused rat liver. Biochem Pharmacol 37:3119–3126

Sorrentino D, Robinson RB, Kiang C-L, Berk PD (1989a) At physiological albumin/oleate concentrations oleate uptake by isolated hepatocytes, cardiac myocytes, and adipocytes is a saturable function of the unbound oleate concentration.

Uptake kinetics are consistent with the conventional theory. J Clin Invest 84:1325–1333
Sorrentino D, Weisiger RA, Bass NM, Licko V (1989b) The hepatocellular transport of sulfobromophthalein-glutathione by clofibrate treated-perfused rat liver. Lipids 24:438–442
Speisky H, Shackel N, Varghese G, Wade D, Israel Y (1990) Role of hepatic γ-glutamyltransferase in the degradation of circulating glutathione: Studies in the intact guinea pig perfused liver. Hepatology 11:843–849
Steele JW, Yagen B, Hernandez O, Cox RH, Smith BR, Bend JR (1981) The metabolism and excretion of styrene oxide-glutathione conjugates in the rat and by isolated perfused liver, lung, and kidney preparations. J Pharmacol Exp Ther 219:35–41
St-Pierre MV, Lee PI, Pang KS (1992) A comparative investigation of hepatic clearance models: predictions of metabolite formation and elimination. J Pharmacokinet Biopharm 20:105–145
Sundheimer DW, Brendel K (1983) Metabolism of harmol and transport of harmol conjugates in isolated rat hepatocytes. Drug Metab Dispos 11:433–440
Sweeny DJ, Reinke LA (1988) Sulfation of acetaminophen in isolated rat hepatocytes. Relationship to sulfate ion concentrations and intracellular levels of 3′-phosphoadenosine-5′-phosphosulfate. Drug Metab Dispos 16:712–715
Tateishi N, Higashi T, Naruse A, Hikita K, Sakamoto Y (1981) Relative contributions of sulfur atoms of dietary cysteine and methionine to rat liver glutathione and proteins. J Biochem 90:1603–1610
Theilmann L, Stollman YR, Arias IM, Wolkoff AW (1985) Does Z-protein have a role in transport of bilirubin and bromosulfophthalein by isolated perfused rat liver? Hepatology 5:923–926
Thurman RG, Kauffman FC, Jungermann K (1987) Regulation of hepatic metabolism. Intra- and intercellular compartmentation. Plenum, New York
Ullrich D, Fisher G, Katz N, Bock KW (1984) Intralobular distribution of UDP-glucuronosyltransferase in livers from untreated, 3-methylcholanthrene- and phenobarbital-treated rats. Chem Biol Interact 48:181–190
Van Anda J, Smith BR, Bend JR (1979) Concentration-dependent metabolism and toxicity of [^{14}C]styrene oxide in the isolated perfused rat liver. J Pharmacol Exp Ther 211:207–212
Wagner JG, DiSanto AR, Gillispie WR, Albert KS (1981) Reversible metabolism and pharmacokinetics. Application to prednisone-prednisolone. Res Commun Chem Pathol Pharmacol 32:387–405
Watari N, Iwai M, Kaneniwa N (1983) Pharmacokinetic study of the fate of acetaminophen and its conjugates. J Pharmacokinet Biopharm 11:245–272
Watkins JB, Klaassen CD (1983) Chemically-induced alteration of UDP-glucuronic acid concentration in rat liver. Drug Metab Dispos 11:37–40
Weisiger RA (1985) Dissociation from albumin: a potentially rate-limiting step in the clearance of substances. Proc Natl Acad Sci USA 82:1563–1567
Weisiger RA, Mendel CA, Cavalieri RR (1986) The hepatic sinusoid is not well-stirred: estimation of the degree of axial mixing by analysis of lobular concentration gradients formed during uptake of thyroxine by the perfused rat liver. J Pharm Sci 75:233–237
Whitsett JL, Dayton PG, McNay TL (1971) The effect of hepatic blood flow on the hepatic removal rate of oxyphenbutazone in the dog. J Pharmacol Exp Ther 177:246–255
Wilkinson GR (1987) Clearance approaches in pharmacology. Pharmacol Rev 39: 1–47
Wilkinson GR, Shand DG (1975) Commentary. A physiological approach to hepatic drug clearance. Clin Pharmacol Ther 18:377–390
Winkler W, Keiding S, Tygstrup N (1973) Clearance as a quantitative measure of structure and function. In: Paumgartner P, Preisig R (eds) The liver: quantitative aspects of structure and function. Karger, Basel, pp 144–155

Winkler K, Bass L, Keiding S, Tygstrup N (1974) The effect of hepatic perfusion on the assessment of kinetic constants. In: Lundquist F, Tygstrup N (eds) Regulation of hepatic metabolism. Munksgaard, Copenhagen, pp 797–807

Wolkoff AW, Goresky CA, Sellin J, Gatmaitan S, Arias IM (1979) Role of ligandin in transfer of bilirubin from plasma into liver. Am J Physiol 236:E638–G648

Wosilait WD, Garten S (1972) Computation of unbound anticoagulant values in plasma. Res Commun Chem Pathol Pharmacol 3:285–291

Xu X, Pang KS (1989) Hepatic modeling of metabolite kinetics in sequential and parallel pathways: salicylamide and gentisamide metabolism in perfused rat liver. J Pharmacokinet Biopharm 17:645–671

Xu X, Tang BK, Pang KS (1990) Sequential metabolism of salicylamide exclusively to gentisamide-5-glucuronide and not gentisamide sulfate conjugates in the single pass in situ perfused rat liver. J Pharmacol Exp Ther 253:965–973

Xu X, Selick P, Pang KS (1993) Nonlinear protein binding and heterogeneity: effect of drug metabolizing enzyme on hepatic drug removal. J Pharmacokinet Biopharm 21:43–74

Zhao Y, Snel CAW, Mulder GJ, Pang KS (1993) Glutathione conjugation of bromosulfophthalein in perfused rat liver: studies with the multiple indicator dilution technique. Drug Metab Dispos 21:1070–1078

CHAPTER 11

Regulation of Drug Conjugate Processing by Hepatocellular Transport Systems

M. VORE

A. Introduction

The present chapter will discuss how polar drugs and/or drug conjugates move across the plasma membrane of the hepatocyte, including movement across the basolateral domain between the plasma and the hepatocyte and across the canalicular domain between the hepatocyte and the bile canaliculus. Since most drug conjugates are anions, i.e., sulfate, glucuronide, or glutathione conjugates, this review will focus on the transport properties of organic anions. Discussion of taurocholate is also essential, since characterization of the transport of this important bile acid has provided the basis for much of our understanding of vectorial transport across the hepatocyte from plasma to bile. Key questions regarding the processing of drug conjugates have included: what determines whether a conjugate formed in the hepatocyte moves across the canalicular domain and is excreted in bile, or moves across the basolateral domain to be excreted in the urine? Is this determined by the presence and substrate specificity of transporters in each membrane domain? How are drug conjugates which are formed in other tissues, such as the intestine, taken up by the liver? Recent advances have provided answers to some of these questions, and the tools to answer the remaining questions are rapidly becoming available.

Like other epithelial cells, the hepatocyte plasma membrane consists of morphologically and functionally distinct domains. Figure 1 shows a schematic view of the hepatocyte plasma membrane domains, the bile canaliculus, and associated transport systems. The *sinusoidal* domain of the hepatocyte is in contact with the intercellular space and represents 37% of the total cell surface. The *lateral* domain accounts for 50% of the membrane surface area and abuts the adjacent cell's plasma membrane. The *canalicular* domain borders the canalicular space and represents the final 13% of the plasma membrane. The sinusoidal–lateral and canalicular domain of the hepatocyte plasma membrane are analogous to the basolateral and apical domains, respectively, of other epithelial cells. Also shown in Fig. 1 are the numerous fenestrations (about 0.1 μm in diameter) in the endothelial cells lining the sinusoid which permit the exchange of albumin and lipoproteins between the sinusoidal space and the space of Disse. Drugs which are tightly bound to albumin thus have direct access to the villous basolateral domain,

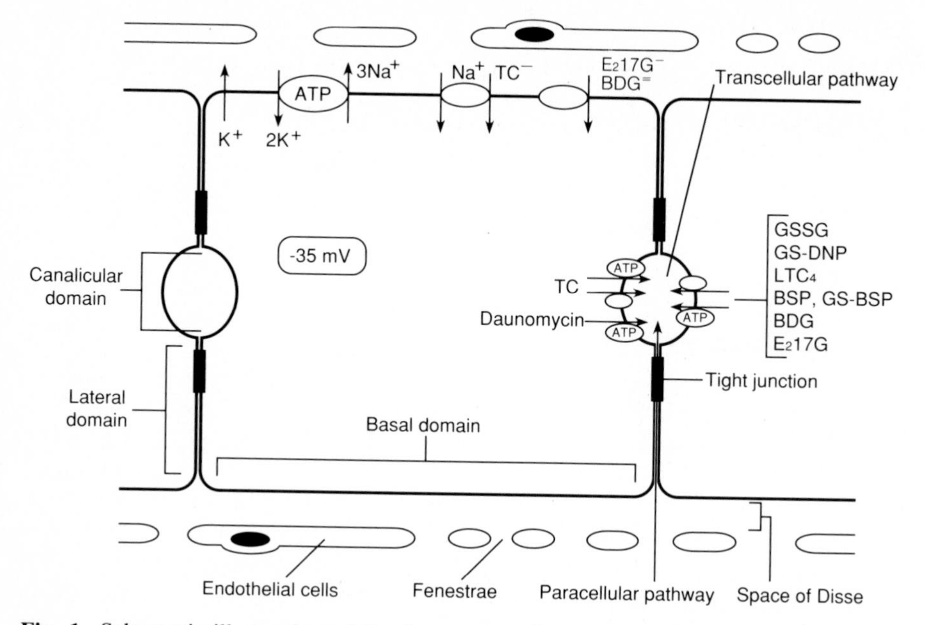

Fig. 1. Schematic illustration of the hepatocyte demonstrating the basal, lateral and canalicular domains of the plasma membrane and transport mechanisms associated with these domains. Endothelial cells lining the sinusoid separate the single layer of hepatocytes from the blood. Fenestrations permit entry of large molecules, such as albumin, and associated drugs to the space of Disse and the plasma membrane. Fluids and small molecules move via the paracellular pathway across the tight junction which separates bile from plasma. Larger molecular weight solutes move across the basolateral and canalicular membranes via the transcellular pathway. Na^+, K^+ATPase extrudes three Na^+ atoms in exchange for two K^+ atoms, which, coupled with a K^+ conductance pathway, creates both an electrical (intracellular negative membrane potential of about 35 mV) and chemical gradient for Na^+, which provides the driving force for the uptake of taurocholate (*TC*). Carrier-mediated, potential-sensitive transport of the non-bile acid organic anions bilirubin diglucuronide (*BDG*) and estradiol-17β(β-D-glucuronide (*$E_2 17G$*) has been demonstrated in the basolateral membrane. TC is secreted into the canaliculus by *ATP*- and voltage-dependent mechanisms. ATP-dependent transport of *daunomycin* across the canalicular plasma membrane via P-glycoprotein has been demonstrated. ATP-dependent transport of several nonbile acid organic anions, i.e., oxidized glutathione (*GSSG*), the glutathione conjugate of 2,4-dinitrobenzene (*GS-DNP*), leukotriene C_4 (*LTC_4*), bromosulfophthalein (*BSP*), BDG, and $E_2$17G, has also been demonstrated in canalicular membranes

making possible their uptake into the hepatocyte. A tight junction separates fluid in the canalicular lumen from that in the extracellular and sinusoidal space; the permeability of this tight junction is intermediate in nature, so that fluid and cationic electrolytes move easily across this barrier, but not compounds of higher molecular weight. There is no evidence for the movement of drugs or their conjugates across the tight junctions via this paracellular pathway under normal physiologic conditions. Rather, these substances must traverse the cell, crossing both the basolateral and canalicular domains of the plasma membrane via the transcellular pathway.

The development of techniques for the preparation of highly purified basolateral and canalicular membrane vesicles made possible the characterization of transport systems in these two major surface domains and showed that these domains are highly specialized, with distinct transport systems localized specifically to the basolateral or canalicular domain (MEIER 1988). Discovery of the exclusive localization of functional Na^+K^+ adenosine triphosphatase (Na^+, K^+-ATPase) to the basolateral domain (SZTUL et al. 1987) was particularly important, since the extrusion of three Na^+ atoms in exchange for two K^+ atoms by this enzyme generates the chemical gradient for Na^+ (extracellular concentration, approximately 140 mM; intracellular concentration, approximately 12 mM). A high basolateral membrane K^+ conductance is largely responsible for the intracellular negative membrane potential difference of −35 mV (BOYER et al. 1992). It is the electrochemical gradient for Na^+ which drives many of the transport systems localized in the basolateral domain, such as the Na^+–taurocholate cotransport system described below, Na^+–H^+ exchange, and the uptake of amino acids such as alanine. Transport systems localized to the canalicular domain include a potential-dependent, Na^+-independent taurocholate transporter and adenosine triphosphate (ATP)-dependent transporters such as P-glycoprotein and those for taurocholate and organic anions. This functional specialization of the transport systems in the basolateral and canalicular domains is essential for the maintenance of vectorial transport of substrates across the hepatocyte.

B. Transport Across the Basolateral Domain

I. Transport from Plasma into the Hepatocyte

1. Na^+–Taurocholate Cotransport – A Multispecific System

Because bile formation is one of the principal functions of the liver, and secretion of bile acids such as taurocholate is a major determinant of bile flow, the transport of taurocholate across the hepatocyte has been investigated in great detail. The transport of taurocholate across the basolateral domain of the hepatocyte has been shown to be carrier-mediated and dependent on an Na^+ gradient. Studies in vivo in the dog (GLASINOVIC et al. 1975a,b), in the isolated perfused rat liver (REICHEN and PAUMGARTNER 1975, 1976), in isolated rat hepatocytes (ANWER et al. 1976; SCHARSCHMIDT and STEPHENS 1981), and in basolateral membrane vesicles (DUFFY et al. 1983; INOUE et al. 1982a; MEIER et al. 1984) have demonstrated saturable uptake of taurocholate and shown that an $Na^+_{out} > Na^+_{in}$ gradient is required for maximal uptake of taurocholate. These data all indicate that the uptake of taurocholate is a secondary active transport system, in which the driving force for the uptake of taurocholate against a concentration gradient is derived from the transmembrane Na^+ gradient. A photoreactive diazirine derivative of taurocholate was used initially to identify a 48- to 50-kDa glycoprotein in basolateral membranes as the putative Na^+–taurocholate cotransporter (VON DIPPE and LEVY 1983; KRAMER et al. 1982; WIELAND et al. 1984). Functional expression cloning of Na^+–taurocholate cotransport in *Xenopus* oocytes has recently identified a cDNA which codes for a glycosylated protein with a molecular weight of 39–41 kDa (HAGENBUCH et al. 1991). The expressed taurocholate transport was strictly dependent on the presence of extracellular Na^+ and was inhibited significantly by taurochenodeoxycholate, bromosulfophthalein (BSP), cholate, and the anionic transport inhibitors bumetanide and probenecid, but not by taurodehydrocholate. The expressed Na^+–taurocholate cotransport system was saturable with a K_m of $25 \mu M$, identical to that reported in isolated hepatocytes (FRIMMER and ZIEGLER 1988) and basolateral plasma membrane vesicles (ZIMMERLI et al. 1989). Sequence and hydropathy analysis revealed five potential *N*-linked glycosylation sites and seven putative transmembrane-spanning domains.

Early studies had suggested that a broad range of amphipathic compounds such as cyclic oligopeptides (e.g., phalloidin, somatostatin analogs), neutral steroids such as ouabain and progesterone, and other drugs were also substrates of the Na^+-coupled taurocholate transport system (FRIMMER and ZIEGLER 1988). ZIMMERLI et al. (1989) rigorously tested the ability of bile acids, steroids and steroid conjugates, drugs, non-bile acid organic anions, and phalloidin to inhibit Na^+–taurocholate cotransport in basolateral plasma membrane vesicles. Many compounds were found to inhibit taurocholate uptake, with no clear structure–activity relationship. Thus, progesterone was a competitive inhibitor, whereas ouabain had no effect; glucuronide and sulfate conjugates of estradiol and estrone at the 3-OH position were effective inhibitors, with estradiol-3-sulfate showing competitive inhibition, whereas estradiol-17-glucuronide was inactive in this regard. Among the drugs tested, both anionic drugs (furosemide, indomethacin, probenecid) and cations (morphine, lidocaine, verapamil) inhibited transport. Detailed kinetic analysis showed that verapamil, furosemide, bumetanide, and phalloidin were competitive inhibitors, whereas BSP, cyclosporin A, and 4,4′-diisothiocyanostilbene-2,2′-disulfonate (DIDS), a classic organic anion transport inhibitor, were noncompetitive inhibitors. These authors concluded that the Na^+–taurocholate cotransport system is in fact a multispecific system, capable of transporting a wide range of drugs and drug conjugates (i.e., estradiol-3-sulfate). Ideally, the transport properties of these putative substrates should be examined in transfected cell lines to establish conclusively that they are true substrates and not merely inhibitors of the Na^+–taurocholate cotransporter. BSP has been shown not to be taken up into *Xenopus* oocytes expressing the Na^+–taurocholate transporter

(JACQUEMIN et al. 1991), consistent with its noncompetitive inhibition of Na^+–taurocholate cotransport in basolateral membrane vesicles.

2. Na^+-Independent Transport Systems

The hepatocellular transport characteristics of a number of non-bile acid organic anions, particularly BSP and bilirubin, have been studied extensively (BERK et al. 1987; WOLKOFF et al. 1987). Carrier-mediated uptake has been demonstrated in the isolated perfused liver, isolated hepatocytes, basolateral membrane vesicles and, most recently, in *Xenopus* oocytes expressing the BSP-uptake system (JACQUEMIN et al. 1991). BSP uptake is independent of Na^+ (BERK et al. 1987) and other cations. However, WOLKOFF et al. (1987) found that in the presence of bovine serum albumin, omission of Cl^- markedly inhibited the uptake of BSP in cultured hepatocytes and the uptake of bilirubin in the isolated perfused rat liver. BSP uptake was not directly coupled to Cl^-, but in the presence of albumin, Cl^- appeared to modulate the affinity of BSP for the transporter (MIN et al. 1991). These studies also showed that BSP uptake was stimulated by an inside-to-outside OH^- gradient, suggestive of a BSP–OH^- exchange or BSP–H^+ cotransport system. The chloride-dependent BSP-uptake system has recently been cloned and functionally expressed in *Xenopus* oocytes (JACQUEMIN et al. 1991, 1992). A 2.8-kb cDNA clone was identified that codes for a 670-amino acid peptide containing three glycosylation sites; in vitro translation experiments yielded a 70-kDa glycoprotein. (It should be noted that the molecular weight of this glycoprotein is quite different from those of other candidate BSP or bilirubin transporters of 37 kDa (TIRIBELLI et al. 1990) and 55 kDa (BERK et al. 1987; WOLKOFF and CHUNG 1980; GOESER et al. 1990).) Interestingly, the chloride dependency for BSP uptake in the presence of albumin was lost when albumin was omitted from the incubation media. No other driving force for the uptake of BSP could be identified in this oocyte expression system. The expressed BSP-uptake system also markedly stimulated the Na^+-independent uptake of taurocholate. This finding is consistent with early results in isolated hepatocytes which identified a saturable Na^+-independent uptake system for taurocholate that is competitively inhibited by BSP and bilirubin (ANWER and HEGNER 1978). Bilirubin, DIDS, and indocyanine green were potent inhibitors of BSP uptake, suggesting that these anions are also substrates of the BSP-transport system (JACQUEMIN et al. 1991).

The transport of bilirubin diglucuronide (ADACHI et al. 1990) and estradiol-17β-glucuronide (E_217G; VORE and HOFFMAN 1993) have been characterized in basolateral membrane vesicles. Both substrates demonstrated saturable uptake that was independent of sodium and inhibited by BSP. The uptake of bilirubin diglucuronide showed strong potential sensitivity in that creation of an inside-negative membrane potential inhibited its uptake. Similarly, the transport of E_217G was markedly stimulated by an inside positive membrane potential. These results, together with the inability to identify a driving force for the transport of these non-bile acid organic anions across the basolateral membrane, suggest that they are taken up as anions by simple carrier-mediated facilitated diffusion.

II. Transport from Hepatocyte to Plasma

How glucuronide, sulfate, and glutathione conjugates, formed in the hepatocyte but excreted in the urine, move across the basolateral membrane from hepatocyte to blood has been a long-standing question. Does this occur by simple diffusion down a concentration gradient, are there transporters which function primarily to mediate the efflux of these organic anions, or are the transporters involved in the uptake of organic anions bidirectional? In view of the polarity of these conjugates, significant diffusion seems unlikely. Evidence for bidirectional transport has been obtained in basolateral membrane vesicles, where both Na^+–taurocholate cotransport (MEIER et al. 1984) and the uptake of bilirubin diglucuronide (ADACHI et al. 1990) showed *trans* stimulation, i.e., incorporation of unlabeled substrate in the vesicles increased the rate of uptake of labeled substrate from the incubation media. In studies with E_217G (VORE and HOFFMAN 1993), we were unable to demonstrate *trans* stimulation of uptake. The phenomenon of *trans* stimulation is attributed to the more rapid reorientation of loaded versus unloaded carrier in the membrane, so that addition of substrate at the opposite (*trans*) face of the membrane increases the rate of reorientation of carrier and thus the number of carriers available for transport of substrate from the *cis* face (STEIN 1990). These observations indicate that both the multispecific Na^+–taurocholate cotransport system and the non-bile acid organic anion transport system are capable of transporting substrate bidirectionally. However, there is still much to be learned regarding the nature of the carrier and how it functions under physiologic conditions. If the non-bile acid organic anions are transported as the charged species, which is most likely, then their efflux would certainly be facilitated by the intracellular negative membrane potential, suggesting that the net movement would be their efflux. However, we do not know whether the substrate-binding sites at the inner and outer face of the membrane are similar or differ with respect to substrate specificities and affinities. We also do not know which conformation of the carrier has the lowest free energy, i.e., is the lowest free energy conformation with the substrate-binding site facing the plasma, ready to transport substrate (e.g., bilirubin) into the liver, or is the lowest free energy conformation one in which the binding site is facing the intracellular milieu, ready to export metabolites formed by the hepatocyte? These are intriguing questions; however, in view of the difficulty in obtaining large quantities of basolateral membrane vesicles, and the lipophilicity and nonspecific binding of many of the substrates, they will not be easily answered.

C. Transport Across the Canalicular Domain

I. Transport Systems from the Hepatocyte into Bile

The liver metabolizes many endogenous and exogenous compounds, usually by oxidation followed by conjugation with glucuronic acid or glutathione, to compounds that are readily excreted in bile. Carrier-mediated transport of these conjugates into bile has long been accepted, based on the demonstration of saturability of transport and competitive inhibition by other substrates (KLAASSEN and WATKINS 1984). However, the features of a compound which make it a substrate for biliary secretion, other than that it must be an amphipathic compound of high molecular weight, have not been well defined. The ability to characterize the transport of glucuronide and glutathione conjugates in canalicular membrane vesicles and the subsequent discovery of ATP-dependent transport systems for these substrates has made it possible to begin to understand the mechanisms of transport, the substrate specificities of the transporters, and their regulation. This section will review the three major ATP-dependent transporter systems and the voltage-dependent transport systems identified in canalicular membranes.

1. P-Glycoprotein

The problem of multidrug resistance (MDR), in which tumors are intrinsically resistant or develop resistance to a broad range of cancer chemotherapeutic agents such as *Vinca* alkaloids, anthracyclines, colchicine, epipodophyllotoxins, and actinomycin D, provided the impetus for the discovery of the first ATP-dependent transporter in canalicular membranes (GOTTESMAN and PASTAN 1988; RONINSON 1992). Early descriptions of the MDR phenotype noted an increased energy-dependent efflux of these drugs associated with increased expression of a 170-kDa glycoprotein termed P-glycoprotein (DANÖ 1973; JULIANO and LING 1976). P-glycoprotein was identified as a product of MDR genes, originally identified as transcribed DNA sequences of unknown nature which were amplified in resistant cell lines (RONINSON et al. 1986; GROS et al. 1986). The ATP-dependent efflux of drugs via P-glycoprotein was soon shown to be the major mechanism for MDR (RIORDAN et al. 1985; UEDA et al. 1987). P-glycoproteins are encoded by a small family of *mdr* genes with two human genes (*MDR1* and *MDR2*) and three murine equivalents (*mdr1*, *mdr2*, and *mdr3*). Transfection of *MDR1*, *mdr1*, or *mdr3*, but not of *MDR2* or *mdr2*, genes into sensitive cells conferred drug resistance (UEDA et al. 1987; ROTHENBERG AND LING 1989). The functions of products of *MDR2* or *mdr2* remain unknown. Human

MDR1 cDNA encodes a 1280-amino acid protein consisting of two halves with a high sequence homology; the amino acid sequences in each half predict six membrane-spanning domains and an ATP-binding domain (GOTTESMAN and PASTAN 1988). AMBUDKAR et al. (1992) recently showed that partially purified P-glycoprotein catalyzes substrate-stimulated ATP hydrolysis when reconstituted in an artificial membrane with vinblastine and doxorubicin as the most potent substrates. Slot-blot analysis of total RNA from normal human tissues using an *MDR1* cDNA probe showed the greatest expression in the adrenal medulla and cortex, with intermediate expression in the colon, small intestine, kidney, and liver (FOJO et al. 1987). CHIN et al. (1989) subsequently showed that *MDR2* is expressed primarily in liver. Immunocytochemical studies using MRK16, an anti-human P-glycoprotein monoclonal mouse antibody that recognizes an external epitope of all mdr gene products, localized hepatic P-glycoprotein to the canalicular membrane (THIEBAULT et al. 1987). KAMIMOTO et al. (1989) subsequently characterized ATP-dependent transport of daunomycin in rat liver canalicular membrane vesicles. ATP-dependent uptake of daunomycin into canalicular vesicles followed Michaelis-Menten kinetics (Table 1), was not present in basolateral membrane vesicles, and was inhibited by MDR substrates such as vinblastine, vincristine, and adriamycin, but not by DIDS or the physiologically relevant bile acids such as taurocholate. These data indicate

Table 1. Comparison of adenosine triphosphate-dependent transport in canalicular liver plasma membranes among different substrates

Substrate	K_m (μM)	V_{max} (pmol/mg per min)[a]	References
Taurocholate	2.1	724	STIEGER et al. (1992)
Taurocholate	7.5	N.R.	MÜLLER et al. (1991)
Taurocholate	26	450	NISHIDA et al. (1991)
Taurocholate	47	810	ADACHI et al. (1991a)
GS-DNP	4	180	KOBAYASHI et al. (1990)
GS-DNP	71	340	AKERBOOM et al. (1991)
LTC_4	0.25	N.R.	ISHIKAWA et al. (1990)
LTD_4	1.5	N.R.	ISHIKAWA et al. (1990)
LTE_4 NAC	5.2	N.R.	ISHIKAWA et al. (1990)
NP-G	20	60	KOBAYASHI et al. (1991)
$E_2$17G	75	598	VORE and HOFFMAN (1992)
BSP	31	33 000	NISHIDA et al. (1992b)
BDG	71	51 000	NISHIDA et al. (1992a)
Daunomycin	49	1 700	KAMIMOTO et al. (1989)

GS-DNP, 2,4-dinitrobenzene-glutathione: NP-G, *p*-nitrophenyl glucuronide; BSP, bromosulfophthalein; $E_2$17G, estradiol-17β(β-D-glucuronide); BDG, bilirubin diglucuronide; LT, leukotriene; LTE_4 NAC, N-acetylleukotriene E_4; N.R., not reported.

[a] V_{max} values were all determined at 37°C. Data reported as pmol/mg per 20 s are expressed as pmol/mg per min for comparative purposes.

that in the rat, and possibly in man, canalicular P-glycoprotein functions as an ATP-dependent transporter with broad specificity for lipophilic, mainly cationic compounds, but not for bile acids or non-bile acid organic anions.

Recent interest has addressed the possible role of *mdr2* and *MDR2* in liver in the transport of endogenous substrates or other xenobiotics into bile. BUSCHMAN et al. (1992) were able to produce antibodies specific for the three P-glycoproteins in mouse encoded by *mdr1*, *mdr2*, and *mdr3* (Mdr1, Mdr2, and Mdr3, respectively), and showed that Mdr2 was present at high levels in canalicular, but not sinusoidal, membrane vesicles from mouse liver. Mdr3 was also expressed in canalicular membranes, but at much lower levels, whereas Mdr1 could not be detected. Mdr3, but not Mdr2, was labeled by [^{125}I]-iodoarylazidoprazosin, a photoactivatable analog which binds to the same site of P-glycoprotein as azidopine (GREENBERGER et al. 1991). Assuming that the distribution of these P-glycoproteins is similar in rat and mouse, these data suggest that Mdr3 is responsible for the transport of daunomycin in rat canalicular membranes, as described by KAMIMOTO et al. (1989). However, the function of Mdr2, the major form expressed in canalicular membranes from normal tissue, remains a mystery. Potential substrates include xenobiotics, perhaps alkaloids present in the diet, or endogenous metabolites such as bilirubin mono- and diglucuronides. Suggestions that bilirubin and/or its conjugates could be endogenous substrates of P-glycoprotein have come from observations in phase I clinical trials in which nontoxic inhibitors of P-glycoprotein have been tested for their ability to reverse MDR by inhibiting P-glycoprotein-mediated efflux of chemotherapeutic agents. In one such study, cyclosporine, an inhibitor of P-glycoprotein, was combined with etoposide; the dose-limiting toxicity of this regimen was hyperbilirubinemia, which was highly correlated with cyclosporine levels (YAHANDA et al. 1992). However, cyclosporine also inhibits taurocholate transport in basolateral and canalicular membranes (MOSELEY et al. 1990) and may simply be a nonselective inhibitor of all of the ATP-dependent transporters in canalicular membranes. NISHIDA et al. (1992a) have shown that the ATP-dependent transport of bilirubin diglucuronide in canalicular membrane vesicles is not inhibited by doxorubicin, a substrate of P-glycoprotein. The disparity between transport studies in canalicular membranes from rat liver and results from clinical trials may be due to significant species differences in the substrate specificities and/or forms of P-glycoprotein between rat and humans. Recent studies by GOSLAND et al. (1993), however, indicate that certain organic anions are substrates for P-glycoprotein. These authors used a human sarcoma cell line, MESSA, and its MDR variant, DX5, to show that $E_2$17G reversed resistance in the DX5 cells to classic MDR substrates such as vinblastine, etoposide and taxol. In the presence of $E_2$17G, DX5 cells accumulated the same amount of ^{3}H-vinblastine as did the MESSA cells. Conversely, DX5 cells accumulated only about 30% as much ^{3}H-$E_2$17G as did MESSA cells, but this defect was reversed in the presence of vinblastine, etoposide or taxol. In contrast, estriol-3-glucuronide did not modulate resistance to MDR substrates. Further structure-activity relationship studies showed that glucuronide conjugates of the steroid D-ring, such as estriol-16α-glucuronide, modulated resistance to MDR, whereas glucuronide conjugates of the steroid A-ring lacked this effect (VORE et al. 1993). Vinblastine and etoposide also significantly inhibited ATP-dependent transport of ^{3}H-$E_2$17G in rat canalicular membrane vesicles. Further studies are clearly needed to sort out the number of ATP-dependent transporters in canalicular membranes and their substrate specificities.

2. Bile Acid Transport Systems

a) Adenosine Triphosphate-Dependent Transport

Shortly after the discovery of ATP-dependent transport of daunomycin in canalicular membrane vesicles, the ATP-dependent transport of taurocholate in these membranes was independently reported by several groups (NISHIDA et al. 1991; ADACHI et al. 1991a; MÜLLER et al. 1991; STIEGER et al. 1992). ATP-dependent taurocholate uptake followed Michaelis-Menten kinetics with an apparent K_m for taurocholate ranging from 2.1 (STIEGER et al. 1992) to 47 μM (ADACHI et al. 1991a; Table 1) and an apparent K_m for ATP of about 0.7 mM (NISHIDA et al. 1991; MÜLLER et al. 1991), although a K_m of 64 μM was reported by ADACHI et al. (1991a). Other nucleotides – guanosine triphosphate (GTP), uridine triphosphate (UTP), and cytidine triphosphate (CTP) – and nonhydrolyzable ATP analogs such as adenosine 5′-(γ-thio)triphosphate did not stimulate taurocholate transport significantly (NISHIDA et al. 1991; STIEGER et al. 1992). Similarly, vanadate, which blocks hydrolysis of the terminal phosphate bond of ATP, also inhibited ATP-dependent uptake of taurocholate, although the sensitivity to inhibition varied among the different laboratories, from 50% inhibition by 5 μM vanadate (MÜLLER et al. 1991) to 20% inhibition by 100 μM vanadate (STIEGER et al. 1992). These data all indicate the importance of hydrolysis of the terminal phosphate bond in mediating transport; however, there is as yet no information on how the hydrolysis of ATP is linked to transport of taurocholate.

Inhibition studies (Table 2) have shown that the conjugated tri- and dihydroxy bile acids are the most potent inhibitors of ATP-dependent taurocholate transport, whereas dehydrocholate and its taurine conjugate had no effect in the same concentration range. Daunomycin, a substrate of P-glycoprotein, did not significantly inhibit taurocholate transport. Neither reduced nor oxidized glutathione inhibited ATP-dependent taurocholate transport, whereas the glutathione conjugates leukotriene C_4 (LTC_4), 2,4-dinitrophenyl-glutathione (GS-DNP), and BSP-glutathione (GS-BSP) were able to inhibit taurocholate transport by up to 50%. As discussed further below, taurocholate was shown to be a competitive inhibitor of ATP-dependent GS-DNP transport, albeit with a very high K_i of 0.61 mM (AKERBOOM et al. 1991). In view of the lack of inhibition of taurocholate

Table 2. Effects of organic compounds on adenosine triphosphate-dependent taurocholate transport in canalicular membrane vesicles

Compound (μM)	Taurocholate Transport (% control)
Bile salts	
Cholate (10)	31 ± 5[a]
Glycocholate (10)	22 ± 7[a]
Cholate (20)	77 ± 13[b]
Taurocholate (20)	39 ± 2[b]
Chenodeoxycholate (20)	46 ± 6[b]
Taurochenodeoxycholate (20)	20 ± 4[b]
Deoxycholate (20)	74 ± 8[b]
Taurodeoxycholate (20)	38 ± 3[b]
Ursodeoxycholate (20)	85 ± 6[b]
Tauroursodeoxycholate (20)	55 ± 4[b]
Dehydrocholate (50)	92 ± 9[b]
Taurodehydrocholate 50	95 ± 7[b]
Other compounds	
GSH (1000)	97 ± 6[b]
GSSG (1000)	97 ± 7[b]
GSSG (3000)	130 ± 13[a]
BSP (10)	50 ± 8[b]
BSP (25)	18 ± 3[a]
GS-BSP (25)	58 ± 2[a]
GS-DNP (25)	102 ± 14[a]
GS-DNP (100)	37 ± 5[c]
LTC_4 (10)	45 ± 4[b]
Bilirubin diglucuronide (10)	74 ± 8[a]
Daunomycin (25)	86 ± 11[a]
Daunomycin (100)	84 ± 13[b]

Data are taken from the indicated sources. The concentration of [^{3}H]taurocholate used in each study is given in parenthesis.
[a] Nishida et al. (1991; 5 μM taurocholate).
[b] Stieger et al. (1992; 2.1 μM taurocholate).
[c] Akerboom et al. (1991; 1 μM taurocholate).
GSH, glutathione; GSSG, glutathione disulfide; BSP, bromosulfophthalein; GS-BSP, bromosulfophthalein glutathione; GS-DNP, 2,4-dinitrophenyl glutathione; LT, leukotriene.

transport by GS-DNP in studies by Nishida et al. (1991), GS-DNP seems at best to be a weak inhibitor of taurocholate transport. Addition of filipin (10–50 μg/mg protein) completely inhibited ATP-dependent taurocholate transport, but had no effect on that of daunomycin or BSP, indicating that these latter compounds are not substrates of the taurocholate transport system (Nishida et al. 1991). Based on the observed inhibition patterns, the conjugated di- and trihydroxy bile acids are most likely the optimal substrates of the ATP-dependent taurocholate transport system, whereas the glutathione conjugates may be relatively poor substrates.

Several approaches have been taken to identify the protein(s) involved in the transport of taurocholate across the canalicular membrane. A photoaffinity probe (7,7-azo-3α,12α-dihydroxy-5β-[3β-^{3}H]cholan-24-oyl)-2'-aminoethane-sulfonate (^{3}H-ATC), was used initially be RUETZ et al. (1987) to label a 110-kDa glycoprotein in canalicular membranes; antiserum against this protein inhibited the voltage-dependent transport of taurocholate in reconstituted proteoliposomes (RUETZ et al. 1988). SIPPEL et al. (1990) used a glycocholate affinity column to purify a 100-kDa protein antigenically similar to that of RUETZ et al. (1988). MÜLLER et al. (1991) used two photoaffinity probes, ^{35}S-adenosine 5'-O-(thiotriphosphate) and ^{3}H-ATC, to identify a 110-kDa protein; ATP stimulated the uptake of taurocholate when the purified protein (termed gp110) was incorporated into proteoliposome vesicles. MÜLLER et al. (1991) argue that gp110 and the 110-kDa protein identified by RUETZ et al. (1987) are the same protein and represents the ATP-dependent taurocholate transporter. They also argue that their protein is similar to that of SIPPEL et al. (1990). Studies by Hubbard and colleagues (MARGOLIS et al. 1990), however, have shown that several highly antigenic glycoproteins isolated from canalicular membranes, i.e., HA4 (BARTLES et al. 1985), pp120 (MARGOLIS et al. 1990), and Ca^{2+}/Mg^{2+}-ecto ATPase (LIN and GUIDOTTI 1989), are in fact identical and that the antibodies to the taurocholate transporter (RUETZ et al. 1988; SIPPEL et al. 1990) also cross-react with HA4 (MARGOLIS et al. 1990). In a recent study by SIPPEL et al. (1993), transfection of Ca^{2+}/Mg^{2+}-ecto-ATPase conferred on COS cells de novo synthesis of a 100 kDa polypeptide which was immunoprecipitated by the antibody to purified canalicular bile acid transport protein. Furthermore, COS cells transfected with the ecto-ATPase cDNA showed taurocholate efflux properties similar those seen in canalicular membrane vesicles. A truncated version of the ecto-ATPase which was missing the cytoplasmic tail did not confer bile acid transport activity; inhibition of protein kinase C-mediated phosphorylation of this cytoplasmic tail blocked taurocholate transport activity. These authors were able to dissociate bile acid transport from ATPase activity, but could not determie if the taurocholate efflux was ATP- or voltage-dependent. Although many questions remain regarding the function of this bile acid transporter/ecto-ATPase, such as its role in cells that do not normally transport bile acids and its similarity/identity to cell adhesion molecule (AURIVILLIUS et al. 1990), the ability to confer taurocholate transport activity in a transfected cell line is an exciting advance in the understanding of canalicular bile acid transport.

b) Voltage-Dependent Transport

Initial studies describing taurocholate transport in canalicular membrane vesicles identified a Na^+-independent, voltage-dependent transport system

(INOUE et al. 1984b; MEIER et al. 1984). The uptake of taurocholate in canalicular vesicles occurred into an osmotically sensitive space, followed saturation kinetics and was *trans* stimulated by taurocholate. Furthermore, an inside negative valinomycin-mediated K^+ diffusion potential inhibited taurocholate uptake and stimulated its efflux from canalicular vesicles. The potential-driven efflux of taurocholate was inhibited by DIDS and could be *cis* inhibited and *trans* stimulated by trihydroxy and conjugated dihydroxy bile acids (MEIER et al. 1987). These data provided convincing evidence that the potential-dependent transport of taurocholate was carrier mediated and most likely also transported other physiologically relevant bile acids. As discussed above, RUETZ et al. (1987, 1988) used ^{3}H-ATC to label a 100-kDa glycoprotein in canalicular membranes; antibodies to this glycoprotein inhibited uptake of taurocholate into canalicular, but not basolateral, vesicles and inhibited taurocholate efflux from canalicular vesicles. When the 100-kDa protein was reconstituted into liposomes, taurocholate uptake was inhibited by DIDS, *trans* stimulated by taurocholate, and stimulated by an inside-positive K^+ diffusion potential (RUETZ et al. 1988).

Studies in isolated hepatocyte couplets have also demonstrated voltage-dependent taurocholate secretion into the canalicular space (WEINMAN et al. 1989). In the past few years, the rat isolated-hepatocyte couplet has been developed as a model system for the study of transport in a preparation that secretes substrates and fluid into the canaliculus (GRAF et al. 1984, 1987; SPRAY et al. 1986; WATANABE et al. 1985). WEINMAN et al. (1989) studied the effect of changes in membrane potential on bile secretion, measured by optically determining the size of the canaliculus, in the presence and absence of taurocholate. In the absence of taurocholate, the secretion rate was 2–4 fl/min and did not change when the hepatocyte was hyperpolarized to -110 mV by intracellular current injection. However, in the presence of 50 μM taurocholate, hyperpolarization increased the fluid secretion rate to 19 fl/min. Taurocholate alone had no effect on the membrane potential of -35 mV. These authors concluded that at a resting membrane potential of -35 mV, the hepatocyte could secrete taurocholate into the canaliculus and concentrate it three- to fourfold.

In view of the similarities between the 100- to 110-kDa glycoprotein(s) identified by RUETZ et al. (1987, 1988), SIPPEL et al. (1990), and MÜLLER et al. (1991), questions have arisen regarding the possible identity of the voltage- and ATP-dependent transport systems. In a recent preliminary report, NISHIDA and ARIAS (1992) presented evidence supporting the hypothesis that the ATP- and voltage-dependent systems share a single carrier system. The K_m value for taurocholate for voltage-dependent transport was decreased in the presence of ATP, and the K_m value for ATP for ATP-dependent taurocholate transport was decreased in the presence of a membrane potential. Furthermore, the V_{max} for taurocholate transport in the presence of both ATP and a membrane potential was less than additive to that of either system alone. Both the ATP- and voltage-dependent systems share similar substrate specificities and inhibitors, and the antibody developed by Sippel et al. (1990) against the voltage-dependent transporter also inhibited ATP-dependent transport. In contrast, Kast et al. (1992) argue, also in a preliminary report, that the voltage-dependent and ATP-dependent transport systems are distinct, based on differences in their subcellular distributions. Thus, endoplasmic reticulum and microsomal subfractions showed marked potential-dependent, saturable, and DIDS-sensitive uptake of taurocholate, but no ATP-dependent transport, whereas canalicular membranes, which were contaminated with endoplasmic reticulum, showed both ATP- and potential-dependent taurocholate uptake. When the canalicular membranes were further purified by free-flow electrophoresis, the potential-dependent taurocholate transport cosegregated with the endoplasmic reticulum. These authors conclude that the voltage-dependent transport identified in canalicular membrane preparations is most likely due to the well-recognized contamination with endoplasmic reticulum and that under physiologic conditions, taurocholate is secreted into the canaliculus solely by an ATP-dependent transport system. Na^+-independent transport of taurocholate has been previously described in smooth microsomal fractions and the Golgi apparatus (Simion et al. 1984; Reuben and Allen 1990) and has been postulated to contribute to the vesicular transport of taurocholate (a relatively minor component of taurocholate transport) across the hepatocyte and into bile. Further studies are clearly needed to resolve this apparent conflict. The increased fluid secretion observed in hepatocyte couplets under hyperpolarized conditions in the presence of taurocholate supports the role of potential-dependent taurocholate transport (Weinman et al. 1989); however, this could possibly be attributed to the increased affinity of ATP for the ATP-dependent transport system under hyperpolarized conditions (Nishida and Arias 1992). It may be that the microsomal transport system represents an "immature" form of the transporter which has not yet acquired an ATP-binding domain or subunit.

3. Nonbile Acid Organic Anion Transport Systems

a) Adenosine Triphosphate-Dependent Transport

Discovery of ATP-dependent transport of glutathione and glucuronide conjugates in canalicular membranes of liver quickly followed discovery of ATP-dependent transport of P-glycoprotein substrates in these membranes. Transport of glutathione conjugates in liver was well known; however, as discussed below, the first studies of transport of glutathione conjugates in canalicular vesicles identified a potential-dependent transport system (Inoue et al. 1984a). ATP-dependent transport of oxidized glutathione (GSSG) and of glutathione S-conjugates was first described in erythrocytes (Sristava and Beutler 1969; Kondo et al. 1980; Board 1981), followed by studies demonstrating GSSG-stimulated ATPase activity and ATP-stimulated GS-DNP transport in rat hepatocyte plasma membrane vesicles (Nicotera et al. 1985;

KOBAYASHI et al. 1988; KUNST et al. 1989). Localization of this activity to the canalicular membrane was greatly facilitated by the discovery of a strain of mutant Wistar rats (TR^-) in which the excretion of glutathione conjugates and other non-bile acid organic anions into bile is defective. The biliary excretion of conjugated bilirubin, sulfated and glucuronidated bile acids, sulfate and glucuronide metabolites of epinephrine, GS-BSP, and GS-DNP, but not of cholate or taurocholate, is markedly inhibited in TR^- rats (JANSEN et al. 1985, 1987; OUDE ELFERINK et al. 1989; KITAMURA et al. 1992). The defect is similar to that described in mutant Corriedale sheep (CORNELIUS et al. 1965) and in human subjects with Dubin-Johnson syndrome (ROY CHOWDHURY et al. 1989). Demonstration of ATP-dependent transport of BSP and GS-BSP (KITAMURA et al. 1990), cysteinyl leukotrienes (ISHIKAWA et al. 1990), BSP (NISHIDA et al. 1992b), and bilirubin glucuronide (NISHIDA et al. 1992a) in canalicular membranes from control, but not TR^-, rats soon followed. ATP-dependent transport of daunomycin was not impaired in TR^- rats, and western blots using C219, an antibody which recognizes an internal epitope of all murine P-glycoproteins, showed similar amounts of P-glycoprotein in both control and TR^- rats (KITAMURA et al. 1990). Likewise, ISHIKAWA et al. (1990) showed that C219 did not inhibit the transport of LTC_4, nor did typical substrates of P-glycoprotein, doxorubicin, daunorubicin, and verapamil, although vincristine and vinblastine were effective inhibitors. These data clearly indicated the presence of an ATP-dependent transport system distinct from P-glycoprotein in canalicular membranes.

The substrate specificity of this nonbile acid organic anion ATP-dependent transport system is quite broad. Thus, LTD_4, LTE_4, N-acetyl-LTE_4, and ω-carboxy-*N*-acetyl-LTE_4 also demonstrated ATP-dependent transport, although at rates less than those for LTC_4, and GS-DNP inhibited ATP-dependent LTC_4 transport (ISHIKAWA et al. 1990). Transport of GS-DNP in canalicular membranes was also shown to be dependent on ATP, saturable, and inhibited by other glutathione and glucuronide conjugates (KOBAYASHI et al. 1990; AKERBOOM et al. 1991). GSH (5 mM) did not inhibit the ATP-dependent uptake of 100 μM GS-DNP, whereas GSSG was shown to be a weak (K_i, 0.4 mM) competitive inhibitor. *S*-(*p*-chlorophenacyl)-glutathione and *S*-(2,4-dinitrophenyl)cys-gly inhibited GS-DNP uptake by 43% and 54% respectively, whereas *S*-(2,4-dinitrophenyl)glu-cys had no effect, indicating the importance of the glycine moiety. The ability of a series of glutathione conjugates, e.g., *S*-methyl-, *S*-propyl-, *S*-butyl-, *S*-pentyl-, and *S*-nonylglutathione, to inhibit ATP-dependent GS-DNP transport was shown to increase with increasing chain length, from no inhibition for the *S*-methyl derivative to 81% inhibition for the *S*-nonylglutathione conjugate (KOBAYASHI et al. 1990). *S*-Hexylglutathione and naphthylglucuronide also competitively inhibited GS-DNP transport, with K_i values of 66 and 420 μM respectively (AKERBOOM et al. 1991). *p*-Nitrophenylglucuronide and ebselen glucuronide inhibited ATP-dependent GS-DNP transport, whereas naphthylsulfate, *p*-nitrophenylsulfate, verapamil, and vinblastine had no effect. These data are consistent with the well-established principle that increases in molecular weight and hydrophobicity of the aglycone increase the transport of substrates into bile and that sulfate conjugates are relatively poor substrates for biliary excretion. AKERBOOM et al. (1991) also demonstrated that taurocholate was a weak (K_i, 0.61 mM) competitive inhibitor of GS-DNP transport, consistent with other data showing that taurocholate at high (500 μM), but not low (25–50 μM), concentrations inhibits the transport of BSP and bilirubin glucuronide (NISHIDA et al. 1992a,b). These data suggest that, at best, taurocholate is a poor substrate of the non-bile acid organic anion transport system. Several glucuronide conjugates have also been shown to be transported by ATP-dependent systems in canalicular membranes. KOBAYASHI et al. (1991) were the first to demonstrate directly the ATP-dependent transport of *p*-nitrophenyl glucuronide (NP-G) in canalicular membrane vesicles. GS-DNP (40 μM) and LTC_4 (4.5 μM) completely inhibited the ATP-dependent transport of 40 μM NP-G, whereas testosterone glucuronide and naphthyl glucuronide (40 μM each) inhibited transport by 66% and 33%, respectively. As shown in Table 1, K_m and V_{max} values for NP-G are significantly less than for other substrates of the non-bile acid organic anion transport system. This may be due to its smaller and less hydrophobic aglycone. We have recently described the ATP-dependent transport of $E_2$17G in canalicular membranes (VORE and HOFFMAN 1992); taurocholate (50–100 μM) did not inhibit ATP-dependent $E_2$17G transport, whereas other steroid glucuronides, particularly estriol-16α-glucuronide, were effective inhibitors. NISHIDA et al. (1992a) have recently described the ATP-dependent transport of bilirubin diglucuronide in canalicular membranes; DIDS and GSSG were effective inhibitors, whereas GSH (5 mM) was a weak inhibitor and doxorubicin had no effect on bilirubin diglucuronide ATP-dependent transport. These studies have clearly established the presence of an ATP-dependent transport system which is distinct from P-glycoprotein and the ATP-dependent bile acid transport system and which can transport both mono- and divalent anions. Further studies will be needed to determine whether more than one transporter exists for all of the non-bile acid organic anions. KOBAYASHI et al. (1991) suggest the presence of more than one system based on the differential inhibition by vanadate of ATP-dependent transport of NP-G (38% inhibition by 500 μM vanadate) versus GS-DNP (IC_{50}, approximately 30 μM; KOBAYASHI et al. 1990).

b) Voltage-Dependent Transport

As indicated above, early studies characterizing the transport of GS-DNP in canalicular membrane vesicles identified a potential-dependent system in which an inside-positive valinomycin-induced K^+-diffusion potential stimulated the uptake of GS-DNP (INOUE et al. 1984a). ADACHI et al. (1991b) have also described the potential-dependent transport of bilirubin diglucuronide in canalicular membranes. In their hands, the transport of bilirubin diglucuronide was stimulated by bicarbonate ion, but not by ATP. Voltage-dependent transport of BSP and bilirubin diglucuronide in canalicular membrane vesicles from TR^- rats which lack the ATP-dependent transport system was identified by NISHIDA et al. (1992a,b), suggesting that these two transport systems differ. Although the rapid association of BSP with the canalicular membranes makes determination of its initial uptake rates difficult, the uptake rates of both BSP and bilirubin diglucuronide in the presence of ATP and a positive-inside membrane potential were additive, further supporting the hypothesis that the ATP- and potential-dependent transport systems are distinct. NISHIDA et al. (1992a) suggest that the low level of excretion of non-bile acid organic anions such as bilirubin glucuronides present in TR^- rats is due to transport via the potential-dependent transport system. However, the molecular mechanism of the deficiency in ATP-dependent transport in TR^- rats is not known, so that definitive data identifying the presence of two distinct transport systems for the non-bile acid organic anions awaits discovery and characterization of the proteins involved.

As mentioned earlier, ATP-dependent transport of GSSG and GS-DNP and ATPase activity stimulated by GSSG and other glutathione conjugates have been identified in erythrocytes (BOARD 1981; KONDO et al. 1980, 1987; SHARMA et al. 1990a). The erythrocyte ATPase has been isolated, characterized, and identified as a protein with a subunit molecular weight of 38 kDa (KONDO et al. 1989; SHARMA et al. 1990b). Similar 37- to 38-kDa proteins were found in human (AWASTHI et al. 1991) and rat (ZIMNIAK et al. 1992) liver which cross-reacted with antibody to the human erythrocyte GS-DNP ATPase. When purified, the human liver protein catalyzed the hydrolysis of ATP in the presence of bilirubin ditaurate (a synthetic model analog of bilirubin diglucuronide), the 3-*O*-sulfate- and 3-*O*-glucuronide conjugates of lithocholic acid, GS-DNP, and the 3-*O*- and 17-*O*-glucuronide conjugates of 17β-estradiol (AWASTHI et al. 1991); the ATPase purified from human erythrocytes behaved similarly (SINGHAL et al. 1991). These data suggest that the erythrocyte and liver canalicular membrane proteins are structurally related. AWASTHI et al. (1991) argue that contamination with erythrocytes cannot explain detection of a similar protein in liver, since the membrane homogenate from human liver contained "barely detectable" amounts of hemoglobin. However, contamination with lysed red cell membranes remains a possibility. The molecular weight of this protein (37–38 kDa) is much lower than P-glycoprotein (170 kDa) or any other known ATP-dependent transporter (HIGGINS 1992), so that it is highly unlikely that it functions alone to mediate transport. Since the 37–38 kDa protein was detected in apparently equal amounts in canalicular membranes from control Wistar and TR^- rats (also termed GY mutants), ZIMNIAK et al. (1992) suggest that the 37- to 38-kDa protein functions as the ATPase domain or subunit of a much larger complex and that the defect in TR^- rats resides in other proteins of the complex. Board et al. (1992) have recently shown that ATP-dependent transport of GS-DNP and GSSG in erythrocytes from TR^- rats and humans with Dubin-Johnson syndrome does not differ from that in normal controls, indicating that the transport systems in the erythrocyte and liver are at least functionally distinct. Clearly, much more work is needed to characterize the erythrocyte and canalicular membrane transport systems and to determine whether and how these systems are related to P-glycoprotein.

II. Transport from Bile into the Hepatocyte

Until recently, the transport of glucuronide and glutathione conjugates, substrates for biliary excretion, from the bile back into the hepatocytes had not been considered likely or of importance. However, recent studies have described a hepatic–biliary recycling system for glutathione conjugates and their degradation products that may be critical for determining the hepatic or extrahepatic toxicity of some glutathione conjugates. The preferential secretion of glutathione conjugates into bile (Wahllander and Sies 1979) coupled with the distribution of γ-glutamyltransferase (GGT) and dipeptidases, both membrane-bound ectoenzymes, in the biliary tree (Albert et al. 1961; Castle et al. 1985; Hinchman and Ballatori 1990) provides the opportunity for extensive metabolism of glutathione and its conjugates within the biliary tree. Ballatori et al. (1986a, 1988) have demonstrated differential reabsorption of the products of glutathione metabolism, i.e., glutamate, cysteine, and glycine, from the biliary tree, and the Na^+-dependent uptake of glutamate (Ballatori et al. 1986b) and glycine (Moseley et al. 1988) in rat liver canalicular membranes has also been demonstrated. The degradation of glutathione *S*-conjugates to cysteine conjugates has been thought to occur primarily in the kidney (Meister and Tate 1976; Moldeus et al. 1978; Orrenius et al. 1983), with some occurring in the small intestine (Bakke et al. 1981; Grafstrom et al. 1979). The cysteine conjugates are then thought to be taken up by the liver (Inoue et al. 1982b, 1984c) or kidney (Green and Elce 1975; Hughey et al. 1978), where they are acetylated to form the mercapturic acid. Most of these studies have been carried out in the rat and mouse, which have low levels of hepatic GGT activity relative to the kidney (Hinchman and Ballatori 1990). However, the guinea pig and probably humans have much higher concentrations of hepatic GGT (Hinchman and Ballatori 1990), so that the concentrations of intact GSH and glutathione conjugates in bile are significantly lower in these species. Hinchman et al. (1991) have recently provided convincing evidence that mercapturic acid formation can occur entirely within the liver. These authors compared the metabolism and biliary excretion of 1-chlor-2,4-dinitrobenzene (CDNB) in isolated perfused rat and guinea pig livers and showed that following a low dose ($0.3\,\mu$mol), the rat liver excreted 55% of total biliary metabolites as the glutathione conjugate and 8.2% as the mercapturic acid, whereas guinea pig livers excreted only 4.8% as the glutathione conjugate and 47% as the mercapturate. Retrograde intrabiliary infusion of acivicin, an inhibitor of GGT, markedly inhibited formation of the mercapturate in both the rat and the guinea pig. These data show clearly that biliary secretion of the glutathione conjugate is followed by degradation within the biliary tree, reabsorption of the cysteine conjugate, *N*-acetylation within the hepatocyte, and finally, secretion of the mercapturic acid into the bile. The extent of the hepatic contribution to mercapturate formation is therefore highly dependent on hepatic GGT levels. This model also requires a transport system for the reabsorption of cysteine conjugates. SIMMONS et al. (1992) have recently described systems for transport of cysteine and *S*-(1,2-dichlorovinyl)-L-cysteine (DCVC) in rat liver canalicular membrane vesicles. ^{35}L-Cysteine uptake consisted of both Na^+-dependent and-independent saturable components; DCVC inhibited uptake of L-cysteine noncompetitively. Uptake of ^{35}*S*-DCVC by rat canalicular membrane vesicles was independent of Na^+, saturable, and inhibited by L-cysteine and other amino acids. K_m values for L-cysteine transport systems were 53 and 1300 μM for the Na^+-dependent systems and 207 μM for the Na^+-independent system; STEIN et al. (1988) reported a concentration of 140 μM cysteine in bile, so that the systems described would be functional at physiologic concentrations. The K_m value for DCVC uptake of 155 μM also indicates that this transport system could function in vivo for the uptake of cysteine *S*-conjugates from bile into the hepatocyte.

DUTCZAK and BALLATORI (1992) have also examined the importance of hepatic GGT on the biliary–hepatic recycling of methyl mercury. Methyl mercury is eliminated from the body primarily through biliary excretion, but undergoes extensive enterohepatic recycling (NORSETH and CLARKSON 1971). Methyl mercury is thought to be excreted in bile primarily as a CH_3Hg-GSH complex (DUTCZAK et al. 1991), so that it also could be subject to degradation by GGT and dipeptidases within the biliary tree followed by reabsorption from bile. Intrabiliary administration of acivicin in the guinea pig increased the biliary excretion of ^{203}Hg, primarily as the $CH_3{}^{203}Hg$-GSH complex (DUTCZAK and BALLATORI 1992). Recovery in bile of ^{203}Hg following intrabiliary administration of $CH_3{}^{203}Hg$ complexes with GSH, cysteine, or albumin was much less for $CH_3{}^{203}Hg$ cysteine than for $CH_3{}^{203}Hg$ albumin or [^{14}C] sucrose. Furthermore, preadministration of intrabiliary acivicin markedly increased the recovery of ^{203}Hg in bile following intrabiliary infusion of $CH_3{}^{203}Hg$-GSH, but had no effect on the recovery of ^{203}Hg following similar infusion of $CH_3{}^{203}Hg$ cysteine. These data support the hypothesis that following its excretion into bile, CH_3Hg-GSH is metabolized by GGT and dipeptidases, followed by reabsorption of CH_3Hg cysteine. DUTCZAK et al. (1991) have also demonstrated significant reabsorption of methyl mercury from the gall bladder in the guinea pig, hamster, and macaque monkey. This biliary–hepatic recycling of methyl mercury undoubtedly contributes to the long biologic half-life and toxicity of methyl mercury.

In summary, these latter studies demonstrate vividly the prominent role which hepatic transport plays in the processing of glutathione conjugates. This is particularly important in view of the ability of the glutathione conjugates of many toxic chemicals, such as the haloalkenes, to induce toxic effects in other tissues particularly the kidney (Monks et al. 1990). The extent to which a glutathione *S*-conjugate is transported across the canalicular membrane will determine its exposure to GGT and dipeptidase ectoenzymes which degrade the glutathione moiety, most importantly to the cysteine *S*-conjugates, which following translocation to the kidney can undergo bioactivation by cysteine conjugate β-lyase to nephrotoxic intermediates (Anders et al. 1988; Dekant et al. 1989). Factors which influence activity of the canalicular transporters involved in transport of conjugates both into and from bile, bile flow, and activity of the enzymes of the biliary tree involved in the degradation of glutathione and its conjugates will influence the toxicity of these conjugates. Some such factors are well known, such as the inhibitory effects of pregnancy and estrogens (Vore 1987) and the stimulatory effects of lactation and prolactin (Liu and Vore 1992; Liu et al. 1992; Ganguly et al. 1993) on canalicular transport and bile flow. Important species differences in the distribution and activity of GGT and dipeptidases in the liver versus the kidney (Hinchman and Ballatori 1990) have already been pointed out. However, inadvertant exposure to environmental pollutants or intentional pretreatment with classic enzyme inducers may have unknown or unappreciated effects. Thus, environmental agents such as chlordecone and mirex influence not only enzymes of the mixed-function oxidase system (Fabacher and Hodgson 1976; Kaminsky et al. 1978; Lewandowski et al. 1989), but also inhibit the transport of taurocholate and several conjugates across the liver (Mehendale 1977, 1981; Curtis and Mehendale 1979; Teo and Vore 1990, 1991). Phenobarbital, commonly used to dissect toxic mechanisms based on its ability to induce xenobiotic-metabolizing enzyme systems, also inhibits the biliary excretion of the glucuronide conjugates of morphine, valproic acid, and acetaminophen and other non-bile acid organic anions (Roerig et al. 1974; Watkins and Klaassen 1982; Rudell et al. 1987; Brouwer and Jones 1990; Gregus et al. 1990; Studenberg and Brouwer 1992). Characterization of transport of drug conjugates in basolateral and canalicular membranes has thus answered many questions regarding how these substrates move across the liver, but has also revealed additional layers of complexity regarding the regulation of these transport systems, the interactions of the substrates with enzymes of the biliary tree, and how these factors influence toxic responses.

References

Adachi Y, Roy-Chowdhury J, Roy-Chowdhury N, Kinne R, Tran T, Kobayashi H, Arias IM (1990) Hepatic uptake of bilirubin diglucuronide: analysis by using sinusoidal plasma membrane vesicles. J Biochem 107:749–754

Adachi Y, Kobayashi H, Kurumi Y, Shouji M, Kitano M, Yamamoto T (1991a) ATP-dependent taurocholate transport by rat liver canalicular membrane vesicles. Hepatology 14:655–659

Adachi Y, Kobayashi H, Kurumi Y, Shouji M, Kitano M, Yamamoto T (1991b) Bilirubin diglucuronide transport by rat liver canalicular membrane vesicles: stimulation by bicarbonate ion. Hepatology 14:1251–1258

Akerboom TPM, Narayanaswami V, Kunst M, Sies H (1991) ATP-dependent S-(2,4-dinitrophenyl)glutathione transport in canalicular plasma membrane vesicles from rat liver. J Biol Chem 266:13147–13152

Albert Z, Orlowski M, Szewczuk A (1961) Histochemical demonstration of gamma-glutamyl transpeptidase. Nature 191:767–768

Ambudkar SV, Lelong IH, Zhang JP, Cardarelli CO, Gottesman MM, Pastan I (1992) Partial purification and reconstitution of the human multidrug-resistance pump – characterization of the drug-stimulatable ATP hydrolysis. Proc Natl Acad Sci USA 89:8472–8476

Anders MW, Lash LH, Dekant W, Elfarra AA, Dohn DR (1988) Biosynthesis and biotransformation of glutathione S-conjugates to toxic metabolites. CRC Crit Rev Toxicol 18:311–341

Anwer MS, Hegner D (1978) Effect of Na^+ on bile acid uptake by isolated rat hepatocytes. Hoppe Seylers Z Physiol Chem 359:181–192

Anwer MS, Kroker R, Hegner D (1976) Cholic acid uptake into isolated rat hepatocytes. Hoppe Seylers Z Physiol Chem 357:1477–1486

Aurivillius M, Hanson OC, Lazrek MV, Bock E, Obrink B (1990) The cell adhesion molecule Cell-CAM 105 is an ecto-ATPase and a member of the immunoglobulin superfamily. FEBS Lett 264:267–269

Awasthi YC, Singhal SS, Gupta S, Ahamd H, Zimniak P, Radominska A, Lester R, Sharma R (1991) Purification and characterization of an ATPase from human liver which catalyzes ATP hydrolysis in the presence of the conjugates of bilirubin, bile acids and glutathione. Biochem Biophys Res Commun 175:1090–1096

Bakke JE, Rafter J, Larsen GL, Gustafsson JA, Gustafsson BE (1981) Enterohepatic circulation of the mercapturic acid and cysteine conjugates of propachlor. Drug Metab Dispos 9:525–528

Ballatori N, Jacob R, Boyer JL (1986a) Intrabiliary glutathione hydrolysis – a source of glutamate in bile. J Biol Chem 261:7860–7865

Ballatori N, Moseley RH, Boyer JL (1986b) Sodium gradient-dependent L-glutamate transport is localized to the canaliuclar domain of liver plasma membranes. Studies in rat liver sinusoidal and canalicular membrane vesicles. J Biol Chem 261:6216–6221

Ballatori N, Jacob R, Barrett C, Boyer JL (1988) Biliary catabolism of glutathione and differential reabsorption of its amino acid constituents. Am J Physiol 254: G1–G7

Bartles JR, Braiterman LT, Hubbard AL (1985) Biochemical characterization of domain-specific glycoproteins of the rat hepatocyte plasma membrane. J Biol Chem 260:12792–12802

Berk PD, Potter BJ, Stremmel W (1987) Role of plasma membrane ligand-binding proteins in the hepatocellular uptake of albumin-bound organic anions. Hepatology 7:165–176

Board PG (1981) Transport of glutathione S-conjugates from human erythrocytes. FEBS Lett 124:163–165

Board PG, Nishida T, Gatmaitan Z, Che M, Arias IM (1992) Erythrocyte membrane transport of glutathione conjugates and oxidized glutathione in the Dubin-Johnson syndrome and in rats with hereditary hyperbilirubinemia. Hepatology 15:722–725

Boyer JL, Graf J, Meier PJ (1992) Hepatic transport systems regulating pH_i, cell volume, and bile secretion. Annu Rev Physiol 54:415–438

Brouwer KLR, Jones JA (1990) Altered hepatobiliary disposition of acetaminophen metabolites after phenobarbital pretreatment and renal ligation: evidence for impaired biliary excretion and a diffusional barrier. J Pharmacol Exp Ther 252:657–664

Buschman E, Arceci RJ, Croop JM, Che M, Arias IM, Housman DE, Gros P (1992) *mdr2* encodes P-glycoprotein expressed in the bile canalicular membrane as determined by isoform-specific antibodies. J Biol Chem 267:18093–18099

Castle JD, Cameron RS, Patterson PL, Ma AK (1985) Identification of high molecular weight antigens structurally related to gamma-glutamyl transferase in epithelial tissues. J Membr Biol 87:13–26

Chin JE, Soffir R, Noonan KE, Choi K, Roninson IB (1989) Structure and expression of the human MDR (P-glycoprotein) gene family. Mol Cell Biol 9:3808–3820

Cornelius CE, Arias IM, Osburn BI (1965) Hepatic pigmentation with photosensitivity: a syndrome in Corriedale sheep resembling Dubin-Johnson syndrome in man. J Am Vet Med Assoc 146:709–713

Curtis LR, Mehendale HM (1979) The effects of kepone pretreatment on biliary excretion of xenobiotics in the male rat. Toxicol Appl Pharmacol 47:295–303

Danö K (1973) Active outward transport of daunomycin in resistant Ehrlich ascites tumor cells. Biochim Biophys Acta 323:466–483

Dekant W, Vamvakas S, Anders MW (1989) Bioactivation of nephrotoxic haloalkenes by glutathione conjugation: formation of toxic and mutagenic intermediates by cysteine conjugate β-lyase. Drug Metab Rev 20:43–83

Duffy MC, Blitzer BL, Boyer JL (1983) Direct determination of the driving forces for taurocholate uptake into rat liver plasma membrane vesicles. J Clin Invest 72:1470–1481

Dutczak WJ, Ballatori N (1992) Gamma-glutamyltransferase-dependent biliary-hepatic recycling of methyl mercury in the guinea pig. J Pharmacol Exp Ther 262:619–623

Dutczak WJ, Clarkson RW, Ballatori N (1991) Biliary-hepatic recycling of a xenobiotic: gallbladder absorption of methyl mercury. Am J Physiol 260:G873–G880

Fabacher DL, Hodgson E (1976) Induction of hepatic mixed-function oxidase enzymes in adult and neonatal mice by kepone and mirex. Toxicol Appl Pharmacol 38:71–77

Fojo AT, Ueda K, Slamon DJ, Poplack DG, Gottesman MM, Pastan I (1987) Expression of a multidrug-resistance gene in human tumors and tissues. Proc Natl Acad Sci USA 84:265–269

Frimmer M, Ziegler K (1988) The transport of bile acids in liver cells. Biochim Biophys Acta 947:75–99

Ganguly T, Hyde JF, Vore M (1993) Prolactin increases Na^+/taurocholate cotransport in isolated hepatocytes from postpartum rats and ovariectomized rats. J Pharmacol Exp Ther 267:82–87

Glasinovic JC, Dumont M, Duval M, Erlinger S (1975a) Hepatocellular uptake of bile acids in the dog: evidence for a common carrier-mediated transport system: an indicator dilution study. Gastroenterology 69:973–981

Glasinovic JC, Dumont M, Duval M, Erlinger S (1975b) Hepatocellular uptake of taurocholate in the dog. J Clin Invest 55:419–426

Goeser T, Nakata R, Braly LF, Sosiak A, Campbell CG, Dermietzel R, Novikoff PM, Stockert RJ, Burk RD, Wolkoff AW (1990) The rat hepatocyte membrane organic anion binding protein is immunologically related to the mitochondrial F_1 adenosine triphosphatase β-subunit. J Clin Invest 86:220–227

Gosland M, Tsuboi C, Hoffman T, Goodin G, Vore M (1993) Estradiol-17β glucuronide: an inducer of cholestasis and a physiological substrate for the multidrug resistance transporter. Cancer Research 53:5382–5385

Gottesman MM, Pastan I (1988) The multidrug transporter, a double-edged sword. J Biol Chem 263:12163–12166

Graf J, Gautam A, Boyer JL (1984) Isolated rat hepatocyte couplets: a primary secretory unit for electrophysiologic studies of bile secretory function. Proc Natl Acad Sci USA 81:6516–6520

Graf J, Henderson RM, Krumpholz B, Boyer JL (1987) Cell membrane and transepithelial voltages and resistances in isolated rat hepatocyte couplets. J Membr Biol 95:241–254

Grafstrom R, Ormstad K, Moldeus P, Orrenius S (1979) Paracetamol metabolism in the isolated perfused rat liver with further metabolism of a biliary paracetamol conjugate by the small intestine. Biochem Pharmacol 28:3573–3579

Green RM, Elce JS (1975) Acetylation of S-substituted cysteines by a rat liver and kidney microsomal N-acetyltransferase. Biochem J 147:283–289

Greenberger LM, Lisanti CJ, Silva JT, Horwitz SB (1991) Domain mapping of the photoaffinity drug-binding sites in P-glycoprotein encoded by mouse *mdr*lb. J Biol Chem 266:20744–20751

Gregus Z, Madhu C, Klaassen CD (1990) Effect of microsomal enzyme inducers on biliary and urinary excretion of acetaminophen metabolites in rats. Decreased hepatobiliary and increased hepatovascular transport of acetaminphen-glucuronide after microsomal enzyme induction. Drug Metab Dispos 18:10–19

Gros P, Croop JM, Roninson IB, Varshavsky A, Houseman DE (1986) Isolation and characterization of DNA sequences amplified in multidrug-resistant hamster cells. Proc Natl Acad Sci USA 83:337–341

Hagenbuch B, Stieger B, Foguet M, Lübbert H, Meier PJ (1991) Functional expression cloning and characterization of the hepatocyte Na^+/bile acid cotransport system. Proc Natl Acad Sci USA 88:10629–10633

Higgins CF (1992) ABC transporters – from microorganisms to man. Annu Rev Cell Biol 8:67–113

Hinchman CA, Ballatori N (1990) Glutathione-degrading capacities of liver and kidney in different species. Biochem Pharmacol 40:1131–1135

Hughey RP, Rankin BB, Elce JS, Curthoys NP (1978) Specificity of a particular rat renal peptidase and its localization along with other enzymes of mercapturic acid synthesis. Arch Biochem Biophys 186:211–217

Inoue M, Kinne R, Tran T, Arias IM (1982a) Taurocholate transport by rat liver sinusoidal membrane vesicles: evidence of sodium cotransport. Hepatology 2:572–579

Inoue M, Okajima K, Morino Y (1982b) Metabolic coordination of liver and kidney in mercapturic acid biosynthesis in vivo. Hepatology 2:311–316

Inoue M, Akerboom TPM, Sies H, Kinne R, Tran T, Arias IM (1984a) Biliary transport of glutathione-S-conjugate by rat liver canalicular membrane vesicles. J Biol Chem 259:4998–5002

Inoue M, Kinne R, Tran T, Arias IM (1984b) Taurocholate transport by rat liver canalicular membrane vesicles. Evidence for the presence of an Na^+-independent transport system. J Clin Invest 73:659–663

Inoue M, Okajima K, Morino Y (1984c) Hepato-renal cooperation in biotransformation, membrane transport, and elimination of cysteine-S-conjugates of xenobiotics. J Biochem (Tokyo) 95:247–254

Ishikawa T, Müller M, Klünemann C, Schaub T, Keppler D (1990) ATP-dependent primary active transport of cysteinyl leukotrienes across liver canalicular membrane. J Biol Chem 265:19279–19286

Jacquemin E, Hagenbuch B, Stieger B, Wolkoff AW, Meier PJ (1991) Expression of the hepatocellular chloride-dependent sulfobromophthalein uptake system in xenopus laevis oocytes. J Clin Invest 88:2146–2149

Jacquemin E, Hagenbuch B, Stieger B, Wolkoff AW, Meier PJ (1992) Cloning and expression of a cDNA encoding the chloride dependent sulfobromophthalein (BSP) uptake system of rat liver. Hepatology 16:89A

Jansen PLM, Peters WH, Lamers WH (1985) Hereditary chronic conjugated hyperbilirubinemia in mutant rats caused by defective hepatic anion transport. Hepatology 5:573–579

Jansen PLM, Groothuis GMM, Peters WHM, Meijer DKF (1987) Selective hepatobiliary transport defect for organic anions and neutral steroids in mutant rats with hereditary conjugated hyperbilirubinemia. Hepatology 7:71–76

Juliano RL, Ling V (1976) A surface glycoprotein modulating drug permeability in Chinese hamster ovary cell mutants. Biochim Biophys Acta 455:152–162

Kamimoto Y, Gatmaitan Z, Hsu J, Arias IM (1989) The function of GP170, the multidrug resistance gene product, in rat liver canalicular membrane vesicles. J Biol Chem 264:11693–11698

Kaminsky LS, Piper LJ, McMartin DN, Fasco MJ (1978) Induction of hepatic microsomal cytochrome P450 by mirex and kepone. Toxicol Appl Pharmacol 43:327–338

Kast C, Stieger B, Meier PJ (1992) Electrogenic and ATP-dependent taurocholate transport exhibit distinct subcellular distributions in rat hepatocytes. Hepatology 16:148A

Klaassen CD, Watkins JB III (1984) Mechanisms of bile formation, hepatic uptake, and biliary excretion. Pharmacol Rev 36:1–67

Kitamura T, Jansen P, Hardenbrook C, Kamimoto Y, Gatmaitan Z, Arias IM (1990) Defective ATP-dependent bile canalicular transport of organic anions in mutant (TR^-) rats with conjugated hyperbilirubinemia. Proc Natl Acad Sci USA 87:3557–3561

Kitamura T, Alroy J, Gatmaitan Z, Inoue M, Mikami T, Jansen P, Arias IM (1992) Defective biliary excretion of epinephrine metabolites in mutant (TR^-) rats: relation to the pathogeneisis of black liver in the Dubin-Johnson syndrome and Corriedale sheep with an analogous excretory defect. Hepatology 15:1154–1159

Kobayashi K, Sogame Y, Hayashi K, Nicotera P, Orrenius S (1988) ATP stimulates the uptake of S-dinitrophenylglutathione by rat liver plasma membrane vesicles. FEBS Lett 240:55–58

Kobayashi K, Sogame Y, Hara H, Hayashi K (1990) Mechanism of glutathione S-conjugate transport in canalicular and basolateral rat liver plasma membranes. J Biol Chem 265:7737–7741

Kobayashi K, Komatsu S, Nishi T, Hara H, Hayashi K (1991) ATP-dependent transport for glucuronides in canalicular plasma membrane vesicles. Biochem Biophys Res Commun 176:622–626

Kondo T, Dale GL, Beutler E (1980) Glutathione transport by inside-out vesicles from human erythrocytes. Proc Natl Acad Sci USA 77:6359–6362

Kondo T, Kawakami Y, Taniguchi N, Beutler E (1987) Glutathione disulfide stimulated Mg^{2+} ATPase of human erythrocyte membranes. Proc Natl Acad Sci USA 84:7373–7377

Kondo T, Myamoto K, Gasa S, Taniguchi N, Kawakimi Y (1989) Purification and characterization of glutathione disulfide-stimulated Mg^{++}-ATPase of human erythrocytes. Biochem Biophys Res Commun 162:1–8

Kramer W, Bickel U, Buscher HP, Gerok W, Kurz G (1982) Bile-salt-binding polypeptides in plasma membranes of hepatocytes revealed by photoaffinity labelling. Eur J Biochem 129:13–24

Kunst M, Sies H, Akerboom TPM (1989) ATP-Stimulated uptake of S-(2,4-dinitrophenyl)glutathione by plasma membrane vesicles from rat liver. Biochim Biophys Acta 983:123–125

Lewandowski M, Levi P, Hodgson E (1989) Induction of cytochrome P450 isozymes by mirex and chlordecone. J Biochem Toxicol 4:195–199

Lin S-H, Guidotti G (1989) Cloning and expression of a cDNA coding for a rat liver plasma membrane ecto-ATPase. J Biol Chem 264:14408–14414

Liu Y, Vore M (1992) Prolactin increases transport of taurocholate in the isolated perfused liver and in basolateral and canalicular membranes. Hepatology 16: 149A

Liu Y, Hyde JF, Vore M (1992) Prolactin regulates maternal bile secretory function post partum. J Pharmacol Exp Ther 261:560–566

Margolis RN, Schell MJ, Taylor SI, Hubbard AL (1990) Hepatocyte plasma membrane ecto-ATPase (pp120/HA4) is a substrate for tyrosine kinase activity of the insulin receptor. Biochem Biophys Res Commun 166:562–566
Mehendale HM (1977) Mirex-induced impairment of hepatobiliary function: suppressed biliary excretion of imipramine and sulfobromophthalein. Drug Metab Dispos 5:56–62
Mehendale HM (1981) Onset and recovery from chlordecone- and mirex-induced hepatobiliary dysfunction. Toxicol Appl Pharmacol 58:132–139
Meier PJ (1988) Transport polarity of hepatocytes. Semin Liver Dis 8:293–307
Meier PJ, St Meier-Abt A, Barrett C, Boyer JL (1984) Mechanisms of taurocholate transport in canalicular and basolateral rat liver plasma membrane vesicles. Evidence for an electrogenic canalicular organic anion carrier. J Biol Chem 259:10614–10622
Meier PJ, Meier-Abt A, Boyer JL (1987) Properties of the canalicular bile acid transport system in rat liver. Biochem J 242:465–469
Meister A, Tate SS (1976) Glutathione and related gamma-glutamyl compounds: biosynthesis and utilization. Annu Rev Biochem 45:559–604
Min AD, Johansen KL, Campbell CG, Wolkoff AW (1991) Role of chloride and intracellular pH on the activity of the rat hepatocyte organic anion transporter. J Clin Invest 87:1496–1502
Moldeus P, Jones DP, Ormstad K, Orrenius S (1978) Formation and metabolism of a glutathione-S-conjugate in isolated rat liver and kidney cells. Biochem Biophys Res Commun 83:195–200
Monks TJ, Anders MW, Dekant W, Stevens JL, Lau SS, van Bladeren PJ (1990) Glutathione conjugate mediated toxicities. Toxicol Appl Pharmacol 106:1–19
Moseley RH, Ballatori N, Murphy SM (1988) Na^+-glycine cotransport in canalicular liver plasma membrane vesicles. Am J Physiol 18:G253–259
Moseley RH, Johnson TR, Morrissette JM (1990) Inhibition of bile acid transport by cyclosporine A in rat liver plasma membrane vesicles. J Pharmacol Exp Ther 253:974–980
Müller M, Ishikawa R, Berger U, Klünemann C, Lucka L, Schreyer A, Kannich C, Reutter W, Kurz G, Keppler D (1991) ATP-dependent transport of taurocholate across the hepatocyte canalicular membrane mediated by a 110-kDa glycoprotein binding ATP and bile salt. J Biol Chem 266:18920–18926
Nicotera P, Moore M, Bellomo G, Mirabelli G, Orrenius S (1985) Demonstration and partial characterization of glutathione disulfide-stimulated ATPase activity in the plasma membrane fraction from rat hepatocytes. J Biol Chem 260: 1999–2002
Nishida T, Arias IM (1992) Evidence for a single ATP-dependent and membrane potential-dependent bile acid transporter in rat canalicular membrane vesicles. Hepatology 16:149A
Nishida T, Gatmaitan Z, Che M, Arias IM (1991) Rat liver canalicular membrane vesicles contain an ATP-dependent bile acid transport system. Proc Natl Acad Sci USA 88:6590–6594
Nishida T, Gatmaitan Z, Roy-Chowdhry J, Arias IM (1992a) Two distinct mechanisms for bilirubin glucuronide transport by rat bile canalicular membrane vesicles. J Clin Invest 90:2130–2135
Nishida T, Hardenbrook C, Gatmaitan Z, Arias IM (1992b) ATP-dependent organic anion transport system in normal and TR^- rat liver canalicular membranes. Am J Physiol 262:G629–G635
Norseth T, Clarkson TW (1971) Intestinal transport of ^{203}Hg-labeled methyl mercury chloride: role of biotransformation in rats. Arch Environ Health 22:568–577
Orrenius S, Ormstad K, Thor H, Jewell S (1983) Turnover and functions of glutathione studied with isolated hepatic and renal cells. Fed Proc 42:3177–3188
Oude Elferink RPJ, Ottenhoff T, Liefting W, de Haan J, Hansen PLM (1989) Hepatobiliary transport of glutathione and glutathione conjugate in rats with hereditary hyperbilirubinemia. J Clin Invest 84:476–483

Reichen J, Paumgartner G (1975) Kinetics of taurocholate uptake by the perfused rat liver. Gastroenterology 68:132–136
Reichen J, Paumgartner G (1976) Uptake of bile acids by the perfused rat liver. Am J Physiol 231:734–742
Reuben A, Allen RM (1990) Taurocholate transport by rat liver Golgi vesicles. Gastroenterology 98:A624
Riordan JR, Deuchars K, Kartner N, Alon N, Trent J, Ling V (1985) Amplification of P-glycoprotein genes in multidrug-resistant mammalian cell lines. Nature 316:817–819
Roerig DL, Hasegawa AT, Peterson RE, Wang RIH (1974) Effect of chloroquine and phenobarbital on morphine glucuronidation and biliary excretion in the rat. Biochem Pharmacol 23:1331–1339
Roninson IB (1992) The role of the *MDR*1 (P-glycoprotein) gene in multidrug resistance in vitro and in vivo. Biochem Pharmacol 43(1):95–102
Roninson IB, Chin JE, Choi K, Gros P, Housman DE, Fojo A, Shen D, Gottesman MM, and Pastan I (1986) Isolation of human *mdr* DNA sequences amplified in multidrug-resistant KB carcinoma cells. Proc Natl Acad Sci USA 83:4538–4542
Rothenberg M, Ling V (1989) Multidrug resistance: molecular biology and clinical relevance. JNCI 81:907–910
Roy Chowdhury F, Wolkoff AW, Arias IM (1989) Hereditary jaundice and disorders of bilirubin metabolism. In: Seriver CR, Beaudet AL, Sly WS, Valle D (eds) The metabolic basis of inherited disease. McGraw-Hill, New York, pp 1367–1408
Rudell U, Foth H, Kahl GF (1987) Eightfold induction of nicotine elimination in perfused rat liver by pretreatment with phenobarbital. Biochem Biophys Res Commun 148:192–198
Ruetz S, Fricker G, Hugentobler G, Winterhalter D, Kurz G, Meier PJ (1987) Isolation and characterization of the putative canalicular bile salt transport system of rat liver. J Biol Chem 262:11324–11330
Ruetz S, Hugentobler G, Meier PJ (1988) Functional reconstitution of the canalicular bile transport system of rat liver. Proc Natl Acad Sci USA 85:6147–6151
Scharschmidt BF, Stephens JE (1981) Transport of sodium, chloride and taurocholate by cultured rat hepatocytes. Proc Natl Acad Sci USA 78:986–990
Sharma R, Gupta S, Ahmad H, Ansari GAS, Awasthi YC (1990a) Stimulation of a human erythrocyte membrane ATPase by glutathione conjugates. Toxicol Appl Pharmacol 104:421–428
Sharma R, Gupta S, Singh SV, Medh R, Ahmad H, LaBelle E, Awasthi Y (1990b) Purification and characterization of dinitrophenyl glutathione ATPase of human erythrocytes and its expression in other tissues. Biochem Biophys Res Commun 171:155–161
Simion FA, Fleischer B, Fleischer S (1984) Two distinct mechanisms for taurocholate uptake in subcellular fractions from rat liver. J Biol Chem 259:10814–10822
Simmons TW, Anders MW, Ballatori N (1992) Cysteine and S-(1,2-dichlorovinyl)-L-cysteine transport in rat liver canalicular membrane vesicles: potential reabsorption mechanisms for biliary metabolites of glutathione and its S-conjugates. J Pharmacol Exp Ther 262:1182–1188
Singhal SS, Sharma R, Gupta S, Ahmad H, Zimniak P, Radominska A, Lester R, Awasthi YC (1991) The anionic conjugates of bilirubin and bile acids stimulate ATP hydrolysis by S-(dinitrophenyl)glutathione ATPase of human erythrocyte. FEBS Lett 281:255–257
Sippel CJ, Ananthanarayanan M, Suchy FJ (1990) Isolation and characterization of the canalicular membrane bile acid transport protein of rat liver. Am J Physiol 258:G728–G737
Sippel DJ, Suchy FJ, Ananthanarayanan M, Perlmutter DH (1993) The rat liver ecto-ATPase is also a canalicular bile acid transport protein. J Biol Chem 268:2083–2091

Spray DC, Ginzbery RD, Morales EA, Gatmaitan Z, Arias IM (1986) Electrophysiological properties of gap junctions between dissociated pairs of rat hepatocytes. J Cell Biol 103:135–144
Srivastava SK, Beutler E (1969) The transport of oxidized glutathione from human erythrocytes. J Biol Chem 244:9–16
Stein AF, Gregus Z, Klaassen CD (1988) Species variations in biliary excretion of glutathione-related thiols and methylmercury. Toxicol Appl Pharmacol 93:351–359
Stein WD (1990) Channels, carriers, and pumps. An introduction to membrane transport. Academic, San Diego
Stieger B, O'Neill B, Meier PJ (1992) ATP-dependent bile-salt transport in canalicular rat liver plasma-membrane vesicles. Biochem J 284:67–74
Studenberg SD, Brouwer KLR (1992) Impaired biliary excretion of acetaminophen glucuronide in the isolated perfused rat liver after acute phenobarbital treatment and in vivo phenobarbital pretreatment. J Pharmacol Exp Ther 261:1022–1027
Sztul ES, Biemesderfer D, Caplan MJ, Kashgarian M, Boyer JL (1987) Localization of Na^+-, K^+-ATPase alpha-subunit to the sinusoidal and lateral but not canalicular membranes of rat hepatocytes. J Cell Biol 104:1239–1248
Teo S, Vore M (1990) Mirex exposure inhibits the uptake of estradiol-17β(β-D-glucuronide), taurocholate and L-alanine into isolated rat hepatocytes. Toxicol Appl Pharmacol 104:411–420
Teo S, Vore M (1991) Mirex inhibits bile acid secretory function in vivo and in the isolated perfused rat liver. Toxicol Appl Pharmacol 109:161–170
Thiebault F, Tsuruo T, Hamada H, Gottesman MM, Pastan I, Willingham MC (1987) Cellular localization of the multidrug-resistance gene product P-glycoprotein in normal human tissues. Proc Natl Acad Sci USA 84:7735–7738
Tiribelli C, Lunazzi GC, Sottocasa GL (1990) Biochemical and molecular aspects of the hepatic uptake of organic anions. Biochim Biophys Acta 1031:261–275
Ueda K, Cardarelli C, Gottesman MM, Pastan I (1987) Expression of a full-length cDNA for the human *mdr*1 gene confers resistance to colchicine, doxorubicin and vinblastine. Proc Natl Acad Sci USA 84:3004–3008
Von Dippe P, Levy D (1983) Characterization of the bile acid transport system in normal and transformed hepatocytes. J Biol Chem 258:8896–8901
Vore M (1987) Estrogen cholestasis. Membranes, metabolites or receptors? Gastroenterology 93:643–649
Vore M, Hoffman T (1992) ATP-dependent transport of estradiol-17β-(β-D-glucuronide) in canalicular plasma membranes. Hepatology 16:146A
Vore M, Hoffman T (1993) Characterization of transport of estradiol-17β(β-D-glucuronide) in rat liver basolateral membrane vesicles. (submitted for publication)
Vore M, Gosland M, Tsuboi C, Hoffman T (1993) Cholestatic steroid glucuronides: Interactions with P-glycoprotein (P-gp). Hepatology 18:139A
Wahllander A, Sies H (1979) Glutathione S-conjugate formation from 1-chloro-2,4-dinitrobenzene and biliary S-conjugate excretion in the perfused rat liver. Eur J Biochem 96:441–446
Watanabe S, Smith CR, Phillips MJ (1985) Coordination of the contractile activity of bile canaliculi. Evidence from calcium microinjection of triplet hepatocytes. Lab Invest 53:275–279
Watkins JB, Klaassen CD (1982) Effect of inducers and inhibitors of glucuronidation on the biliary excretion and choleretic action of valproic acid in the rat. J Pharmacol Exp Ther 220:305–310
Weinman SA, Graf J, Boyer JL (1989) Voltage-driven, taurocholate-dependent secretion in isolated hepatocyte couplets. Am J Physiol 256:G826–G832
Wieland T, Nassal M, Kramer W, Fricker G, Bickel U, Kurz G (1984) Identity of hepatic membrane transport systems for bile salts, phalloidin, and antamanide by photoaffinity labeling. Proc Natl Acad Sci USA 81:5232–5236

Wolkoff AW, Chung CT (1980) Identification, purification, and partial characterization of an organic anion binding protein from rat liver cell plasma membrane. J Clin Invest 65:1152–1161
Wolkoff AW, Samuelson AC, Johnsen KL, Nakata R, Withers DM, Sosiak A (1987) Influence of Cl^- on organic anion transport in short-term cultured rat hepatocytes and isolated perfused rat liver. J Clin Invest 79:1259–1268
Yahanda AM, Adler KM, Fisher GA, Brophy NA, Halsey J, Hardy RI, Gosland MP, Lum BL, Sikic BI (1992) Phase I trial of etoposide with cyclosporine as a modulator of multidrug resistance. J Clin Oncol 10:1624–1634
Zimmerli B, Valantinas J, Meier PJ (1989) Multispecificity of Na^+-dependent taurocholate uptake in basolateral (sinusoidal) rat liver plasma membrane vesicles. J Pharmacol Exp Ther 250:301–308
Zimniak P, Ziller SA, Panfil I, Radominska A, Wolters H, Kuipers F, Sharma R, Saxena M, Moslen MT, Vore M, Vonk R, Awasthi YC, Lester R (1992) Identification of an anion-transport ATPase that catalyzes glutathione conjugate-dependent ATP hydrolysis in canalicular plasma membranes from normal rats and rats with conjugated hyperbilirubinemia (GY mutant). Arch Biochem Biophys 292:534–538

Section III
Pharmacology and Toxicology of Drug Conjugates

CHAPTER 12

Biologically Active Conjugates of Drugs and Toxic Chemicals

F.C. KAUFFMAN, J. ZALESKI, R.G. THURMAN, and G.Y. KWEI

A. Introduction

Conjugation reactions associated with metabolism of drugs and xenobiotics function primarily as detoxification pathways (CALDWELL 1982); however, they also serve to convert drug metabolites either to compounds that are biologically active per se or to prodrugs that serve as carriers of biological activity to various tissues. This chapter reviews important examples of the role of phase II reactions in generating biologically active compounds. Among the earliest examples of this phenomenon is the formation of potent carcinogenic compounds by conjugation. In the late 1960s, the Millers and their colleagues found that sulfation of *N*-hydroxy-*N*-2-fluorenylacetamine generated a reactive electrophile that caused cancer in rodents (MILLER et al. 1974). This and similar findings with the glucuronide (IRVING 1971; MAHER and REUTER 1973) led to the concept that metabolic activation is required for the generation of a wide range of carcinogens and toxic chemicals. Newer aspects of the role of phase II conjugation reactions in drug toxicity and carcinogenesis are reviewed in Chaps. 14, 15, and 16 of this volume. Phase II reactions that either directly activate drugs to biologically active compounds or to forms that enhance their availability to extrahepatic tissues are described below. Some drug conjugates produced in the liver and transported to various target tissues must be hydroloyzed to forms that are either directly active or require further metabolism to active compounds. Drug conjugates may be made tissue specific by targeting various hydrolytic enzymes. A novel approach of using monoclonal antibodies to deliver hydrolytic enzymes to tumor cell surfaces (HELLSTROM and SENTER 1992) that facilitate hydrolysis of drug conjugates to toxic compounds at these sites is an exciting extension of the use of conjugates as prodrugs. The increasing awareness of drug conjugates as biologically active products has stimulated the recent publication of several reviews (MULDER 1992) and symposia (OLSON et al. 1992; KAUFFMAN 1992) on this subject.

B. Biologically Active Drug Conjugates

Drug development entails optimizing the chemical structure of drugs to enhance ionic and hydrophobic interactions at drug receptor sites. Thus, it is not unexpected that hydrophilic conjugates formed in vivo are most often considered inactivation products. Addition of hydrophilic glucuronide or sulfate groups to phenolic parent compounds or products of phase I metabolism most often leads to loss of activity at critical sites and to enhanced elimination in bile or urine. This prevailing view has been challenged recently by findings that morphine-6-glucuronide is several orders of magnitude more potent as a μ-opioid receptor agonist than morphine itself and by the finding that the antihypertensive drug minoxidil is only active as a sulfate conjugate.

I. Morphine-6-Glucuronide

Morphine has two nucleophilic sites that may be conjugated, a 3-hydroxy group on an aromatic ring and an alcoholic 6-hydroxy group (Fig. 1). Conjugation of the 3-hydroxy group with glucuronic acid occurs in many

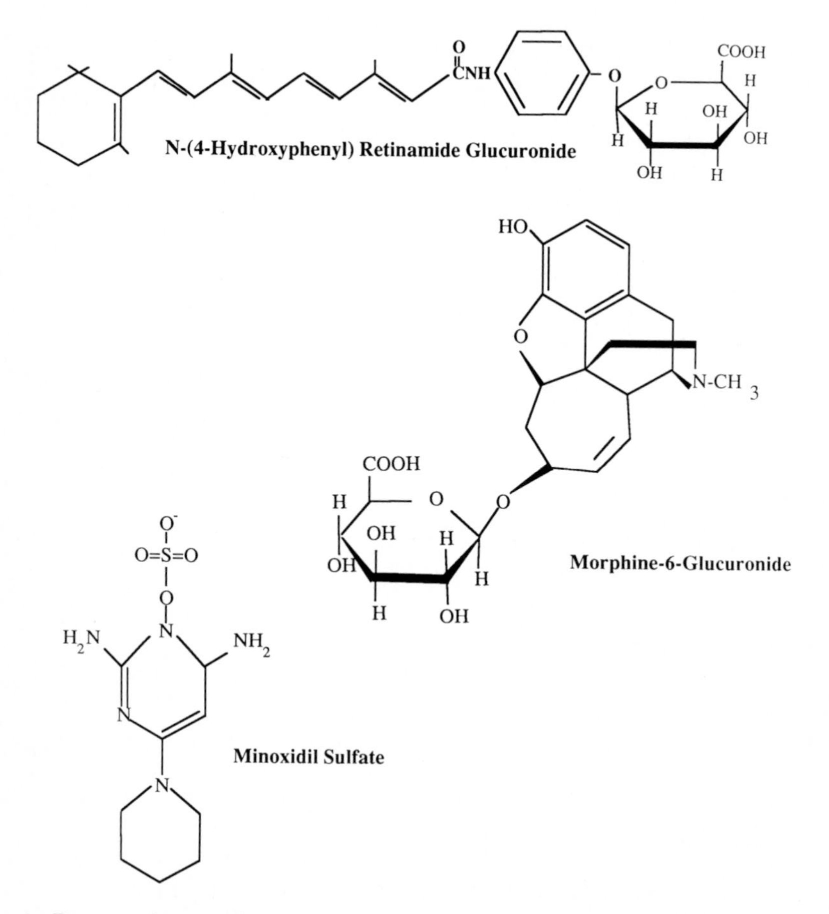

Fig. 1. Drug conjugates that are biologically active

mammalian species, while glucuronidation at the 6 position appears to be unique to man (PAUL et al. 1989; PORTENOY et al. 1991; MULDER 1992). Morphine-6-glucuronide is a major metabolite of morphine in humans (PAUL et al. 1989) and accumulates in blood with chronic dosing to values greater than morphine (PAUL et al. 1989). Although the analgesic potency of morphine-6-glucuronide has been recognized for more than two decades (YOSHIMURA et al. 1973), the potential clinical use of the 6-glucuronide conjugate has only been explored recently (HAND et al. 1987; PORTENOY et al. 1991). Morphine-6-glucuronide, but not the 3-glucuronide, binds to μ_1 and μ_2 receptors with affinities similar to morphine in mouse brain (PAUL et al. 1989; MULDER 1992). Based on the pharmacodynamic action and the area under the curve of subcutaneous doses of drug, the 6-glucuronide conjugate is more than three times more active than an equimolar subcutaneous dose of morphine in mice (PAUL et al. 1989). Cross-tolerance develops between morphine and its 6-glucuronide metabolite.

Recent clinical studies in cancer patients given morphine-6-glucuronide indicated that useful analgesic effects are achieved with an absence of nausea and vomiting (OSBORNE et al. 1992). Thus, this agent may have a significant advantage over intravenous morphine, which causes nausea and vomiting. However, because of its long-term use, oral morphine will likely remain the major component of narcotic analgesic therapy. Amounts of morphine-6-glucuronide generated by first-pass hepatic metabolism remains poorly defined. The isoform of uridine diphosphate (UDP) glucuronosyl transferase that forms the 6-glucuronide has not been identified, and it is not clear whether morphine-6-glucuronide is formed in the brain or enters the brain from the blood. Recent work (PORTENOY et al. 1991) has confirmed that morphine-6-glucuronide present in plasma is distributed into the cerebral spinal fluid of humans, but only one tenth that of morphine. The potency of morphine-6-glucuronide is in part explained by unexpectedly high lipophilicity of the folded form of the molecule. Recent studies (CARRUPT et al. 1991) using force-field and quantum mechanical calculations indicate that the glucuronide conjugates of morphine can exist in conformational equilibrium between extended and folded forms. The extended conformer, which predominates in aqueous media, is highly hydrophilic because it efficiently exposes polar groups of the molecule to surrounding aqueous media. On the other hand, the folded conformers mask part of these polar groups and are much more lipophilic. The folded forms likely predominate in media of low polarity such as biological membranes (CARRUPT et al. 1991).

The 6-sulfate conjugate of morphine is also analgesic (OGURI et al. 1987), suggesting that anionic interactions may be involved in receptor activation. In addition to anionic properties, other structural features of the molecule must also be involved, since the 3-sulfate, but not the 3-glucuronide, conjugate is analgesic (YAKSH and HARTY 1988). MULDER (1992) has speculated that addition of a hydrophilic group improves the biological action of low molecular weight ligands at peptide receptor sites. Conjugation with glucuronic acid, activated sulfate, or glutathione may yield such compounds.

Although morphine-3-glucuronide is not analgesic, it is a potent μ-opioid receptor antagonist (Smith et al. 1990). When administered to rats via intracerebroventricular injection, the 3-glucuronide conjugate antagonized the action of either morphine or its 6-glucuronide conjugate, irrespective of whether it was given 15 min prior to or 15 min after administration of the two agonists. The 3-glucuronide also resembles morphine in that it causes allodynia, a condition in which an ordinarily innocuous stimulus is perceived as painful (Yaksh and Harty 1988). Both the 3-glucuronide and 3-sulfate conjugates of morphine are 10–50 times more potent than the parent compound in causing allodynia (Yaksh and Harty 1988). In summary, a number of recent studies indicate clearly that conjugated metabolites of morphine formed largely in the liver are biologically active.

II. Minoxidil Sulfate

Minoxidil is a compound widely used as a direct acting vasodilator in the treatment of hypertension and to treat alopecia. Both of these therapeutic activities are mediated by the *N*-sulfate conjugate (Fig. 1) of minoxidil rather than the parent compound. Studies concerning the action of minoxidil and its *N*-sulfate conjugate, a major metabolite (Johnson et al. 1982), on vascular smooth muscle in vitro show clearly that the *N*-sulfate, but not minoxidil, causes relaxation. Further, minoxidil is slow in producing a hypotensive effect in vivo, while the sulfate conjugate directly impairs norepinephrine-induced contractures of arterial smooth muscle (Bray and Quast 1991).

Many endogenous and pharmacological vasodilators hyperpolarize vascular smooth muscle by increasing conductance of potassium ions (Brayden et al. 1991). Membrane hyperpolarization can, in turn, close voltage-dependent calcium channels and thereby lead to vasodilatation (Nelson et al. 1988). Minoxidil sulfate is a potent smooth muscle relaxant which opens K^+ channels, as demonstrated by electrophysiological (Leblanc et al. 1989; Meisheri et al. 1988; Newgreen et al. 1990) and ion flux studies (Bray and Quast 1991). Recent investigations (Meisheri et al. 1991; Groppi et al. 1990) raise the possibility that minoxidil sulfate modifies K^+-channel activity by sulfating a critical component of the K^+ channel in vascular smooth muscle.

A role for increased K^+ permeability in minoxidil sulfate-induced vasodilatation was demonstrated by the action of the compound on isolated rabbit superior mesenteric artery (Meisheri et al. 1988). For example, minoxidil sulfate ($5 \times 10^{-6} M$) relaxed maximal contractions induced by norepinephrine ($5 \times 10^{-6} M$), but failed to impair contractions induced by

80 m*M* K^+. Tetraethylammonium, a potassium channel blocker, inhibited minoxidil sulfate-induced relaxation of rabbit mesenteric artery (MEISHERI et al. 1988). Finally, minoxidil sulfate enhanced ^{42}K efflux from mesenteric arteries preloaded with ^{42}K. The ability of minoxidil sulfate to open potassium channels is unique among clinically used vasodilators. Comparison of the vascular relaxant effects of minoxidil sulfate with another vasodilator that opens K^+ channels, BRL-34915 (chromakalim), indicated that minoxidil sulfate action was irreversible, while the effects of BRL-34915 on rabbit mesenteric artery were readily reversed by washing with normal saline (MEISHERI et al. 1991).

The possibility that protein sulfation is involved in the action of minoxidil sulfate is indicated by studies of radioactive sulfate incorporation into rabbit mesenteric artery preparations treated with either [^{35}S]-labeled minoxidil sulfate or [^{3}H]-minoxidil sulfate (label on the piperidine ring; MEISHERI et al. 1991). More than 30% of ^{35}S was retained after 2 h of washing mesenteric artery strips with saline, while virtually no ^{3}H was retained (Fig. 2). Analyses of proteins labeled with ^{35}S indicated that predominant labeling occurred in a 116-kDa and a 43-kDa protein. The 116-kDa fraction is a membrane component, while the 43-kDa protein appears to be actin (MEISHERI et al. 1991). The function of the 116-kDa protein is not known. The close temporal relationship between labeling of this component and alterations in K^+ permeability suggest that the long-term hypotensive effects of minoxidil sulfate are indeed related to sulfation of a

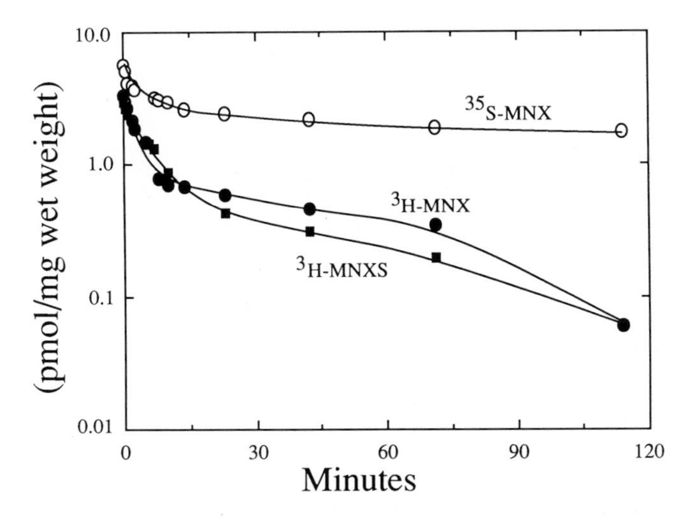

Fig. 2. Washout efflux of radiolabeled minoxidil sulfate (*MNXS*) and minoxidil (*MNX*) from mesenteric artery; a semilogarithmic plot showing the time course of washout efflux of the radiolabeled drug. The data are presented as the amount of drug (picomoles per milligram of wet weight) associated with the tissue at a given time during the washout efflux. From MEISHERI et al. (1991)

protein component of the K^+ channel. Minoxidil sulfate is very active chemically and able to donate sulfate groups to nucleophiles, as suggested by the ability of [^{35}S]minoxidil sulfate to sulfate proteins and peptides nonenzymatically in vitro (GROPPI et al. 1990). The enzymatic and nonenzymatic sulfation mechanisms in the biological actions of minoxidil have been reviewed recently (MEISHERI et al. 1993).

A number of commonly prescribed drugs, including clomiphene, testosterone, donnatal, ibuprofen, chlorpheniramine, and dimenhydrinate are known inhibitors of sulfotransferase (BAMFORTH et al. 1992) and may thus alter the biological activity of compounds such as minoxidil when coadministered with this drug. Sulfate conjugates are generally quite hydrophobic and thus able to diffuse across cell membranes and bind intracellular constituents. Sulfate conjugates also generally bind proteins to a greater extent than other drug conjugates. For example, sulfate conjugates of 4-nitrophenol and 1-naphthol bind to serum albumin much more effectively than unconjugated compounds (MIZUMA et al. 1991). Catecholamine sulfates regulate blood pressure. For example, dopamine 3-*O*-sulfate is known to inhibit adrenocortical secretion of aldosterone in vitro (KUCHEL et al. 1986). Sulfated catecholamines also have unusually long plasma half-lives and thus may serve as storage forms of parent compounds that modulate blood pressure. Accordingly, compounds that modify the formation of sulfate conjugates, either in the liver or in target tissues, would be expected to modify the biological activity of minoxidil sulfate and possibly other compounds that are converted to biological active sulfate conjugates.

III. Other Drug Conjugates

1. Retinoid Glucuronides

The potential use of retinoids as cancer chemopreventive agents has been appreciated for more than 70 years, since it was observed that a deficiency in vitamin A led to metaplastic changes in respiratory tract epithelium (MORI 1922). The development of retinoid deficiency-related squamous metaplasia resembles changes induced by various chemical carcinogens. Thus, there has been a great deal of interest in developing analogs of retionids as useful cancer chemopreventive agents. Studies carried out over the last decade have shown that retinoids, in particular the synthetic retinoid *N*-(4-hydroxyphenyl) retinamide (HPR; Fig. 1), markedly inhibit the growth of chemically induced mammary tumors in rodents (MOON et al. 1979; SPORN and ROBERTS 1983).

Studies of natural metabolites of retinoic acid indicated that retinoyl glucuronide has greater biological activity than parent vitamin A and is significantly less toxic (OLSON et al. 1992). Both retinyl and retinoyl *β*-glucuronides have been isolated in bile, plasma, and tissues of many species including humans given retinoic acid (OLSON et al. 1992; DUNAGIN et al.

1966). Retinoid β-glucuronides can undergo oxidation to the 4-hydroxy and 4-oxo derivatives and can be hydrolyzed to the parent compound. Both retinyl and retinoyl β-glucuronides are as active as the parent compound in stimulating rat growth; however, in some systems, marked differences occur between conjugates of retinoic acid and retinol. For example, retinyl glucuronide is much more effective than retinoyl glucuronide in stimulating granulocytic differentiation in HL-60 cells (JANICK-BUCKNER et al. 1991). Both conjugates are less toxic than the parent compounds in inducing cytolysis in the HL-60 cell system. Glucuronide conjugates of both retinoic acid and retinol are more active than their parent compounds in inhibiting prolactin-induced DNA biosynthesis in explant cultures of mouse mammary glands, both with and without addition of steroids (MEHTA et al. 1993). Findings with the glucuronide conjugates of retinoic acid and retinol stimulated the biosyntheses of a number of other congeners including retinoyl glucose, retinyl glucose, retinoly-adenine, retinoyl-adenosine, and retinoyl-α-glucuronide. Except for retinyl glucose, all these derivatives were active in stimulating the differentiation of HL-60 cells; however, their activity varied widely and most were more toxic than the β-glucuronide conjugates (JANICK-BUCKNER et al. 1991). A recent review (OLSON et al. 1992) compares the relative biological activities of some of these retinoid derivatives.

There is at least one report indicating that dietary glucurate, which is converted to D-glucaro-1,4-lactone, an inhibitor of β-glucuronidase, enhance the capacity of the synthetic retinoid HPR to inhibit the induction of rat mammary tumors by 7,12-dimethylbenz(a)anthracene (ABOU-ISSA et al. 1988). The interaction between glucurate and HPR led to further evaluation of HPR-*O*-glucuronide in suppressing breast tumors. A recent study of the influence of this conjugate on the growth of MCF-7 human breast cancer cells in vitro showed that the glucuronide had slightly greater potency and much less cytotoxicity than the free HPR retinoid (BHATNAGAR et al. 1991). The mechanism of action of retinoid glucuronides is not established. A novel action of the conjugate is suggested, because the glucuronides do not bind to cellular retinoic acid-binding proteins or to nuclear receptors for retinoic acid (SANI et al. 1992). Only intact HPR-*O*-glucuronide is detected in MCF-7 breast tumor cells treated with this compound, and very low activities of β-glucuronidase are found in these cells (BHATNAGAR et al. 1991). Similar results have been observed in HL-60 cells treated with retinoyl glucuronide, i.e., virtually no hydrolysis of the conjugate and very low levels of β-glucuronidase (ZILE et al. 1987). Further work to clarify the mechanism of action of glucuronide conjugates of retinoic acid derivatives is clearly warranted.

2. Fatty Acid Conjugates

A major problem in cancer chemotherapy is the lack of sufficient selectivity of cytotoxic drugs for tumors. Attempts to overcome this problem have involved conjugating chemotherapeutic agents to targeting macromolecules such as enzymes (HELLSTROM and SENTER 1992) and antibodies raised against cancer-specific antigens (CHOSE and BLAIR 1978) or by entrapping them in liposomes conjugated with antibodies (BARBET et al. 1981). A novel approach coupling a fatty acid to a cytotoxic drug has recently been introduced. Entry of fatty acids into cells is facilitated, in part, by α-fetoprotein (AFP) through the interaction of this protein with specific receptors which are particularly high in neoplastic cells of varied origin (URIEL et al. 1987). Covalent conjugates of chlorambucil and fatty acids with different degrees of unsaturation (Fig. 3) have been prepared and tested for cytotoxicity against two lymphoma cell lines and mitogen-activated normal human lymphocytes in vitro (ANEL et al. 1990). The results showed that the coupling of chlorambucil with polyunsaturated fatty acid improves its cytotoxicity and its selectivity against malignant lymphocytes. Recently, 2-deoxy-5-fluorouridine (5dFU) has been coupled to oleic (18:1) and docosahexaenoic (22:6) acids.

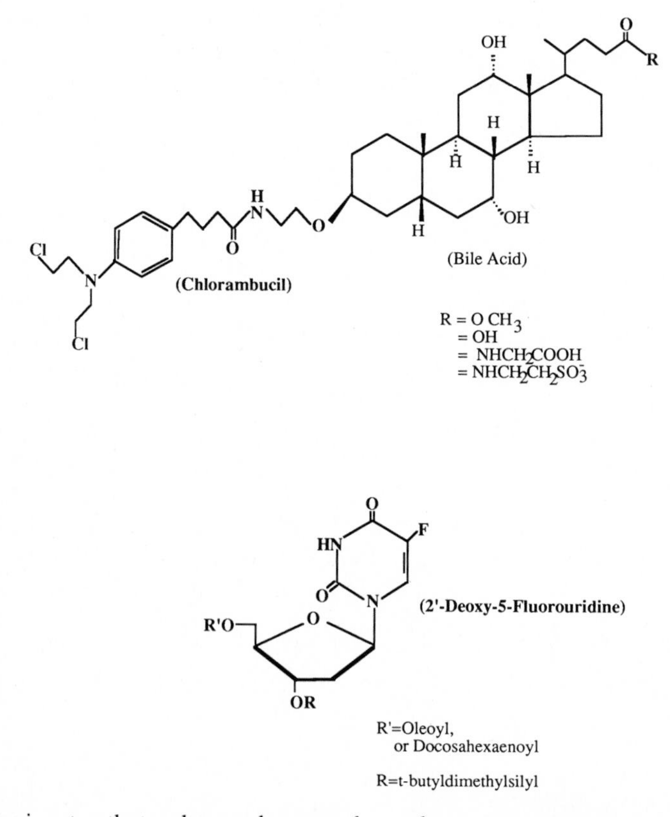

Fig. 3. Conjugates that enhance drug uptake and transport. Structure for bile acid conjugates (*top*) was adapted from KRAMER et al. (1992) and structure for fatty acid conjugates (*bottom*) has been adopted from HALMOS et al. (1992)

The cytotoxicity of the drugs and their fatty acid conjugates were evaluated using a colon carcinoma cell line of human origin (HT-29) (HALMOS et al. 1992). Over a 2-h incubation, both fatty acid conjugates showed dose-dependent (10–200 μM) cytotoxicity, while the parent compound was not toxic. Similar results were obtained when the conjugates were tested against HT-29 cells over 24 and 48 h. 5dFU by itself was virtually not effective, while the two fatty acid conjugates, particularly the docosahexaenoic acid derivative, were highly toxic (HALMOS et al. 1992). The results are similar to those noted with fatty acid conjugates of chlorambucil (ANEL et al. 1990) and suggest that further work to improve the selectivity of cytotoxic drugs using this approach may be fruitful. Although the mechanism of fatty acid uptake into cells is generally considered to occur by simple diffusion, there is evidence that the transfer of fatty acids into cells may also involve membrane receptors for fatty acids and for serum carrier proteins such as albumin and AFP (SORENTINO et al. 1988).

3. Acyl-Linked Glucuronides

Many carboxylic acids are conjugated by UDP-glucuronosyl-transferase to form 1-*O*-acyl glucuronides, which are activated esters. Members of this class of compounds are known to undergo a variety of spontaneous chemical reactions in vitro and in vivo, including hydrolysis and nucleophilic transacylation (STOGNIEW and FENSELAU 1982; VANBREEMEN and FENSELAU 1985; BRADOW et al. 1989). The ester-linked glucuronides are not hydrolysed by β-glucuronidase; thus, measurements employing this hydrolytic enzyme will often underestimate amounts of glucuronide metabolites. Factors governing the production of this class of conjugates and some of their physiological functions are reviewed in Chap. 13 of this volume. Because of their established biological activity, they are only discussed briefly here. The finding that the 1-*O*-acyl glucuronide conjugate of clofibric acid reacted non-enzymatically with ethanethiol, while the free acid and ethyl ester did not, led to the suggestion that necrosis and carcinogenicity caused by clofibrate was due to the reactivity of the acyl-linked glucuronide (STOGNIEW and FENSELAU 1982). FENSELAU and her colleagues have proposed that the transacylation of activated 1-*O*-acyl glucuronide provides a novel mechanism for the interaction of lipophilic xenobiotics with a variety of biopolymers (BRADOW et al. 1989). Such interaction may be involved in immunogenicity, transport and clearance, receptor binding, and cytotoxicity (OLSON et al. 1992).

4. Bile Acid Conjugates

A recent study (KRAMER et al. 1992) demonstrated that conjugates formed by covalent linkage of a drug to a modified bile acid molecule facilitates its uptake into liver and the ileum via the Na^+-dependent bile acid uptake system. Bile acids are synthesized from cholesterol within hepatocytes and undergo enterohepatic circulation after secretion into bile. The occurrence of very active, Na^+-dependent bile acid transport systems in sinusoidal membranes of hepatocytes (ANWER et al. 1976) and the brush border membrane of ileal enterocytes (BURCKHARDT et al. 1983) indicated that bile acids may serve as carriers for drugs to the liver and improve intestinal absorption of poorly absorbed drugs. The possibility of using this approach was tested by examining the biological activity of the alkylating cytotoxic drug chlorambucil and a peptide inhibitor of prolyl 4-hydroxylase, either alone or as bile acid conjugates (KRAMER et al. 1992).

Chlorambucil, as well as other drugs, was attached to the bile acid molecule either via an ester or peptide bond and a modified bile acid linker conserving the negatively charged side chain of natural bile acids (KRAMER et al. 1992) (Fig. 3). These conjugates were made to optimize features required for optimal Na^+-dependent bile acid transport by liver and small intestine, which include a negative charge in the side chain of the bile acid molecule and at least one hydroxyl group in position 3, 7, or 12 of the steroid moiety (HARDISON et al. 1991). The biological activity of the chlorambucil bile acid conjugate was demonstrated by inhibition of [^{3}H]taurocholate uptake into isolated rat hepatocytes and by inhibition of phalloidin hepatotoxicity. In contrast, equimolar amounts ($10\,\mu M$) of chlorambucil were without effect (KRAMER et al. 1992). Uptake of the bile acid conjugate into liver, but not free chlorambucil was indicated by the appearance of the conjugate only in bile after injection of the compounds into a peripheral mesenteric vein of an anesthetized rat. Phalloidin, a toxin from the poison mushroom, *Amanita phalloides*, is taken up selectively into hepatocytes by the multispecific hepatic bile acid transporter (BUSCHER et al. 1986). Hepatoxicity of the mushroom poison is indexed by protrusions from the hepatocyte surface. The bile acid conjugate of chlorambucil, but not the free drug, inhibited the toxicity of phalloidin.

To evaluate the pharmacokinetic behavior of peptides and their bile acid conjugates, a fluorescent oxoprolyl-peptide and its bile acid conjugate were synthesized. Both the parent peptide and its bile acid conjugate inhibit prolyl hydroxylase. After injection of these compounds into a peripheral mesenteric vein of anesthetized rats and subsequent thin-layer chromatography of bile, the peptide bile acid conjugate was found unchanged in the bile, whereas the parent compound was not found (KRAMER et al. 1992). Thus, the conjugate, but not the parent peptide, underwent hepatobiliary transport. The time-dependent appearance of bile acid conjugates of chlorambucil and the peptide inhibitor of prolyl hydroxylase indicates that drugs covalently linked to bile acids are handled like a bile acid molecule. Perhaps even more significantly, peptide-derived drugs, which are easily cleaved by membrane-bound proteases in the liver and intestine, may escape membrane proteolysis after covalent conjugation with bile acids. The selective transport of bile acid conjugates by the liver and small intestine may have special significance for pharmaceutical agents, e.g., developing liver-specific drugs and improving intestinal absorption of drugs that are either poorly absorbed or not absorbed at all. A problem remaining to be resolved is how to limit the biliary excretion of such drug conjugates.

5. Polymeric Conjugates

A number of examples exist indicating that biopolymers are activated by conjugation. It has long been known that folates and certain antifolates are metabolized to polyglutamate conjugates that are more active than parent folic acid. The length of the polyglutamate chain varies from the triglutamate in bacteria to nonaglutamates in mammalian tissues (SHANE 1989). The metabolism of some antifolates to polyglutamates in sensitive tissues is believed to play an important role in their cytotoxicity. Polyglutamate conjugates apparently have greater affinity than unconjugated antifolates for intracellular binding sites including target enzymes and consequently are retained within cells to a much greater extent than parent compounds. A recent study (MCCLOSKEY et al. 1992) showed that resistance of several human leukemia cell lines to methotrexate involves decreased ability of these cells to form polyglutamate derivatives of the antifolate. Further studies are needed to determine whether this is an important mechanism of resistance to antifolates used clinically.

Chondroitin sulfate, a soluble glucuronic acid-rich mucopolysaccharide, while not strictly a drug conjugate, has been used recently as a drug delivery vehicle. The sulfated polymer serves as a substrate for colonic bacteria and consequently may act to deliver drugs specifically to the colon (RUBINSTEIN et al. 1992). By formulating various cross-linked polymers containing indomethacin, the rate of release of the compound in the presence of colonic bacteria could be controlled in a precise manner (RUBINSTEIN et al. 1992). Another application of chondroitin sulfate is the delivery of drugs and diagnostic agents to the reticuloendothelial system. While colloid carbon inhibits the reticuloendothelial system competitively, chondroitin sulfate formulations do not. In a multidose study (ISHIDA et al. 1992) in which chondroitin sulfate iron colloid was administered to rabbits, uptake of the complex by cells of the reticuloendothelial system was reflected by dose-dependent increases in blood iron levels. Thus, the chondroitin sulfate iron colloid may be a useful analytical agent to monitor function of the reticuloendothelial system in a noninvasive manner.

A final example of the polymeric drug conjugate is pentosansulfate, an exogenous polysaccharide, which may be useful in preventing acrolein-induced bladder injury (KALOTA et al. 1992). Acrolein is an active metabolite of the antineoplastic drug cyclophosphamide, which often causes dose-dependent hemorrhagic cystitis and limits the utility of this potent anticancer drug. Damage to the transitional epithelium of the bladder by acrolein, evaluated by measuring trypan blue uptake and urea transport in rabbit bladder epithelial cells, was reduced by approximately 50%. The polymer also reduced the cytotoxicity of acrolein against a human epithelial cell in culture. The above tests suggest that pentosansulfate forms a protective barrier and might be a useful adjunct to other regimens in reducing cyclophosphamide toxicity.

C. Steroids

Both glucuronide and sulfate conjugates of certain sterols are biologically active. A brief overview of these compounds is given below.

I. Glucuronides

There are a number of examples illustrating that both glucuronide and sulfate conjugates of steroids are biologically active. Vitamin D glucuronides and related glucosides increase intestinal Ca^{2+} transport and bone Ca^{2+} mobilization in vitamin D-deficient rats when given intravenously (LONDOWSKI et al. 1985). Ethinyl estradiol-17β-glucuronide conjugates are potent cholestatic agents in the rat (VORE et al. 1983) and apparently act by increasing permeability of hepatocellular tight junctions (KAN et al. 1989).

II. Sulfates

Sulfation is a major route of metabolism of many endogenous and exogenous steroids. Studies are emerging which indicate that a number of sulfate conjugates in particular represent biologically active products of steroid metabolism.

1. Pregnenolone Sulfate

Pregnenolone and pregnenolone sulfate are steroids that are active at the γ-aminobutyric acid (GABA)-benzodiazepine-chloride receptor complex (MELCHIOR and ALLEN 1992; KREUGER and PAPADOPOULOS 1992). Pregnenolone is a barbituate-like agonist, whereas its sulfate conjugate acts as a picrotoxin-like antagonist. The behavioural effects of both steroids either alone or in combination with pentobarbital or ethanol, which also act at benzodiazepine receptors, were recently studied in male C57Bl/6 mice (MELCHIOR and ALLEN 1992). When pregnenolone was given in combination with either pentobarbital or ethanol, it enhanced hypothermia, sleep time, and depressed motor activity. In contrast, pregnenolone sulfate enhanced hypothermia caused by ethanol but did not affect motor activity or sleep time, suggesting different sites of action for the parent compound and the conjugate.

Pregnenolone sulfate formed in glial cells may be related to the biological activity of a new class of compounds called 2-phenylindole-3-acetamides that interact with mitochondrial benzodiazepine receptors (KREUGER and

Papadopoulos 1992). This group of receptors is present in tissues that have a high capacity for steroidogenesis such as the adrenal cortex and Leydig cells of the testes (Buhl et al. 1990; Iorizzi et al. 1990), as well as glial cells, and are apparently regulated by diazepam-binding inhibitor (DBI) receptors localized on the outer membrane of mitochondria (Kreuger and Papadopoulos 1992). DBI is a neuropeptide in the cytosol of glial cells that binds with high affinity to mitochondrial DBI receptors and modulates local steroidogenesis. A scheme depicting the DBI receptor as a potential new drug target is shown in Fig. 4. DBI receptors apparently regulate the transfer of cholesterol to the inner mitochondrial membrane, where it serves

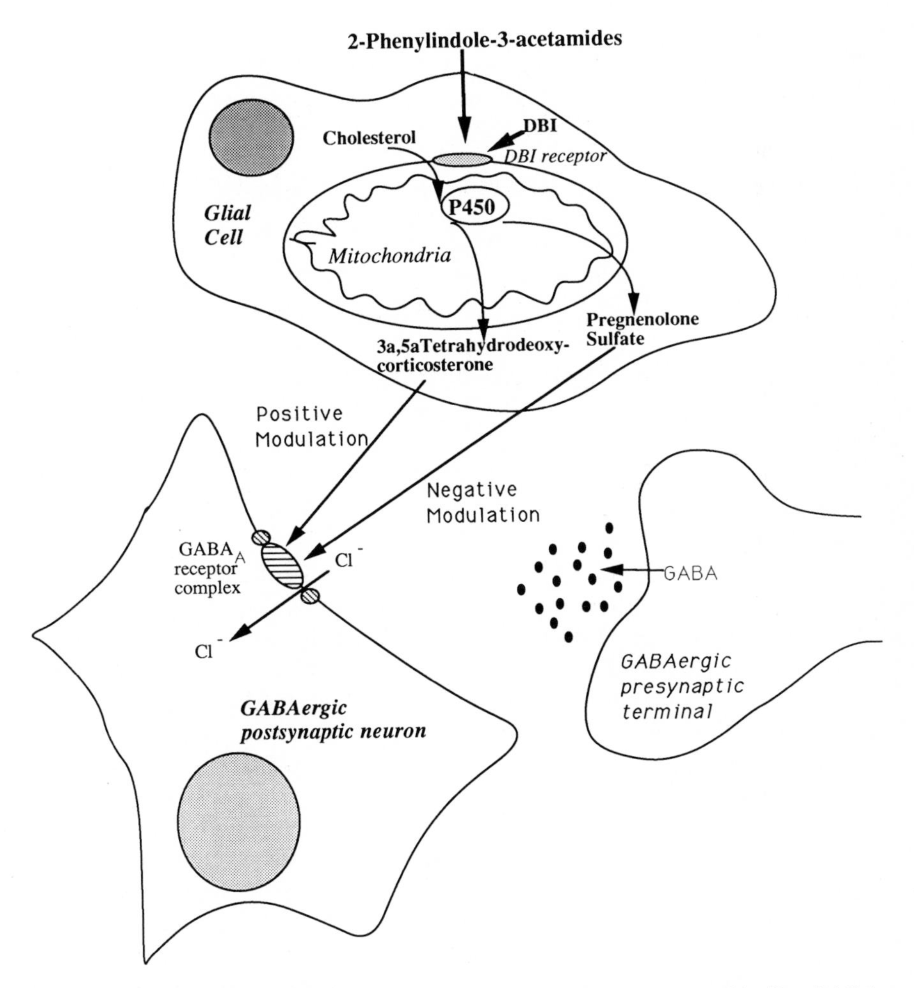

Fig. 4. Scheme depicting the coupling of mitochondrial diazepam-binding inhibitor (*DBI*) receptors to the formation of pregnenolone sulfate. Adapted from Kreuger and Papadropoulos (1992)

as a substrate for cytochrome P450-dependent enzymes that participate in steroidogenesis (KREUGER and PAPADOPOULOS 1992). Binding of 2-phenylindole-3-acetamides to DBI receptors stimulates glial cells to produce "neurosteroids" such as pregnenolone sulfate, which in turn regulates GABA receptors on neurons. Thus, pregnenolone sulfate appears to be a key component in a novel mechanism whereby a new class of pharmaceutical agents indirectly regulate GABA receptors in the central nervous system. The isoform of sulfotransferase that generates pregnenolone sulfate in glial cells and its regulation remain to be determined. Interestingly, pregnenolone sulfate also modulates the activity of central NMDA receptors, and it has been suggested that it is somehow involved in the balance between excitation and inhibition in the central nervous system (WU et al. 1991). Further work to test this hypothesis and to further define the actions of steroid sulfates is clearly warranted, based on the neuromodulatory role that has been demonstrated for pregnenolone sulfate. Interestingly, relatively high concentrations of pregnenolone sulfate and fatty acid esters of this steroid are found in sciatic nerves (MORFIN et al. 1992), suggesting a potential role for these conjugates in regulating the activity of peripheral nerve.

2. Dehydroepiandrosterone Sulfate

Another steroid that has received attention as a potential prohormone or as a compound possessing biological activity of its own is dehydroepiandrosterone sulfate (DHEAS). DHEAS concentrations are at least 300- to 500-fold higher than those of the parent steroid, dehydroepiandrosterone (DHEA; GORDON et al. 1991). Circulating levels of these steroids reach peak levels in individuals of both sexes at about 25 years of age and subsequently decline continuously (ORENTREICH et al. 1984). The marked decline in these steroids with age has stimulated studies concerning relationships between serum levels of DHEA and DHEAS and age-related diseases such as cancer and atherosclerosis. Although this area is controversial, epidemiological studies indicate that the risk of developing some forms of cancer (SONKA et al. 1973) and increased mortality from cardiovascular disease (BARRETT-CONNOR et al. 1986) are accompanied by abnormally low serum and urinary levels of DHEAS. Hyperinsulinemia, which promotes microvascular disease, also reduces serum DHEA and DHEAS (NESTLER et al. 1992). A recent study (GORDON et al. 1991) supports a role for DHEA and DHEAS in preventing bladder cancer. Serum levels of both steroids were determined in 35 individuals who donated serum to a community-based serum bank in Maryland in 1974 and who subsequently developed bladder cancer, and in 69 matched controls from the same cohort of volunteers. Prediagnostic serum concentrations of DHEA and DHEAS were significantly lower in individuals who subsequently developed bladder cancer than those measured in controls. The observed association between bladder cancer risk and blood levels of the two steroids was not affected by adjustments for smoking or the time interval between serum collection and diagnosis. While these results imply a chemoprotective role for DHEA and DHEAS, it is necessary to determine whether these findings can be replicated in animal studies and other epidemiological investigations.

The mechanism by which DHEAS may prevent bladder cancer is by no means clear. One possibility that has been suggested is that DHEAS serves as a prohormone that is further processed to potent estrogens and androgens that inhibit the progression of cancer in target tissues. In this regard, it is important to note that bladder cancer is more common and more aggressive in men. The possibility that vascular DHEAS serves as a precursor of ovarian androgens was convincingly demonstrated in a recent study involving local infusion of [^{3}H]DHEAS into women undergoing surgery (HANING et al. 1991). The formation of [^{3}H] androgens in ovarian tissue indicated clearly that DHEAS can serve as a prohormone.

D. Toxic Conjugates Formed and Released from Liver

There is growing appreciation that conjugates of metabolites derived from toxic xenobiotics such as bromobenzene vicinyl halides and polycyclic aromatic hydrocarbons (PAHs) are biologically active. The role of conjugation–deconjugation reactions in the metabolism of toxic xenobiotics is discussed extensively in Chaps. 14–16 of this volume. The purpose of this section is to emphasize the role of the liver in forming toxic conjugates and to underscore the importance of "metabolite trafficking" between the liver and extrahepatic tissues.

I. Polycyclic Aromatic Hydrocarbons

It is estimated that consumption of certain foods may introduce an order of magnitude more benzo(a)pyrene, a procarcinogen, into the body than would be inhaled by an adult in a polluted, winter urban environment assumed to have outdoor concentrations of approximately 5 μg PAH/m^3 (GREENBERG et al. 1990). Since the liver is the major site of PAH metabolism, it is logical to consider relationships between hepatic metabolism of PAHs and cancer in sensitive extrahepatic tissues. Recent studies employing orthotopic liver transplantation tested the possibility that the liver serves as a reservoir of potential carcinogenic metabolities (WALL et al. 1991). Livers that had been preloaded in vivo with benzo(a)pyrene were transplanted into control rats, and release of benzo(a)pyrene metabolites was monitored (WALL et al. 1991). This study indicated unequivocally that stable conjugates of benzo(a) pyrene phase I metabolites were released from the transplanted livers and were transported to extrahepatic tissues, where they accounted for virtually all of the DNA binding observed (WALL et al. 1991). These important findings indicate that the liver cannot be viewed solely as a site of PAH detoxification. Rather, the liver also produces PAH conjugates that travel to target tissues, where they are further processed to reactive intermediates.

There are several mechanisms by which metabolites of benzo(a)pyrene released from the liver may be carcinogenic to target tissues. Direct-acting carcinogens such as the (+)anti-benzo(a)pyrene-7,8-dihydrodiol-9,10-epoxide (BPDE) may be released from the liver and transported to target organs in association with various plasma proteins that offer protection from hydrolysis. A second mechanism involves transport of stable conjugates of benzo(a)pyrene metabolites, generally considered detoxification products, to target organs, where they are taken up and hydrolyzed to products that either bind directly to critical sites or are further metabolized by monooxygenases to reactive electrophiles. Since stable glutathione, glucuronide, and sulfate conjugates are, by far, the major fraction of benzo(a)pyrene metabolites released from the liver (ZALESKI et al. 1991; KWEI et al. 1992), factors regulating the release, transport, and processing of these products by target organs have long been overlooked and now require critical evaluation.

Monooxygenation of PAHs gives rise to a variety of products, some of which are biologically inactive. However, others are highly reactive, bind covalently to cellular nucleophiles, and are mutagenic and carcinogenic (CONNEY 1967; MILLER et al. 1974; THAKKER et al. 1985). It is well established that benzo(a)pyrene requires activation by microsomal monooxygenases to reactive electrophilic species to cause cell mutation and cancer (MILLER et al. 1974; MILLER 1970; CONNEY 1967; COOPER et al. 1983). Monooxygenase activity in the liver is clearly orders of magnitude higher than in tissues where PAHs cause tumors (CONNEY 1967; KWEI et al. 1991). It is difficult, however, to envision how highly reactive electrophiles formed from benzo(a)pyrene leave the liver and travel to target tissues. It is generally assumed that reactive metabolites such as BPDE are formed in target tissues. Several lines of evidence support the idea that specific conjugates of benzo(a)pyrene metabolites are carriers of carcinogenic activity. For example, glucuronide conjugates of benzo(a)pyrene phenols are mutagenic (KARI et al. 1984; BOCK 1991), and inhibition of β-glucuronidase in vivo prevents PAH-induced tumors in animals (WALASZEK 1990). Importantly, radioactive benzo(a)pyrene administered to rats in vivo binds covalently to brain tissue, which is virtually devoid of monooxygenase activity (WALL et al. 1991). Work reviewed in Chap. 15 of this volume demonstrates that the sulfate conjugate of 6-hydroxymethyl benzo(a)pyrene (SURH et al. 1990a,b) and a benzo(a)pyrene bay region sulfonate (GREEN and REED 1990) induce tumors in infant mice. The possibility that sulfation of benzo(a)pyrene phenols is critical in tumorogenesis is supported by the finding that pentachlorophenol, an inhibitor of sulfotransferase, prevented tumor formation from 6-hydroxymethyl benzo(a) pyrene in vivo (SURH et al. 1990a,b). Interestingly, benzo(a)pyrene-1-sulfate has recently been found to be mutagenic in the Ames test (IRWIN et al. 1992). Data from studies in animals and humans (BAUER et al. 1979; REDDY and WYNDER 1973; REDDY 1981) imply a link between hydrolysis of carcinogenic glucuronide conjugates via β-glucuronidase and intestinal cancer. An inhibitor of β-glucuronidase, an analog of the known β-glucuronidase inhibitor D-glucaro-1,4-lactone, present in natural diets markedly diminished breast tumors produced by 7,12-dimethylbenzanthracene (WALASZEK 1990). Glucuronides of benzo(a)pyrene that are excreted via bile and effluent perfusate from perfused livers are mutagenic in the Ames test (KARI et al. 1984, 1985). Further, intermediates formed from hydrolysis of 3-hydroxy benzo(a)pyrene-glucuronide via β-glucuronidase is more active in binding DNA than benzo(a)pyrene-3-hydrophenol (KINOSHITA and GELBOIN 1978). These data raise the interesting possibility that nonphenolic intermediates formed via hydrolysis of benzo(a) pyrene conjugates are carcinogenic. Further work to test this hypothesis is clearly needed.

It is generally assumed that BPDE is the ultimate carcinogen arising from benzo(a)pyrene metabolism. Work by A. Conney, D. Jerina, and their collaborators (BUENING et al. 1978) identified BPDE as an ultimate carcinogen by administration of this compound to infant mice and determination of the frequency of tumors after 30–37 weeks. All mice given a total of 14 nmol BPDE in three intraperitoneal doses over 15 days after birth developed lung tumors. Although it is clear that BPDE is a powerful mutagen and induces tumors in vivo, alternative interpretations of this experiment exist. For example, BPDE is extremely reactive and it is difficult to envision its absorption, transport through the liver, and uptake by lung without further metabolism. It is possible that BPDE could reach the lung protected by serum proteins (GINSBERG and ATHERHOLT 1989; ROCHE et al. 1985); however, data described below indicate that only a small fraction of BPDE is likely to reach target tissues as such (i.e., it is largely conjugated). Thus, how injected BPDE causes lung tumors in vivo remains unclear.

When $\pm[^{14}C]$BPDE (approximately the same dose of the enantiomer used to induce lung tumors) or $[^{3}H]$benzo(a)pyrene was given to 15-day-old mice and blood, liver, and lung were examined for metabolites (KWEI et al. 1992), more than 90% of metabolites recovered after administration of either BPDE or benzo(a)pyrene were stable conjugates (Fig. 5). Glutathione (metabolite 1), glucuronide (metabolite 2), and sulfate conjugates (metabolite 4) accounted for most of the conjugates generated from benzo(a) pyrene. Glucuronides were the most abundant conjugate formed from benzo(a)pyrene and BPDE (Fig. 5). The finding that more than 90% of the circulating metabolites of BPDE were in the form of stable metabolites suggests that conjugates formed from BPDE or its metabolites in the liver may be involved in the induction of lung tumors noted after injection of ±BPDE. Since less than 0.02% of the injected dose of BPDE remained in the serum as direct-acting electrophilic material at 1 h, the possibility that carcinogenesis was due to small amounts of BPDE reaching the lung cannot be ruled out. It is very important to identify the chemical structures of conjugates formed from BPDE and test their mutagenic and carcinogenic

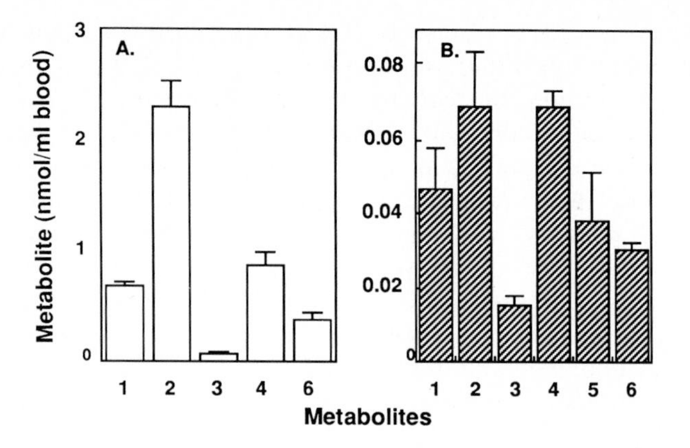

Fig. 5A,B. Benzo(a)pyrene metabolites in blood of mice injected with (±)antibenzo (a)pyrene-7,8-dihydrodiol-9,10-epoxide (BPDE) **A** or benzo(a)pyrene **B**. Fifteen-day-old Swiss Webster mice were injected with 39 nmol BPDE or 10 nml benzo(a) pyrene. Blood was collected 2 h after i.p. injection and analyzed for conjugates after separation on thin-layer chromatography plates (ZALESKI et al. 1991). Data are means ± S.E.M. of five animals per group. *1*, glutathione conjugates; *2*, glucuronide conjugates; *3*, unknown; *4*, sulfate conjugates and tetrols; *5*, dihydrodiols; *6*, benzo (a)pyrene-diolepoxide **A** or benzo(a)pyrene **B**

potential. Findings discussed above also emphasize the importance of considering the role of hydrolysis of phase II metabolites in chemical carcinogenesis.

II. Glutathione Conjugates

Various mechanisms exist by which glutathione conjugation can enhance the biological activity of toxic compounds. Briefly, these mechanisms include: (a) the formation of direct-acting glutathione conjugates of vicinal dihaloethanes, (b) generation of conjugates that undergo β-lyase-dependent bioactivation, e.g., haloalkenes, (c) generation of glutathione conjugates that serve as transport molecules, and (d) glutathione-dependent release of toxic metabolites from the liver (OLSON et al. 1992). Example of each of these mechanisms are reviewed extensively in Chap. 16 of this volume. Formation of glutathione conjugates in the liver is central to each of the above mechanisms. One of the best examples of the formation of a transport form involves the glutathione conjugates of bromohydroquinone, which are generated from bromobenzene in the liver and are highly nephrotoxic (MONKS et al. 1985). Glutathione conjugates of bromohydroquinones are released from the liver and travel in the blood stream to tissues such as kidney which are particularly rich in γ-glutamyl transpeptidase. Reversible glutathione conjugate formation has been noted with allyl and benzylisothiocyanates (OLSON et al. 1992). Glutathione conjugates of these types of compounds serve as transport forms of thiocarbamoylating or carbamoylating groups (PEARSON et al. 1990). *N*-Propylisothiocyanate is a potential metabolite of the oral-hypoglycemic agent chlorpropamide that has been implicated in inhibition of aldehyde dehydrogenase and enhanced susceptibility to ethanol intoxication in individuals receiving the drug (SHIROTA et al. 1992). Substitution of *N'*-nitrogen of chlorpropamide with allyl groups generates alkylcarbamoylating species that inhibit yeast and liver aldehyde dehydrogenase. Paradoxically, elevation of intracellular glutathione with cysteine prodrugs enhanced rather than inhibited aldehyde dehydrogenase (SHIROTA et al. 1992), due possibly to protection of -SH groups on the enzyme. Additional research to test this interesting possibility is needed.

E. Activation of Drug Conjugates by Targeted Enzymes

A great deal of research has been aimed at utilizing monoclonal antibodies (MAbs) that bind to tumor-associated antigens to target low molecular weight drugs (THORPE 1985) or toxic proteins (VITETTA et al. 1987) to cancer cells. The rationale behind this approach is that therapy with MAb conjugates limits toxicity at nontarget tissues while enhancing drug delivery to cancer cells that bind the conjugates. While this approach has been useful in some cases, it has generally not been successful in the treatment of solid tumors. Many cytotoxins have low potency, heterogeneity in antigens expression can lead to populations of tumor cells that are not exposed to cytotoxic quantities of the targeted agent, and most MAb–cytotoxic drug complexes are not delivered to intracellular sites of action. An alternative strategy that is currently being developed to circumvent these problems is to target MAb–hydrolytic enzyme complexes to the surface of tumors that convert relatively nontoxic prodrug conjugates into active drugs (HELLSTROM and SENTER 1992; SENTER 1990). Theoretically, a simple hydrolytic enzyme targeted for tumor cells should be capable of generating large amounts of active drug at these sites. Several enzymes of both mammalian and nonmammalian origin are being explored for the activation of a variety of prodrug conjugates. One of the first examples of the use of targeted enzymes in cancer chemotherapy involved the use of MAb-alkaline phosphatase to convert etoposide phosphate to the active cancer drug etoposide (SENTER et al. 1988). Direction of drug derivatives to target tissues including mitomycin phosphate and doxorubicin phosphate were also explored using MAb-alkaline phosphatase derivatives. While targeted enzyme prodrugs showed promise as therapeutically useful agents, the maximum tolerated doses of both the parent and phosphate-conjugated prodrugs were comparable, due possibly to hydrolysis of the conjugates at nontarget sites by endogenous alkaline phosphatase. The bacterial enzyme carboxypeptidase G2 (CPG2) from *Psuedomonas spp*. has been complexed with tumor-specific MAbs and used to activate conjugates of nitrogen mustards and methotrexate (SPRINGER et al. 1991). Three novel bifunctional alkylating agents were conjugated with glutamic acid. Hydrolysis of glutamic acid from each of these conjugates by MAb–CPG2 complexes targeted for human chariocarcinoma was quite effective with K_m values ranging between 4.5 and 12 μM (SPRINGER et al. 1991). Athymic Nu/No mice with palpable transplanted human choriocarcinoma xenografts, which are resistant to conventional chemotherapy, were pretreated with enzyme MAb complexes 24–72 h prior to administering the glutamic acid prodrugs. Significant increases in survival of up to four times that of control animals were noted in mice given one course of treatment (SPRINGER et al. 1991). These experiments clearly demonstrate the utility of carboxypeptidase complexed to tumor-specific MAb as an approach having considerable therapeutic potential. Other enzymes that have been tested in antibody-directed enzyme prodrug therapy include penicillin amidase, β-lactamase, cytosine deaminase, nitroreductase (HELLSTROM and SENTER 1992; SENTER 1990), and β-glucuronidase (SPRINGER et al. 1991). A wide variety of glucuronide prodrugs may be synthesized that can be hydrolyzed by targeted enzymes. In addition, glucuronide prodrugs appear less toxic than sulfate or phosphate antitumor prodrugs (BUKHARI et al. 1972), and any activated drug not taken up by tumor cells may be converted back to glucuronide prodrug by hepatic glucuronosyltransferase. One of the earliest examples of the formation of a glucuronide prodrug in the liver involved the unique action of aniline mustard and related analogs in curing mice bearing advanced plasma cell tumors (CONNORS and WHISSON 1966). This relatively nontoxic prodrug, *P*-hydroxyaniline mustard glucuronide, is formed in vivo in the liver of mice treated with aniline mustard and subsequently converted to highly cytotoxic aniline mustard by β-glucuronidase in murine tumors. Unfortunately, most human tumors do not have high activities of β-glucuronidase, and clinical trials using aniline mustard alone have been disappointing (KYLE et al. 1973). Recent studies demonstrating that the activity of glucuronide prodrugs can be greatly enhanced by targeting β-glucuronidase–MAb complexes to several different human tumor cell lines (ROFFLER et al. 1991; WANG et al. 1992) while maintaining low toxicity of the prodrug. Clearly, this interesting class of agents raises the possibility that other prodrugs may be targeted for specific sites in the body using targeted enzymes that hydrolyze conjugates.

F. Conclusions

Work reviewed in this chapter indicates that phase II conjugating reactions serve important roles in both the enhancement of biological activity and inactivation of a wide array of compounds. Based on new data that have emerged showing that conjugates such as morphine glucuronide, minoxidil sulfate, and retinoid glucuronides possess greater biological activity than their parent compounds, it is important that more attention than has been given previously be directed at the activity of drug conjugates during the process of drug development. Indeed, some drug conjugates may be considerably more active and specific than unconjugated drugs. Conjugates may also serve as important carriers of biological activity from the liver to target tissues and may be utilized as very useful prodrugs. Coupling of antibody-linked hydrolases to enhance the availability of active drugs delivered from inactive drug conjugates is a field that holds considerable promise. Finally, the possibility of drug interactions at sites of conjugation and deconjugation needs to be considered both in terms of potentiation of pharmacological activity as well as loss of activity in the case of biologically active drug conjugates.

Acknowledgement. Our work on the conjugation of benzo(a)pyrene metabolites and their biological activity was supported by grant CA-20807 from the National Cancer Institute, U.S. Department of Health and Human Services. The authors are grateful to Marybeth Sarsfield for her expert assistance in assembling the manuscript.

References

Abou-Issa HM, Duruibe VA, Minton JP, Larroya S, Dwivedi C, Webb TE (1988) Putative metabolites derived from dietary combinations of calcium glucarate and N-(4-hydroxyphenyl) retinamide act synergistically to inhibit the induction of rat mammary tumors by 7,12-dimethylbenz(a)anthracene. Proc Natl Acad Sci USA 85:4181–4184

Anel A, Halmos T, Torres JM, Antonakas K, Uriel J (1990) Cytotoxicity of chlorambucil-fatty acid complexes against normal human lymphocytes and human lymphoma cell lines. Biochem Pharmacol 40:1193–1200

Anwer MS, Kroker R, Hegner D (1976) Cholic acid uptake into isolated rat hepatocytes. Hoppe-Seyler's Z Physiol Chem 375:1477–1486

Bamforth KJ, Dalgliesh K, Coughtrie MWH (1992) Inhibition of human liver steroid sulfotransferase activities by drugs: a novel mechanism of drug toxicity? Eur J Pharmacol 228:15–21

Barbet J, Machy P, Leserman LD (1981) Monoclonal antibody coupled to liposomes: specific targeting to cells. J Supramol Struct Cell Biochem 16:243–258

Barrett-Connor E, Khaw K-T, Yen SSC (1986) A prospective study of dehydroepiandrosterone sulfate, mortality, and cardiovascular disease. N Engl J Med 315:1519–1524

Bauer HG, Asp N-G, Oste R, Dahlquist A, Fredlund PE (1979) Effect of dietary fiber on the induction of colorectal tumors and fecal β-glucuronidase activity. Cancer Res 39:3752–3756

Bhatnagar R, Abou-Issa H, Curley RW Jr, Koolemans-Beynen A, Moeschberger ML, Webb TE (1991) Growth suppression of human breast carcinoma cells in culture by *N*-(4-hydroxyphenyl) retinamide and its glucuronide and through synergism with glucarate. Biochem Pharmacol 41:1471–1477

Bock KW (1991) Roles of UDP-glucuronosyltransferases in chemical carcinogenesis. Crit Rev Biochem Mol Biol 26:129–150

Bradow G, Kan L, Fenselau C (1989) Studies of intramolecular rearrangements of acyl-linked glucuronides using salicylic acid, flufenamic acid, and [S]- and [R]-benoxaprofen and confirmation of isomerization in acyl-linked delta-9-11-carboxytetrahydrocannabinol glucuronide. Chem Res Toxicol 2:316–324

Bray K, Quast U (1991) Some degree of overlap exists between the K^+-channels opened by chromakalim and those opened by minoxidil sulphate in rat isolated aorta. Arch Pharmacol 344:351–359

Brayden JE, Quayle JM, Standen NB, Nelson MT (1991) Role of potassium channels in the vascular response to endogenous and pharmacological vasodilators. Blood Vessels 28:147–153

Buening MK, Wislocki PG, Levin W, Yagi H, Thakker DR, Akagi H, Koreeda M et al. (1978) Tumorigenicity of the optical enantiomers of the diastereomeric benzo(a)pyrene, 7,8-diol-9,10-epoxides in newborn mice: exceptional activity of (+)-7b,8a-dihydroxy-9a,10a-epoxy-7,8,9,10-tetrahydrobenzo(a)pyrene. Proc Natl Acad Sci USA 75:5358–5361

Buhl AE, Waldon DJ, Baker CA, Johnson GA (1990) Minoxidil sulfate is the active metabolite that stimulates hair follicles. J Invest Dermatol 95:553–557

Bukhari MA, Everett JL, Ross WCJ (1972) Aryl-2-halogenoalkylamines-XXVI. Glucuronic, sulphuric and phosphoric esters of *p*-di-2-chloroethylamino-phenol. Biochem Pharmacol 21:963–967

Burckhardt G, Kramer W, Kurz G, Wilson FA (1983) Inhibition of bile salt transport in brush-border membrane vesicles from rat small intestine by photoaffinity labeling. J Biol Chem 258:3618–3622

Buscher HP, Fricker G, Gerok W, Kramer W, Kurz G, Muller M, Schneider S (1986) In: Greten H, Windler E, Beisiegel U (eds) Receptor-mediated uptake in the liver. Springer, Berlin Heidelberg New York, pp 189–199

Caldwell J (1982) Conjugation reactions in the metabolism of xenobiotics. In: Arias I, Popper H, Schacter D, Shafritz DA (eds) The liver: biology and pathobiology. Raven, New York, pp 281–295

Carrupt P-A, Testa B, Bechalany A, El Tayar N, Descas P, Perrissoud D (1991) Morphine 6-glucuronide and morphine 3-glucuronide as molecular chameleons with unexpected lipophilicity. J Med Chem 34:1272–1275

Chose TI, Blair AH (1978) Antibody-linked cytotoxic agents in the treatment of cancer: current status and future prospects. J Natl Cancer Inst 657:657–676

Conney AH (1967) Pharmacological implications of microsomal enzyme induction. Pharmacol Rev 19:317–366

Coonors TA, Whisson ME (1966) Cure of mice bearing advanced plasma cell tumours with aniline mustard: the relationship between glucuronidase activity and tumour sensitivity. Nature 210:866–867

Cooper CS, Grover PL, Sims P (1983) The metabolism and activation of benzo(a) pyrene. Prog Drug Metab 7:295–395

Dunagin PE Jr, Zachman RD, Olson JA (1966) The identification of metabolites of retinol and retinoic acid in rat bile. Biochim Biophys Acta 124:71–85

Ginsberg GL, Atherholt TB (1989) Transport of DNA-adducting metabolites in mouse serum following benzo(a)pyrene administration. Carcinogenesis 10:673–679

Gordon GB, Helzlsouer KJ, Comstock GW (1991) Serum levels of dehydroepiandrosterone and its sulfate and the risk of developing bladder cancer. Cancer Res 51:1366–1369

Green JL, Reed GA (1990) Benzo(a)pyrene bay-region sulfonates, a novel class of reactive intermediates. Chem Res Toxicol 3:59–64

Greenberg A, Luo S, Hsu C-H, Creighton P, Waldman J, Lioy P (1990) Benzo(a) pyrene in composite prepared meals: results from the THEES (Total Human Exposure to Environmental Substances) Study. Polycyclic Aromatic Compounds 1:221–231

Groppi VE, Burnett BA, Maggoria L (1990) Protein sulfation: a unique mechanism of action of minoxidil sulfate. J Invest Dermatol 194:522

Halmos T, Moroni R, Antonakis K, Uriel J (1992) Fatty acid conjugates of 2′deoxy-5-fluorouridine as prodrugs for the selective delivery of 5-fluorouracil to tumor cells. Biochem Pharmacol 44:149–155

Hand CW, Blunnie WP, Claffey LP, McShane AJ, McQuay HJ, Moore RA (1987) Potential analgesic contribution from morphine-6-glucuronide in CSF. Lancet ii:1207–1208

Haning RV Jr, Flood CA, Hackett RJ, Loughlin JS, McClure N, Longcope C (1991) Metabolic clearance rate of dehydroepiandrosterone sulfate, its metabolism to testosterone, and its intrafollicular metabolism to dehydroepiandrosterone, androstenedione, testosterone, and dihydrotestosterone in vivo. J Clin Endocrinol Metab 72:1088–1095

Hardison WGM, Heasley VL, Shellhamer DF (1991) Specificity of hepatocyte Na(+)-dependent taurocholate transporter: influence of side-chain length and change. Hepatology 13:68–72

Hellstrom KE, Senter PD (1992) Activation of prodrugs by targeted enzymes. Eur J Cancer 27:1342–1343

Iorizzi M, Minale L, Riccio R (1990) Starfish saponins, 45. Novel sulfated steroidal glycosides from the starfish *Astropecten scoparius*. J Nat Prod 53:1225–1233

Irving CC (1971) Metabolic activation of *N*-hydroxy compounds by conjugation. Xenobiotica 1:387–398

Irwin SE, Kwei GY, Blackburn GR, Thurman R, Kauffman FC (1992) Mutagenicity of benzo(a)pyrenyl-1-sulfate in the Ames test. Environ Mol Mutagen 19:235–243

Ishida H, Tsujinaka T, Kido Y, Kan K, Iijima S, Sakaue M, Ebisui C et al. (1992) Establishment of a multi-dose study of chondroitin sulfate iron colloid for evaluation of the reticuloendothelial system function. J Biochem Biophys Methods 25:25–35

Janick-Buckner D, Barua AB, Olson JA (1991) Induction of HL-60 cell differentiation by water soluble and nitrogen-containing conjugates of retinoic acid and retinol. FASEB J 5:320–325

Johnson GA, Barsuhn KJ, McCall JM (1982) Sulfation of minoxidil by liver sulfotransferase. Biochem Pharmacol 31:2949–2954

Kalota SJ, Stein PC, Parsons CL (1992) Prevention of acrolein-induced bladder injury by pentosanpolysulfate. J Urol 148:163–166

Kan KS, Monte MJ, Parslow RA, Coleman R (1989) Oestradiol 17β-glucuronide increases tight-junctional permeability in rat liver. Biochem J 261:297–300

Kari FW, Kauffman FC, Thurman RG (1984) Characterization of mutagenic glucuronide formation from benzo(a)pyrene in the nonrecirculating perfused rat liver. Cancer Res 44:5073–5078

Kari FW, Kauffman FC, Thurman RG (1985) Effect of bile salts on rates of formation, accumulation and export of mutagenic benzo(a)pyrene metabolites by the perfused rat liver. Cancer Res 45:1621–1627

Kaufman FC (1992) Biologically active drug conjugates. Pharmacoloist 34:126–127

Kinoshita N, Gelboin HV (1978) β-Glucuronidase catalyzed hydrolysis of benzo(a) pyrene-3-glucuronide and binding to DNA. Science 1999:307–309

Kramer W, Wess G, Schubert G, Bickel M, Girbig F, Gutjar U, Kowalewski S et al. (1992) Liver-specific drug targeting by coupling to bile acids. J Biol Chem 267:18598–18604

Kreuger KE, Papadopoulos V (1992) Mitochondrial benzodiazepine receptors and the regulation of steroid biosynthesis. Annu Rev Pharmacol Toxicol 32:211–237

Kuchel O, Buu NT, Racz K, De Lean A, Serri O, Kyncl J (1986) Role of sulfate conjugation of catecholamines in blood pressure regulation. Fed Proc 45: 2254–2259

Kwei GY, Zaleski GY, Thurman RG, Kauffman FC (1991) Enzyme activities associated with carcinogen metabolism in liver and nonhepatic tissues of rats maintained on high-fat and food-restricted diets. J Nutr 121:131–137

Kwei GY, Zaleski J, Irwin SE, Thurman RG, Kauffman FC (1992) Conjugation of benzo(a)pyrene 7,8-dihydrodiol-9,10-epoxide in infant Swiss-Webster mice. Cancer Res 52:1639–1642

Kyle RA, Costa G, Cooper MR, Ogawa M, Silver RT, Glidewell O, Holland JF (1973) Evaluation of aniline mustard in patients with multiple myeloma. Cancer Res 33:956–960

Leblanc N, Wilde DW, Keef KD, Hume JR (1989) Electrophysiological mechanisms of minoxidil sulfate-induced vasodilitation of rabbit portal veins. Circ Res 65:1102–1111

Londowski JM, Kost SB, Gross M, Labler L, Meier W, Kumar R (1985) Biologic activity of 3βD-glucopyranoside of vitamin D compound. J Pharmacol Exp Ther 234:25–29

Maher VM, Reuter MA (1973) Mutations and loss of transforming activity of DNA caused by the *O*-glucuronide conjugate of the carcinogen, *N*-hydroxy-2-aminofluorene. Mutat Res 21:63–71

McCloskey DE, Mcguire JJ, Russell CA, Rowan BG, Pizzorno G, Mini E (1992) Decreased folypolyglutamate synthetase activity as a mechanism of methotrexate resistance in CCRF-CEM human leukemia sublines. J Biol Chem 266:6181–6187

Mehta RB, Barua AB, Olson JA, Moon RC (1993) Effects of retinoid glucuronides on mammary gland development in organ culture. Oncology (in press)

Meisheri KD, Cipkus LA, Taylor CJ (1988) Mechanism of action of minoxidil sulfate-induced vasodilation: a role for increased K^+ permeability. J Pharmacol Exp Ther 245:751–760

Meisheri KD, Oleynek JL, Puddington L (1991) Role of protein sulfation in vasodilation induced by minoxidil sulfate, a K^+ channel opener. J Pharmacol Exp Ther 258:1091–1097

Meisheri KD, Johnson GA, Puddington L (1993) Enzymatic and nonenzymatic sulfation mechanisms in the biological actions of minoxidil. Biochem Pharmacol 45:271–279

Melchior CL, Allen PM (1992) Interaction of pregnanolone and pregnenolone sulfate with ethanol and pentobarbital. Pharmacol Biochem Behav 42:605–611

Miller EC, Miller JA (1974) In: Bush H (ed) Molecular biology of cancer. Academic, New York, pp 301–402

Miller JA (1970) Carcinogenesis by chemicals: an overview. Cancer Res 30:559–576

Mizuma T, Komori M, Horikoshi I (1991) Sulphate conjugation enhances reversible binding of drug to human serum albumin. J Pharm Pharmacol 43:446–448

Monks TJ, Lau SS, Highet RJ, Gillette JR (1985) Glutathione conjugates of 2-bromoquinone are nephrotoxic. Drug Metab Dispos 13:553–559

Moon RC, Thompson HJ, Becci PJ, Grubbs CJ Gander RJ, Newton DL, Smith JM et al. (1979) N-(4-Hydroxyphenyl) retinamide, a new retinoid for prevention of breast cancer in the rat. Cancer Res 39:1339–1346

Morfin R, Young J, Corpéchot C, Egestad B, Sjövall J, Baulieu E-E (1992) Neurosteroids: pregnenolone in human sciatic nerves. Proc Natl Acad Sci USA 89:6790–6793

Mori S (1922) The changes in the paraocular glands which follow administration of diets low in fat soluble A with notes of the effects of the same diets on the salivary glands and the mucosa of the larynx and trachea. Bull Johns Hopkins Hosp 33:357

Mulder GJ (1992) Pharmacological effects of drug conjugates: is morphine 6-glucuronide an exception? Trends Pharmacol Sci 13:302–304

Nelson MT, Standen NB, Brayden JE, Worley JF (1988) Noradrenalin contracts arteries by activating voltage-dependent calcium channels. Nature 336:383–385

Nestler JE, Clore JN, Blackard WG (1992) Dehydroepinadrosterone: the "missing link" between hyperinsulinemia and atherosclerosis? FASEB J 6:3073–3075

Newgreen DT, Bray KM, McHarg AD, Weston AH, Duty S, Brown BS, Kay PB et al. (1990) The action of diazoxide and minoxidil sulfate on rat blood vessels; a comparison with chromakalim. Br J Pharmacol 100:605–613

Oguri K, Yamada-Mori I, Shigezane J, Hirano T, Yoshimura H (1987) Enhanced binding of morphine to opioid delta receptor by glucuronate and sulfate conjugations at the 6-position. Life Sci 41:1457–1464

Olson JA, Moon RC, Anders MW, Fenselau C, Shane B (1992) Enhancement of biological activity by conjugation reactions. J Nutr 122:614–624

Orentreich N, Brind JL, Rizer RL, Vogelman JH (1984) Age changes and sex differences in serum DHEA-sulfate concentrations throughout adult-hood. J Clin Endocrinol Metab 59:551–555
Osborne R, Thompson P, Joel S, Trew D, Patel N, Slevin M (1992) The analgesic activity of morphine-6-glucuronide. Br J Clin Pharmacol 34:130–138
Paul D, Standifer KM, Inturrisi CE, Pasternak GW (1989) Pharmacological characterization of morphine-6β-glucuronide, a very potent morphine metabolite. J Pharmacol Exp Ther 251:477–483
Pearson PG, Slatter JG, Rashed MS, Han D-H, Grillo MP, Baillie TA (1990) S-(N-methylcarbamoyl) glutathione: a reactive S-linked metabolite of methyl isocyanate. Biochem Biophys Res Commun 166:245–250
Portenoy RK, Khan E, Layman M, Lapin J, Malkin MG, Foley KM, Thaler HT et al. (1991) Chronic morphine therapy for cancer pain: plasma and cerebrospinal fluid morphine and morphine-6-glucuronide concentrations. Neurology 41: 1457–1461
Reddy B (1981) Dietary fat and its relationship to large bowel cancer. Cancer Res 41:3700–3705
Reddy BS, Wynder EL (1973) Large bowel carcinogenesis. Fecal constituents of populations with diverse incidence rates of colon cancer. J Natl Cancer Inst 50:1437–1442
Roche CJ, Zinger D, Geacintov NE (1985) Enhancement of stability of 7β,8(a)-dihyroxy-9(a)epoxybenzo(a)pyrene by complex formation with serum albumin. Cancer Biochem Biophys 8:35–40
Roffler SR, Wang SM, Chern Ji-W, Yeh M-Y, Tung E (1991) Anti-neoplastic glucuronide prodrug treatment of human tumor cells targeted with a monoclonal antibody-enzyme conjugate. Biochem Pharmacol 42:2062–2065
Rubinstein A, Nakar D, Sintov A (1992) Chondroitin sulfate: a potential biodegradable carrier for colon-specific drug delivery. Int J Pharmacol 84:141–150
Sani BP, Barua AB, Hill TW, Shih TW, Olson JA (1992) Retinoyl beta-glucuronide: lack of binding to receptor proteins of retinoic acid as related to biological activity. Biochem Pharmacol 43:919–922
Senter PD, Saulnier MG, Schreiber GJ, Hirschberg DL, Brown JP, Hellstrom I, Hellstrom KE (1988) Anti-tumor effects of antibody-alkaline phosphatase conjugates in combination with ectoposide phosphate. Proc Natl Acad Sci USA 85:4842–4946
Senter PD (1990) Activation of prodrugs by antibody-enzyme conjugates: a new approach to cancer therapy. FASEB J 4:188–193
Shane B (1989) Folylpolyglutamate synthesis and role in the regulation of one carbon metabolism. Vitam Horm 45:263–335
Shirota FN, Elberling JA, Nagasawa HT, DeMaster EG (1992) Failure of glutathione and cysteine prodrugs to block the chlorpropamide-induced inhibition of aldehyde dehydrogenase in vivo. Biochem Pharmacol 43:916–918
Smith MT, Watt JA, Cramond T (1990) Morphine-3-glucuronide – a potent antagonist of morphine analgesia. Life Sci 47:579–585
Sonka J, Vitkova M, Gregorova I, Tomsova Z, Higertova J, Stas J (1973) Plasma and urinary dehydroepiandrosterone in cancer. Endokrinologie 62:61–68
Sorentino D, Stump D, Potter BJ, Robinson RB, White R, Kiang Ch, Berk PD (1988) Oleate uptake by cardiac myocytes is carrier mediated and involves a 40 kD plasma membrane fatty acid binding protein similar to that in liver, adipose tissue, and gut. J Clin Invest 82:928–935
Sporn MB, Roberts AB (1983) The role of retinoids in differentiation and carcinogenesis. Cancer Res 43:3034–3039
Springer CJ, Bagshawe KD, Sharma SK, Searle F, Boden JA, Antoniw P, Burke PJ et al. (1991) Ablation of human choriocarcinoma xenografts in nude mice by antibody-directed enzyme prodrug therapy (ADEPT) with three novel compounds. Eur J Cancer 11:1361–1366

Stogniew M, Fenselau C (1982) Electrophilic reactions of acyl-linked glucuronides. Drug Metab Dispos 10:609–613
Surh Y, Liem A, Miller EC, Miller JA (1990a) The strong hepatocarcinogenicity of the electrophilic and mutagenic metabolite 6-sulfooxymethylbenzo[a]pyrene and its formation of benzylic DNA adducts in the livers of infant male B6C3F1 mice. Biochem Biophys Res Commun 172:85–91
Surh Y-J, Blomquist JC, Liem A, Miller EC, Miller JA (1990b) Metabolic activation of 9-hydroxymethyl-10-methylanthracene and 1-hydroxymethylpyrene to electrophilic, mutagenic and tumorigenic sulfuric acid esters by rat hepatic sulfotransferase activity. Carcinogenesis 11:1451–1460
Thakker DR, Yagi H, Levin W, Wood AW, Conney AH, Jerina DM (1985) Polycyclic aromatic hydrocarbons: metabolic activation to ultimate carcinogens. In: Anders MW (ed) Bioactivation of foreign compounds. Academic Press, Orlando, pp 177–242
Thorpe PE (1985) Antibody carriers of cytotoxic agents in cancer therapy, a review. In: Pinchera A, Doria G, Dammacco F, Bargellesi A (eds) Monoclonal antibodies '84: biological and clinical applications. Editrice Kurtis, Milan, pp 475–506
Uriel J, Naval J, Laboradora J (1987) AFP-mediated transfer of arachadonic acid into cultured cloned cells deriver from a rat rhabdhomyosarcoma. J Biol Chem 262:3579–3585
vanBreemen RB, Fenselau C (1985) Acylation of albumin by 1-O-acyl glucuronides. Drug Metab Dispos 13:318–320
Vitetta ES, Fulton RJ, May RD, Till M, Uhr JW (1987) Redesigning nature's poisons to create anti-tumor reagents. Science 238:1098–1104
Vore M, Hadd H, Slikker W Jr (1983) Ethynylestradiol-17β D-ring glucuronide conjugates are potent cholestatic agents in the rat. Life Sci 32:2989–2993
Walaszek Z (1990) Potential use of D-glucaric acid derivatives in cancer prevention. Cancer Lett 54:1–8
Wall KL, Gao WS, te Koppele JM, Kwei GY, Kauffman FC, Thurman RG (1991) The liver plays a central role in the mechanism of chemical carcinogenesis due to polycyclic aromatic hydrocarbons. Carcinogenesis 12:783–786
Wang S-M, Chern J-W, Yeh M-Y, Ng JC, Tung E, Roffler SR (1992) Specific activation of glucuronide prodrugs by antibody-targeted enzyme conjugates for cancer therapy. Cancer Res 52:4484–4491
Wu FS, Gibbs TT, Farb DH (1991) Pregnenolone sulfate: a positive allosteric regulator of the NMDA receptor. Mol Pharmacol 40:333–336
Yaksh TL, Harty GJ (1988) Pharmacology of the allodynia in rats evoked by high does intrathecal morphine. J Pharmacol Exp Ther 244:501–507
Yoshimura H, Ida S, Oguri K, Tsukamoto H (1973) Biochemical basis for analgesic activity of morphine-6-glucuronide-I: penetration of morphine-6-glucuronide in the brain of rats. Biochem Pharmacol 22:1423–1430
Zaleski J, Kwei GY, Thurman RG, Kauffman FC (1991) Suppression of benzo(a) pyrene metabolism by accumulation of triacylglycerols in rat hepatocytes: effect of high-fat and food-restricted diets. Carcinogenesis 12:2073–2079
Zile MH, Cullum ME, Simpson RU, Barua AB, Swartz DA (1987) Induction of differentiation of human promyelocytic leukemia cell line HL-60 by retinoyl glucuronide, a biologically active metabolite of vitamin A. Proc Natl Acad Sci USA 84:2208–2212

CHAPTER 13

Acyl Glucuronides as Chemically Reactive Intermediates

C. FENSELAU

A. Acyl Glucuronides as Chemically Reactive Intermediates

Virtually all types of xenobiotic acids form 1-*O*-acyl glucuronides. Many other xenobiotic compounds are metabolized to carboxylic acids, which subsequently undergo phase II conjugation with glucuronic acid. Often such a conjugate constitutes the major metabolite. Many examples are found among the hypolipidemic agents, diuretic agents, and nonsteroidal antiinflammatory drugs. Most herbicides are metabolized in this manner by fish, birds and mammals. 1-*O*-Acyl glucuronides are also formed from endogenous lipids such as retinoic acid, lithocholic acid and bilirubin. The major site of conjugation in humans is the liver. 1-*O*-Acyl glucuronides are excreted through the bile duct and the kidney, and many of these conjugates have been shown to circulate in plasma.

The glycosidic bond formed between glucuronic acid and a xenobiotic is a result of a UDP-glucuronyltransferase mediated reaction that requires cellular energy (DUTTON 1966). This reaction may occur with alcohols, acids, amines, thiols, and electrophilic carbon atoms to produce corresponding ether, ester, amide, or thioester glucuronide conjugates. In particular, the ester glucuronides are known to be chemically labile, owing to the facile displacement of the glucuronic acid moiety by nucleophilic species (Fig. 1). This ester hydrolysis is thermodynamically favored and proceeds via a tetrahedral intermediate, proposed by FISCHER (1920) for glycosidic esters and confirmed by subsequent mechanistic studies (DOERSCHUK 1952; BONNER 1959). This and other features of carbohydrate chemistry have become familiar to pharmacologists in the last 20 years, as advances in physicochemical tools have made it easy to characterize and study intact glucuronides (BAX et al. 1984; FENSELAU and YELLE 1986; VAN BREEMEN et al. 1988; ABRAMSON 1990; FENSELAU 1992). Depending on the nature of the reacting nucleophile, the tetrahedral intermediate described above results in either hydrolysis to the aglycon carboxylic acid, intramolecular rearrangement to regioisomeric esters, or covalent adduct formation. These three reaction products are depicted in Fig. 2 and have been extensively documented in the literature.

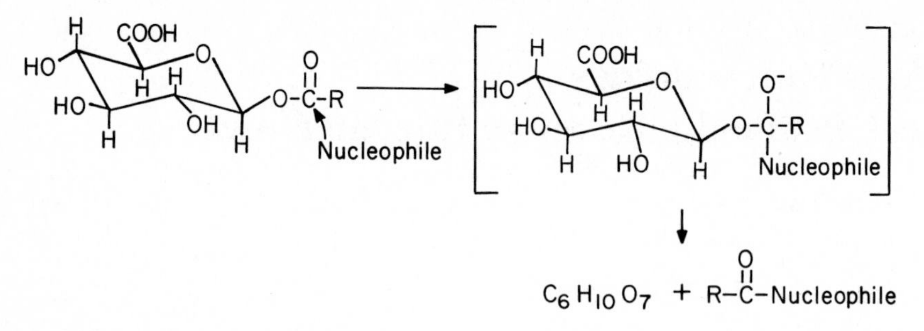

Fig. 1. Nucleophilic displacement of glucuronic acid from the 1-*O*-acyl glucuronide linkage via a tetrahedral intermediate

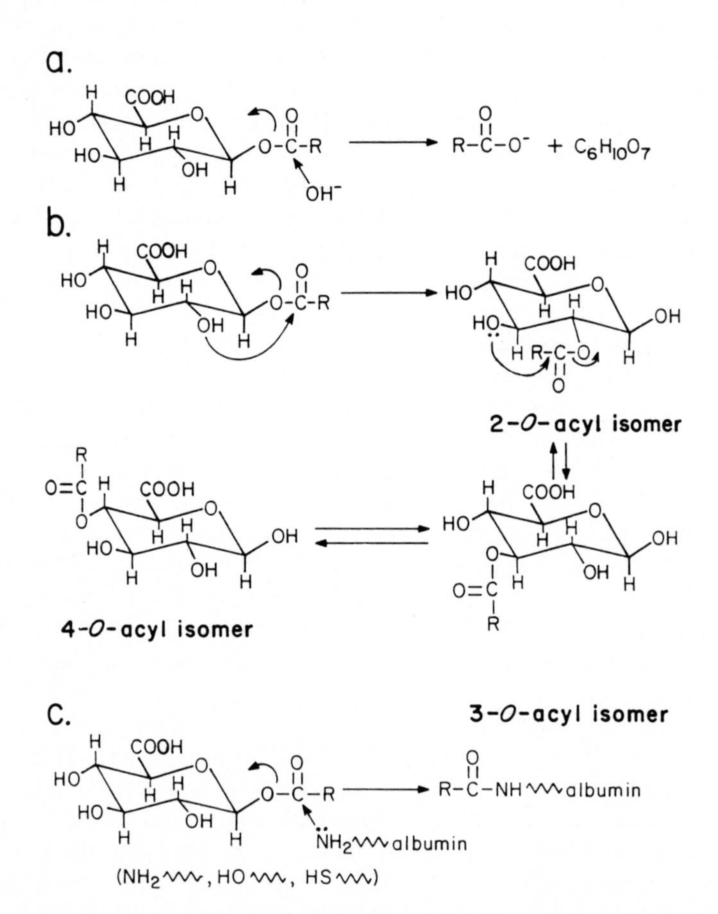

Fig. 2a–c. Examples of nucleophilic displacement. **a** Base-catalyzed hydrolysis; **b** intramolecular acyl migrations; **c** intermolecular transacylation illustrated with *albumin*

In the absence of strong nucleophiles, the 1-*O*-acyl glucuronides that have been studied kinetically undergo apparent first-order degradation. Closer examination shows that the products are usually mixtures of hydrolytically released drug (Fig. 2a) and isomers of the glucuronide conjugate formed by intramolecular rearrangement (Fig. 2b). Typical results are shown in Fig. 3. in which the concentration of tolmetin, its acyl glucuronide, and three ester isomers in human urine adjusted to pH 7.4 are measured through 24 h at 37°C (HYNECK et al. 1988). The 1-*O*-acyl conjugate of tolmetin disappears rapidly at pH 7.4 (Table 1), undergoing both hydrolysis and intramolecular rearrangement. The ester isomers also undergo hydrolysis (and further rearrangement) and at 24 h the hydrolysis products predominate.

Rates of degradation of 1-*O*-acyl glucuronides depend on both the nature of the acidic aglycon and the pH of the solution. Half-lives published for some of these metabolites are collected in Table 1 and illustrate well the variability between conjugates of different aglycons, including diastereomeric glucuronides, in the pH range 7.0–7.4. Examination of a smaller set of samples indicates that the stabilities of 1-*O*-acyl conjugates do not correlate with the rank order of pK values for the acidic aglycons, and the influence of steric factors has been suggested (VAN BREEMEN and FENSELAU 1985). The pH at which each glucuronide is most stable also varies from one compound to another, although generally speaking most are more stable in mildly acidic solutions and unstable in basic solutions. The dramatic effect of

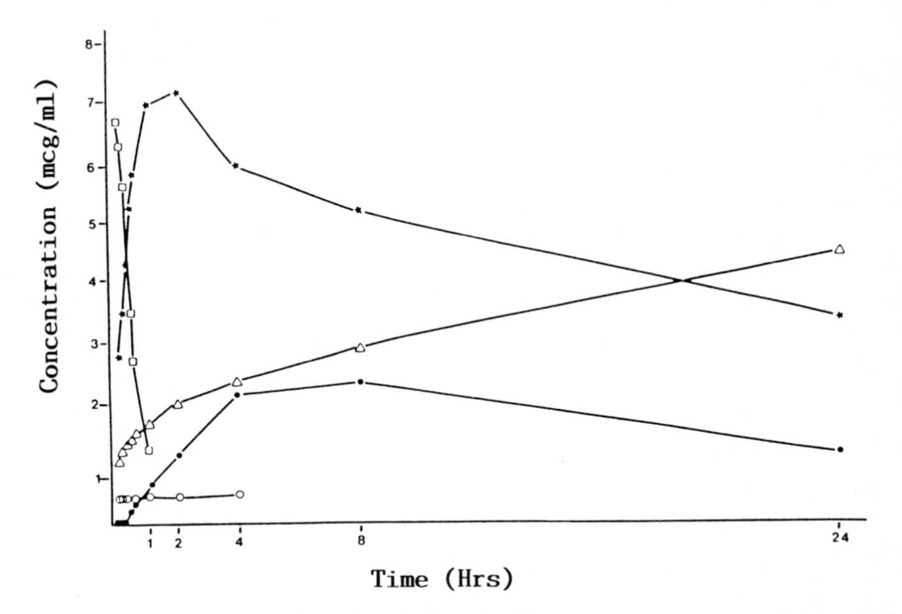

Fig. 3. Time-dependent degradation of the 1-*O*-acyl glucuronide of tolmetin at pH 7.4, 37°C in urine. □, 1-*O*-Acyl glucuronide; ● ○ ★, three ester isomers; △, tolmetin. Reproduced with permission from HYNECK et al. (1988)

Table 1. Half-lives for degradation of some 1-*O*-acyl glucuronides in aqueous solutions at pH 7.4, 37°C

Drug	Half-life (h)	References
Tolmetin	0.26	MUNOFO et al. (1990)
Wy-18251	0.38	RUELIUS et al. (1985)
Probenecid	0.40	HANSEN-MOLLER and SCHMIT (1991)
Zomepirac	0.45	SPAHN-LANGGATH and BENET (1992)
Diflunisal	0.57	WATT and DICKINSON (1990)
Oxaprozin	1.3	RUELIUS et al. (1985)
Indomethacin	1.4	VAN BREEMEN et al. (1986)
R-Fenoprofen	1.0	VOLLAND et al. (1991)
S-Fenoprofen	2.0	VOLLAND et al. (1991)
R-Carprofen	1.7	SPAHN-LANGGATH and BENET (1992)
S-Carprofen	1.9	SPAHN-LANGGATH and BENET (1992)
R-Benoxaprofen	2.0	SPAHN et al. (1989)
S-Benoxaprofen	4.1	SPAHN et al. (1989)
R-Flunoxaprofen	4.5	SPAHN (1988)
S-Flunoxaprofen	8.0	SPAHN (1988)
Furosemide	5.3	RACHMEL et al. (1985)
Flufenamic acid	7.0	VAN BREEMEN et al. (1986)
Clofibric acid	7.3	VAN BREEMEN et al. (1986)
Wy-41770	14.0	RUELIUS et al. (1985)
Etodolac	20.6	SMITH et al. (1992)
Valproic acid	79.0	WILLIAMS et al. (1992)

Table 2. Half-lives of 1-*O*-acyl glucuronides at various pH values[a,b]

pH	Flufenamic acid glucuronide	Indomethacin glucuronide	Clofibric acid glucuronide
2.0	1109 h	71.1 ± 39 h	124 ± 53 h
4.0	495 h	146 ± 20.3 h	49.5 ± 7.0 h
6.0	70.7 ± 2.9 h	21.0 ± 1.4 h	48.4 ± 10.7 h
7.4	6.96 ± 0.02 h	1.41 ± 0.01 h	7.26 ± 0.61 h
10.0	4.8 ± 0.1 min	<1 min	<2 min

[a] Buffered aqueous solution, 37°C; $n = 3$.
[b] VAN BREEMEN et al. (1986).

pH on hydrolysis and rearrangement of several conjugates is illustrated in Table 2. Half-lives can also vary when they are measured in buffered aqueous solution, in urine or in plasma (for example, SMITH et al. 1985; MUNAFO et al. 1990; WATT and DICKINSON 1990; HANSEN-MOLLER and SCHMIT 1991; WILLIAMS et al. 1992).

In addition to facile chemical hydrolysis, the 1-*O*-acyl conjugates are susceptible to hydrolysis by *β*-glucuronidase and by some esterases. Albumin is reported to catalyze hydrolysis of some 1-*O*-acyl glucuronides (WELLS et al. 1987; VOLLARD et al. 1991; SMITH et al. 1992; HAYBALL et al. 1992).

Overall, both the chemical lability and susceptibility to enzymatic cleavage of acyl glucuronides provide an important mechanism for the enterohepatic curculation of many carboxylic acid compounds in vivo (CALDWELL et al. 1983; FAED 1984; RUELIUS et al. 1985; MUSSON et al. 1985; SALLUSTIO et al. 1989; DICKINSON et al. 1991; SPAHN-LANGGUTH 1992; KOMURA et al. 1992). Several drugs, such as valproic acid, carprofen, and tolmetin, are known to undergo extensive recirculation via their enzyme-sensitive acyl glucuronide conjugates. These are excreted in bile primarily as intact conjugates. In the intestinal lumen the 1-*O*-acyl glucuronide is hydrolyzed to parent drug, which is subsequently reabsorbed into the systemic circulation. A comparison of the area under the plasma concentration versus time curve in intact and bile duct catheterized rats provides an estimation of the fraction of the total administered dose that undergoes recirculation. The ability of the acyl glucuronide to undergo intremolecular rearrangement to β-glucuronidase resistant isomers in the biliary tree serves to decrease the amount of compound that undergoes recirculation (KOMURA et al. 1992).

B. Intramolecular Rearrangements

The products of isomeric rearrangement (Fig. 2b) are formed by intramolecular transacylation across a broad pH range in vitro. Isomerization of 1-*O*-acyl glucuronides is most conveniently characterized by high pressure liquid chromatography (HPLC). A typical result is shown in Fig. 4, in which rat bile containing an acyl-linked glucuronide is analyzed by reverse phase HPLC at 0, 15, and 30 min after collection (JANNSEN et al. 1982). The glycosidic conjugate (peak 1) is the major peak at 0 min and steadily decreases in proportion as three other isomers appear. The application of mass spectrometry can rapidly provide supporting evidence that such families of HPLC peaks comprise multiple isomers (BLANKAERT et al. 1978; HIGNITE et al. 1981; JANNSEN et al. 1982). However, for rigorous assignment of the position of esterification, two-dimensional nuclear magnetic resonance (NMR) spectroscopy must be used (SMITH and BENET 1986; HANSEN-MOLLER et al. 1988; BRADOW et al. 1989). As has been demonstrated in earlier carbohydrate studies (BAX et al. 1984). NMR can readily identify which hydroxyl group is esterified and recognises epimerization at C-1 and changes in ring structure. In one demonstration of the analytical utility of NMR, isomer structures were assigned and their formation from flufenamic acid glucuronide was followed in situ in a 300 mHz NMR. The results of this experiment are illustrated in Fig. 5, where it can be seen that the isomers appear in order of the proximity of each ester group to the original 1-glycosidic linkage, i.e., the 2-hydroxy ester is detected first, followed by the 3-hydroxy ester, and finally the 4-hydroxy ester. The tetrahedral intermediate proposed in Fig. 1 was not detected in this study, in which signals

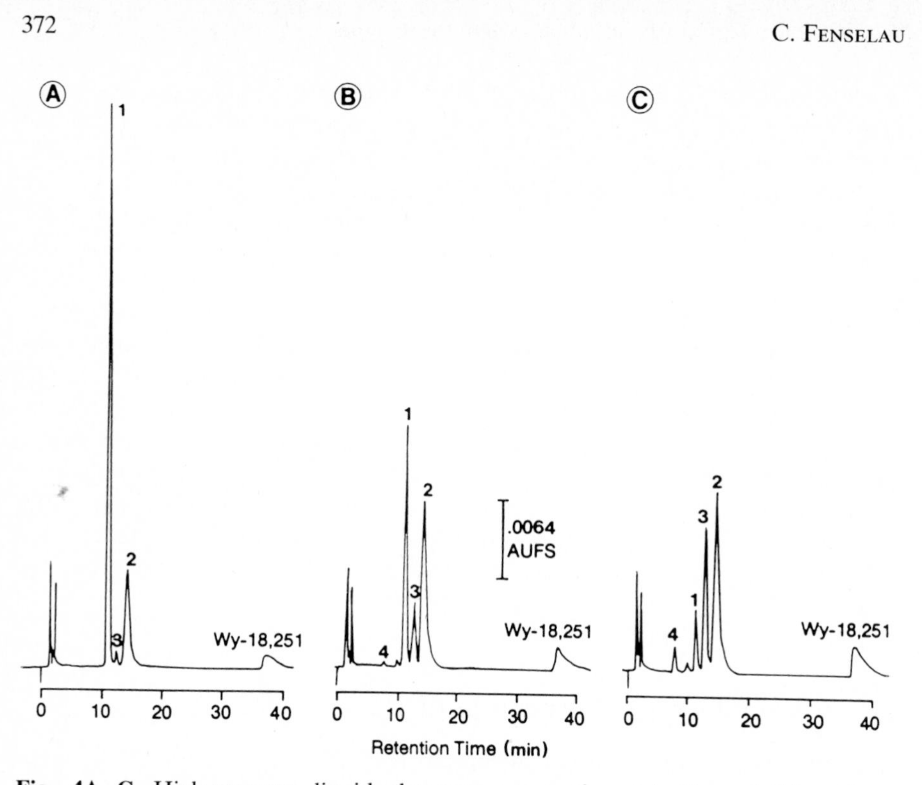

Fig. 4A–C. High-pressure liquid chromatograms of metabolites of 3-(*p*-chlorophenyl) thiazolo[3,2,-*a*]benzimidazole-2-acetic acid (*Wy-18251*) in rat bile collected by cannulation and allowed to stand for 0 min (**A**), 15 min (**B**), and 30 min (**C**). *Peak 1* was identified as the 1-*O*-acyl glucuronide. *Peaks 2, 3, and 4* are intramolecular rearrangement products. Reproduced with permission from JANSSEN et al. (1982)

were integrated through 5 min for each point on the curve. This order of appearance has been rigorously assigned in at least four cases (HANSEN-MOLLER et al. 1988; SMITH and BENET 1986; BRADOW et al. 1989), which all support the assumption that is generally used for assigning HPLC peaks to otherwise uncharacterized isomers. When one of the three ester isomers of an acyl glucuronide is purified, it will rearrange to a new mixture of ester isomers. However, the highly endothermic reformation of the 1-*O*-acyl glycosidic isomer does not occur. Epimerization or mutarotation can further elaborate the mixture of isomers detectable by HPLC and NMR; however, these can be reduced by controlling the pH.

The rates and the product distributions of intramolecular rearrangements differ from one acyl glucuronide to another and also differentiate diastereomers (BRADOW et al. 1989; SPAHN-LANGGUTH and BENET 1992). Not all acyl-linked glucuronides rearrange at physiologic pH; lithocholic acid glucuronide, for example, is reported to be stable (PANFIL et al. 1992).

This variability and its dependence on pH, temperature, time, and medium can seriously complicate pharmacokinetic assays. The resistance of

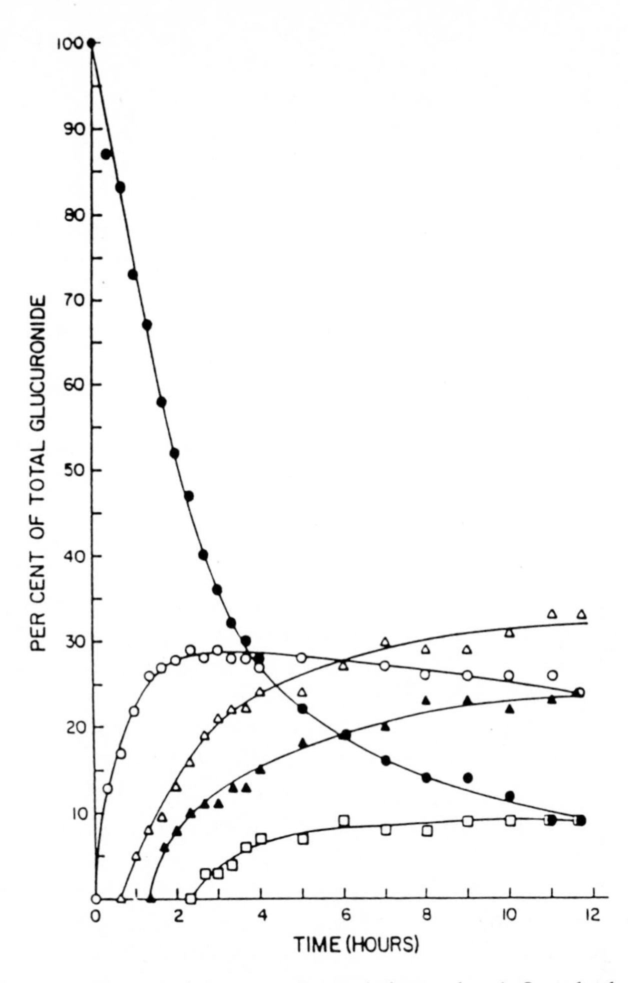

Fig. 5. Relative amounts of isomers formed from the 1-*O*-acyl glucuronide of flufenamic acid in situ in a 300 mHz nuclear magnetic resonance instrument through 12 h. ●, 1-*O*-Acyl; ○, 2-ester; △, 3-ester; ▲, 4-ester; □, hydrolyzed glucuronic acid. Reproduced with permission from BRADOW et al. (1989)

ester isomers to hydrolysis by β-glucuronidases is also significant, since many assays employ this reaction to release conjugated metabolites for quantitation. Indeed, the compromise of pharmacokinetic studies provided much of the incentive to understand the source and nature of the isomers (FAED 1984). Basic hydrolysis can be used to recover aglycon from both the glucuronide and its ester isomers.

Ester isomers have been shown to be formed in vivo and, in some cases, to circulate in plasma (for example, BLANCKAERT et al. 1978; RUELIUS et al. 1985; MUSSON et al. 1985; HYNECK et al. 1987; WATT et al. 1991). The more chemically stable ester isomers may be susceptible to further biotransformation. For example, ester isomers of diflunisal glucuronide are conjugated with a second molecule of glucuronic acid (KING and DICKINSON 1991). Ester isomers of oxaprozin glucuronide are substrates for hydrolysis by caecum esterases (RUELIUS et al. 1985). The ester isomers are capable of further spontaneous chemical reactions via the unblocked reducing terminus (aldehyde or cryptaldehyde) of the carbohydrate moiety. Their reactions with methoxyamine (COMPERNOLLE et al. 1978) and *p*-anisidine (JANNSEN et al. 1982) provide convenient methods to detect these species in biological samples.

C. Nucleophilic Displacement

Cleavage of the activated C-1 ester bond by nucleophilic reagents other than water (one example of which is shown in Fig. 3c) was observed more than 20 years ago by groups studying the metabolism of retinoic acid and of bilirubin. Exposure of retinoyl glucuronide (LIPPEL and OLSON 1968) or bilirubin acyl glucuronides (SALMON et al. 1975) to methanol rapidly leads to formation of methyl esters. Reactivities of other acyl glucuronides with methanol vary widely; however, use of that solvent in the chromatographic separation of 1-*O*-acyl glucuronides will be inappropriate in many cases. Ammonia has also been shown to displace acyl-linked glucuronic acid from bilirubin to produce amides characterized by mass spectrometry (COMPERNOLLE et al. 1970). Amides and methyl esters produced this way have been used as derivatives to distinguish conjugated from unconjugated bilirubin. Methanol also forms methyl esters by rapid transacylation of lithocholic acid glucuronide (PANFIL et al. 1992).

The 1-*O*-acyl glucuronide metabolite of the hypolipidemic clofibrate has been shown to react directly with ethanethiol to produce a well-characterized thio ester (STOGNIEW and FENSELAU 1982). Interestingly, the glucuronide did not react readily with glutathione at physiologic pH, but required catalysis by glutathione transferase.

Nucleophilic displacement has also been used as the basis of a color test to screen specifically for acyl-linked glucuronides on thin-layer chromatographic (TLC) plates (VAN BREEMEN and FENSELAU 1985). Reaction with the highly reactive nucleophile 4-(*p*-nitrobenzyl)pyridine (NBP) produces, under base catalysis, a dark blue product, visualized as a blue spot on the TLC plate. The investigator can determine the presence of glucuronides in a metabolic mixture by using the naphthoresorcinol color test for glycosiduronic acids and then distinguish acyl-linked glucuronides by reaction with NBP and rearranged ester isomers by the color reaction with *p*-anisidine (BRADOW et al. 1989). The chromophorogenic reaction with NBP has also been used to study the kinetics of transacylation of acyl glucuronides (VAN BREEMEN and FENSELAU 1985). Table 3 indicates that although there is wide variability in the alkylation rates of the glucuronides studied, their rates are

Table 3. Relative rate constants for alkylation of 4-(*p*-nitrobenzyl) pyridine[a,b]

	Rate constant (min^{-1})
Flufenamic 1-*O*-acyl glucuronide	0.436 ± 0.135
Indomethacin 1-*O*-acyl glucuronide	0.709 ± 0.081
Clofibric 1-*O*-acyl glucuronide	1.08 ± 0.23
Chlorambucil	137 ± 6

[a] Standard deviations were calculated for ⩾3 rate determinations
[b] VAN BREEMEN et al. (1986)

approximately two orders of magnitude lower than the alkylation rate of the chemotherapeutic agent chlorambucil. Conjugates of more than 50 endogenous and xenobiotic organic acids have been observed to undergo nucleophilic displacement to date, based on the NBP color test or other analyses.

Although the rates that have been measured for nucleophilic displacement, e.g., by NBP, are relatively low, the reactions of activated metabolites in vivo can accumulate throughout the time of exposure. With a drug such as clofibrate that is administered daily over long periods of time, nucleophilic groups in proteins and tissues will be exposed to the slowly reacting glucuronide metabolite through many years of dosage.

D. Covalent Bonding to Biopolymers

Covalent bonding between acyl-linked glucuronides and proteins and tissues has become well established through the last 11 years. Albumin has been studied most extensively, because it is physiologically relevant and readily available. Covalent bonding of drugs to albumin was initially demonstrated in vitro using glucuronides of radioisotope(^{14}C)-labeled clofibrate, indomethacin, benoxaprofen, and flufenamic acid (VAN BREEMEN and FENSELAU 1984). The covalent attachment summarized in Table 4 resulted from incubation of 2:1 molar ratios of glucuronide to bovine serum albumin for 12 h at pH 7.4 and 37°C. The most reactive glucuronide (benoxaprofen) bound about 5% of the albumin molecules in this short incubation. More than a dozen acyl glucuronides have now been shown to form covalently bound products with human and bovine serum albumin in vitro. Covalent attachment has also been demonstrated to α-casein (SMITH et al. 1990) and polylysine (MUNAFO et al. 1990).

In vivo covalent bonding was first recognized for the nono- and diglucuronides of bilirubin with human serum albumin (GAUTAM et al. 1984; McDONAUGH et al. 1984; VAN BREEMEN et al. 1986; YOSHIDA et al. 1987). This product was characterized by the distinctive spectroscopic properties of

Table 4. Acylation of bovine serum albumin by 1-*O*-acyl glucuronides[a,b]

Reagent	Aglycon-bound/ bovine serum albumin (mmol/mol)	95% Confidence level	Standard deviation
[^{14}C]Flufenamic acid (control)	1.75	±0.15	±0.06
[^{14}C]Flufenamic glucuronide	31.9	±1.3	±0.5
[^{14}C]Indomethacin (control)	5.04	±0.28	±0.11
[^{14}C]Indomethacin glucuronide	43.0	±1.3	±0.5
[^{14}C]Colfibric acid (control)	8.00	±0.29	±0.18
[^{14}C]Colfibric glucuronide	14.4	±0.3	±0.3
[^{14}C]Benoxaprofen (control)	11.1	±0.5	±0.3
[^{14}C]Benoxaprofen glucuronide	58.5	±7.4	±3.0

[a] Error values are determined for experiments where $n \geq 3$.
[b] VAN BREEMEN and FENSELAU (1985).

bilirubin. Subsequently, the list of xenobiotic conjugates shown to form covalent bonds with plasma proteins in vivo has been expanded to include (among others) the hypolipidemic clofibrate (SALLUSTIO et al. 1991), the antiepileptic valproic acid (WILLIANS et al. 1992), the uricosuric probenecid (MCKINNON and DICKINSON 1989; HANSEN-MOLLER and SCHMIT 1991), and the anti-inflammatory drugs tolmetin (HYNECK et al. 1988), zomepirac (SMITH et al. 1986), diflunisal (MCKINNON and DICKINSON 1989), and fenoprofen (VOLLAND et al. 1991) and ketoprofen (HAYBILL et al. 1992). The last two references report diastereomeric selectivity in vivo in protein bonding by acyl glucuronides and esters.

Figure 6 summarizes concentrations of diflunisal, diflunisal acyl glucuronide, and diflunisal covalently bound to plasma proteins, measured in plasma from five subjects who received multiple oral doses through 132 h (MCKINNON DICKINSON 1989). Concentrations of parent drug, acyl glucuronide, and plasma protein–drug adduct increased throughout the course of diflusinal administration. The subsequent curve for elimination of protein-bound diflunisal was significantly extended compared to clearance of the other two metabolites. The inset in Fig. 6 shows in more detail the biphasic clearance of diflunisal covalently bound to plasma proteins in all five subjects. If all the protein were albumin, about 1.4% of the albumin molecules would have carried one covalently attached diflunisal molecule. In this study, covalently bound diflunisal was assayed by HPLC after being released from the protein by treatment with 1 *M* NaOH overnight at 65°C. The authors pointed out that in the absence of verification with radioisotopes, it was not clear that all covalently bound drug is recovered by this procedure. In particular, it was unlikely that carboxylic acid-containing drugs bonded as amides (by the mechanism in Fig. 3a) would have been released quantitatively.

The correlation observed by MCKINNON and DICKINSON (1989) between the level of covalent bonding of plasma protein and the exposure of patients

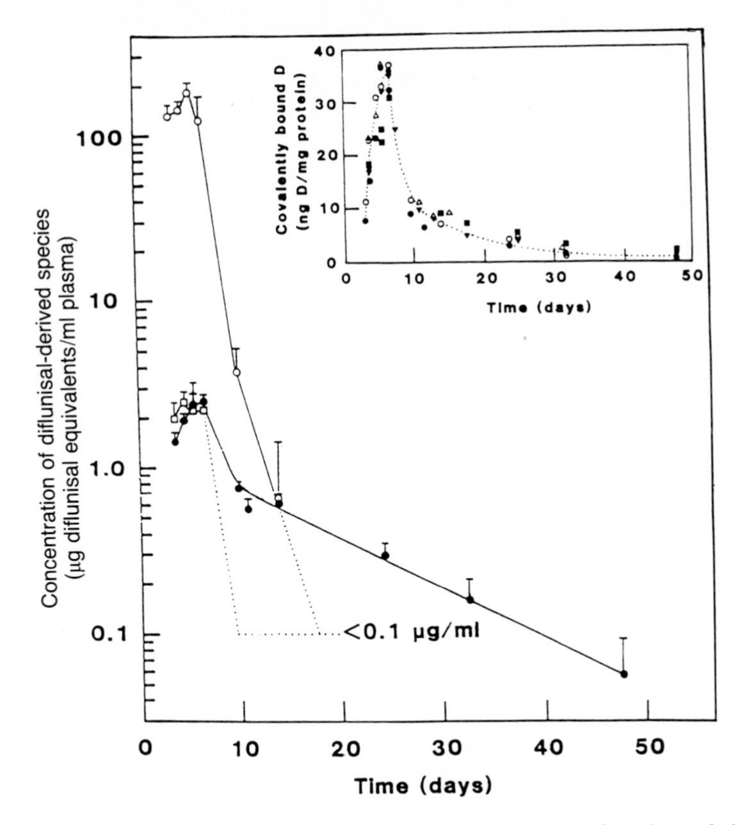

Fig. 6. Mean plasma concentrations from five volunteers as a function of time. ○, Diflunisal; □, diflunisal glucuronide; ●, covalently bound diflunisal released from plasma proteins by base hydrolysis. Diflunisal was administered 0–132 h; probenecid was administered 96–132 h. The *inset* shows individual values for diflunisal (*D*) released by base hydrolysis in the five subjects. Reproduced with permission from McKinnon and Dickinson (1989)

to the drug in terms of dosage levels and time, as well as impaired clearance, is consistent with other clinical studies (for example, Gautam et al. 1984; Smith et al. 1986; Hyneck et al. 1988; Volland et al. 1991; Sallustio et al. 1991). Evidence suggests that the extent of plasma protein and tissue bonding need not correlate with plasma concentrations of either acyl glucuronides or their corresponding isomeric esters (Sallustio et al. 1991; Spahn-Langguth and Benet 1992; King and Dickinson 1993).

Evidence for covalent binding of clofibrate to rat liver proteins in vivo has been presented recently (Sallustio et al. 1991). The authors propose that the acyl glucuronide is the alkylating species, however, they point out that thioesters formed with coenzyme A cannot be excluded in these experiments in whole animals. Acyl glucuronides have also been implicated in covalent attachment of diclofenac to liver proteins (Pumford et al. 1993) and diflunisal to liver, kidney, intestine (King and Dickinson 1993).

I. Albumin as Nucleophile

The reaction of oxaprozin 1-*O*-acyl glucuronide with human serum albumin (HSA) is summarized in Fig. 7 (WELLS et al. 1987). During the 8 h study, radioisotope labeled oxaprozin became covalently bound to HSA, ester isomers were formed, and free oxaprozin was formed by hydrolysis. The abundances of these products are shown in the figure as a function of time. The experiment was carried out at pH 7.0 and 37°C, with a molar ratio of approximately 1:3, glucuronide to albumin. After about 3 h, hydrolyzed oxaprozin is the dominant species.

Albumin is a fairly complex molecule to us as the nucleophilic partner in studies of the reactions of 1-*O*-acyl glucuronides (PETERS 1985; HE and CARTER 1992). It has been difficult to correlate covalent bonding of albumin with hydrolysis, isomerization or other chemical properties (VAN BREEMEN

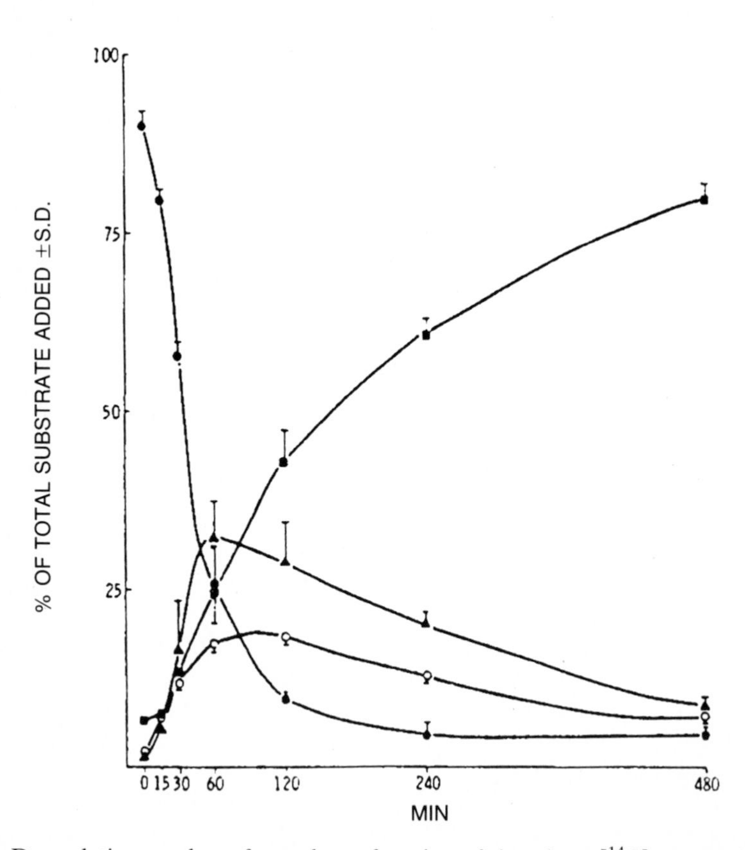

Fig. 7. Degradation products formed as a function of time from [^{14}C]-oxaprozin 1-*O*-acyl glucuronide in aqueous solution pH 7.0, 37°C in the presence of human serum albumin, 1:1 molar ratio. ●, Oxaprozin 1-*O*-acyl glucuronide; ▲, ester isomers; ■, oxaprozin; ○, oxaprozin covalently bound to albumin. Reproduced with permission from WELLS et al. (1987)

and FENSELAU 1985; CALDWELL et al. 1988). The reactivities of the many amino, hydroxyl and thiol groups in albumin can be masked by its tertiary structure and accentuated by several high affinity binding sites that have selectivities for different kinds of organic compounds. Both reversible binding and covalent bonding by drug metabolites can be reduced if fatty acids or other lipophiles are already complexed. Human serum albumin has been reported to catalyze degradation of some acyl glucuronides (for example, RUELIUS et al. 1986; VOLLAND et al. 1991) and to stabilize others (MUNAFO et al. 1990; WATT and DICKINSON 1990). HANSEN-MOLLER and SCHMIT (1991) report that HSA both stabilizes rearrangement of probenecid 1-*O*-acyl glucuronide and catalyses its hydrolysis. They suggest that this reflects the steric restrictions of a tight binding site.

A role for high-affinity reversible binding in the mechanism of covalent bonding was first suggested by the kinetic study presented in Fig. 8, in which time courses are shown for the acylation by flufenamic glucuronide of bovine serum albumin and albumin in which the sulfhydryl group on Cys-34

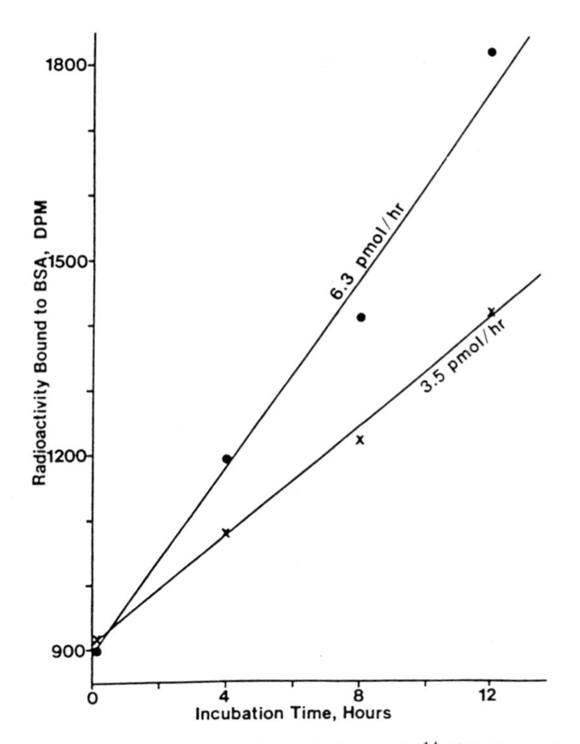

Fig. 8. Covalent attachment as a function of time of [^{14}C]flufenamic acid to bovine serum albumin (*dots*) and sulfhydryl-blocked bovine serum albumin (*X*) incubated with [^{14}C]flufenamic 1-*O*-acyl glucuronide at pH 7.4, 37°C, with a 1.7:1 molar ratio of glucuronide to albumin. Reproduced with permission from VAN BREEMEN and FENSELAU (1984)

is blocked (numbering follows HIRAYAMA et al. 1990). Rapid initial reaction occurred in both incubations, as measured at the first time point ($t < 3$ min), and was attributed to reaction at a specific binding site (VAN BREEMEN and FENSELAU 1985). The second part of the biphasic curves may reflect nonspecific reactions and indicates a nonexclusive role for the free sulfhydryl group.

Studies with inhibitors of reversible binding further support the important role of reversible binding in the process of covalent bonding. Covalent bonding by oxaprozin glucuronide, for example, is inhibited by prior complexation of HSA with unconjugated oxaprozin or decanoic acid (RUELIUS et al. 1986). Prior complexation of aspirin has no effect on the covalent reaction of HSA with oxaprozin glucuronide (RUELIUS et al. 1986), but reduces the covalent bonding of zomepirac glucuronide by about 20% (SMITH et al. 1990). Chiral selectivities in reversible binding of acyl glucuronides (e.g., IWAKAWA et al. 1990), in covalent transacylation (KURONA et al. 1983), and in covalent bonding of acyl glucuronides (e.g., VOLLAND et al. 1991) further support the important role of selective binding pockets.

The extent to which thiol, phenol, hydroxyl, and amino groups on albumin are involved in covalent bonding of acyl glucuronides has been probed to some extent by selective pretreatment. Thus, blockage of the single free sulfhydryl group (Cys-34) provided only limited reduction of bonding by flufenamic acid glucuronide (Fig. 8). However, derivatization of the phenol group in Tyr-411 significantly reduced attachment of oxaprozin glucuronide (RUELIUS et al. 1986). Ultimately, the variety of protein nucleophiles involved will best be addressed by direct analyses of proteins modified by different conjugates.

II. Four Reagents and Three Mechanisms

Both 1-*O*-acyl glucuronides and their ester isomers have been shown to undergo covalent reactions with biopolymers. Transacylation of 1-*O*-acyl glucuronides has been demonstrated with a number of small nucleophilic reagents, as discussed above, to lead to well-characterized esters, thio esters, and amides. It should be pointed out that transacylation by amino groups on a protein will form amide bonds, which can be broken only under chemical or enzymatic conditions that will also cleave protein backbone amides. The most compelling evidence for transacylation of 1-*O*-acyl glucuronides by proteinaceous, functional groups (Fig. 1c) was reported by RUELIUS et al. (1986), in which human serum albumin was found to be irreversibly radiolabeled by reaction with [^{14}C]oxaprozin glucuronide, but not by oxaprozin [^{14}C]glucuronide. These experiments demonstrated that the drug was covalently attached to albumin, but not the glucuronic acid moiety, consistent with the mechanism presented in Fig. 1c. The results of this study are summarized in Table 5 and indicate that limited attachment is also observed

Table 5. Covalent binding of oxaprozin to human albumin[a,b]

Substrate	% Radioactivity bound
[^{14}C]Oxaprozin glucuronide	22.0
Oxaprozin [^{14}C]Glucuronide	0.6
[^{14}C]Oxaprozin C-2 isomer	2.1
[^{14}C]Oxaprozin	1.0

[a] Binding determined after 1 h at pH 7.0.
[b] RUELIUS et al. (1986).

with the radioisotope-labeled C-2 isomer. The use of radioisotopes provides a sensitive and definitive method for both qualitative and quantitative analysis of protein bond products formed in vivo and in vitro and has historically been the method of choice (MACLAUF et al. 1980; POHL and BRANCHWATER 1981; WELL et al. 1988; CALDWELL et al. 1988).

The three ester isomers of 1-*O*-acyl glucuronides provide two additional mechanisms for covalent linkage of xenobiotic acids with proteins. In the mechanism illustrated in Fig. 9a, the aglycon is displaced from the (unactivated) ester linkages by functional groups on the HSA polymer, analogous to the transacylations by albumin reported with acetylsalicylate, *p*-nitrophenylacetate, and *N-trans*-cinnamoylimidazoles (PETERS 1985). Either esters or amides could be formed, and previous studies of reactions of this kind have implicated the amino group on Lys-199 and the phenol group on Tyr-411 (numbering follows TAKAHASHI et al. 1987).

In the third mechanism, the unblocked reducing terminus of the sugar group undergoes covalent bonding with nucleophilic amine groups on the protein (Fig. 9b). This glycation reaction has been well established as occurring between glucose and specific residues in albumin (GARLICK and MAZER 1983; ROBB et al. 1989), other proteins, and nucleic acids (LEE and CERAMI 1989). It proceeds with reversible formation of unstable aldimines. The most direct evidence that albumin is glycosylated by ester isomers of 1-*O*-acyl glucuronides has been provided by DING et al. (1993) working with ester isomers of tolmetin glucuronide. These workers displaced the reaction equilibrium to favor aldimine products stabilized by reduction with sodium cyanoborohydride. They then mapped the modified protein to locate glycosylated lysines and confirmed attachment of tolmetin via the ester isomer using mass spectrometry. At least half a dozen residues were found to be modified (Table 6). About 60% of the trapped tolmetin adduct was attached to residues 195 and 199. This was suggested by the authors to be consistent with inhibition of zomepirac bonding by preincubation with acetylsalicylate. Reduction or trapping of aldimines in situ allows these adducts to be isolated; however, the amounts of trapped products may not reflect the extent of alkylation in situ or in vivo since the aldehyde/aldimine (off/on) equilibria have been disrupted.

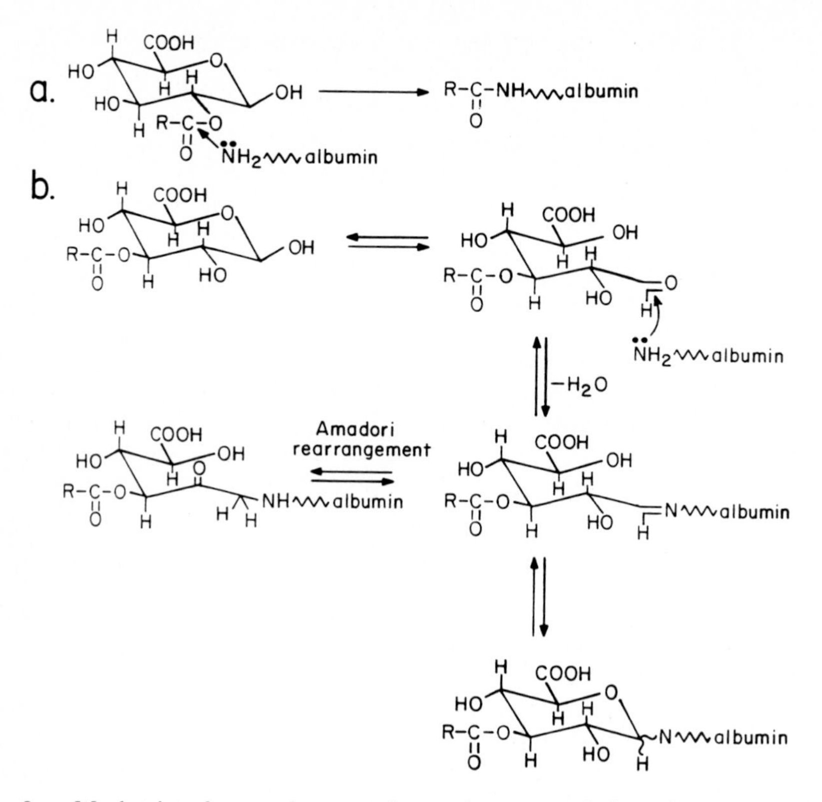

Fig. 9. **a** Mechanism for covalent attachment by transacylation of ester isomers; **b** mechanism for covalent attachment of ester isomers by glycosylation: the aldimine, the glycosylamine, and the *Amadori rearrangement* product (available to 3-esters and 4-esters)

Table 6. Sites for glycosylation of human serum albumin by ester isomers of tolmetin 1-*O*-acyl glucuronide[a]

Amino acid	Percent of total
Lys-137	2
Lys-195	20
Lys-199	40
Lys-351	9
Lys-525	14
Lys-541	6

[a] DING et al. (1993).

Although most are readily hydrolyzed, some fraction of the aldimines formed between amines and reducing sugars undergoes reversible rearrangements to form the more stable aminoglycoside and aminoketone (Amadori) products shown in Fig. 9b (HARDING 1985). The rates and equilibrium positions are sensitive to buffers and cosolvents, distinguishing studies in vitro from the situation in vivo, and they vary from one amino group to another, even on the same protein. The Amadori rearrangement can be catalyzed by proximal acid or base groups (BAYNES et al. 1989), and it is proposed that the carboxyl group of glucuronic acid facilitates that rearrangement in the aldimines under discussion here (SPAHN-LANGGUTH and BENET 1992).

A number of studies have undertaken to distinguish the contributions of the various mechanisms by comparing the extents of covalent bonding by selected 1-*O*-acyl glucuronides with those of their respective ester isomers. The definitive comparison by RUELIUS et al. (1986) with radioisotope-labeled oxaprozin conjugates has already been described (Sect. D.II). Evidence was obtained for reactions of both the 1-*O*-acyl and C-2-ester conjugates, in about a 10:1 ratio (Table 5). Other comparisons have relied on base-catalyzed hydrolysis to release bound drug. The thoroughness of this procedure has not been proven, for example, by application to radioisotope-labeled adducts. In particular, it is not clear how well amide bonds are hydrolyzed, if at all. Nonetheless, this approach has provided evidence for covalent bonding with proteins by both 1-*O*-acyl glucuronides and ester isomers. For example, the reaction of 1-*O*-acyl zomepirac glucuronide was found to produce 60% more base-hydrolyzable covalent product with HSA than a comparable 6-h reaction with a mixture of ester isomers (SMITH et al. 1986). On the other hand, ester isomers of diflunisal (DICKINSON and KING 1991) and suprofen glucuronides (SMITH and LIU 1993) formed base-hydrolyzable adducts with HSA to a larger extent than the corresponding glucuronides. Although the ester isomers did, the 1-*O*-acyl glucuronide of valproic acid did not form base-hydrolyzable products with albumin at physiologic pH (WILLIAMS et al. 1992).

III. Product Stabilities

The stabilities of these protein-bound adducts have implications for both their mechanisms of adduction and their physiologic effects. Bilirubin-albumin (biliprotein), assayed using double radioisotope techniques, was found to have a turnover rate in Sprague-Dawley rats indistinguishable from that of unmodified serum albumin (REED et al. 1988). The albumin adduct of radioisotope-labeled oxaprozin can be seen in Fig. 7 to peak around 90 min and then to decompose slowly through the next 6 h. A number of studies have used base hydrolysis to measure the durability of susceptible adducts. For example, elimination of base-hydrolyzable plasma protein adducts of diflunisal in humans was found to be biphasic, and the second, slow phase (half-life about 10 days) was suggested to reflect the composite clearance rates of several plasma proteins (MCKINNON and DICKINSON 1989).

E. Implications

The sum of the evidence supports the operation of both the transacylation and the glycation mechanisms, in relative proportions that probably vary from one aglycon to another and between different proteins. Since these are both spontaneous chemical reactions, the availability of the reagents will be a major determinant of which reaction takes place in vivo. This will reflect the rate of intramolecular migration of each glucuronide. Sites of covalent attachment, particularly with albumin, will be influenced by the selectivities of reversible binding sites for glucuronides and isomers of different shapes, sizes, and charge distributions. Presently, little is known about product stabilities. However, these will also be important qualitative and quantitative determinants of the population of covalent adducts in vivo. Reactions of 1-*O*-acyl glucuronides with nucleophilic functional groups in other biopolymers such as nucleotides have not yet been reported, but are likely to occur.

Metabolic implications of the chemical reactivity of 1-*O*-acyl glucuronides are summarized in Fig. 10. Experimental observations that support the transformations of 1-*O*-acyl glucuronides and of ester isomers in Fig. 10 have been discussed in this chapter. Potential relationships suggested in Fig. 10 between covalent bonding of proteins and benign or malignant physiologic consequences are harder to document experimentally, and as yet no toxicity

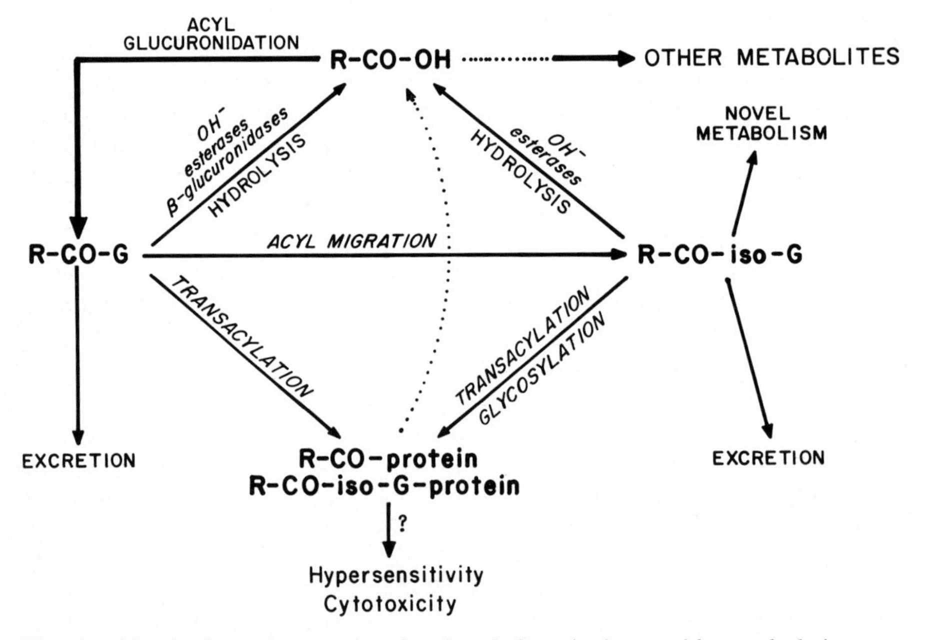

Fig. 10. Metabolic pathways that involve 1-*O*-acyl glucuronides and their ester isomers. *R-CO-G*, 1-*O*-acyl glucuronide; *R-CO-iso-G*, ester isomers of 1-*O*-acyl glucuronide. R.G. Dickinson is acknowledged for providing this figure

of an acyl glucuronide or ester isomer has been reported to result from protein adduct formation.

Some of the potential physiologic implications of the spontaneous chemical reactivities of this widely occurring class of metabolites were pointed out 10 years ago (STOGNIEW and FENSELAU 1982; FAED 1984). Transacylation offers a new mechanism for the interaction of endogenous and xenobiotic lipophilic acids with biopolymers, analogous to activation by thioester (coenzyme A) intermediates.

Formation of covalent bonds in vivo by transacylation and glycation may provide a molecular mechanism for cytotoxicity, carcinogenicity, and mutagenicity, as well as idiosyncratic immunologic responses. Clofibrate, whose major glucuronide metabolite is discussed here, was withdrawn from the U.S. market when serious diseases of the liver, kidney, gall bladder, and intestines were found to be associated with chronic use. Benoxaprofen and zomepirac, whose major metabolites are also acyl glucuronides, have also been withdrawn from the market because of acute hepatotoxicity. Ideopathic allergies, analgesic nephropathy, and other toxicities are occasionally associated with the administration of nonsteroidal anti-inflammatory drugs. Although a causal link between protein modification and allergy or other disease has not been established, the recent availability of in vitro immunosorbent assays (for example, PUMFORD et al. 1993) may allow the hypothetical relationship to be tested experimentally.

Benign biological consequences are also possible and include effects on transport and clearance, reversible covalent bonding to receptors, and signal transduction. Certainly the covalent attachment of bilirubin to serum proteins provides an alternate (though slower) mechanism for clearing that toxic substance in pathological circumstances. As another example, studies are underway to determine, whether the biologically active acyl glucuronide formed from retinoic acid might provide a mechanism for covalent bonding to carrier or receptor proteins (OLSON et al. 1992; SANI et al. 1992).

Acknowledgement. I thank Dr. Deanne Dulik for reading this chapter and for helpful discussions, and the National Institutes of Health and the National Science Foundation for support.

References

Abramson FP (1990) Mass spectrometry in pharmacology. In: Saulter CH, Watson JT (eds) Biomedical applications of mass spectrometry. Wiley, New York, pp 289–347 (Methods of biochemical analysis, vol 34)

Bax A, Egan W, Kovac P (1984) New NMR techniques for structure determination and resonance assignments of complex carbohydrates. J Carbohyd Chem 3:593–611

Baynes JW, Watkins NG, Fisher CI, Hull CJ, Patrick JS, Amhed MU, Dunn JA, Thorpe SR (1988) The Amadori product on protein: structure and reactions. In: Baynes JW, Monnier VM (eds) Maillard reaction in aging, diabetes, and nutrition. Liss, New York, pp 43–67

Blanckaert N, Compernolle F, Leroy P, Van Houtte R, Fevery J, Heirwegh KPM (1978) The fate of bilirubin-IXα glucuronide in cholestasis and during storage in vitro intermolecular rearrangement to positional isomers of glucuronic acid. Biochem J 171:203–214

Bonner WA (1959) C1–C2 acetyl migration on methylation of the anomeric 1,3,4,6-tetra-O-acetyl-D-glucopyranoses. J Org Chem 24:1388–1390

Bradow G, Kan LS, Fenselau C (1989) Studies of intramolecular rearrangements of acyl-linked glucuronides using salicylic acid, flufenamic acid, and (S)- and (R)-benoxaprofen and confirmation of isomerization in acyl-linked Δ^9-11-carboxytetrahydrocannabinol glucuronide. Chem Res Toxicol 2:316–324

Caldwell J, Hutt AJ, Marsh MV, Sinclair KA (1983) Isolation and characterization of amino acid and sugar conjugates of xenobiotic carboxylic acids. In: Reid E, Leppard EP (eds) Drug metabolite isolation and determination. Plenum, New York, pp 161–178

Caldwell J, Grubb N, Sinclair KA, Hutt AJ, Weil A, Fournel-Gigleux S (1988) Structural and sterochemical aspects of acyl glucuronide formation and reactivity. In: Siest G, Magdalou J, Burchell B (eds) Cellular and molecular aspects of glucuronidation. Libbey, Paris, pp 185–192

Compernolle F, Jansen FH, Heirwegh PM (1970) Mass-spectrometric study of the azopigments obtained from bile pigments with diazotized ethyl anthranilate. Biochem J 120:891–894

Compernolle F, Van Hees GP, Blanckaert N, Heirwegh KP (1978) Glucuronic acid conjugates of bilirubin-IXα in normal bile compared with post-obstructive bile transformation of the 1-O-acylglucuronide into 2-, 3-, and 4-acylglucuronides. Biochem J 171:185–201

Dickinson RG, King AR (1991) Studies on the reactivity of acyl glucuronides-II: interactions of diflunisal acyl glucuronide and its isomers with human serum albumin in vitro. Biochem Pharmacol 42:2301–2306

Dickinson RG, Verbeeck RK, King AR, Restifo AC, Pond SM (1991) Diflunisal and its conjugates in patients with renal failure. Br J Clin Pharmacol 31:546–550

Ding A, Ojingwa JC, McDonagh AF, Burlingame AL, Benet LZ (1993) Evidence for Covalent Binding of Acyl Glucuronides to Serum Albumin via an Imine Mechanism as Revealed by Tandem Mass Spectrometry. Proc Nat Acad Sci USA 90:3797–3801

Doerschuk AP (1952) Acyl migrations in partially acylated, polyhydroxylic systems. J Am Chem Soc 74:4202–4207

Dutton GJ (1966) Glucuronic acid free and combined. Academic, New York

Faed EM (1984) Properties of acyl glucuronides: implications for studies of the pharmacokinetics and metabolism of acidic drugs. Drug Metab Rev 15:1213–1249

Fenselau C (1992) Tandem mass spectrometry: the competitive edge for pharmacology. Annu Rev Pharmacol Toxicol 32:555–578

Fenselau C, Yelle L (1986) Analysis of glucuronides, sulfates and glutathione conjugates by mass spectrometry. In: Paulson GD, Caldwell J, Watson DH, Menn JJ (eds) Xenobiotic conjugation chemistry. ACS Symposium Series. American Chemical Society, Washington, pp 159–176

Fischer E (1920) Wanderung von Acyl bei den Glyceriden. Chem Ber 53:1621–1633

Garlick RL, Mazer JS (1983) The principal site of nonenzymatic glycosylation of human serum albumin in vivo. J Biol Chem 258:6142–6146

Gautam A, Sellgson H, Gordon ER, Sellgson D, Boyer JL (1984) Irreversible binding of conjugated bilirubin to albumin in cholestatic rats. J Clin Invest 73:873–877

Hansen-Moller J, Cornett C, Dalgaard L, Hansen SH (1988) Isolation and identification of the rearrangement products of diflunisal 1-O-acyl glucuronide. J Pharm Belg 6:229–240

Hansen-Moller J, Schmit U (1991) Rapid high-performance liquid chromatographic assay for the simultaneous determination of probenecid and its glucuronide in urine. Irreversible binding of probenecid to serum albumin. J Pharm Belg 9:65–73

Harding JJ (1985) Nonenzymatic covalent post-translational modification of proteins in vivo. Adv Prot Chem 37:247–334

Hayball PJ, Nation RL, Bochner F (1992) Stereoselective interactions of ketoprofen glucuronides with human plasma protein and serum albumin. Biochem Pharmacol 44:291–299

He XM, Carter DC (1992) Atomic structure and chemistry of human serum albumin. Nature 358:209–215

Hignite CE, Tschanz C, Lemons S, Wiese H, Azarnoff DL, Huffman DH (1981) Glucuronic acid conjugates of clofibrate: four isomeric structures. Life Sci 28:2077–2081

Hirayama K, Akashi S, Furuya M, Fukuhara KI (1990) Rapid confirmation and revision of the primary structure of bovine serum albumin by ESIMS and FRIT-FAB LC/MS. Biochem Biophys Res Commun 173:639–646

Hyneck ML, Smith PC, Unseld E, Benet LZ (1987) High-performance liquid chromatographic determination of tolmetin, tolmetin glucuronide and its isomeric conjugates in plasma and urine. J Chromatogr 420:349–356

Hyneck ML, Munafo A, Benet LZ (1988) Effect of pH on acyl migration and hydrolysis of tolmetin glucuronide. Drug Metab Dispos 16:322–324

Iwakawa S, Spahn H, Benet LZ, Lin ET (1990) Stereoselective binding of the glucuronide conjugates of carprofen enantiomers to human serum albumin. Biochem Pharmacol 39:949–953

Janssen FW, Kirkman SK, Fenselau C, Stogniew M, Hofmann BR, Young EM, Ruelius HW (1982) Metabolic formation of N- and O-glucuronides of 3-(p-chlorophenyl) thiazolo[3,2-a] benzimidazole-2-acetic acid rearrangement of the 1-O-acyl glucuronide. Drug Metab Dispos 10:599–604

King AR, Dickinson RG (1991) Studies on the reactivity of acyl glucuronides-I phenolic glucuronidation of isomers of diflunisal acyl glucuronide in the rat. Biochem Pharmacol 42:2289–2299

King AR, Dickinson RG (1993) Studies on the reactivity of acyl glucuronides-IV covalent binding of diflunisal to tissues of the rat. Biochem Pharmacol 45:1043–1047

Komura H, Fukui H, Sasaki H, Morino A (1992) Pharmacokinetic analysis of enterohepatic circulation of 4-[2-(4-isopropylbenzamido) ethoxy] benzoic acid. Drug Metab Disp 20:585–591

Kurono Y, Kondo T, Ikeda K (1983) Esterase-like activity of human serum albumin: enantioselectivity in the burst phase of reaction with p-nitrophenyl α-methoxyphenyl acetate. Arch Biochem 227:339–341

Lee AT, Cerami A (1989) Nonenzymatic glycosylation of DNA by reducing sugars. In: Baynes JW, Monnier VM (eds) Maillard reaction in aging, diabetes, and nutrition. Liss, New York, pp 291–299

Lippel K, Olsen JA (1968) Origin of some derivatives of retinoic acid found in rat bile. J Lipid Res 9:580–586

Maclouf J, Kindahl H, Granstrom E, Samuelsson B (1980) Interactions of prostaglandin H_2 and thromboxane A_2 with human serum albumin. Eur J Biochem 109:561–566

McDonagh AF, Palma LA, Lauff JJ, Wu TW (1984) Origin of mammalian biliprotein and rearrangement of bilirubin glucuronides in vivo in the rat. J Clin Invest 74:763–770

McKinnon GE, Dickinson RG (1989) Covalent binding of diflunisal and probenecid to plasma protein in humans: persistence of the adducts in the circulation. Res Commun Chem Pathol Pharmacol 66:339–354

Munafo A, McDonagh AF, Smith PC, Benet LZ (1990) Irreversible binding of tolmetin glucuronic acid esters to albumin in vitro. Pharm Res 7:21–27

Musson DG, Lin JH, Lyon KA, Tocco DJ, Yek KC (1985) Assay methodology for quantification of the ester and ether glucuronide conjugates of diflunisal in human urine. J Chromatogr 337:363–378

Olson JA, Moon RC, Anders MW, Fenselau C, Shane B (1992) Enhancement of biological activity by conjugation reactions. J Nutr 122:615–624

Panfil I, Lehman PA, Zimniak P, Ernst B, Franz T, Lester R, Radominska A (1992) Biosynthesis and chemical synthesis of carboxyl-linked glucuronide of lithocholic acid. Biochim Biophys Acta 1126:221–228

Peters T (1985) Serum albumin. In: Anfinsen CB, Edsall JT, Richards FM (eds) Advances in protein chemistry, vol 37. Academic, Orlando, pp 161–245

Pohl LR, Branchflower RV (1981) Covalent binding of electrophilic metabolities to macromolecules. Methods Enzymol 77:43–50

Pumford NR, Meyers TG, Davila JC, Highet RJ, Pohl LR (1993) Immunochemical detection of liver protein adducts of the non steroidal antiinflammatory drug diclofenac. Chem Res Toxicol 6:147–150

Rachmel A, Hazelton GA, Yergey AL, Liberato DJ (1985) Furosemide 1-O-acyl glucuronide in vitro biosynthesis and pH-dependent isomerization to β-glucuronidase-resistant forms. Drug Metab Dispos 13:705–710

Reed RG, Davidson LK, Burrington CM, Peters T Jr (1988) Non-resolving jaundice: bilirubin covalently attached to serum albumin circulates with the same metabolic half-life as albumin. Clin Chem 34:1992–1994

Robb DA, Olufemi OS, Williams DA, Midgley JM (1989) Identification of glycation at the N-terminus of albumin by gas chromatography-mass spectrometry. Biochem J 261:871–878

Ruelius HW, Young EM, Kirkman SK, Schillings RT, Sisenwine SF, Janssen FW (1985) Biological fate of acyl glucuronides in the rat the role of rearrangement, intestinal enzymes and reabsorption. Biochem Pharmacol 34:451–452

Ruelius HW, Kirkman SK, Young EM, Fanssen FW (1986) Reactions of oxaprozin-1-O-acyl glucuronide in solutions of human plasma and albumin. Adv Exp Med Biol 197:431–441

Sallustio BC, Puride YJ, Birkett DJ, Meffin PJ (1989) Effect of renal dysfunction on the acyl-glucuronide futile cycle. J Pharmacol Exp Ther 251:288–294

Sallustio BC, Knights KM, Roberts BJ, Zacest R (1991) In vivo covalent binding of clofibric acid to human plasma proteins and rat liver proteins. Biochem Pharmacol 42:1421–1425

Salmon M, Fenselau C, Cukier JO, Odell GB (1975) Rapid transesterification of bilirubin glucuronides in methanol. Life Sci 15:2069

Sani BP, Barua AB, Hill DL, Shih TW, Olson JA (1992) Retinoyl β-glucuronide: lack of binding to receptor proteins of retinoic acid as related to biological activity. Biochem Pharmacol 43:919–922

Smith PC, Benet LZ (1986) Characterization of the isomeric esters of zomepirac glucuronide by proton NMR. Drug Metab Dispos 14:503–505

Smith PC, Hasegawa J, Langendijk NJ, Benet LZ (1985) Stability of acyl glucuronides in blood, plasma, and urine: studies with zomepirac. Drug Metab Dispos 13:110–112

Smith PC, McDonagh AF, Benet LZ (1986) Irreversible binding of zomepirac to plasma protein in vitro and in vivo. J Clin Invest 77:934–939

Smith PC, Benet LZ, McDonagh AF (1990) Covalent binding of zomepirac glucuronide to proteins: evidence for a schiff base mechanism. Drug Metab Dispos 18:639–644

Smith PC, Song WQ, Rodriguez RJ (1992) Covalent binding of etodolac acyl glucuronide to albumin in vitro. Drug Metab Disp 20:962–965

Spahn H (1988) Assay method for product formation in in vitro enzyme kinetic studies of uridine diphosphate glucuronyltransferases: 2-arylpropionic acid enantiomers. J Chromotogr 430:368–375

Spahn H, Iwakawa S, Lin ET, Benet LZ (1989) Procedures to properly characterize in vivo and in vitro enantioselective glucuronidation: studies with benoxaprofen glucuronides. Pharmacol Res 6:125–132

Spahn-Langguth H, Benet LZ (1992) Acyl glucuronides revisited: is the glucuronidation process a toxification as well as a detoxification mechanism? Drug Metab Rev 24:5–48

Stogniew M, Fenselau C (1982) Electrophilic reactions of acyl-linked glucuronides formation of clofibrate mercapturate in humans. Drug Metab Dispos 10:609–613

Takahashi N, Takahashi Y, Blumberg BS, Putnam FW (1987) Amino acid substitutions in genetic variants of human serum albumin and in sequences inferred from molecular cloning. Proc Natl Acad Sci USA 84:4413–4417

van Breemen RB, Fenselau C (1984) Acylation of albumin by 1-O-acyl glucuronides. Drug Metab Dispos 13:318–320

van Breemen RB, Fenselau CC (1985) Reaction of 1-O-acyl glucuronides with 4-(p-nitrobenzyl) pyridine. Drug Metab Dispos 14:197–201

van Breeman RB, Fenselau C, Mogilevsky W, Odell GB (1986) Reaction of bilirubin glucuronides with serum albumin. J Chromatogr 383:387–392

van Breeman RB, Stogniew M, Fenselau C (1988) Characterization in acyl-linked glucuronides by electron impact and fast atom bombardment mass spectrometry. Biomed Environ Mass Spectrom 17:97–103

Volland C, Sun H, Dammeyer J, Benet LZ (1991) Stereoselective degradation of the fenoprofen acyl glucuronide enantiomers and irreversible binding to plasma protein. Drug Metab Dispos 19:1080–1086

Watt JA, Dickinson RG (1990) Reactivity of diflunisal acyl glucuronide in human and rat plasma albumin solutions. Biochem Pharmacol 39:1067–1075

Watt JA, King AR, Dickinson RG (1991) Contrasting systemic stabilities of the acyl and phenolic glucuronides of diflunisal in the rat. Xenobiotica 21:403–415

Weil A, Guichard JP, Caldwell J (1988) Interactions between fenofibryl glucuronide and human serum albumin or human plasma. In: Siest G, Magdalou J, Burchell B (eds) Cellular and molecular aspects of glucuronidation. Colloque INSERM/John Libbey Eurotext 173, pp 233–236

Wells DS, Janssen FW, Ruelius HW (1987) Interactions between oxaprozin glucuronide and human serum albumin. Xenobiotica 17:1437–1449

Williams AM, Worrall S, De Jersey J, Dickinson RG (1992) Studies on the reactivity of acyl glucuronides: III. Glucuronide-derived adducts of valproic acid and plasma protein and anti-adduct antibodies in humans. Biochem Pharmacol 43: 745–755

Yoshida H, Inagaki T, Hirano M, Sugimoto T (1987) Analyses of azopigments obtained from the delta fraction of bilirubin from mammalian plasma (mammalian biliprotein). Biochem J 248:79–84

CHAPTER 14

Roles of Uridine Diphosphate Glucuronosyltransferases in Chemical Carcinogenesis

K.W. BOCK and W. LILIENBLUM

A. Introduction

Roles of isozymes of the uridine diphosphate (UDP)-glucuronosyltransferase (UGT) family (EC 2.4.1.17) will be discussed in the light of recent concepts of carcinogenesis. Glucuronides may be transport forms of carcinogens that play a major role in determining the target of carcinogenicity, for example, in urinary bladder or colon epithelium. Roles of UGT isozymes can be best appreciated in the context of overall xenobiotic metabolism. In addition to preventing accumulation of lipid-soluble compounds, "xenobiotic" or drug-metabolizing enzymes may also fulfill important roles in controlling endogenous signal compounds such as hormones (NEBERT 1991).

Reviews are mostly selective, and hence, a number of items and important contributions are often not included. The present review emphasizes the role of individual UGT isozymes and their regulation and also tackles extrapolations from the enzyme to the cellular level and from experimental animals to man. The reader is referred to other chapters of this volume and to comprehensive reviews on the role of other drug-metabolizing enzymes in carcinogenesis (MANNERVIK and DANIELSON 1988; COLES and KETTERER 1990; GUENGERICH 1990) and on other aspects of UGTs (DUTTON 1980; JANSEN et al. 1992; MULDER 1992).

I. Control of Nucleophilic Metabolites by Glucuronidation Preventing their Conversion to Electrophilic, Reactive Metabolites

A large number of exogenous and endogenous lipophilic chemicals are converted by phase I enzymes of drug metabolism to a variety of nucleophilic and electrophilic metabolites (Fig. 1). It has been demonstrated that the interaction of the chemically reactive, electrophilic metabolites with critical cellular macromolecules often initiates toxicity and plays an essential role in the multistage carcinogenic process (MILLER and MILLER 1981). Electrophiles may react with DNA and thereby activate critical genes, such as the c-Ha-*ras* protooncogene (MILLER and MILLER 1986; WISEMAN et al. 1986). Electrophilic metabolites are largely controlled in phase II by a family of glutathione *S*-transferases and, in the case of epoxides, by epoxide hydrolases. However, the more stable and more abundant nucleophilic metabolites

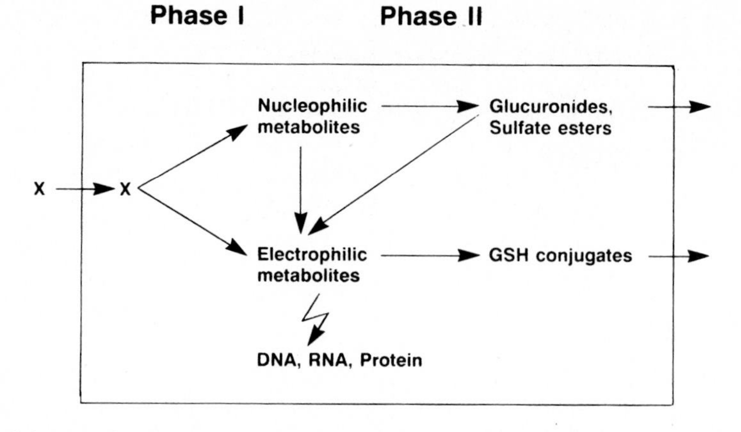

Fig. 1. Scheme of cellular xenobiotic metabolism. *GSH*, glutathione

can also be converted to reactive metabolites. For example, phenols can be oxidized to radicals, polyphenols, semiquinones, and quinones. Quinones may undergo quinone–quinol redox cycles with the generation of reactive oxygen species (Lorentzen and Ts'o 1977; Lorentzen et al. 1979; Lilienblum et al. 1985). In addition, N-oxidized aromatic amines can be converted to electrophiles via sulfation and acetylation (Miller and Miller 1986; Shinohara et al. 1989). Therefore, the control of nucleophiles (phenols, quinols, aromatic amines, and their N-oxidized metabolites, etc.) by glucuronidation (in concert with other reactions) may be as important as the control of electrophiles. It is the balance between phase I and phase II enzymes which is responsible for detoxication of reactive metabolites in tissues.

II. Initiation of Carcinogenesis by Reactive Metabolites

The multistage nature of preneoplastic development has been demonstrated during carcinogenesis in numerous organs in both experimental animals and humans (Pitot 1990; Pitot et al. 1991). Two early stages can be distinguished: initiation and promotion. At the stage of initiation, genotoxic lesions may lead to alterations of genes critical for cellular growth control, such as the activation of the cellular protooncogene c-Ha-*ras* (Wiseman et al. 1986). These lesions may lead to heritable changes in the base sequence of cellular DNA (Zarbl et al. 1985; Weinberg 1989; Bishop 1991). However, persistent alterations of at least two cooperating protooncogenes have been shown to be required for transformation (Land et al. 1983). Inactivation of tumor suppressor genes may also be involved, as shown in the heritable predisposition to cancer (Knudson 1985; Bishop 1991). At the second stage (tumor promotion), cells containing critical genotoxic lesions ("initiated cells") have to be clonally expanded. Hence, epigenetic (nongenotoxic) factors altering growth control may be critical at this stage. Cell proliferation markedly influences several steps in carcinogenesis (Fig. 2; MOOLGAVKAR 1989; COHEN and ELLWEIN 1990). In this model, a normal cell (N), possibly a stem cell, is converted by genotoxic lesions into a preneoplastic "initiated" cell (I). The rate of conversion of N to I (μ_I) is influenced by both the mitotic rate of normal cells (α_1) and by terminal differentiation or death of normal cells (β_1). Similarly, the size of the population of initiated cells (I) is determined by its mitotic rate (α_2) and its death rate (β_2). The size of the population of initiated cells will be a major determinant of the rate of conversion (μ_T) of initiated cells to transformed cells (T). Proliferation of initiated cells can be markedly influenced by nongenotoxic agents, frequently termed tumor promoters. The process of tumor promotion is mostly determined by the formula $\alpha_2 - \beta_2$. It has to be distinguished from transformation, which is often determined by a second genotoxic lesion.

III. Tumor Promotion and Reactive Metabolites

Nongenotoxic agents can be subdivided into: (a) those compounds reacting with receptors that may directly affect growth control (such as steroid hormones) and (b) reactive metabolites that indirectly affect growth control through cytotoxicity and subsequent regenerative growth of neighboring cells. Reactive metabolites may also affect tumor promotion by more subtle effects such as mitoinhibition. Hence, the formation of reactive metabolites in cells not only determines initiation through formation of genotoxic lesions, but also tumor promotion through generation of cytotoxic metabolites, leading either to cell death (stimulating regenerative growth of neighboring cells) or more subtle adverse effects such as mitoinhibition. In fact, in the case of "complete carcinogens," the same ultimate toxins may be responsible for both genotoxicity and cytotoxicity. In future, it may be advisable to characterize complete carcinogens on the basis of their relative genotoxic and cytotoxic activities (SCHWARZ et al. 1984). This distinction may be important for low-dose extrapolation and risk assessment in toxicology.

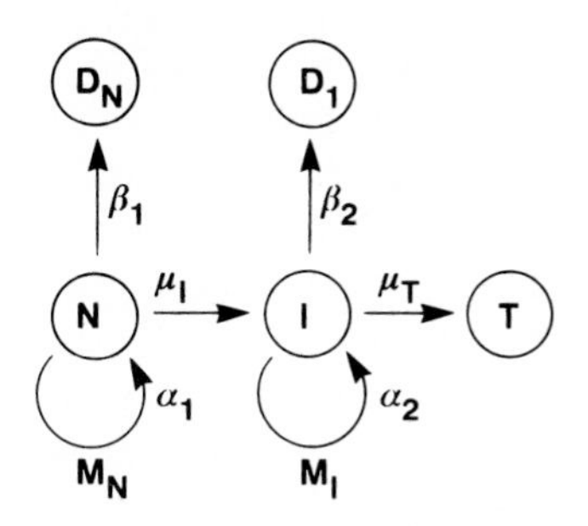

Fig. 2. Two-stage model of carcinogenesis (MOOLGAVKAR 1989; COHEN and ELLWEIN 1990). See text for explanation

Regenerative proliferation may affect both initiation and promotion. At the stage of initiation, cell proliferation predisposes the cell to genotoxic actions of carcinogens, since it has been demonstrated that the liver is particularly vulnerable to genotoxic agents in the early S-phase of the cell cycle (Rabes 1983). At the stage of promotion, cytotoxicity may stimulate selective growth of initiated cells. Initiated cells often have the "toxin-resistance phenotype" (Farber 1984; see below). Death of normal hepatocytes may lead to selective growth of toxin-resistant, initiated hepatocytes, i.e., to their selective proliferation. In this context, it is interesting to note that carcinogens such as polycyclic aromatic hydrocarbons may affect carcinogenicity in multiple ways: (a) by the generation of genotoxic and cytotoxic reactive metabolites and (b) by directly stimulating components of growth-signal pathways, for example by activating the Ah receptor, a nuclear transcription factor, discussed later (Poland and Knutson 1982; Nebert 1991).

The brief discussion of recent concepts of carcinogenesis aimed at emphasizing the multiple ways in which the balance between activating and inactivating drug-metabolizing enzymes by xenobiotic metabolizing enzymes (including UGTs) may influence neoplastic transformation of cells. In the following, two roles of glucuronidation in the control of carcinogens will be discussed: (1) glucuronidation of metabolites of aromatic amines as transport forms of proximate carcinogens determining the target of carcinogenicity and (2) its major role in detoxication of aromatic hydrocarbons and aromatic amines. In addition, after a brief discussion of various factors affecting glucuronide formation in the cell, the role of UGT isozymes in the metabolism of carcinogens will be discussed, in particular regulation of UGT1A1 (a phenol UGT of the 1A family) by the Ah receptor and its persistent alteration at cancer prestages.

B. Glucuronides as Transport Forms of Carcinogens

I. Bladder Carcinogenesis

Aromatic amines were widely used in the dye industry in the mid-nineteenth century. Accordingly, aromatic amines were among the first chemicals to be recognized as human carcinogens. As early as 1895, a German physician, Ludwig Rehn (1895), suggested that cancers of the urinary bladder found in dyestuff workers were due to chemical exposure to certain aniline dyes. In 1938, Hueper and coworkers demonstrated the urinary bladder carcinogenicity of 2-naphthylamine in dogs (Fig. 3; Hueper et al. 1938). Aromatic amines such as 2-naphthylamine and 4-aminobiphenyl are found in nanogram amounts in cigarette smoke (Patrianakos and Hoffmann 1979). These compounds (among others) may account for the positive correlation between cigarette smoking and the incidence of bladder cancer in humans (Wynder

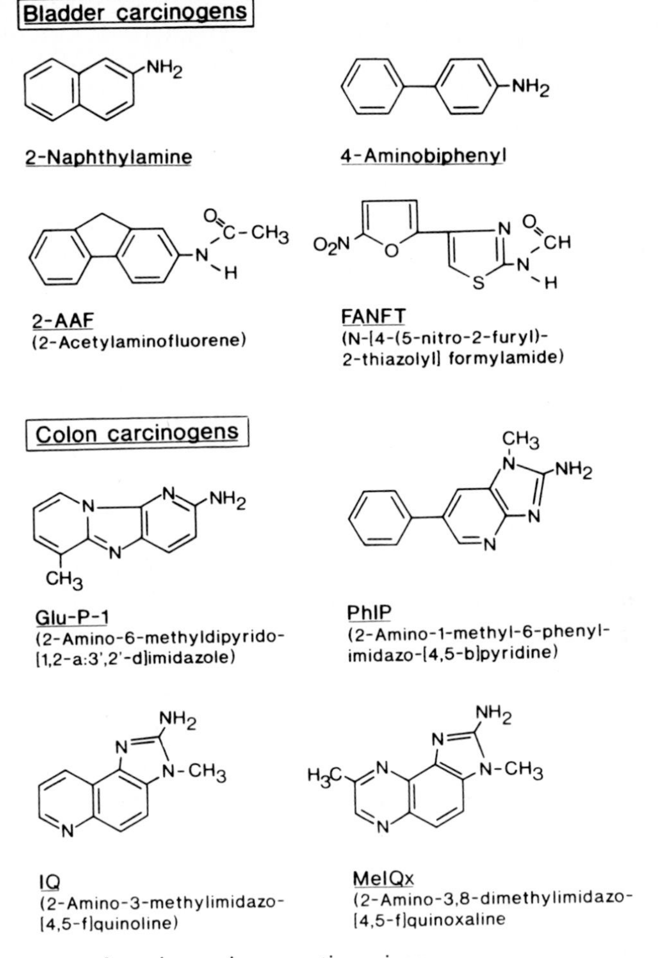

Fig. 3. Structures of carcinogenic aromatic amines

and GOLDSMITH 1977; MOOLGAVKAR and STEVENS 1981; MOMMSEN and AAGAARD 1983). These observations have led to intensive studies on the metabolism of arylamines.

In 1941, 2-acetylaminofluorene (2-AAF; Fig. 3), a proposed insecticide, was shown to be carcinogenic to the liver, mammary gland, and urinary bladder of rats after dietary administration (WILSON et al. 1941). Subsequently, the *N*-hydroxy metabolite of 2-AAF was found to be more carcinogenic than the parent compound (MILLER and MILLER 1981). This provided the first evidence for the concept of metabolic activation and of the formation of a more "proximate carcinogen." It was later found that sulfation and acetylation/deacetylation reactions led to even more reactive intermediates which formed covalent adducts with DNA (ultimate carcinogens).

Glucuronidation led to the formation of the *N-O*-glucuronide of the corresponding *N*-hydroxy-2-AAF. *N*-Hydroxy-2-naphthylamine and *N*-hydroxy-4-aminobiphenyl have been shown to be converted to the corresponding *N*-glucuronides (KADLUBAR et al. 1977; RADOMSKI et al. 1977; POUPKO et al. 1979). Thsee *N*-glucuronides are semistable transport forms which are excreted via the blood into the urinary system. In the case of 2-naphthylamine, the corresponding *N*-hydroxy-*N*-glucuronide has been shown to decompose at the slightly acidic pH of urine to the hydroxylamine and to its protonated nitrenium ion, which readily reacts with DNA, thereby initiating bladder cancer (Fig. 4; KADLUBAR et al. 1981; MILLER and MILLER 1981). In the case of *N*-hydroxy-4-aminobiphenyl, both the glucuronide and most of the unconjugated hydroxylamine enter the bladder (BELAND and KADLUBAR 1990). The resulting DNA adducts have been identified in exfoliated urothelial cells of the dog, a method which may be useful to monitor adduct levels in humans (TALASKA et al. 1990).

In addition to being N-oxidized in the liver and transported to the bladder as the *N*-hydroxy-*N*-glucuronide, 2-naphthylamine is converted to 6-hydroxy- and 1-hydroxy-2-naphthylamine in the liver. The latter can be further oxidized in the bladder epithelium to the corresponding electrophilic iminoquinone by peroxidases, such as prostaglandin H synthase (BELAND and KADLUBAR 1990). This may be an alternative way to form DNA adducts.

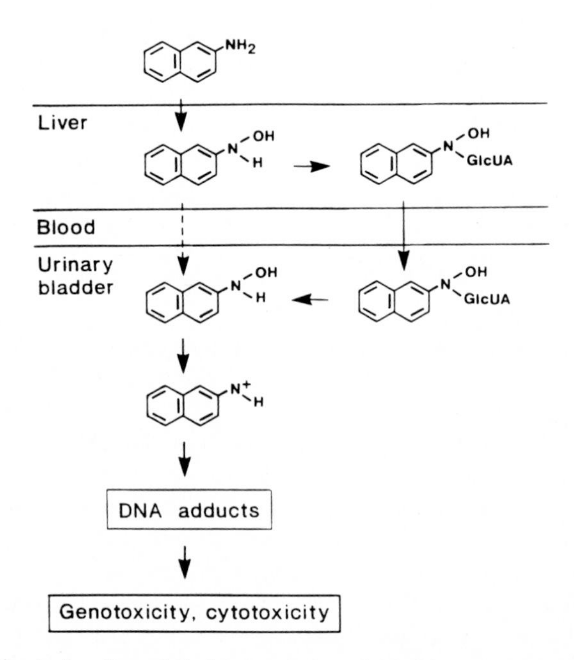

Fig. 4. Hypothesis for 2-naphthylamine-induced bladder cancer (KADLUBAR et al. 1981)

1-Naphthylamine, in contrast to 2-naphthylamine, has not been found to be a bladder carcinogen in experimental animals and humans (RADOMSKI et al. 1980; PURCHASE et al. 1981). This is due to lack of N-oxidation of 1-naphthylamine (BELAND and KADLUBAR 1990), in addition to rapid glucuronidation to the *N*-glucuronide (LILIENBLUM and BOCK 1984; GREEN and TEPHLY 1987; ORZECHOWSKI et al. 1992).

II. Colon Carcinogenesis

Recently, mutagenic heterocyclic arylamines have been discovered which are formed at trace levels in foods such as meat and fish in typical household cooking practices (Fig. 3; SUGIMURA and SATO 1983; SUGIMURA 1986; GERHARDSSON DE VERDIER et al. 1991). In experimental animals, these heterocyclic amines have been found to be involved in colon carcinogenicity. Their appearance in a wide variety of daily food may pose a significant risk for human health. Cancer of the colon and rectum accounted in USA for an estimated 61 300 deaths in 1989, ranking second only to lung cancer. A number of factors have been suggested to be responsible for colorectal cancer risk. For example, this risk was found to be increased by dietary fat and decreased by dietary fiber intake (REDDY et al. 1987; HENDERSON et al. 1991). As described for arylamines involved in bladder carcinogenicity, heterocyclic arylamines have to be N-oxidized (as well as C-oxidized) in liver and are subsequently conjugated with glucuronic acid (Fig. 5; LUKS et al. 1989; WALLIN et al. 1989; TURESKY et al. 1990; ALEXANDER et al. 1991; TURESKY et al. 1991). High molecular weight glucuronides are secreted via the bile into the intestine and the corresponding hydroxylamines and phenolic metabolites may be liberated in the colon by bacterial β-glucuronidases (WEISBURGER 1971). It should be noted, however, that the molecular weight is not the only factor responsible for biliary secretion. Our knowledge about the carriers responsible for biliary secretion of glucuronides and of the properties of these carriers is still very limited.

It has been learned from studies on the metabolism of 2-AAF that O-acetylation of *N*-hydroxy arylamines leads to reactive *N*-acetoxy metabolites. They spontaneously decompose to arylnitrenium ion intermediates, which may be the ultimate reactants with DNA of colon epithelial cells. Recently it was shown that *N*-hydroxy-2-amino-3-methylimidazo-[4,5-*f*] quinoline and *N*-hydroxy-2-amino-1-methyl-6-phenylimidazo-[4,5-*b*]pyridine (Fig. 3) can react in vitro with DNA. At acidic pH, the level of DNA binding was increased, suggesting potential formation of reactive arylnitrenium ions (TURESKY et al. 1991). It has also been shown that N-oxidized arylamines can be further activated by acetyltransferases in human colon (KIRLIN et al. 1991; ILETT et al. 1991). The importance of O-acetylation in the colon is underscored by recent epidemiological evidence showing that the "rapid acetylator" phenotype (about 50% of the Caucasian population) appears to be associated with a higher risk of colorectal cancer (ILETT et al. 1987;

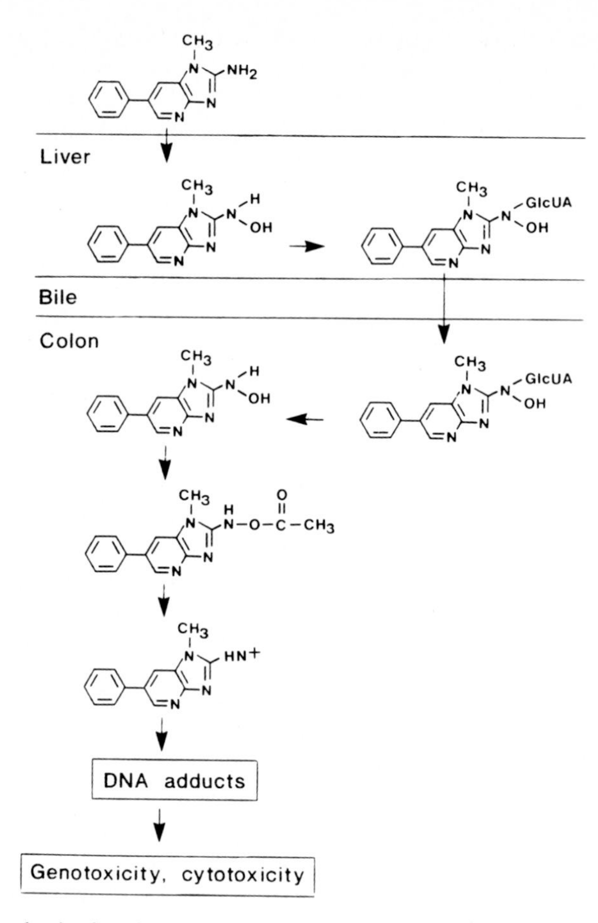

Fig. 5. Hypothesis for 2-amino-1-methyl-6-phenyl-imidazo-[4,5-*b*]pyridine-induced colon cancer (ALEXANDER et al. 1991)

WOHLLEB et al. 1990). In contrast, slow acetylators are at higher risk of developing bladder cancer (BELAND and KADLUBAR 1990; WEBER and HEIN 1985; HEIN 1988). Association of colon carcinogenesis with the acetyltransferase polymorphism is remarkable because of the many factors involved in initiation, promotion, and progression of carcinogenesis.

In contrast to activating reactions such as sulfation and acetylation, the competing glucuronidation reaction may be an important detoxication factor within the cell, as discussed below. This function has to be distinguished from the role of glucuronidation in the formation of transport forms of proximal carcinogens.

C. Role of Glucuronidation in Detoxication of Carcinogens

I. Aromatic Hydrocarbons

Since the discovery of polycyclic aromatic hydrocarbons (PAHs) in chimney soot and coal tar, extensive studies have been conducted on the metabolic activation of these compounds to their ultimate carcinogens (CONNEY 1982; HALL and GROVER 1990). Besides its role in transport of proximal carcinogens (discussed above), glucuronidation must be regarded mostly as a detoxication mechanism. Only selected aspects linking glucuronidation with detoxication of benzo(a)pyrene, benzene, and 2-hydroxybiphenyl will be discussed here.

1. Benzo(a)pyrene

The relationship between inhibition of glucuronidation (and sulfation) by salicylamide and increased covalent binding has been studied in isolated hepatocytes (BURKE et al. 1977) and in perfused liver (BOCK et al. 1981). The liver plays a major role in benzo(a)pyrene metabolism (WALL et al. 1991). Indirect evidence for the role of glucuronidation in the inactivation of genotoxic benzo(a)pyrene metabolites also stems from mutagenicity studies. Several laboratories have shown that addition of UDP-glucuronic acid to the Ames test reduces benzo(a)pyrene mutagenicity (NEMOTO et al. 1978; OWENS et al. 1979; BOCK et al. 1984). In particular, the mutagenicity of benzo(a) pyrene-3,6-quinone in the Ames test was found to be reduced by addition of UDP-glucuronic acid when liver homogenates from 3-methylcholanthrene-treated rats were used as the enzyme source (BOCK et al. 1990a). The mechanism leading to mutagenicity is still unclear. In contrast, increased benzo(a)pyrene mutagenicity has been observed at high benzo(a)pyrene concentrations in the presence of UDP-glucuronic acid (NEMOTO et al. 1978; BOCK et al. 1984). The latter effect is probably due to the removal of quinones which inhibit benzo(a)pyrene metabolism at high concentrations (SHEN et al. 1979). Removal of quinones by glucuronidation of quinols enhances benzo(a)pyrene monooxygenase activity (BOCK 1978) and DNA binding of metabolites (SHEN et al. 1979).

Metabolic pathways of benzo(a)pyrene to ultimate carcinogens include nucleophilic metabolites which can be inactivated by glucuronidation. The degree of inactivation varies considerably. For example, the pathway leading to bay region dihydrodiol epoxides (CONNEY 1982) appears to be poorly inhibited. Dihydrodiols seem to be poor substrates of UGTs (BOCK et al. 1980a). On the other hand, quinone/quinol redox cycles between benzo(a) pyrene-3,6-quinone and benzo(a)pyrene-3,6-quinol are efficiently inhibited (LORENTZEN et al. 1979; LILIENBLUM et al. 1985; LIND 1985; SEGURA-AQUILAR et al. 1986). This may be due in part to efficient conjugation of quinols. For example, benzo(a)pyrene-3,6-quinol is conjugated to both mono- and diglucuronides by phenol UGTs (see Table 3). Benzo(a)pyrene-3,6-quinol diglucuronide has recently been detected in rat bile after intratracheal instillation of benzo(a)pyrene (Bevan and Sadler 1992). It is intriguing why several enzymes involved in detoxication of quinones (NAD(P)H quinol oxidoreductase, glutathione transferases Ya, UGT1A1, etc.) are induced by a common receptor, the Ah receptor (see below).

2. Benzene

Earlier findings indicated that addition of UDP-glucuronic acid to a benzene-oxidizing system reduced covalent binding of metabolites to protein (Tunek et al. 1978). In addition, studies of the influence of enzyme inducers on benzene-induced bone marrow toxicity demonstrated a temporary protective effect of treatment with 3,3′,4,4′-tetrachlorobiphenyl (a 3-methylcholanthrene- or dioxin-type inducer), which was paralelled by an induction of hepatic UGT (Greenlee and Irons 1981). There is growing evidence that the liver is the primary site of bioactivation of benzene (Fig. 6). Metabolites are generated in liver (phenol, hydroquinone, etc.) which may be transported to the bone marrow. Partial hepatectomy or inhibition of hepatic benzene metabolism resulted in a pronounced reduction of myelotoxicity (Sammett et al. 1979). In support of a role of glucuronidation in the inactivation of toxic intermediates, it has been shown that 3-methylcholanthrene treatment leads to a marked shift in the conjugation of phenol sulfation to glucuronidation in isolated hepatocytes (Schrenk and

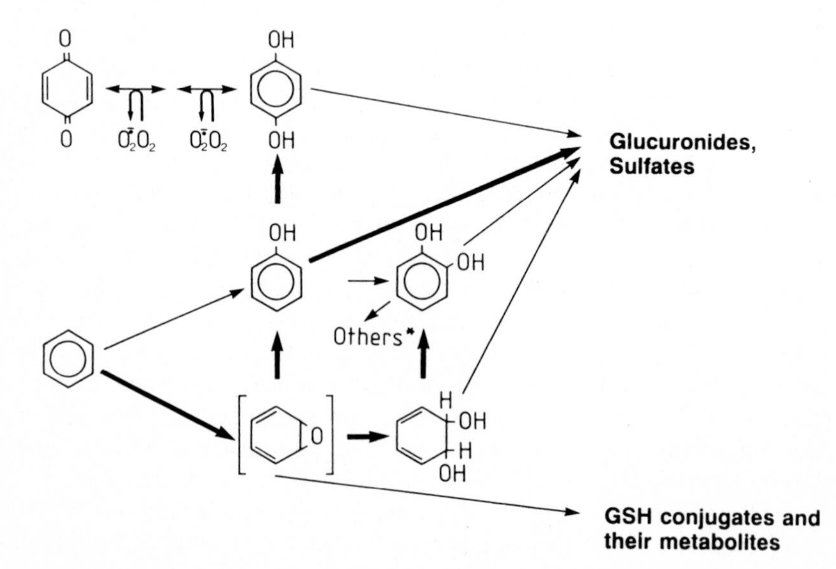

Fig. 6. Selected pathways of benzene metabolism in hepatocytes. *Others include trans, trans-muconaldehyde and the corresponding acid as well as 1,2,4-benzenetriol (for references see Schrenk and Bock 1990). *GSH*, glutathione

Bock 1990). The shift was shown to be due to induction of phenol UGT. Phenol sulfate and sulfuric acid esters of other phenolic benzene metabolites are known to be less stable than the corresponding glucuronides and may liberate the parent compound by chemical or enzymatic hydrolysis at the target of toxicity. In this context, the rate-limiting step of benzene oxidation by P4502E1 should not be forgotten (Johansson and Ingelman-Sundberg 1988; Schrenk et al. 1992).

3. 2-Hydroxybiphenyl

2-Hydroxybiphenyl is widely used as an antimicrobial agent to protect edible crops, and hence the human population may be exposed to it. It is assumed, however, that this human exposure does not lead to a significant health hazard. At low doses, 2-hydroxybiphenyl is mostly excreted as the glucuronide and sulfate ester and no toxicity is observed. At high doses, conjugation pathways are saturated and the compound is further oxidized to the corresponding hydroquinone and semiquinone, metabolites which are probably responsible for covalent binding, genotoxicity, and initiation of bladder cancer (Reitz et al. 1983). This example demonstrates that saturation of glucuronidation leads to the accumulation of phenols and to their further oxidation to reactive metabolites.

II. Aromatic Amines

1. 2-Acetylaminofluorene

2-AAF is one of the most extensively studied chemical carcinogens (Fig. 3). As with other aromatic amines, N-oxidation (catalyzed mainly by P4501A2; Hammons et al. 1985; Butler et al. 1989) is the initial activation step, followed in liver by deacetylation and sulfuric acid conjugation. The resulting unstable conjugate decomposes and leads (in long-term feeding studies) to the only DNA adduct, *N*-(deoxyguanosine-8-yl)-2-aminofluorene, which may be responsible for initiation of hepatocarcinogenesis by 2-AAF (Miller and Miller 1981; Beland and Kadlubar 1990). Glucuronidation competes with sulfuric acid conjugation. Conflicting results have been published about the reactivity of *N-O*-glucuronides of *N*-hydroxy-2-AAF. The *N-O*-glucuronide has been reported to react with DNA under in vitro conditions (Cardona and King 1975; Irving 1977). However, whereas *N*-glucuronides of arylhydroxylamines induce repair synthesis of DNA in cultured urothelial cells of several species, the *N-O*-glucuronide of *N*-hydroxy-AAF does not induce DNA repair synthesis in the absence of β-glucuronidase (Wang et al. 1984), suggesting that no reactive metabolites are formed under in vivo conditions. These observations indicate that formation of *N-O*-glucuronides of arylhydroxylamines may be a detoxication mechanism. Moreover, an inverse relationship was found between the carcinogenicity of 2-naphthylamine,

4-acetylaminobiphenyl, and 2-AAF and the ease of glucuronidation of their hydroxamic acid derivatives, suggesting that glucuronidation may play an important role in determining the carcinogenicity of arylamines and arylacetamides in the rat (WANG et al. 1985). There are other examples suggesting a role of glucuronidation in detoxication. Enhanced glucuronidation of *N*-hydroxy-2-AAF in hepatocyte nodules may be involved in the "toxin-resistance phenotype" of these cells in the Solt-Farber model (SPIEWAK RINAUDO et al. 1989), discussed below. Further support for the role of glucuronidation in detoxication of carcinogens stems from studies of the mutagenicity of 2-naphthylamine (BOCK-HENNIG et al. 1982). Addition of UDP-glucuronic acid to the Ames test led to a marked reduction of 2-naphthylamine mutagenicity.

Knowledge about glucuronidation of *N*-hydroxy-2-AAF is scarce in human tissues. Studies with primary cultures of human hepatocytes demonstrated that the cells conjugated 2%–52% (up to 51% glucuronides and 12% sulfates) of 2-AAF over a thousand-fold concentration range. The C-hydroxylated AAF metabolites were conjugated to glucuronides more efficiently than *N*-hydroxy-2-AAF and deacetylated aminofluorene metabolites (MONTEITH et al. 1990).

In addition to the competition between sulfotransferases and UGTs, the relationship between *N*-acetyltransferases and UGTs in determining the reactivity of N-oxidized arylamines is intriguing. Depending on the hepatic N-acetylation and N-deacetylation capacities, these metabolites appear mainly as the glucuronic acid conjugates of hydroxylamines or *N*-arylacetohydroxamic acids. The *N-O*-glucuronide of *N*-hydroxy-2-AAF is not carcinogenic when injected subcutaneously to the rat, and it does not induce DNA repair synthesis in cultured urothelial cells unless in the presence of β-glucuronidase (WANG et al. 1984). Depending on the species, the deglucuronidated hydroxamic acids can be activated by urothelial cells through N-deacetylation or *N,O*-acetyl transfer and produce DNA repair synthesis in cultured urothelial cells secondary to modification of DNA. Because of the low level of β-glucuronidase in the urine, *N-O*-glucuronides are subject to little metabolic activation in the bladder and are, therefore, considered as detoxified metabolites. However, since both the *N*-glucuronides and free hydroxylamines induce DNA repair synthesis in cultured urothelial cells, the semistable *N*-glucuronides of hydroxylamines are considered to be responsible for the induction of bladder tumors. This has been demonstrated by instillation of the *N*-glucuronide of *N*-hydroxy-2-aminofluorene in the heterotopic bladder of rats (WANG et al. 1987).

2. Others

The heterocyclic amine *N*-[4-(5-nitro-2-furyl)-2-thiazolyl]formylamide (FANFT) (Fig. 3) is a model compound used to study bladder cancer in rats, mice, and hamsters. However, guinea pigs are resistant to FANFT-induced bladder cancer (DAWLY et al. 1991). A more proximate carcinogen in FANFT-induced bladder cancer is thought to be ANFT, a deformylated FANFT. ANFT *N*-glucuronide was shown to be a major metabolite in guinea pigs, but not in rats. The glucuronide was produced by liver and kidney microsomes of guinea pigs, which appears to be responsible (at least in part) for the reduced amount of free ANFT excreted in guinea pigs compared with rats. The reduced levels of urinary ANFT observed in guinea pigs may partially explain the resistance of this species to FANFT-induced bladder cancer.

The role of glucuronidation in the formation of water-soluble excretory products of arylamines can be very complex, as demonstrated in studies of benzidine metabolism (LYNN et al. 1984). In addition to the formation of biologically inactive glucuronides, "reactive" acyl-linked glucuronides have also been demonstrated (STOGNIEW and FENSELAU 1982; VAN BREEMEN and FENSELAU 1986; SPAHN-LANGGUTH and BENET 1992); the latter will be dealt with in another chapter of this volume.

D. Metabolism of Carcinogens by Isozymes of the Uridine Diphosphate Glucuronosyltransferase Enzyme Superfamily

I. Factors Controlling Glucuronide Formation in the Intact Cell

Comprehensive reviews on various factors affecting glucuronide formation have recently been published (JANSEN et al. 1992; MULDER 1992). In addition to the pattern of UGT isozymes (reviewed in Sect. D.II and Chap. 1 of this volume), the following factors have been discerned:

1. The Uridine Diphosphate Glucuronic Acid Level

Although influenced by various pretreatments, the cellular level of UDP-glucuronic acid is generally held constant in hepatocytes (0.3 μmol/g tissue wet weight; BOCK and WHITE 1974; ULLRICH and BOCK 1984a). This is mainly due to the fact that, despite the varying demands for glucuronidation, regeneration of UDP-glucuronic acid appears to be quite high in the liver of fed rats.

2. Localization of Uridine Diphosphate Glucuronosyltransferase: Latency

Evidence derived from the gene structure of UGTs suggests that the active site of UGT is located on the luminal site of the endoplasmic reticulum (IYANAGI et al. 1986; JANSEN et al. 1992). This transmembrane topology implies that UDP-glucuronic acid, synthesized in the cytoplasm, has to be transported through the membrane to the active site. There is indirect evidence for carriers of UDP-glucuronic acid (HAUSER et al. 1988; VANSTAPEL and Blanckaert 1988; Milla et al. 1992). The nature of the rate-limiting steps remains unclear. Maximal glucuronidation can be achieved, for example by adding detergents to microsomes, which leads to membrane perturbation. The ratio of UGT activities in disrupted versus intact microsomes is operationally called "latency." Latency is less apparent at low substrate concentrations (Table 1). For example, latency of UGT activity towards 1-naphthol is about 26 at 0.5 m*M*, but only 3 at 0.002 m*M*. In contrast, the level of UDP-glucuronic acid does not affect the latency of membrane-bound UGTs.

UDP-*N*-Acetylglucosamine has been implicated as an activator of UGTs facilitating transport of UDP-glucuronic acid from the cytosol to the active site of UGT via the microsomal carrier of UDP-glucuronic acid (Hauser et al. 1988). Hence, in vivo UGT appears to operate neither in the fully activated state (corresponding to detergent-treated microsomes) nor in the fully latent state (corresponding to the enzyme in intact microsomes). UGT activity in intact microsomes in the presence of UDP-*N*-acetylglucosamine may be close to that operating in vivo (Bock and White 1974; Otani et al. 1976; Ullrich and Bock 1984b).

Table 1. Influence of 1-naphthol and the uridine diphosphate (UDP)-glucuronic acid (UDPGlcUA) level on UDP-glucuronosyltransferase (UGT) activity in intact and detergent-treated microsomes

Substrate (m*M*)	UGT activity (nmol/min per mg protein)		Latency
	Intact microsomes	Detergent-treated microsomes	
1-Naphthol (3 m*M* UDPGlcUA)			
0.002	1.2	3.2	2.7
0.005	1.3	5.9	4.5
0.01	1.6	11.0	6.9
0.02	1.9	17.0	8.9
0.05	2.1	32.0	15.0
0.1	2.3	44.0	19.0
0.2	2.6	58.0	22.0
0.5	2.6	65.0	26.0
UDPGlcUA (0.5 m*M* 1-naphthol)			
0.1	0.8	20	25
0.2	1.3	32	25
0.3	1.7	40	24
0.6	2.4	49	20
3.0	2.8	68	24

UGT activity was determined in liver microsomes from untreated rats (Bock and White 1974). Data represent means of three determinations.

3. Interaction of Uridine Diphosphate Glucuronosyltransferases with Phospholipids

When phospholipids are totally removed from purified UGT preparations, very little activity is left. The type of phospholipid is rather critical. A structure–activity study of 1-palmitoyl-sn-glycero-3-phosphocholines suggested that negatively charged phospholipids are inhibitory, whereas neutral or positively charged phospholipids are activating (ZAKIM et al. 1988). Addition of phospholipds leads to conformational changes of purified UGTs (SINGH et al. 1982).

Interpretation of the phenomenon of latency has led to a lot of controversy in UGT research in the past, because latency can be viewed both as the result of the removal of a permeability barrier for UDP-glucuronic acid (as discussed above) or as a constraint imposed on the enzyme by the interaction with phospholipids (ZAKIM and DANNENBERG 1992). Investigators have been divided into two camps for a long time: the "compartmentationalists," who believe that activation opens the compartment of restricted accessibility (e.g., the access of water-soluble glucuronic acid to the microsomal lumen) and the "conformationalists," who believe that activation removes constraints that prevent full expression of enzyme activity. So far the controversy has not yet been fully resolved. In fact, the interpretation of latency represents one of the major unsolved questions in glucuronidation research.

4. Sequestration of Substrates in the Microsomal Membrane

Sequestration of UGT substrates has been described in many laboratories (ILLING and BENFORD 1976; ZAKIM and VESSEY 1977). For example, octanol/water partition coefficients of a selected series of simple phenols differ by more than 50-fold (Table 2). The concentration in microsomal membranes increases accordingly. UGT activity towards these substrates (tested with microsomes from 3-methylcholanthrene-treated rats) increases with increasing lipophilicity, but reached saturation at octanol/water coefficients greater than 100 (Fig. 7). Similar findings are obtained using microsomes from untreated rats, suggesting that the properties described are independent of the pattern of UGT isozymes (described below). The influence of lipophilicity appears to be less pronounced with intact microsomes (in the presence or absence of UDP-*N*-acetylglucosamine) than with detergent-activated microsomes. Since substrate lipophilicity determines substrate sequestration, amphiphilic substrates such as phenol or paracetamol may reach lower concentrations in the membrane. For paracetamol, an octanol/water partition coefficient of 6.2 has been reported (RAAFIAUB 1986). When drawing conclusions from UGT studies at the microsomal level to glucuronide formation in the cell, transport of UDP-glucuronic acid from the cytoplasm to the active site of UGT in the lumen of microsomes has to be

Table 2. Partitioning of a series of simple phenols between octanol/buffer or liver microsomes/buffer

No.	Substrate	Partition coefficient (octanol/water)	Concentration in microsomes (nmol/mg protein)
1	4-Dimethylaminophenol	15 ± 2[a]	19 ± 3
2	4-Methoxyphenol	24 ± 1	22 ± 4
3	Phenol	32 ± 2	23 ± 4
4	4-Nitrophenol	33 ± 2	33 ± 4
5	Umbelliferone	35 ± 3	27 ± 5
6	3-Methoxyphenol	36 ± 4	27 ± 2
7	4-Methylumbelliferone	94 ± 12	48 ± 6
8	3-Methylphenol	99 ± 9	38 ± 2
9	3-Nitrophenol	101	n.d.
10	4-Methylphenol	104 ± 8	41 ± 4
11	4-Ethylphenol	240[b]	74 ± 6
12	4-Chlorophenol	272 ± 29	130 ± 10
13	3-Chlorophenol	359 ± 30	100 ± 10
14	4-Bromophenol	390	n.d.
15	2-Naphthol	690[b]	300 ± 30
16	1-Naphthol	1009 ± 34	440 ± 20

Octanol/buffer coefficients were determined as described by Illing and Benford (1976). Conditions for partitioning between microsomes/buffer and methods used to measure the concentrations of phenols were the same as those described in Fig. 7.
n.d., not determined.
[a] Data represent means ± S.D. of four experiments.
[b] Taken from Fujita et al. (1964).

taken into account as a possible rate-limiting step. This rate limitation may be particularly important with high turnover substrates, including highly lipophilic substrates such as 1-naphthol (Table 1).

II. Functions of Uridine Diphosphate Glucuronosyltransferase Isozymes

1. Uridine Diphosphate Glucuronosyltransferase Enzyme Superfamily

Many lines of evidence suggested multiplicity of UGTs in the past, for example their differential inducibility by 3-methylcholanthrene or phenobarbital (Bock et al. 1973; Lucier et al. 1975; Wishart 1978; Lilienblum et al. 1982). The existence of a supergene family of isozymes has recently been established by their purification to apparent homogeneity (Falany and Tephly 1983; Bock et al. 1979, 1988) and in particular by cloning, sequencing, and expression of the cDNAs in cultured cells. Information of the current state of knowledge about the UGT superfamily and its nomenclature is given in Chap. 1 of this volume.

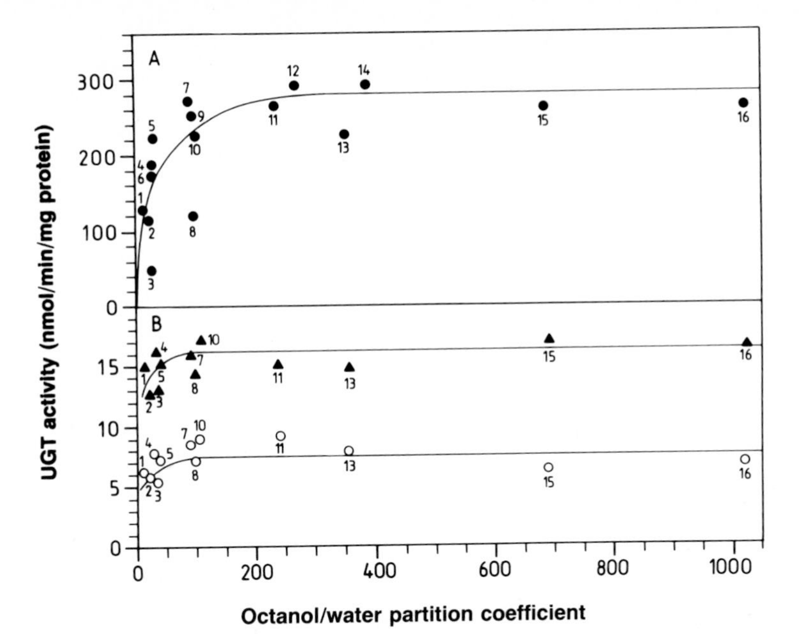

Fig. 7A,B. Influence of substrate lipophilicity on microsomal uridine diphosphate (UDP) glucuronosyltransferase (UGT) activity. **A** ●, Detergent-treated microsomes. **B** Intact microsomes without (○) and with (▲) 3 m*M* UDP-*N*-acetylglucosamine. Substrates are numbered as in Table 1. UGT activities were determined at a substrate concentration of 0.5 m*M* and with microsomes from 3-methylcholanthrene-treated rats (0.5 mg protein per ml). UGT activity toward most substrates was determined from the disappearance of substrate (ILLING and BENFORD 1976), with the exception of substrates 1, 5, 7, 15, and 16 (assays described by LILIENBLUM et al. 1982) and of substrates 4 and 19 (assays described by BOCK et al. 1973). Data represent means of four experiments

More than 26 distinct cDNAs in five mammalian species have been sequenced to date (BURCHELL et al. 1991). A nomenclature system for UGTs has been proposed similar to that developed for P450 isozymes (NEBERT and GONZALEZ 1987). Comparison of the deduced amino acid sequences leads to the definition of two families and a total of three subfamilies. For naming each gene, the root symbol UGT was proposed, to be followed by an Arabic number denoting the family, a letter designating the subfamily, and an Arabic number representing the individual gene, for example, or izozyme within the family or subfamily. Family 1 consists of one subfamily. All its members appear to be derived from one gene, the rat and human phenol/bilirubin UGT gene complex (Fig. 8; IYANAGI 1991; JANSEN et al. 1992; RITTER et al. 1992a). The four human isozymes sequenced to date share exons 2–5 and are characterized by their unique exons 1. mRNAs with different 5′-ends are formed by alternative splicing. Each exon 1 is preceded by its own promotor. Four human isozymes of the gene

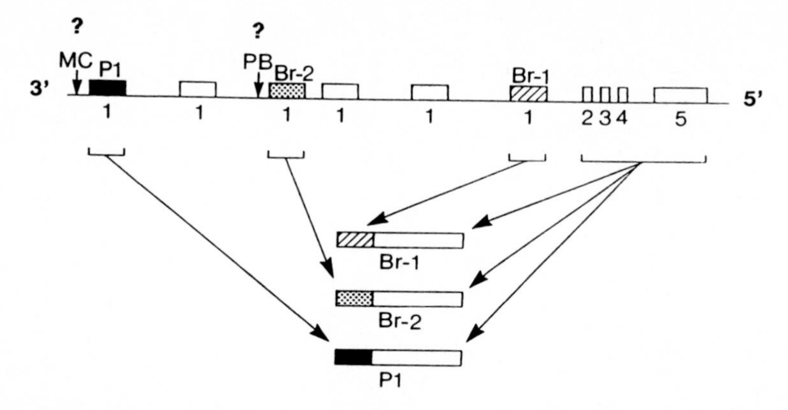

Fig. 8. Organization of the human phenol/bilirubin uridine diphosphate glucuronosyltransferase (UGT) gene complex (Ritter et al. 1992a; Jansen et al. 1992). The data are consistent with the existence of a large gene (>110 kb) in which at least six independently regulated alternative first exons share four common 3′-exons to form mRNAs with different 5′-ends by alternative splicing. *P1*, exon 1 for HlugP1 (UGT1A1); *Br-2*, exon 1 for bilirubin-UGT2; *Br-1*, exon 1 for bilirubin-UGT1. Each of the unique exons is preceded by its own TATA box promoter and regulatory region. P1 is probably inducible by 3-methylcholanthrene (*MC*) and Br-2 by phenobarbital (*PB*)

complex have been identified: (1) HlugP1 (also termed phenol UGT1*6 or human UGT1A1), conjugating planar phenols; (2) HlugP4, conjugating bulky phenols, and (c) and (d) two bilirubin UGTs, Br-1 (UGT1*1) and Br-2 (UGT1*4; Ritter et al. 1992a). Individual genes of the gene complex appear to be differentially regulated; UGT1A1, for example, by 3-methylcholanthrene-type inducers (discussed below), Br-2 by phenobarbitaltype inducers (Ritter et al. 1992a). Family 2 consists of two subfamilies. Subfamily 2A consists of a unique olfactory UGT present in support cells of the olfactory epithelium. This UGT2A1 is probably involved in the inactivation of odorous signals such as eugenol and borneol, but also conjugates standard phenols such as 4-methylumbelliferone (Lazard et al. 1991). Subfamily 2B is composed of multiple steroid UGTs. Overlap of substrate specificity not only includes steroids, but also xenobiotics. For example, phenobarbital-inducible testosterone/chloramphenicol UGT (UGT2B1) is involved in 4-hydroxybiphenyl glucuronidation (Mackenzie 1987), and androsterone UGT (UGT2B2) has been shown to conjugate 4-aminobiphenyl (Falany and Tephly 1983).

Some UGT isozymes have not been completely sequenced, such as rat and human UGTs toward morphine (Puik and Tephly 1986 and Thomassin et al. 1991, respectively) and rat UGTs toward digitoxigenin-monodigitoxoside (von Meyerinck et al. 1985) and toward 4-hydroxybiphenyl (Styczynski et al. 1991). It remains to be elucidated to what extend these UGTs are involved in the metabolism of toxins.

It is interesting that closely related isozymes (considered to be orthologs) have been found in different species, for example human and rat UGT1A1 and bovine and rat UGT2A1 (see BURCHELL et al. 1991). The pattern of UGT isozymes in various tissues is quite different. For example, UGT1A1 appears to be almost ubiquitously distributed in tissues (BOCK et al. 1980a). More work is needed to characterize the enzyme pattern in different tissues.

2. Substrate Specificity of Phenol Uridine Diphosphate Glucuronosyltransferases in Family 1A

Investigations on the substrate specificity of various UGTs, purified to apparent homogeneity, provided a lot of information on their substrate specificity (BOCK et al. 1979; FALANY and TEPHLY 1983). However, due to the instability of purified UGTs (even in the presence of phospholipids), studies of substrate specificity using purified UGT isozymes are tedious. Stable transfection of UGT cDNAs offers a great opportunity in this respect, in particular in studies of low-turnover substrates (FOURNEL-GIGLEUX et al. 1991; BOCK et al. 1992).

Knowledge about glucuronidation of carcinogens and their metabolites by individual UGT isozymes is limited. Therefore, only phenol UGT isozymes of rat and human liver will be discussed here. It was already known that simple phenols (used frequently as standard substrate in UGT assays) are overlapping substrates for several UGTs (FALANY and TEPHLY 1983). Simple phenols are substrates of 3-methylcholanthrene-inducible UGTs (BOCK et al. 1973, 1979; FALANY and TEPHLY 1983). Therefore, inducibilty has been used to assign substrates to inducible or constitutive UGT isozymes.

On the basis of high induction factors (about tenfold), phenols of PAHs have been suggested to be more selective substrates of 3-methylcholanthrene-inducible rat UGT1A1 (LILIENBLUM et al. 1985, 1987; BOCK 1991). Particularly high induction factors were found with diglucuronide formation of 3,6-dihydroxybenzo(a)pyrene and -chrysene (40- and 310-fold, respectively; LILIENBLUM et al. 1985; BOCK et al. 1992).

cDNAs of UGT isozymes which have been stably transfected into cells may offer an opportunity to study the substrate specificity of individual isozymes. The utility of such studies is demonstrated by comparing three transfected isozymes of family 1A, rat UGT1A1 (BOCK et al. 1992), its human ortholog HlugP1 (FOURNEL-GIGLEUX et al. 1991), and HlugP4 (WOOSTER et al. 1991). Arylamines and their N-oxidized metabolites and phenolic metabolites of benzo(a)pyrene and 6-hydroxychrysene (the latter selected as a stable and safe representative of PAH phenols) are compared with standard substrates and a widely used analgetic drug, paracetamol (Table 3). This drug was chosen since paracetamol has been used as an in vivo test to screen

Table 3. Glucuronide formation of xenobiotics with transfected uridine diphosphate glucuronosyltransferases (UGTs)

Substrate	Glucuronide formation (nmol/min per mg protein)		
	HlugP1	HlugP4	$UGT1A1_{rat}$
Standard substrates			
4-Methylumbelliferone	9.3 ± 2.6	1.7 ± 0.5	12.1 ± 0.4
1-Napthol	10.2 ± 3.0	0.4	9.0 ± 0.4
Arylamines			
1-Naphthylamine	11.1	1.8	7.2 ± 1.0
2-Naphthylamine	0.4	0.7	1.5
N-Hydroxy-2-naphthylamine	2.3 ± 0.3	4.6	5.8 ± 0.8
PAH phenols			
3-Hydroxybenzo(a)pyrene	–	0.3 ± 0.03	0.07 ± 0.01
6-Hydroxychrysene	1.9	1.6 ± 0.2	0.27 ± 0.02
3,6-Dihydroxybenzo(a)pyrene			
(6-monoglucuronidation	2.2 ± 0.7	6.6 ± 0.5	1.5 ± 0.2
(diglucuronidation)	0.2 ± 0.2	0.04 ± 0.01	0.09 ± 0.03
Others			
Paracetamol	0.3 ± 0.02	0.03 ± 0.01	0.08 ± 0.01

Methods used to obtain stable transfectants have been described: HlugP1 (Fournel-Gigleux et al. 1991), HlugP4 (Wooster et al. 1991), and $UGT1A1_{rat}$ (Bock et al. 1992). Described methods were used for the assay of UGT activity toward 1-naphthol, *N*-hydroxy-2-naphthylamine, and 3-hydroxybenzo(a)pyrene (Bock et al. 1979), toward 4-methylumbelliferone (Lilienblum et al. 1982), toward 1-naphthylamine (Lilienblum and Bock 1984), toward 3,6-dihydroxybenzo(a)pyrene (Lilienblum et al. 1985), toward 6-hydroxychrysene (Bock et al. 1992), and toward paracetamol (Bock et al. 1993). Data represent means ± S.D. (n = 4) or means of two determinations.
PAH, polycyclic aromatic hydrocarbon.

for the glucuronidation capacity in population studies (Bock et al. 1987). With cell-expressed UGT isozymes, relative UGT activities toward various substrates can be compared (absolute values obviously depend on the efficiency of transfection). As shown in Table 3, the two human phenol UGTs and the rat UGT1A1 are able to catalyze the conjugation of the chosen substrates. HlugP1 and $UGT1A1_{rat}$ appear to be more efficient in conjugating simple phenols (including paracetamol), whereas HlugP4 appears to be more efficient in catalyzing the conjugation of the larger PAH phenols. The isozymes are also able to catalyze both mono- and diglucuronide formation of 3,6-dihydroxybenzo(a)pyrene. These observations are substantiated by kinetic analysis showing that HlugP4 reveals a lower K_m for 6-hydroxychrysene, whereas HlugP1 has the lower K_m for paracetamol (Table 4).

The chosen enzymes also catalyze the conjugation of aromatic amines, such as 1- and 2-naphthylamine, and *N*-hydroxy-2-naphthylamine (Orzechowski et al. 1992), confirming earlier suggestions based on induc-

Table 4. Kinetic analysis of transfected uridine diphosphate glucuronosyltransferases (UGTs) (BOCK et al. 1993)

Isozyme Substrate	K_M (mM)	V_{max} (nmol/min per mg protein)	V_{max}/K_M
HlugP1			
4-Methylumbelliferone	0.15	14.00	93.00
6-Hydroxychrysene	0.14	2.50	18.00
Paracetamol	2.00	0.40	0.20
HlugP4			
4-Methylumbelliferone	0.02	1.80	90.00
6-Hydroxychrysene	0.02	1.68	84.00
Paracetamol	~50.00	1.90	0.04
$UGT1A1_{rat}$			
4-Methylumbelliferone	0.18	25.50	142.00
6-Hydroxychrysene	0.10	0.60	6.00
Paracetamol	2.70	0.20	0.07

Data represent means of three experiments.

tion studies and studies using purified rat UGT1A1 (BOCK et al. 1979; LILIENBLUM and BOCK 1984).

Much more work is needed using diverse endogenous and exogenous substrates to delineate the substrate specificity of UGT isozymes. On the basis of induction studies, it has been suggested that *R*-naproxen (EL MOUELHI and BOCK 1991; EL MOUELHI et al. 1993; note that the *S*-enantiomer is used as an anti-inflammatory drug), thyroxin (BEETSTRA et al. 1991), and *all-trans* retinoic acid (BANK et al. 1989) are substrates of 3-methylcholanthrene-inducible UGT isozymes. Assignment to particular UGTs cannot be done until studies with transfected isozymes have been carried out. It is difficult to characterize the substrate specificity of UGTs, since UGT isozymes with similar substrate specificity appear to have evolved, as suggested from comparative studies with HlugP1 and HlugP4 (see below) and from studies on different steroid UGTs conjugating hyodeoxycholic acid and certain estrogen derivatives (RITTER et al. 1992b).

E. Regulation of Uridine Diphosphate Glucuronosyltransferase Isozymes

I. General Features

Similar to P450 isozymes, rodent liver UGT isozymes are known to be differentially requlated by prototype inducers, such as phenobarbital and 3-methylcholanthrene (LUCIER et al. 1975; WISHART 1978; FALANY and TEPHLY

1983; Iyanagi et al. 1986; Bock et al. 1973, 1979, 1988), pregnenolone 16α-carbo-nitril (Watkins et al. 1982; von Meyerinck et al. 1985), clofibric acid (Lilienblum et al. 1982; Sato et al. 1990), and antioxidants (Bock et al. 1980b; Prochaska and Talalay 1988). All these inducers appear to switch on regulatory programs including transcriptional activation of a number of genes. Interestingly, antioxidants to not induce P450 isozymes. A *cis*-acting regulatory element has been characterized in the upstream region of glutathione *S*-transferase Ya (Rushmore and Pickett 1990). The pattern of enzyme induction – including NAD(P)H oxidoreductase$_1$ (DT-diaphorase), UGT1A1, and glutathione *S*-transferase Ya – is reminiscent of an "oxidative stress" response (Nebert et al. 1990; Liang et al. 1992). The two-electron reduction of quinones by NAD(P)H-quinone oxidoreductase$_1$ and the conjugation reactions of hydroquinones are part of the antioxidant defense (Sies 1991). In this sense, phenol UGTs may be called ancillary antioxidant enzymes.

As with other genes, it is probably the interaction of multiple *cis*-regulatory elements with a variety of *trans*-acting factors that controls the cell-specific expression of UGT isozymes (Mackenzie and Rodbourn 1990). These factors may function with different elements at different developmental stages. In non-expressing cells, some of these factors may be absent or modified to prevent the interactions necessary for efficient transcription. Post-transcriptional mechanisms may also have to be taken into account. Two kinds of transcriptional mechanisms will be discussed in detail: (1) regulation of phenol UGTs by the Ah receptor and (2) persistent increase of phenol UGT expression at cancer prestages.

II. Regulation of Phenol Uridine Diphosphate Glucuronosyltransferases by the Ah Receptor

Earlier genetic evidence indicated that mouse liver phenol UGT is regulated by the Ah receptor (Owens 1977). This result in the mouse model was supported in rat liver by induction studies using Ah receptor ligands differing in induction potencies by a factor of more than 100000-fold (Fig. 9; Bock et al. 1990a; Bock 1991; Schrenk et al. 1991b). Dose–response curves indicate that P4501A1 and UGT1A1 activities are induced at the same concentration of inducers differing in potency by over 100000-fold. Potencies of PCDDs have been calculated from the IC_{50} values (i.e., the concentration of PCDD leading to 50% of the induction maximum). These findings, together with those observed with other 2,3,7,8-substituted PCDDs in both primary cultures of hepatocytes and H4IIE hepatoma cells (Bock 1991), suggest that both enzymes are induced by a common receptor, the Ah receptor.

In man, there is also some evidence for UGT isozymes responsive to 3-methylcholanthrene-type inducers. Glucuronidation of paracetamol is increased in heavy smokers (presumably exposed to 3-methylcholanthrene-type inducers; Mucklow et al. 1980; Bock et al. 1987). Paracetamol has

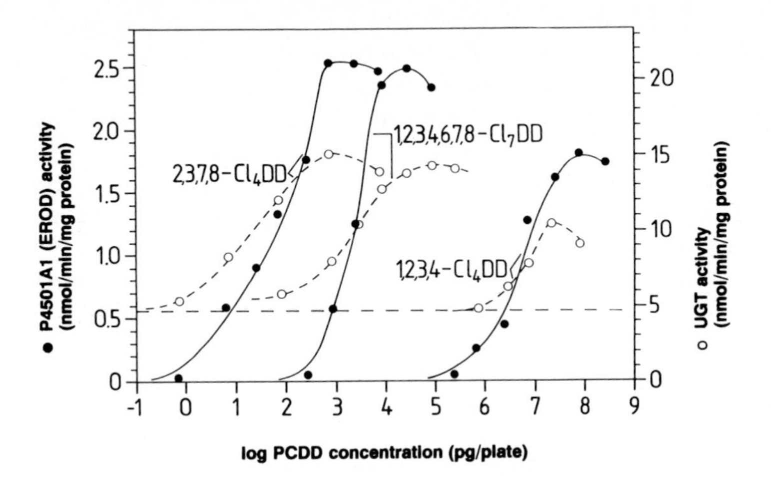

Fig. 9. Dose-response curves of P4501A1-dependent 7-ethoxyresorufin-*O*-deethylase (*EROD*) and of phenol uridine diphosphate glucuronosyltransferase (UGT) activity toward 4-methylumbelliferone (Bock et al. 1990a). Primary cultures of rat hepatocytes were incubated for 48 h with various concentrations of polychlorinated dibenzo-*p*-dioxins (PCDDs). PCDDs are designated by the position and number of chlorine atoms; for example, 2,3,7,8-tetrachlorodibenzo-*p*-dioxin is termed 2,3,7,8-Cl_4DD. Incubation for 48 h resulted in maximal induction of a P4501A1-dependent enzyme activity, EROD, and of phenol UGT activity towards 4-methylumbelliferone. The data are shown as dose–response curves. The *dashed line* indicates the level of phenol UGT in the absence of inducers

been shown to be a high-affinity substrate of human UGT1A1 or HlugP1 and other phenol UGTs (Table 3; Bock et al. 1993). Moreover, in a population study, a high correlation ($r = 0.85$) was found between the caffeine test (Campbell et al. 1987; suggesting induction of P4501A2) and paracetamol glucuronidation in male heavy smokers (Jansen et al. 1992).

The Ah or dioxin receptor is a soluble protein which binds planar, halogenated aromatic compounds (for example 2,3,7,8-tetrachlorodibenzo-*p*-dioxin, TCDD) with high affinity (k_D-TCDD $\approx 7 \times 10^{-12} M$; Bradfield and Poland 1988). Ligands of the Ah receptor include PAHs (such as benzo(a)pyrene and 3-methylcholanthrene), polyhalogenated hydrocarbons and related compounds, photo-oxidation products of L-tryptophan, and a large number of plant constituents such as rutaecarpine alkaloids (Gillner et al. 1989). Recently, indolo[3,2-*b*]carbazole has been demonstrated to be a high-affinity ligand for the Ah receptor (Rannug et al. 1987; Bjeldanes et al. 1991). These tryptamine derivatives can be formed under the acid conditions of the stomach from indole-3-carbinol present in cabbage, Brussels sprouts, etc. (Wattenberg 1992). Furthermore, heterocyclic amines found in broiled foods (described above) have also been discovered as ligands of the Ah receptor (Kleman et al. 1990).

The ligand-free form of the Ah receptor is found in the cytosol in complex with 90-kDa heat-shock proteins (hsp90; Perdew 1988; Wilhelmsson et al. 1990). After ligand binding (leading to detachment of hsp90), the complex is transferred to the nucleus. Nuclear transfer and DNA binding requires association with a second protein, the Ah receptor nuclear translocator protein (Arnt; Hoffman et al. 1991). It has been shown that the Ah receptor binds to DNA sequences in the upstream region of a number of genes, known as xenobiotic responsive elements (XRE; Fujisawa-Sehara et al. 1986; Whitlock 1990; Landers and Bunce 1991). Evidence has been obtained that the Ah receptor binds to XREs as a heterodimeric complex with Arnt (Reyes et al. 1992). Preliminary evidence suggests that the DNA-binding activity of the Ah receptor is regulated by phosphorylation (Pongratz et al. 1991).

Because of the similarity between ligand-activated transcription by the Ah receptor and by members of the steroid hormone receptor superfamily (Evans et al. 1988), many researchers have speculated that the Ah receptor may be a member of that family. The Ah receptor has recently been cloned (Burbach et al. 1992; Ema et al. 1992). However, the sequence of the Ah receptor was not related to the steroid receptor superfamily, but to the Arnt protein and to two developmental regulatory proteins of Drosophila, per and sim (Nambu et al. 1991). Unlike the steroid receptor superfamily which uses zinc finger motives for DNA binding, the Ah receptor uses instead a basic region helix–loop–helix motive (Weintraub et al. 1991). Recently, a consensus sequence for binding of the AhR to XRE (TNGCGTG) has been found in the 5′ regulatory region of P4501A1 and P4501A2 (Nebert and Jones 1989; Whitlock 1990). It has also been found in other human genes, such as NAD(P)H quinone oxidoreductase$_1$ (NQO$_1$; Jaiswal 1991), plasminogen activator inhibitor 2 (PAI-2; Sutter et al. 1991), and UGT1*6 or UGT1A1 (Münzel et al. 1994). However, for UGT1*6 the functional role of the consensus sequence still needs to be established.

The physiological ligand of the Ah receptor is unknown. In view of the similarities between the Ah receptor and steroid hormone receptor superfamily systems, it is conceivable that the physiological ligand for the Ah receptor is a yet unidentified hormone. By analogy to retinoic acid, TCDD is able to modulate differentiation processes. Thus, it is possible that the endogenous ligand may represent an unknown morphogen. However, it cannot be excluded that physiological ligands of the Ah receptor are xenobiotics occurring in the plant diet. In addition, PAHs from forest fires have always been present in the environment. It is, therefore, conceivable that the Ah receptor fulfills two functions: (1) important roles in detoxication and elimination of lipid-soluble environmental and dietary products and (2) regulatory mechanisms which may control the steady state levels of effector molecules involved in growth and differentiation pathways (Nebert 1991).

III. Persistent Alterations of Phenol Uridine Diphosphate Glucuronosyltransferase in Preneoplastic Liver

The multiple mechanisms leading to drug resistance have recently been reviewed (HAYES and WOLF 1990). Similar to persistent alterations of other drug-metabolizing enzymes (FARBER 1984; PITOT 1990), phenol UGT is increased in preneoplastic liver lesions such as hepatocyte foci (FISCHER et al. 1983, 1985) and hepatocyte nodules (BOCK et al. 1982; YIN et al. 1982). Alterations of UGT are heterogeneous, including both UGT-positive and -negative foci (BOCK 1991; BOCK et al. 1989, 1991). Interestingly, UGT-positive foci are preponderant in the rat, whereas UGT-negative foci are preponderant in mice. Investigation of a number of hepatocyte nodules and differentiated hepatocellular carcinomas, produced by feeding 2-AAF, suggested that one phenol UGT isozyme, UGT1A1, was selectively enhanced. Bilirubin UGT and testosterone UGT were not increased (BOCK et al. 1982). Northern blot analysis using a selective cDNA fragment of UGT1A1 demonstrated increased expression of UGT1A1 under these conditions. However, immunoblot analysis using antibodies to UGT1A1 led to conflicting results. Whereas in some nodules or carcinomas the regular 55-kD UGT1A1 peptide was increased, in others a 53-kD peptide was preponderant (BOCK et al. 1990b). It has been demonstrated that UGT1A1 represents a glycoprotein containing high mannose-type carbohydrate moieties, with a relative molecular mass of about 2 kDa (IYANAGI et al. 1986). It is therefore conceivable that the 53-kDa phenol UGT polypeptide found in hepatocyte nodules is produced by post-transcriptional modification (i.e., differential glycosylation) of UGT1A1.

Adaptive induction of UGT1A1 by 3-methylcholanthrene-type inducers has to be clearly distinguished from the persistent alterations of this isozyme observed in preneoplastic liver lesions. The persistent alterations of UGT1A1 contribute to the "toxin-resistance phenotype" of preneoplastic cells (Table 5). This phenotype denotes an altered pattern of drug-metabolizing enzymes observed in different carcinogenesis models (FARBER 1984). It includes decreased P4501A1 and decreased sulfotransferase IV (RINGER et al. 1990), increased glutathione *S*-transferase P, and increased phenol UGT as well as increased expression of the multidrug-resistance gene product P-glycoprotein (THORGEIRSSON et al. 1987). The toxin-resistance phenotype may explain selective growth of preneoplastic cells under the conditions of the Solt-Farber model (SPIEWAK RINAUDO et al. 1989), as discussed below.

In the evaluation of focal alterations, the putative progenitor cells of hepatocytes have to be considered. Mitoinhibitory agents such as 2-AAF are known to stimulate growth of oval cells (SELL 1990; EVARTS et al. 1989; HIXSON and ALLISON 1985; GERMAIN et al. 1988). Moreover, frequently studied rat liver epithelial cells (a heterogenous group of cells including

Table 5. Permanent alterations of enzymes involved in drug metabolism and disposition in rat liver nodules[a]

Enzyme	Relative nodular activity[a]
Phase I	
Cytochromes P450	0.2
Aryl hydrocarbon hydroxylase	0.05–0.3
NAD(P)H quinone oxidoreductase$_1$ = NQO$_1$ (cytosol)	13
Aldehyde hehydrogenase (cytosol)	40
Phase II	
Phenol sulfotransferase IV	0.06
UGT1A1	5–10
Epoxide hydrolase (microsomal)	5
Glutathione *S*-transferases	5
Glutathione *S*-transferase P	34
Others	
γ-Glutamyltranspeptidase	100–170
Glycoprotein-P (mdr gene product)	Increased

[a] Data represent the ratios between uridine diphosphate glucuronosyltransferase (UGT) activities in nodular tissue and in normal liver. They are taken from references Bock et al. (1982 and 1989).

precursors of bile duct cells and hepatocytes) show some characteristics of oval cells (McMahon et al. 1986). They also display a pattern of drug-metabolizing enzymes similar to the toxin-resistance phenotype (Schrenk et al. 1991a). Whereas P450 activities were found to be lower in rat liver epithelial cells, phenol UGT activities were comparable to those found in differentiated hepatocytes.

A toxin-resistance phenotype, including increased UGT activity, is also found in human tumor cells, in particular after treatment with chemotherapeutic agents (Cowan et al. 1986; Akman et al. 1990; Gessner et al. 1990), and may explain therapeutic failure after long-term treatment with these agents.

Molecular mechanisms underlying the persistent alterations of proteins (including UGT1A1) in preneoplastic hepatocyte foci remain unknown. It is unlikely that they result from genotoxic lesions of the individual genes which are increased in their expression. It is more likely that they reflect persistent changes of regulatory genes. Hepatocyte foci have attracted wide interest as biochemical markers associated with preneoplastic stages during hepatocarcinogenesis in rodents (Pitot 1990). Findings from different laboratories indicate a marked phenotypic heterogeneity of hepatocellular foci in rodents, reflecting subpopulations of clonally expanding hepatocytes. However, a direct correlation has been observed between the complexity of the enzymatic phenotype (i.e., the number of enzymatic changes) and the growth behaviour of the clones (Peraino et al. 1988; Schwarz et al. 1989; Bock 1991; Buchmann et al. 1992). Hence, apart from being useful preneoplastic markers, the persistent preneoplastic enzyme alterations may guide us to intriguing regulatory mechanisms. There is a good correlation between the number and size of enzyme-altered foci and subsequent malignancy of the rat liver, and it is widely accepted that at least some of these foci are premalignant. Thus, the persistent enzyme alterations may be considered as surrogate (and by no means perfect) markers of initiation. In the future, it will be important to analyze a time sequence of the growth and disappearance of altered clones (LUEBECK et al. 1991).

F. Conclusions

UGTs play a major role in the elimination of nucleophilic metabolites of carcinogens such as phenols and quinols of PAHs. In this way they prevent their further oxidation to electrophiles which may react with DNA, RNA, and protein. They also inactivate carcinogenic, N-oxidized metabolites of aromatic amines. As the quantitatively most important reaction, glucuronidation fulfills a major role in the defense system against the accumulation of lipid-soluble xenobiotics and their conversion to reactive electrophiles. The latter affect carcinogenesis by genotoxic and cytotoxic damage of cells at the stages of initiation, promotion, and progression.

Two roles of glucuronides are emphasized: (1) their role as transport forms excreted via the biliary or urinary tract, thereby liberating the ultimate carcinogen at the target of carcinogenicity and (2) their role in sequestering proximate carcinogens, leading to their detoxication. For example, glucuronidation of quinols (readily formed from quinones) is important, since they are readily autoxidized to reactive semiquinones and quinones and undergo toxic redox cycles with the generation of reactive oxygen species. Arylacetohydroxamic acids are inactivated by glucuronidation instead of being activated by sulfation and acetylation.

Isozymes of the UGT enzyme superfamily have been identified which control the glucuronidation of phenols and quinols of aromatic hydrocarbons and of carcinogenic N-oxidized aromatic amines. In particular, phenol UGTs such as UGT1*6 or UGT1A1 are coinduced with P4501A1 and other drug-metabolizing ezymes via the Ah or dioxin receptor and play a major role in the control of various proximate carcinogens. The rat UGT1A1 is persistently increased at cancer prestages in rat hepatocarcinogenesis models and contributes to the altered enzyme pattern leading to the toxin-resistance phenotype.

Knowledge about the isozymes of this enzyme superfamily in different species, their tissue distribution, and regulation will improve extrapolation of drug and carcinogen metabolism data from experimental animals to man as well as risk assessment of carcinogens. In particular, regulatory properties of some isozymes, such as the control of UGT1A1 by the Ah receptor and its persistent alterations at cancer prestages, will open new avenues to understand higher-order, pleiotropic regulatory programs.

Acknowledgements. The authors' work referred to in this review was supported by the Deutsche Forschungsgemeinschaft and the Forschungsschwerpunkt Baden-Württemberg. Secretarial help by Mrs. A. von Bank and Mrs. E. Schenk is gratefully acknowledged.

References

Akman SA, Forrest G, Fong-Fong C, Esworthy RC, Doroshow JH (1990) Antioxidant and xenobiotic-metabolizing enzyme gene expression in doxorubicin-resistant MCF-7 breast cancer cells. Cancer Res 50:1397–1402

Alexander J, Wallin H, Rossland OJ, Solberg KE, Holme JA, Becher G, Andersson R, Grivas S (1991) Formation of a glutathione conjugate and a semistable transportable glucuronide conjugate of N^2-oxidized species of 2-amino-1-methyl-6-phenylimidazo [4,5-b] pyridine PhIP in rat liver. Carcinogenesis 12:2239–2245

Bank PA, Salyers KL, Zile MH (1989) Effect of tetrachlorodibenzo-p-dioxin (TCDD) on the glucuronidation of retinoic acid in the rat. Biochim Biophys Acta 993:1–6

Beetstra JB, van Engelen JGM, Karels P, van der Hoek HJ, de Jong M, Docter R, Krenning EP, Hennemann G, Brouwer A, Visser TJ (1991) Thyroxine and 3,3′,5-triiodothyronine are glucuronidated in rat liver by different uridine diphosphate-glucuronosyltransferases. Endocrinology 128:741–746

Beland FA, Kadlubar FF (1990) Metabolic activation and DNA adducts of aromatic amines and nitroaromatic hydrocarbons. In: Cooper CS, Grover PL (eds) Chemical carcinogenesis and mutagenesis I. Springer, Berlin Heidelberg New York, pp 267–325

Bevan DR, Sadler VM (1992) Quinol diglucuronides are predominant conjugated metabolites found in bile of rats following intratracheal instillation of benzo(a) pyrene. Carcinogenesis 13:403–407

Bishop JM (1991) Molecular themes in oncogenesis. Cell 64:235–248

Bjeldanes LF, Kim J-Y, Grose KR, Bartholomew JC, Bradfield CA (1991) Aromatic hydrocarbon responsiveness-receptor agonists generated from indole-3-carbinol in vitro and in vivo: comparisons with 2,3,7,8-tetrachlorodibenzo-p-dioxin. Proc Natl Acad Sci USA 88:9543–9547

Bock KW (1978) Increase of liver microsomal benzo(a)pyrene monooxygenase activity by subsequent glucuronidation. Naunyn-Schmiedebergs Arch Pharmacol 304:77–79

Bock KW (1989) Conjugation reactions in carcinogen metabolism and their permanent alterations after initiation of hepatocarcinogenesis. In: Bannasch P, Keppler D, Weber G (eds) Liver cell carcinoma. MTP Press, Lancaster, pp 251–259

Bock KW (1991) Roles of UDP-glucuronosyltransferases in chemical carcinogenesis. CRC Crit Rev Biochem Mol Biol 26:129–150

Bock KW, White INH (1974) UDP-glucuronyltransferase in perfused rat liver and in microsomes: influence of phenobarbital and 3-methylcholanthrene. Eur J Biochem 46:451–459

Bock KW, Fröhling W, Remmer H, Rexer B (1973) Effects of phenobarbital and 3-methylcholanthrene on substrate specificity of rat liver microsomal UDP-glucuronyltransferase. Biochim Biophys Acta 327:46–56

Bock KW, Josting D, Lilienblum W, Pfeil H (1979) Purification of rat liver microsomal UDP-glucuronyl-transferase. Eur J Biochem 98:19–26

Bock KW, von Clausbruch UC, Kaufmann R, Lilienblum W, Oesch F, Pfeil H, Platt KL (1980a) Functional heterogeneity of UDP-glucuronyltransferase in rat tissues. Biochem Pharmacol 29:495–500

Bock KW, Kahl R, Lilienblum W (1980b) Induction of rat hepatic UDP-glucuronyltransferase by dietary ethoxyquin. Naunyn-Schmiedebergs Arch Pharmacol 310:249–252

Bock KW, Bock-Henning BS, Lilienblum W, Volp RF (1981) Release of mutagenic metabolites of benzo(a)pyrene from the perfused rat liver after inhibition of glucuronidation and sulfation by salicylamide. Chem Biol Interact 36:167–177

Bock KW, Lilienblum W, Pfeil H, Eriksson LC (1982) Increased uridine diphosphate-glucuronyltransferase activity in preneoplastic liver nodules and Morris hepatomas. Cancer Res 42:3747–3752

Bock KW, Bock-Henning BS, Fischer G, Lilienblum W, Ullrich D (1984) Role of glucuronidation and sulfation in the control of reactive metabolites. In: Greim H, Jung R, Kramer M, Marquardt H, Oesch F (eds) Biochemical basis of chemical carcinogenesis. 13th Workshop Conference Hoechst. Raven, New York, pp 13–22

Bock KW, Wiltfang J, Blume R, Ullrich D, Bircher J (1987) Paracetamol as a test drug to determine glucuronide formation in man. Effects of inducers and of smoking. Eur J Clin Pharmacol 31:677–683

Bock KW, Schirmer G, Green MD, Tephly TR (1988) Properties of a 3-methylcholanthrene-inducible phenol UDP-glucuronosyltransferase from rat liver. Biochem Pharmacol 37:1439–1443

Bock KW, Kobusch AB, Fischer G (1989) Heterogeneous alterations of UDP-glucuronosyltransferases in mouse hepatic foci. J Cancer Res Clin Oncol 115: 285–289

Bock KW, Lipp HP, Bock-Hennig BS (1990a) Induction of drug-metabolizing enzymes by xenobiotics. Xenobiotica 20:1101–1111

Bock KW, Münzel PA, Röhrdanz E, Schrenk D, Eriksson LC (1990b) Persistently increased expression of a 3-methylcholanthrene-inducible phenol UDP-glucuronosyl-transferase in rat hepatocyte nodules and hepatocellular carcinomas. Cancer Res 50:3569–3573

Bock KW, Kobusch AB, Lipp HP, Münzel PA, Röhrdanz E, Schrenk D, Eriksson LC (1991) Regulation of rat phenol UDP-glucuronosyltransferase and its persistently increased expression at liver cancer prestages. In: Bock KW, Gerok W, Matern S, Schmid R (eds) Hepatic metabolism and disposition of endo- and xenobiotics. Kluwer Academic, Dordrecht, pp 217–228

Bock KW, Gschaidmeier H, Seidel A, Baird S, Burchell B (1992) Mono- and diglururonide formation of chrysene and benzo(a)pyrene phenols by 3-methylcholanthrene-inducible phenol UDP-glucuronosyltransferase (UGT1A1). Mol Pharmacol 42:613–618

Bock KW, Forster A, Gschaidmeier H, Brück M, Münzel P, Schareck W, Fournel-Gigleux, Burchell B (1993) Paracetamol glucuronidation by recombinant rat and human phenol UDP-glucuronosyltransferases. Biochem Pharmacol 45: 1809–1814

Bock-Henning BS, Ullrich D, Bock KW (1982) Activating and inactivating reactions controlling 2-naphthylamine mutagenicity. Arch Toxicol 50:259–266

Bradfield CA, Poland A (1988) A competitive binding assay for 2,3,7,8-tetrachlorodibenzo-p-dioxin and related ligands of the Ah receptor. Mol Pharmacol 34:682–688

Buchmann A, Bock KW, Schwarz M (1992) Enzyme and immunohistochemical phenotyping of diethylnitrosamine-induced liver lesions of male C3H/He, B6C3F1 and C57BL/6J mice. Carcinogenesis 13:691–697

Burbach KM, Poland A, Bradfield CA (1992) Cloning of the Ah-receptor cDNA reveals a distinctive ligand-activated transcription factor. Biochemistry 89: 8185–8189

Burchell B, Nebert DW, Nelson DR, Bock KW, Iyanagi T, Jansen PLM, Lancet D, Mulder GJ, Roy Chowdhury J, Siest G, Tephly TR, Mackenzie PI (1991) The UDP glucuronosyltransferase gene superfamily. Suggested nomenclature based on evolutionary divergence. DNA Cell Biol 10:487–494

Burke MD, Vadi H, Jernström B, Orrenius S (1977) Metabolism of benzo[a]pyrene with isolated hepatocytes and the formation and degradation of DNA-binding derivates. J Biol Chem 252:6424–6431

Butler MA, Iwasaki M, Guengerich FP, Kadlubar FF (1989) Human cytochrome P-450_{PA} (P-4501A2), the phenacetin O-deethylase, is primarily responsible for the hepatic 3-demethylation of caffeine and N-oxidation of carcinogenic arylamines. Proc Natl Acad Sci USA 86:7696–7700

Campbell ME, Spielberg SP, Kalow W (1987) A urinary metabolite ratio that reflects systemic caffeine clearance. Clin Pharmacol Ther 42:157–165

Cardona RA, King CM (1975) Activation of the O-glucuronide of the carcinogen N-hydroxy-N-2-fluorenyl-acetamide by enzymatic deacetylation in vitro: formation of fluorenylamine-tRNA adducts. Biochem Pharmacol 25:1051–1056

Cohen SM, Ellwein LB (1990) Cell proliferation in carcinogenesis. Science 249: 1007–1011

Coles B, Ketterer B (1990) The role of glutathione and glutathione transferases in chemical carcinogenesis. Crit Rev Biochem Mol Biol 25:47–70

Conney AH (1982) Induction of microsomal enyzmes by foreign chemicals and carcinogenesis by polycyclic aromatic hydrocarbons: G.H.A. Clowes memorial lecture. Cancer Res 42:4875–4917

Cowan KH, Batist G, Tulpule A, Sinha BK, Myers C (1986) Similar biochemical changes associated with multidrug resistance in human breast cancer cells and carcinogen-induced resistance to xenobiotics in rats. Proc Natl Acad Sci USA 83:9328–9332

Dawley RM, Zenser TV, Mattammal MB, Lakshmi VM, Hsu FF, Davis BB (1991) Metabolism and disposition of bladder carcinogens in rat and guinea pig: possible mechanism of guinea pig resistance to bladder cancer. Cancer Res 51: 514–520

Denison MS, Fisher JM, Whitlock J (1988) The DNA-recognition site for the dioxin-Ah receptor complex. J Biol Chem 263:17221–17224

Dutton GJ (1980) Glucuronidation of drugs and other compounds. CRC Press, Boca Raton, pp 23–28

El Mouelhi M, Bock KW (1991) Stereoselective (S)- and (R)-naproxen glucuronosyltransferase of rat liver. Drug Metab Dispos 19:304–308

El Mouelhi M, Beck S, Bock KW (1993) Stereoselective glucuronidation of (R)- and (S)-naproxen by recombinant rat phenol UDP-glucuronosyltransferase (UGT1A1) and its human orthologue. Biochem Pharmacol 46:1298–1300

Ema M, Sogawa K, Watanabe N, Chujoh Y, Matsushita N, Gotoh O, Funae Y, Fujii-Kuriyama Y (1992) cDNA Cloning and structure of mouse putative Ah receptor. Biochem Biophys Res Commun 184:246–253

Evans RM (1988) The steroid and thyroid hormone receptor superfamily. Science 240:889–895

Evarts RP, Nagy P, Nakatsukasa H, Marsden E, Thorgeirsson SS (1989) In vivo differentiation of rat liver oval cells into hepatocytes. Cancer Res 49:1541–1547

Falany CN, Tephly TR (1983) Separation, purification and characterization of three isoenzymes of UDP-glucuronosyltransferase from rat liver microsomes. Arch Biochem Biophys 227:248–258

Farber E (1984) Cellular biochemistry of the stepwise development of cancer with chemicals. Cancer Res 44:5463–5474

Fischer G, Ullrich D, Katz N, Bock KW, Schauer A (1983) Immunohistochemical and biochemical detection of uridine-diphosphate-glucuronyltransferase (UDP-GT) activity in putative preneoplastic liver foci. Virchows Arch 42:193–200

Fischer G, Ullrich D, Bock KW (1985) Effects of N-nitrosomorpholine and phenobarbital on UDP-glucuronyltransferase in putative preneoplastic foci of rat liver. Carcinogenesis 6:605–609

Fournel-Gigleux S, Sutherland L, Sabolovic N, Burchell B, Siest G (1991) Stable expression of two human UDP-glucuronosyltransferase cDNAs in V79 cell cultures. Mol Pharmacol 39:177–183

Fujisawa-Sehara A, Sogawa K, Yamane M, Fujii-Kuriyama Y (1987) Characterization of xenobiotic responsive elements upstream from the drug-metabolizing cytochrome P-450c gene: a similarity to glucocorticoid regulatory elements. Nucl Acids Res 15:4179–4191
Fujita T, Iwasa J, Hansch C (1964) A new substitution constant, II, derived from partition coefficient. J Am Chem Soc 86:5175–5180
Gerhardsson de Verdier M, Hagman U, Peters RK, Steineck G, Övervik E (1991) Meat, cooking methods and colorectal cancer: a case-referent study in Stockholm. Int J Cancer 49:520–525
Germain L, Noel M, Gourdeau H, Marceau N (1988) Promotion of growth and differentiation of ductular oval cells in primary culture. Cancer Res 48:368–378
Gessner T, Vaughan LA, Beehler BC, Bartels CJ, Baker RM (1990) Elevated pentose cycle and glucuronyltransferase in daunorubicin-resistant P388 cells. Cancer Res 50:3921–3927
Gillner M, Bergman J, Cambillau C, Gustafsson J-A (1989) Interactions of rutaecarpine alkaloids with specific binding sites for 2,3,7,8-tetrachlorodibenzo-p-dioxin in rat liver. Carcinogenesis 10:651–654
Green MD, Tephly TR (1987) N-Glucuronidation of carcinogenic aromatic amines catalyzed by rat hepatic microsomal preparations and purified rat liver uridine 5′-diphosphate-glucuronosyltransferases. Cancer Res 47:2028–2031
Greenlee WF, Irons RD (1981) Modulation of benzene-induced lymphocytopenia in the rat by 2,4,5,2′,4′,5′-hexachlorobiphenyl and 3,4,3′,4′-tetrachlorobiphenyl. Chem Biol Interact 33:345–360
Guengerich FP (1990) Enzymatic oxidation of xenobiotic chemicals. Crit Rev Biochem Mol Biol 25:97–153
Hall M, Grover PL (1990) Polycyclic aromatic hydrocarbons: metabolism, activation and tumour initiation. In: Cooper CS, Grover PL (eds) Chemical carcinogenesis and mutagenesis I. Springer, Berlin Heidelberg New York, pp 327–372
Hammons GJ, Guengerich FP, Weis CC, Beland FA, Kadlubar FF (1985) Metabolic oxidation of carcinogenic arylamines by rat, dog, and human hepatic microsomes and by purified flavin-containing and cytochrome P-450 monooxygenases. Cancer Res 45:3578–3585
Hauser SC, Ziurys JC, Gollan JL (1988) A membrane transporter mediates access of uridine 5′-diphosphoglucuronic acid from the cytosol into the endoplasmic reticulum of rat hepatocytes: implications for glucuronidation reactions. Biochim Biophys Acta 967:149–157
Hayes JD, Wolf CR (1990) Molecular mechanisms of drug resistance. Biochem J 272:281–295
Hein DW (1988) Acetylator genotype and arylamine-induced carcinogenesis. Biochim Biophys Acta 948:37–66
Henderson BE, Ross RK, Pike MC (1991) Toward the primary prevention of cancer. Science 254:1131–1138
Hixson DC, Allison JP (1985) Monoclonal antibodies recognizing oval cells induced in the liver of rats by N-2-fluorenylacetamide or ethionine in a choline-deficient diet. Cancer Res 45:3750–3760
Hoffman EC, Reyes H, Chu F-F, Sander F, Conley LH, Brooks BA, Hankinson O (1991) Cloning of a factor required for activity of the Ah (dioxin) receptor. Science 252:954–958
Hueper WC, Wiley FH, Wolfe HD, Ranta KE, Leming MF, Blood FR (1938) Experimental production of bladder tumors in dogs by administration of β-naphthylamine. J Ind Hyg Toxicol 20:46–84
Ilett KF, David BM, Detchon P, Castleden WM, Kwa R (1987) Acetylation phenotype in colorectal carcinoma. Cancer Res 47:1466–1469
Ilett KF, Reeves PT, Minchin RF, Kinnear BF, Watson HF, Kadlubar FF (1991) Distribution of acetyltransferase activities in the intestines of rapid and slow acetylator rabbits. Carcinogenesis 12:1465–1469

Illing JPA, Benford D (1976) Observations on the accessibility of acceptor substrates to the active centre of UDP-glucuronosyltransferase in vitro. Biochim Biophys Acta 429:768–779

Irving CC (1977) Influence of the aryl group on the reaction of glucuronides of N-arylacethydroxamic acids with polynucleotides. Cancer Res 37:524–528

Iyanagi T (1991) Molecular basis of multiple UDP-glucuronosyltransferase isoenzyme deficiencies in the hyperbilirubinemic rat (Gunn rat). J Biol Chem 266: 24048–24052

Iyanagi T, Haniu M, Sogawa K, Fujii-Kuriyama Y, Watanabe S, Shively JE, Anan KF (1986) Cloning and characterization of cDNA encoding 3-methylcholanthrene inducible rat mRNA for UDP-glucuronosyltransferase. J Biol Chem 261: 15607–15614

Jaiswal AK (1991) Human NAD(P)H: quinone oxidoreductase (NQO_1) gene structure and induction by dioxin. Biochemistry 30:10647–10653

Jansen PLM, Mulder GJ, Burchell B, Bock KW (1992) New developments in glucuronidation research: report of a workshop on "Glucuronidation, its role in health and disease". Hepatology 15:532–544

Johansson I, Ingelman-Sundberg M (1988) Benzene metabolism by ethanol-, acetone-, and benzene-inducible cytochrome P-450 (IIE1) in rat and rabbit liver microsomes. Cancer Res 48:5387–5390

Kadlubar FF, Miller JA, Miller EC (1977) Hepatic microsomal N-glucuronidation and nucleic acid binding of N-hydroxy arylamines in relation to urinary bladder carcinogenesis. Cancer Res 37:805–814

Kadlubar FF, Unruh LE, Flammang TJ, Sparks D, Mitchum RK, Mulder GJ (1981) Alteration of urinary levels of the carcinogen, N-hydroxy-2-naphthylamine, and its N-glucuronide in the rat by control of urinary pH, inhibition of metabolic sulfation, and changes in biliary excretion. Chem Biol Interact 33:129–147

Kirlin WG, Ogolla F, Andrews AF, Trinidad A, Ferguson RJ, Yerokun T, Mpezo M, Hein DW (1991) Acetylator genotype-dependent expression of arylamine N-acetyltransferase in human colon cytosol from non-cancer and colorectal cancer patients. Cancer Res 51:549–555

Kleman M, Övervik E, Mason G, Gustafsson J-A (1990) Effects of the food mutagens MeIQx and PhIP on the expression of cytochrome P450IA proteins in various tissues of male and female rats. Carcinogenesis 11:2185–2189

Knudson AG (1985) Hereditary cancer, oncogenes, and anti-oncogenes. Cancer Res 45;1437–1443

Land H, Parada LF, Weinberg RA (1983) Tumorigenic conversion of primary embryo fibroblasts requires at least wo cooperating oncogenes. Nature 304: 596–602

Landers JP, Bunce NJ (1991) The Ah receptor and the mechanism of dioxin toxicity. Biochem J 276:273–287

Lazard D, Zupko K, Poria Y, Nef P, Lazarovits J, Horn S, Khen M, Lancet D (1991) Odorant signal termination by olfactory UDP glucuronosyl transferase. Nature 349:790–793

Liang H-CL, Shertzer HG, Nebert DW (1992) "Oxidative stress" response in liver of an untreated newborn mouse having a 1.2-centimorgan deletion on chromosome 7. Biochem Biophys Res Commun 182:1160–1165

Lilienblum W, Bock KW (1984) N-Glucuronide formation of carcinogenic aromatic amines in rat and human liver microsomes. Biochem Pharmacol 33:2041–2046

Lilienblum W, Walli AK, Bock KW (1982) Differential induction of rat liver microsomal UDP-glucuronosyltransferase activities by various inducing agents. Biochem Pharmacol 31:907–913

Lilienblum W, Bock-Hennig BS, Bock KW (1985) Protection against toxic redox cycles between benzo(a)pyrene-3,6-quinone and its quinol by 3-methylcholanthrene-inducible formation of the quinol mono- and diglucuronide. Mol Pharmacol 27:451–458

Lilienblum W, Platt KL, Schirmer G, Oesch F, Bock KW (1987) Regioselectivity of rat liver microsomal UDP-glucuronosyltransferase activities towards phenols of benzo(a)pyrene and dibenzo(a,h)anthracene. Mol Pharmacol 32:173–177
Lind C (1985) Formation of benzo(a)pyrene-3,6-quinol mono- and diglucuronides in rat liver microsomes. Arch Biochem Biophys 240:226–235
Lorentzen RJ, Ts'o POP (1977) Benzo(a)pyrenedione/benzo(a)pyrenediol oxidation–reduction couples and the generation of reactive reduced molecular oxygen. Biochemistry 16:1467–1473
Lorentzen RJ, Lesko SA, McDonald K, Ts'o POP (1979) Toxicity of metabolic benzo(a)pyrenediones to cultured cells and the dependence upon molecular oxygen. Cancer Res 39:3194–3198
Lucier GW, McDaniel OS, Hook GER (1975) Nature of the enhancement of hepatic uridine diphosphate glucuronyltransferase activity by 2,3,7,8-tetrachlorodibenzo-p-dioxin in rats. Biochem Pharmacol 24:325–334
Luebeck EG, Moolgavkar SH, Buchmann A, Schwarz M (1991) Effects of polychlorinated biphenyls in rat liver: quantitative analysis of enzyme-altered foci. Toxicol Appl Pharmacol 111:469–484
Luks HJ, Spratt, TE, Vavrek MT, Roland SF, Weisburger JH (1989) Identification of sulfate and glucuronic acid conjugates of the 5-hydroxy derivative as major metabolites of 2-amino-3-methyl-imidazo[4,5-f]quinoline in rats. Cancer Res 49:4407–4411
Lynn RK, Garvie-Gould CT, Milam DF, Scott KF, Eastman CL, Ilias AM, Rodgers RM (1984) Disposition of the aromatic amine, benzidine, in the rat: characterization of mutagenic urinary and biliary metabolites. Toxicol Appl Pharmacol 72:1–14
Mackenzie PI (1987) Rat liver UDP-glucuronosyltransferase. Identification of cDNAs encoding two enzymes which glucuronidate testosterone, dihydrotestosterone and β-estradiol. J Biol Chem 262:9744–9749
Mackenzie PI, Rodbourn L (1990) Organization of the rat UDP-glucuronosyltransferase, UDPGTr-2, gene and characterization of its promoter. J Biol Chem 265:11328–11332
Mannervik B, Danielson UH (1988) Glutathione transferases – structure and catalytic activity. Crit Rev Biochem 23:283–337
McMahon JB, Richards WL, del Campo AA, Song MH, Thorgeirsson SS (1986) Differential effects of transforming growth factor-β on proliferation of normal and malignant rat liver epithelial cells in culture. Cancer Res 46:4665–4671
Milla ME, Clairmont CA, Hirschberg CB (1992) Reconstitution into proteoliposomes and partial purification of the golgi apparatus membrane UDP-galactose, UDP-xylose, and UDP-glucuronic acid transport activities. J Biol Chem 267:103–107
Miller EC, Miller JA (1981) Searches for ultimate chemical carcinogens and their reactions with cellular macromolecules. Cancer 47:2327–2345
Miller A, Miller EC (1986) Electrophilic sulfuric acid ester metabolites as ultimate carcinogens. Adv Exp Med Biol 197:583–595
Mommsen S, Aagaard J (1983) Tobacco as a risk factor in bladder cancer. Carcinogenesis 4:335–338
Monteith DK, Michalopoulos G, Strom SC (1990) Conjugation of chemical carcinogens by primary cultures of human hepatocytes, Xenobiotica 20:753–763
Moolgavkar SH (1989) Multistage models for cancer risk assessment. In: Travis CT (ed) Biologically based methods for cancer risk assessment. Plenum, New York, pp 9–20
Moolgavkar SH, Stevens RG (1981) Smoking and cancers of bladder and pancreas: risks and temporal trends. J Natl Cancer Inst 67:15
Mucklow JC, Fraser HS, Bulpitt CJ, Kahn C, Mould G, Dolery CT (1980) Environmental factors affecting paracetamol metabolism in London factory and office workers. Br J Clin Pharmacol 10:67–74

Münzel PA, Brück M, Bock KW, Owens IS, Ritter JK (1994) Transcriptional regulation of the human phenol UDP-glucuronosyltransferase (UGT1*6) gene in the A549 lung carcinoma cell line. Naunyn-Schmiedeberg's Arch Pharmacol, in press

Mulder GJ (1992) Glucuronidation and its role in regulation of biological activity of drugs. Annu Rev Pharmacol Toxicol 32:25–49

Nambu JR, Lewis JO, Wharton KA, Crews ST (1991) The Drosophila single-minded gene encodes a helix–loop–helix protein that acts as a master regulator of CNS midline development. Cell 67:1157–1167

Nebert DW (1991) Proposed role of drug-metabolizing enzymes: regulation of steady state levels of the ligands that effect growth, homeostasis, differentiation, and neuroendocrine functions. Mol Endocrinol 5:1203–1214

Nebert DW, Gonzalez FJ (1987) P450 genes: structure, evolution, and regulation. Annu Rev Biochem 56:945–993

Nebert DW, Jones JE (1989) Regulation of the mammalian cytochrome P_1-450 (CYP1A1) gene. Int J Biochem 21:243–252

Nebert DW, Petersen DD, Fornace AJ (1990) Cellular responses to oxidative stress: the [Ah] gene battery as a paradigm. Environ Health Perspect 88:13–25

Nemoto N, Takayama S, Nagao M, Umezawa K (1978) Modification of the mutagenicity of benzo(a)pyrene on bacteria by substrates of enzymes producing water soluble conjugates. Toxicol Lett 2:205–211

Orzechowski A, Schrenk D, Bock KW (1992) Metabolism of 1- and 2-naphthylamine in isolated rat hepatocytes. Toxicol Lett [Suppl] 126

Otani G, Abou-El-Makarem MM, Bock KW (1976) UDP-glucuronyltransferase in perfused rat liver and in microsomes. III. Effects of galactosamine and carbon tetrachloride on the glucuronidation of 1-naphthol and bilirubin. Biochem Pharmacol 25:1293–1297

Owens IS (1977) Genetic regulation of UDP-glucuronosyl-transferase induction by polycyclic aromatic compounds in mice. J Biol Chem 252:2827–2833

Owens IS, Koteen GM, Legraverend C (1979) Mutagenesis of certain benzo[a]pyrene phenols in vitro following further metabolism by mouse liver. Biochem Pharmacol 28:1615–1629

Patrianakos C, Hoffmann D (1979) Chemical studies on tobacco smoke, LXIV. On the analysis of aromatic amines in cigarette smoke. J Anal Toxicol 3:150–154

Peraino C, Carnes BA, Stevens FJ, Staffeldt EF, Russell JJ, Prapuolenis A, Blomquist JA, Vesselinovitch SD, Maronpot RR (1988) Comparative developmental and phenotypic properties of altered hepatocyte foci and hepatic tumors in rats. Cancer Res 48:4171–4178

Perdew GH (1988) Association of the Ah receptor with the 90-kDA heat shock protein. J Biol Chem 263:13802–13805

Pitot HC (1990) Altered hepatic foci: their role in murine hepatocarcinogenesis. Annu Rev Pharmacol Toxicol 30:465–500

Pitot HC, Dragan Y, Sargent L, Xu Y-H (1991) Biochemical markers associated with the stages of promotion and progression during hepatocarcinogenesis in the rat. Environ Health Perspect 93:181–189

Poland A, Knutson JC (1982) 2,3,7,8-Tetrachlorodibenzo-p-dioxine and related halogenated hydrocarbons: examination of the mechanism of toxicity. Annu Rev Pharmacol Toxicol 22:517–554

Pongratz I, Strömstedt P-E, Mason GGF, Poellinger L (1991) Inhibition of the specific DNA binding activity of the dioxin receptor by phosphatase treatment. J Biol Chem 266:16813–16817

Poupko JM, Hearn WL, Radomski JL (1979) N-Glucuronidation of N-hydroxy aromatic amines: a mechanism for their transport and bladder-specific carcinogenicity. Toxicol Appl Pharmacol 50:479–484

Prochaska HJ, Talalay P (1988) Regulatory mechanisms of mono-functional and bifunctional anticarcinogenic enzyme inducers in murine liver. Cancer Res 48: 4776–4782

Puik JF, Tephly TR (1986) Isolation and purification of rat liver morphine UDP-glucuronosyltransferase. Mol Pharmacol 30:558–565
Purchase IFH, Kalinowski AE, Ishmael J, Wilson J, Gore CW, Chart IS (1981) Lifetime carcinogenicity study of 1- and 2-naphthylamine in dogs. Br J Cancer 44:892–901
Raaflaub J (1986) Pharmacokinetik. Ein Leitfaden für Autodidakten. Roche, Basel, p 17
Rabes HM (1983) Development and growth of early preneoplastic lesions induced in the liver by chemical carcinogens. J Cancer Res Clin Oncol 106:85–92
Radomski JL, Hearn WL, Radomski T, Moreno H, Scott WE (1977) Isolation of the glucuronic acid conjugate of N-hydroxy-4-aminobiphenyl from dog urine and its mutagenic activity. Cancer Res 37:1757–1762
Radomski JL, Deichmann WB, Altman NH, Radomski T (1980) Failure of pure 1-naphthylamine to induce bladder tumors in dogs. Cancer Res 40:3537–3539
Rannug A, Rannug U, Rosenkranz HS, Winqvist L, Westerholm R, Agurell E, Grafström A-K (1987) Certain photooxidized derivatives of tryptophan bind with very high affinity to the Ah receptor and are likely to be endogenous signal substances. J Biol Chem 262:15422–15427
Reddy BS, Sharma C, Simi B, Engle A, Laakso K, Puska P, Korpela R (1987) Metabolic epidemiology of colon cancer: effect of dietary fiber on fecal mutagens and bile acids in healthy subjects. Cancer Res 47:644–648
Rehn L (1895) Blasengeschwülste bei Fuchsin-Arbeitern. Arch Klin Chir 50:588–600
Reitz RH, Fox TR, Quast JF, Hermann EA, Watanabe PG (1983) Molecular mechanisms involved in the toxicity of orthophenylphenol and its sodium salt. Chem Biol Interact 43:99–119
Reyes H, Reisz-Porszasz S, Hankinson O (1992) Identification of the Ah receptor nuclear translocator protein (Arnt) as a component of the DNA binding form of the Ah receptor. Science 256:1193–1195
Ringer DP, Norton TR, Howell BA (1990) 2-Acetyl-aminofluorene-mediated alteration in the level of liver arylsulfotransferase IV during rat hepatocarcinogenesis. Cancer Res 50:5301–5307
Ritter JK, Chen F, Sheen YY, Tran HM, Kimura S, Yeatman MT, Owens IS (1992a) A novel complex locus UGT1 encodes human bilirubin, phenol and other UDP-glucuconosyltransferase isozymes with identical carboxyl termini. J Biol Chem 267:3257–3261
Ritter JK, Chen F, Sheen YY, Lubet RA, Owens IS (1992b) Two human liver cDNAs encode UDP-glucuconosyltransferases with 2 log differences in activity toward parallel substrates including hyodeoxycholic acid and certain estrogen derivatives. Biochemistry 31:3409–3414
Rushmore TH, Pickett CB (1990) Transcriptional regulation of the rat glutathione S-transferase Ya subunit gene. J Biol Chem 265:14648–14653
Sammett D, Lee EW, Kocsis JJ, Snyder R (1979) Partial hepatectomy reduces both metabolism and toxicity of benzene. J Toxicol Environ Health 5:785–792
Sato H, Koiwai O, Tanabe K, Kashiwamata S (1990) Isolation and sequencing of rat liver bilirubin UDP-glucuronosyltransferase cDNA: possible alternate splicing of a common primary transcript. Biochem Biophys Res Commun 169:260–264
Schrenk D, Bock KW (1990) Metabolism of benzene in rat hepatocytes: influence of inducers on phenol glucuronidation. Drug Metab Dispos 18:720–725
Schrenk D, Eisenmann-Tappe I, Gebhardt R, Mayer D, El Mouelhi M, Röhrdanz E, Münzel P, Bock KW (1991a) Drug metabolizing enzyme activities in rat liver epithelial cells, hepatocytes and bile duct cells. Biochem Pharmacol 41: 1751–1757
Schrenk D, Lipp HP, Wiesmüller T, Hagenmaier H, Bock KW (1991b) Assessment of biological activities of mixtures of polychlorinated dibenzo-p-dioxins: comparison between defined mixtures and their constituents. Arch Toxicol 65: 114–118

Schrenk D, Ingelman-Sundberg M, Bock KW (1992) Influence of P-4502E1 induction on benzene metabolism in rat hepatocytes and on biliary metabolite excretion. Drug Metab Dispos 20:137–141

Schwarz M, Pearson D, Port R, Kunz W (1984) Promoting effect of 4-dimethylaminoazobenzene on enzyme altered foci induced in rat liver by N-nitrosodiethanolamine. Carcinogenesis 5:725–730

Schwarz M, Buchmann A, Schulte M, Pearson D, Kunz W (1989) Heterogeneity of enzyme-altered foci in rat liver. Toxicol Lett 49:297–317

Segura-Aquilar JE, Barreiro V, Lind C (1986) Dicoumarol-sensitive glucuronidation of benzo(a)pyrene metabolites in rat liver microsomes. Arch Biochem Biophys 251:266–275

Sell S (1990) Is there a liver stem cell? Cancer Res 50:3811–3815

Shen AL, Fahl WE, Wrighton SA, Jefcoate CR (1979) Inhibition of benzo[a]pyrene and benzo[a]pyrene-7,8-dihydrodiol metabolism by benzo[a]pyrene quinones. Cancer Res 39:4123

Shinohara A, Saito K, Yamazoe Y, Kamataki T, Kato R (1989) Acetyl coenzyme A dependent activation of N-hydroxy derivatives of carcinogenic arylamines: mechanism of activation, species difference, tissue distribution, and acetyl donor specificity. Cancer Res 46:4362–4367

Sies H (1991) Oxidative stress: from basic research to clinical application. Amer J Medicine 91 [Suppl 3C]:31S–38S

Singh OMP, Graham AB, Wood GC (1982) The phospholipid dependence of UDP-glucuronosyltransferase: conformation/reactivity studies with purified enzyme. Biochem Biophys Res Commun 107:345–349

Spahn-Langguth H, Benet LZ (1992) Acyl glucuronides revisited: Is the glucuronidation process a toxification as well as a detoxication mechanism? Drug Metab Rev 24:5–48

Spiewak Rinaudo JA, Eriksson LC, Roomi MW, Farber E (1989) Kinetics of excretion of 2-acetylaminofluorene in normal and xenobiotic-treated rats and in rats with hepatocyte nodules. Lab Invest 60:399–408

Stogniew M, Fenselau C (1982) Electrophilic reactions of acyl-linked glucuronides. Formation of clofibrate mercapturate in humans. Drug Metab Disp 10:609–613

Styczynski P, Green M, Puig J, Coffman B, Tephly T (1991) Purification and properties of a rat liver phenobarbital-inducible 4-hydroxybiphenyl UDP-glucuronosyltransferase. Mol Pharmacol 40:80–84

Sugimura T (1986) Past, present, and future of mutagens in cooked foods. Environ Health Perspect 67:5–10

Sugimura T, Sato S (1983) Mutagens–carcinogens in foods. Cancer Res [Suppl] 43:2415s–2421s

Sutter TR, Guzman K, Dold KM, Greenlee WF (1991) Targets for dioxin: genes for plasminogen activator inhibitor-2 and interleukin-1β. Science 254:415–418

Talaska G, Dooley KL, Kadlubar FF (1990) Detection and characterization of carcinogen-DNA adducts in exfoliated urothelial cells from 4-aminobiphenyl-treated dogs by ^{32}P-postlabeling and subsequent thin-layer and high-pressure liquid chromatography. Carcinogenesis 11:639–646

Thomassin J, Styczynski P, Coffman B, Green M, Tephly T (1991) Studies on human liver microsomal morphine and tertiary amine UDP-glucuronosyltransferases: photoaffinity labelling and immunoinhibition. In: Bock KW, Gerok W, Matern S, Schmid R (eds) Hepatic Metabolism and disposition of endo- and xenobiotics. Kluwer Academic, Dordrecht, pp 133–139

Thorgeirsson SS, Huber BE, Sorrell S, Fojo A, Pastan I, Gottesman MM (1987) Expression of the multidrug-resistant gene in hepatocarcinogenesis and regenerating rat liver. Science 236:1120–1122

Tunek A, Platt KL, Bentley P, Oesch F (1978) Microsomal metabolism of benzene to species irreversibly binding to microsomal protein and effects of modifications of this metabolism. Mol Pharmacol 14:920–929

Turesky RJ, Bracco-Hammer I, Markovic J, Richli U, Kappeler AM, Welti DH (1990) The contribution of N-oxidation to the metabolism of the food-borne carcinogen 2-amino-3,8-dimethylimidazo[4,5-f]quinoxaline in rat hepatocytes. Chem Res Toxicol 3:524–535

Turesky RJ, Lang NP, Butler MA, Teitel CH, Kadlubar FF (1991) Metabolic activation of carcinogenic heterocyclic aromatic amines by human liver and colon. Carcinogenesis 12:1839–1845

Ullrich D, Bock KW (1984a) Glucuronide formation of various drugs in liver microsomes and in isolated hepatocytes from phenobarbital- and 3-methylcholanthrene-treated rats. Biochem Pharmacol 33:97–101

Ullrich D, Bock KW (1984b) Inhibition of glucuronide formation by D-galactosone or D-galactosamine in isolated hepatocytes. Biochem Pharmacol 33:1827–1830

Vanstapel F, Blanckaert N (1988) Topology and regulation of bilirubin UDP-glucuronyltransferase in sealed native microsomes from rat liver. Arch Biochem Biophys 263:216–225

Van Breemen RB, Fenselau CC (1986) Reaction of 1-O-acyl glucuronides with 4-(p-nitrobenzyl)pyridine. Drug Metab Dispos 14:197–201

von Meyerinck L, Coffman BL, Green MD, Kirkpatrick RB, Schmoldt A, Tephly TR (1985) Separation, purification, and characterization of digitoxigenin-monodigitoxoside UDP-glucuronosyltransferase activity. Drug Metab Dispos 13:700–704

Wall KL, Gao W, te Koppele JM, Kwei GY, Kauffman FC, Thurman RG (1991) The liver plays a central role in the mechanism of chemical carcinogenesis due to polycyclic aromatic hydrocarbons. Carcinogenesis 12:783–786

Wallin H, Holme JA, Becher G, Alexander J (1989) Metabolism of the food carcinogen 2-amino-3,8-dimethylimidazo[4,5-f]quinoxaline in isolated rat liver cells. Carcinogenesis 10:1277–1283

Wang CY, Christensen B, Zukowski K, Morton KC, Lee MS (1984) Induction of DNA repair synthesis in human urothelial cells by the N-hydroxy metabolites of carcinogenic arylamines. J Natl Cancer Inst 72:847–852

Wang CY, Zukowski K, Lee MS (1985) Glucuronidation of carcinogenic arylamine metabolites by rat liver microsomes. Biochem Pharmacol 34:837–841

Wang CY, Zukowski K, Lee MS, Imaida K (1987) Production of urothelial tumors in the heterotopic bladder of rats by instillation of N-glucuronosyl or N-acetyl derivates of N-hydroxy-2-aminofluorene. Cancer Res 47:3406–3409

Watkins JB, Gregus Z, Thompson TN, Klaassen CD (1982) Induction studies on the functional heterogeneity of rat liver UDP-glucuronsyltransferases. Toxicol Appl Pharmacol 64:439–446

Wattenberg LW (1992) Inhibition of carcinogenesis by minor dietary constituents. Cancer Res [Suppl] 52:2085s–2091s

Weber WW, Hein DW (1985) N-Acetylation pharmacogenetics. Pharmacol Rev 37:25–79

Weinberg RA (1989) Oncogenes, antioncogenes, and the molecular basis of multistep carcinogenesis. Cancer Res 49:3713–3721

Weintraub H, Davis R, Tapscott S, Thayer M, Krause M, Benezra R, Blackwell K, Turner D, Rupp R, Hollenberg S, Zhuang Y, Lassar A (1991) The myoD gene family: nodal point during specification of the muscle cell lineage. Science 251:761–766

Weisburger JH (1971) Colon carcinogens: their metabolism and mode of action. Cancer 28:60–70

Whitlock JP (1990) Genetic and molecular aspects of 2,3,7,8-tetra-chlorodibenzo-p-dioxin action. Annu Rev Pharmacol Toxicol 30:251–277

Wilhelmsson A, Cuthill S, Denis M, Wikström A-C, Gustafsson J-A, Poellinger L (1990) The specific DNA binding activity of the dioxin receptor is modulated by the 90 kd heat shock protein. EMBO J 9:69–76

Wilson RH, DeEds F, Cox AJ Jr (1941) The toxicity and carcinogenic activity of 2-acetaminofluorene. Cancer Res 1:595–608
Wiseman RW, Stowers SJ, Miller EC, Anderson MW, Miller JA (1986) Activating mutations of the c-Ha-ras protooncogene in chemically induced hepatomas of the male B6C3F_1 mouse. Proc Natl Acad Sci USA 83:5825–5829
Wishart GJ (1978) Demonstration of functional heterogeneity of hepatic uridine diphosphate glucuronosyltransferase activities after administration of 3-methylcholanthrene and phenobarbital to rats. J Biochem 174:671–672
Wohlleb JC, Hunter CF, Blass B, Kadlubar FF, Chu DZJ, Lang NP (1990) Aromatic amine acetyltransferase as a marker for colorectal cancer: environmental and demographic associations. Int J Cancer 46:22–30
Wooster R, Sutherland L, Ebner T, Clarke D, Da Cruz e Silva O, Burchell B (1991) Cloning and stable expression of a new member of the human liver phenol/bilirubin: UDP-glucuronosyltransferase cDNA family. Biochem J 278:465–469
Wynder EL, Goldsmith R (1977) The epidemiology of bladder cancer, A second look. Cancer 40:1246–1268
Yin Z, Sato K, Tsuda H, Ito N (1982) Changes in activities of uridine diphosphate-glucuronyltransferase during chemical hepatocarcinogenesis. Gann 73:239–248
Zakim D, Vessey DA (1977) Membrane-bound estrone as substrate for microsomal UDP-glucuronyltransferase. J Biol Chem 252:7534–7537
Zakim D, Cantor M, Eibl H (1988) Phospholipids and UDP-glucuronosyltransferase. Structure/function relationships. J Biol Chem 263:5164–5169
Zakim D, Dannenberg AJ (1992) How does the microsomal membrane regulate UDP-glucuronosyltransferases? Biochem Pharmacol 43:1385–1393
Zarbl H, Sukumar S, Arthur AV, Martin-Zanca D, Barbacid M (1985) Direct mutagenesis of Ha-*ras*-1 oncogenes by N-nitroso-N-methylurea during initiation of mammary carcinogenesis in rats. Nature 315:382–385

Note added in proof:

In a recent modification of the UGT nomenclature system UGT1 family proteins are identified by the position of their exon 1 upstream of the 4 conserved exons (Fig. 8). Hence, the major human bilirubin UGT (Br-1) will be designated UGT1.1h, and the phenol UGT conjugating planar phenols (P1 = UGT1A1) will be UGT1.6h. The corresponding 3-methylcholanthrene-inducible rat orthologue will be UGT1.6r. The phenobarbital-inducible rat testosterone/chloramphenicol UGT (UGT2B1) will be UGT2.01r.

CHAPTER 15

Sulfonation in Chemical Carcinogenesis

J.A. MILLER and Y.-J. SURH

A. Introduction

"Sulfonation" is the term we use – in place of the commonly used, but less precise, term "sulfation" – for the sulfotransferase-catalyzed transfer of the sulfo group ($-SO_3H$, $-SO_3^-$; BENKOVIC and HEVEY 1970) from the cofactor 3′-phospho-adenosine-5′-phosphosulfate (PAPS; ROBBINS and LIPMANN 1957) to the oxygen and nitrogen atoms of -C-OH, -N-OH, and -NH groups in physiological and foreign substrates (MULDER and JAKOBY 1990). The products of these transfers are sulfuric acid esters (also variously called sulfates, or sulfooxy or sulfonyloxy derivatives) or sulfamides (sulfamates). Sulfate transfer is apparently unknown in biology. Were it to occur, the products in most cases would be peroxysulfates. We suggest that "sulfonation" be used to describe the conjugation of substrates by sulfotransferases and PAPS.

In animal cells, *O*- and *N*-sulfonation generate many endogenous water-stable sulfuric acid esters and amides (chondroitin sulfate, heparin, cerebrosulfatides, estrogen sulfates, etc.; MULDER and JAKOBY 1990). Likewise, it has long been known that many foreign compounds are detoxified in mammals by metabolism to water-stable sulfates to facilitate their passage across membranes and excretion in urine (WILLIAMS 1959). More recently, however, the metabolism of certain chemical carcinogens has been found to include toxification as well as detoxification by the sulfonation pathway. For several classes of chemical carcinogens, a principal pathway of activation for carcinogenesis is the formation of toxic and water-unstable (short half-life) sulfuric acid esters. In water, heterolytic cleavage generates sulfate ion and highly reactive electrophiles that combine covalently with nucleophilic groups in cellular macromolecules to form adducts. The adducts in cellular DNA may initiate mutagenic and carcinogenic processes. The biochemical and biological properties of these water-unstable sulfuric acid metabolites of various chemical carcinogens are the subject of this review.

In the studies described below, the nature of all but one of the nucleophilic substitutions with the water-unstable sulfuric acid esters is not known. Allusions to "nitrenium ions" or "carbocations" suggest that the reactions are thought to be SN1 in nature. However, in one instance (SMITH et al. 1985, 1986), the evidence is in favor of a SN2 reaction. Similarly, isolation of the unstable sulfuric acid esters from tissue preparations was generally not attempted, although this was accomplished in one instance (WATABE et al. 1986). Instead, indirect evidence for the formation of these esters was obtained by the isolation and characterization of adducts in DNA, RNA, protein, or components of these macromolecules in reactions that were dependent on PAPS and showed inhibitions of the sulfotransferase activities by pentachlorophenol (PCP), 2,6-dichloro-4-nitrophenol (DCNP), or dehydroepiandrosterone (DHEA). Likewise, sulfonation-dependent toxicities, mutagenicities, and carcinogenicities were demonstrated through the use of these inhibitors. Use was also made of brachymorphic mice (see BOBERG et al. 1983), which have a genetic impairment in the synthesis of PAPS. The sulfotransferases for foreign chemicals and various physiological compounds reside predominantly in the cytosols of mammalian tissues and include the phenol sulfotransferases that are inhibited by PCP and DCNP and the hydroxy-steroid sulfotransferases that are not inhibited by these compounds, but are inhibited by DHEA, a competitive substrate. These enzymes are discussed in detail in Chap. 2 of this volume.

B. Metabolic Activation of Chemical Carcinogens by Sulfonation

I. Aromatic Amides and Amines

1. 2-Acetylaminofluorene

The versatile carcinogen 2-acetylaminofluorene (AAF) is one of the most studied chemical carcinogens (KRIEK 1992; BELAND and KADLUBAR 1990). While the ring-hydroxy metabolites of AAF proved to be inactive as carcinogens in the rat, the *N*-hydroxy metabolite was found to be more carcinogenic than the parent amide in the liver and other tissues in this species (E.C. MILLER et al. 1961). This was the first example of a *proximate* carcinogenic metabolite (i.e., closer to the final active metabolite) of a chemical carcinogen. It was also the first example of the metabolic *N*-hydroxylation of an aromatic amide (CRAMER et al. 1960). *N*-Hydroxy-AAF also produced greater amounts of covalently bound adducts to the hepatic nucleic acids and proteins in the rat in vivo than did AAF, but this metabolite did not react with these macromolecules in vitro (see DEBAUN et al. 1968, 1970). The key to the nature of the activation of *N*-hydroxy-AAF was provided by concurrent investigations on *N*-methyl-4-aminoazobenzene (MAB), a hepatocarcinogenic dye in the rat that was known to produce covalently bound dye adducts in the liver nucleic acids and proteins. The *N*-hydroxy derivative of MAB proved to be difficult to synthesize and the synthetic derivative *N*-benzoyloxy-MAB was prepared as a possible precursor of the *N*-hydroxy derivative in vivo. Unexpectedly, this water-unstable benzoic acid ester was found to react directly with nucleic acids and proteins to give covalently bound adducts in these macromolecules (POIRIER et al. 1967). With this clue, synthetic esters of *N*-hydroxy-AAF such as *N*-acetoxy-AAF and *N*-sulfooxy-AAF (AAF-*N*-sulfate) were prepared and found to be water unstable and highly electrophilic. They reacted directly with nucleic acids and proteins in vitro to form covalently-bound adducts of AAF in these macromolecules (see E.C. MILLER and MILLER 1981). The first nucleic acid adduct of AAF to be characterized was *N*-(guanosin-8-yl)-AAF (KRIEK et al. 1967). AAF-*N*-Sulfate was shown to be a metabolite of rat hepatic sulfotransferase activity on *N*-hydroxy-AAF by two groups (DEBAUN et al. 1968; KING and PHILLIPS 1968). These observations established AAF-*N*-sulfate as the first water-unstable and electrophilic sulfuric acid ester metabolite of a carcinogen. These findings depended on PAPS-dependent bindings of AAF residues to added DNA and RNA, and to endogenous protein in rat liver cytosols. Synthetic AAF-*N*-sulfate was also found to be mutagenic in *Bacillus subtilis*-transforming DNA (MAHER et al. 1968). AAF-*N*-Sulfate was thus considered at that time to be an ultimate carcinogenic metabolite of AAF in the livers of rats. However, further studies in several laboratories showed that the metabolism of AAF was quite complex. At present, it is recognized that AAF, via *N*-hydroxy-AAF, forms multiple electrophiles in rat and mouse livers that generate three guanine adducts in DNA, as shown in Fig. 1 (see LAI et al. 1985; BELAND and KADLUBAR 1990). Two of the five

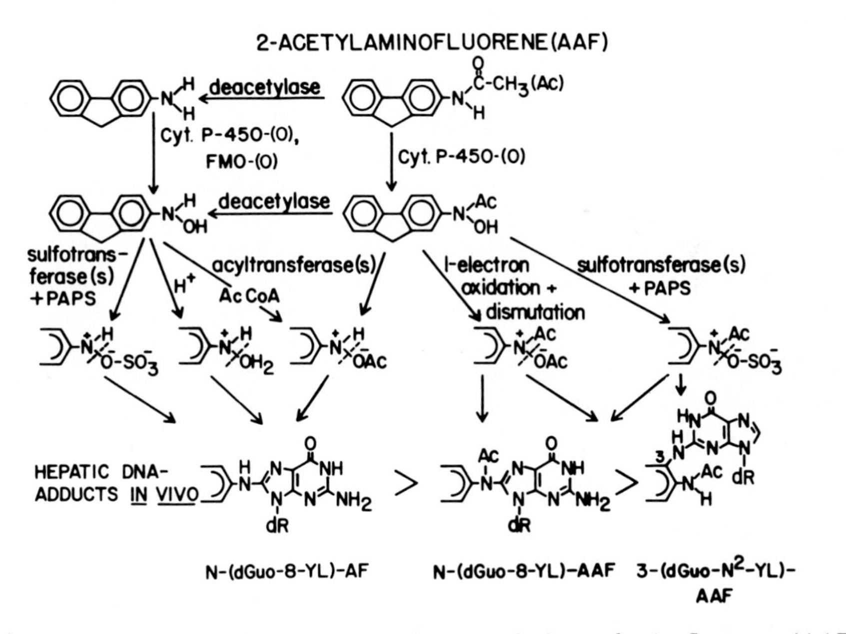

Fig. 1. The metabolic activation pathways of *2-acetylaminofluorene (AAF)* and 2-aminofluorene (*AF*) in the rat and mouse. *PAPS*, 3′-phosphoadenosine-5′-phosphosulfate

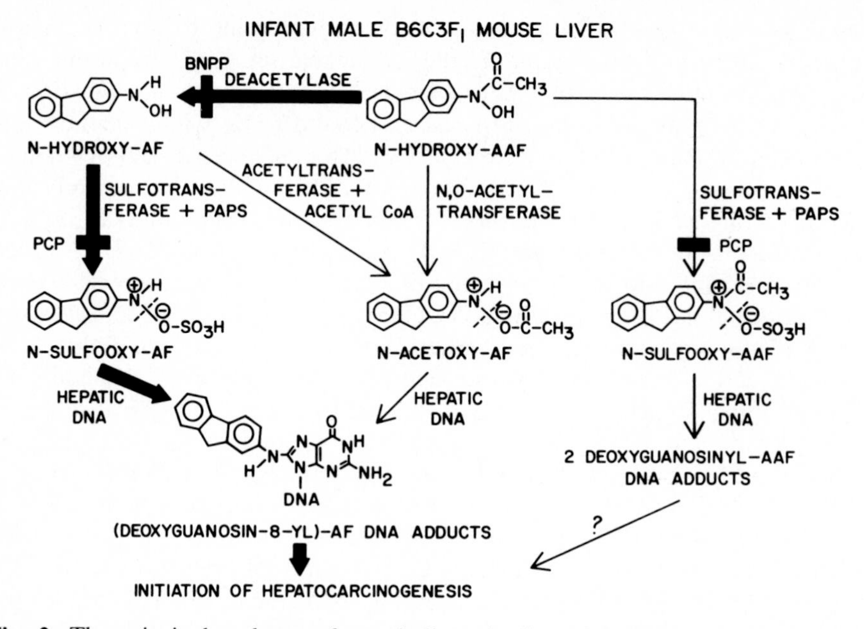

Fig. 2. The principal pathway of metabolic activation of *N*-hydroxy-2-acetylaminofluorene (*N-hydroxy-AAF*) and *N*-hydroxy-2-aminofluorene (*N*-hydroxy-AF) in the *infant male $B6C3F_1$ mouse liver* (LAI et al. 1988). *BNPP*, bis(*p*-nitrophenyl)phosphate; *PCP*, pentachlorophenol; *PAPS*, 3′-phosphoadenosine-5′-phosphosulfate

known pathways of activation of *N*-hydroxy-AAF are sulfotransferase-dependent sulfonations of *N*-hydroxy-AAF and *N*-hydroxy-2-aminofluorene (*N*-hydroxy-AF). The role of AAF-*N*-sulfate in carcinogenesis is undecided (BELAND and KADLUBAR 1990). However, AF-*N*-sulfate is clearly a major ultimate carcinogenic metabolite of *N*-hydroxy-AAF and *N*-hydroxy-AF in the livers of infant male B6C3F1 mice (Fig. 2; LAI et al. 1985, 1987, 1988) and forms only one DNA adduct, *N*-(deoxyguanosin-8-yl)-AF. The decisive observations that support this conclusion are that *N*-hydroxy-AF is *not* *N*-acetylated in vivo and that PCP greatly inhibits the formation of the hepatic DNA adduct *and* the induction of liver tumors by this hydroxylamine in the infant male B6C3F1 mouse.

2. 4-Acetylaminobiphenyl

The amide 4-acetylaminobiphenyl (AABP), despite its close structural similarity to AAF, is not carcinogenic in the livers of male rats, but like AAF it is highly carcinogenic in the mammary glands of female rats (E.C. MILLER et al. 1956). AABP is readily *N*-hydroxylated in the rat (presumably in the liver) and, like AAF, *N*-hydroxy-AABP (as a glucuronide) is a urinary metabolite (J.A. MILLER et al. 1961). *N*-Hydroxy-AABP is O-sulfonated by male rat liver sulfotransferase activity, but AABP-*N*-sulfate is less reactive than AAF-*N*-sulfate (DeBaun et al. 1970). Since rat mammary gland tissue does not contain sulfotransferase activity for *N*-hydroxy-AAF (Irving et al. 1971), it seems likely that AABP-*N*-sulfate is not important in mammary carcinogenesis with AABP; possibly *N*-acetoxy-4-aminobiphenyl is the relevant electrophile in this tissue (see Beland and Kadlubar 1990). AABP is readily deacetylated in vivo to 4-aminobiphenyl (ABP), and this amine is a strong urinary bladder carcinogen in the dog and human (IARC 1972). However, no evidence has been obtained that *O*-sulfonation is involved in the activation of *N*-hydroxy-ABP in the urinary bladder tissue of these species (Beland and Kadlubar 1990).

3. 4-Acetylaminostilbene

The aromatic amide 4-acetylaminostilbene (AAS) induces primarily ear duct gland and mammary gland tumors in rats (Andersen et al. 1964). Its *N*-hydroxy metabolite is more carcinogenic than AAS. The synthetic electrophilic ester *N*-acetoxy-AAS has been used in generating DNA adducts in vitro for characterization studies. These adducts result from nucleophilic substitution of the -CH=CH- group joining the aromatic rings (see Beland and Kadlubar 1990). No evidence has been reported that sulfonation is involved in the formation of DNA adducts of radiolabeled AAS in vivo in the rat.

4. 2-Acetylaminophenanthrene

Leukemia and tumors of the mammary glands, ear duct glands, and small intestine are induced in the rat by the aromatic amide 2-acetylaminophenanthrene (AAP; Miller et al. 1956). It is not hepatocarcinogenic in the rat. *N*-Hydroxy-AAP is a metabolite of AAP in the rat and is more carcinogenic than AAP (E.C. Miller et al. 1966). AAP-*N*-sulfate has been synthesized for studies on DNA adducts formed in vitro (Scribner and Naimy 1975), but no studies have been reported on its formation by sulfotransferase activity in vitro or in vivo.

5. Phenacetin

Phenacetin (PA) is an analgesic that was widely used in humans before it was found that patients who abused this drug and were sensitive to its nephrotoxic effects had a high incidence of renal pelvic cancer (Johansson et al. 1984; IARC 1987). PA induces tumors of the nasal cavity and the urinary tract in rats (Isaka et al. 1979) and renal cell tumors in B6C3F1 mice (Nakanishi et al. 1982). The *N*-hydroxy metabolite was more carcinogenic than PA and induced a high incidence of liver tumors in rats (Calder et al. 1976). PA-*N*-sulfate can be generated by rat cytosolic hepatic sulfotransferase activity (Mulder et al. 1978). It apparently reacts with protein via the formation of a *N*-acetylimidoquinone. Other *O*-conjugates also give rise to this reactive intermediate.

6. 4-Aminoazobenzene, *N*-Methyl-4-Aminoazobenzene, and *N*,*N*-Dimethyl-4-Aminoazobenzene

N,*N*-dimethyl-4-aminoazobenzene (DAB) and *N*-methyl-4-aminoazobenzene (MAB) have long been known to be strong dietary hepatocarcinogens in the rat, while 4-aminoazobenzene (AB) shows little or no carcinogenicity in the liver of this species (J.A. MILLER and MILLER 1953). Demethylation of DAB to MAB and of MAB to AB occurs in the livers of rats and mice. More recently, these three aminoazo dyes were found to have equal high hepatocarcinogenicities after single i.p. injections in infant male B6C3F1 mice (DELCLOS et al. 1984). MAB and AB are N-hydroxylated in the livers of rats and mice (SATO et al. 1966; KADLUBAR et al. 1976a), and the *N*-hydroxy metabolites are O-sulfonated by hepatic sulfotransferase activities (KADLUBAR et al. 1976b; DELCLOS et al. 1986). MAB-*N*-sulfate gives rise to two guanine adducts and one adenine adduct in rat liver DNA in vivo (BELAND et al. 1980), while AB-*N*-sulfate forms only the *N*-(deoxyguanosin-8-yl)-AB DNA adduct in the mouse liver (DELCLOS et al. 1986). In the mouse, the formation of this hepatic DNA adduct, the hepatic sulfotransferase activity for *N*-hydroxy-AB, and the formation of hepatomas by *N*-hydroxy-AB are all partially inhibited to approximately the same extent by treatment with PCP (DELCLOS et al. 1986; Fig. 3). The level of the AB adduct in the liver DNA of male brachymorphic mice given AB was only 12% of that found in their similarly treated phenotypically normal littermates. Likewise, hepatoma formation in the brachymorphic mice was only 10% of that produced in their normal littermates. These data are consistent with a strong role of AB-*N*-sulfate in hepatocarcinogenesis by AB in the mouse (Fig. 3).

7. Benzidine

The amine benzidine (4,4′-diaminobiphenyl) is carcinogenic in the urinary bladders of dogs and humans and in the livers of rats, mice, and hamsters (see BELAND and KADLUBAR 1990). It is metabolically activated in part by *N*-acetylation and *N*-hydroxylation followed by *O*-sulfonation. The *N*-acetyl, *N*′-acetyl-*N*′-sulfooxy-benzidine metabolite forms a guan-8-yl adduct in the hepatic DNA of rats. Other pathways of activation of benzidine have been found, and it is not known to what extent the *N*-sulfate contributes to the carcinogenicity of benzidine in the rat.

8. Heterocyclic Aromatic Amines

Heterocyclic aromatic amines may be formed in the cooking of food and are derived from certain amino acids, sometimes with creatinine and sugars as

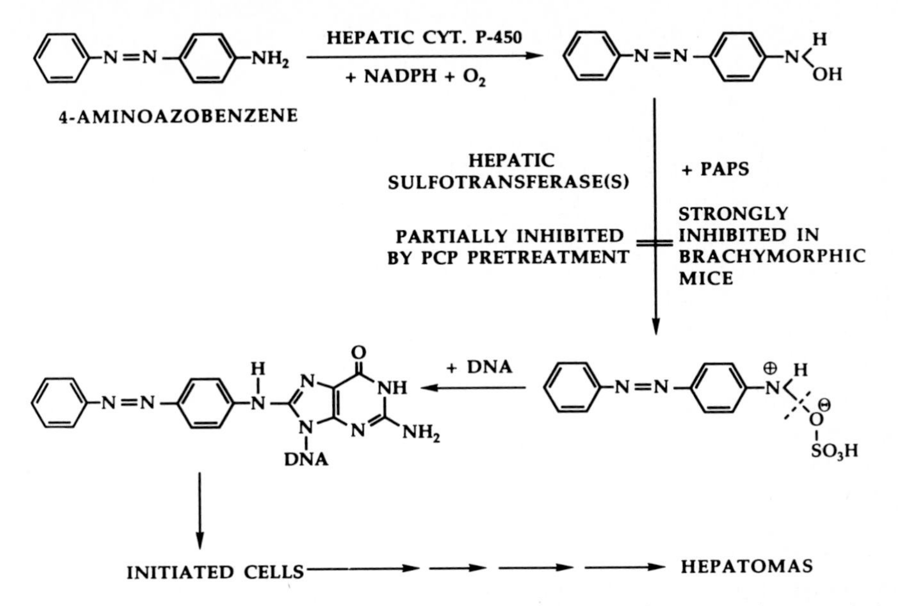

Fig. 3. The metabolic activation of *4-aminoazobenzene* in hepatocarcinogenesis in infant male B6C3F_1 mice. *PCP*, pentachlorophenol; PAPS, 3′-phosphoadenosine-5′-phosphosulfate; *NADPH*, reduced nicotinamide adenine dinucleotide phosphate

coprecursors (SUGIMURA 1986). The following four compounds are representative of these amines: (1) 2-amino-3-methylimidazo(4,5-*f*)quinoline (IQ); (2) 2-amino-1-methyl-6-phenylimidazo(4,5-*b*)pyridine (PhIP); (3) 2-amino-6-methyl-dipyrido(1,2-*a*:3′,2′-*d*)imidazole (Glu-P-1); and (4) 3-amino-1-methyl-5*H*-pyrido-(4,3-*b*)indole (Trp-P-2). These compounds are very potent mutagens (KATO 1986; FELTON et al. 1988) and carcinogens (SUGIMURA 1986; FELTON and KNIZE 1990; DOOLEY et al. 1992). *N*-Hydroxylation appears to be a necessary step in the metabolic activation of these amines (KATO 1986; KATO and YAMAZOE 1987). *O*-Sulfonation. *O*-acetylation, and *O*-prolylation of these *N*-hydroxy metabolites appear to be important pathways of activation in mutagenesis and presumably in carcinogenesis by these amines (BUONARATI et al. 1990; BELAND and KADLUBAR 1990).

9. Hydroxylamine-*O*-Sulfonic Acid

KAWAZOE and HUANG (1972) noted the ability of the simplest synthetic *N*-sulfate, H_2N-O-SO_3H, to react with guanosine at pH 2–4 and 70°C to produce a 20% yield of 8-aminoguanosine. This C_8 amination of guanosine closely resembles the reactivity of the sulfuric acid and acetic acid ester metabolites of aromatic hydroxylamines to arylaminate the C_8 atoms of guanyl bases in DNA at pH 7 and 37°C (see BELAND and KADLUBAR 1990). At pHs above 7, hydroxylamine-*O*-sulfonic acid aminates the N^1 atom of guanosine.

II. Alkenylbenzenes

1. Safrole and Estragole

Safrole (1-allyl-3,4-methylenedioxybenzene) is one of many closely related alkenylbenzenes that occur naturally in a variety of plant species that are sources of essential oils and spices (LEUNG 1980). Safrole is a major component of oil of sassafras and a minor constituent of several other essential oils and spices. It is a weak to moderately active hepatocarcinogen in rats and mice (E.C. MILLER et al. 1983). The related spice constituents estragole (1-allyl-4-methoxybenzene) and methyleugenol (1-allyl-3,4-dimethoxybenzene) have carcinogenic activities similar to that of safrole, but more extensively substituted alkenylbenzenes have shown little or no carcinogenic activity (E.C. MILLER et al. 1983).

Microsomal cytochrome P-450 activities in mouse and rat liver hydroxylate safrole and estragole at the benzylic 1′ position of the allyl groups in these compounds (SWANSON et al. 1981). The 1′-hydroxy metabolites are more potent carcinogens than the parent alkenylbenzenes and are thus proximate carcinogens (BORCHERT et al. 1973a,b: DRINKWATER et al. 1976; E.C. MILLER et al. 1983). These 1′-hydroxy metabolites are further metabolized by liver enzymes to three kinds of electrophiles: 1′-esters of sulfuric acid, 2′,3′-epoxides, and 1′-oxo derivatives (OSWALD et al. 1971; WISLOCKI et al. 1976, 1977; FENNELL et al. 1984). Only the sulfuric acid esters appear to form adducts in the liver DNA in vivo (PHILLIPS et al. 1981a,b). The same adducts are formed in vitro in reactions of DNA or deoxyguanosine and deoxyadenosine with the synthetic electrophilic ester 1′-acetoxysafrole (WISEMAN et al. 1985). Entirely analogous results were obtained with 1′-hydroxyestragole and 1′-acetoxyestragole (PHILLIPS et al. 1981a; WISEMAN et al. 1985).

In view of the presence of sulfotransferase activity for 1′-hydroxysafrole in rat and mouse liver (WISLOCKI et al. 1976), the inhibitor PCP and brachymorphic mice were used to probe the role of 1′-sulfooxysafrole in the formation of DNA adducts and hepatomas in mouse liver (BOBERG et al. 1983). The levels of DNA adducts in the livers of male 12-day-old $B6C3F_1$ mice given a dose of radiolabeled 1′-hydroxysafrole 45 min after a single dose of 0.04_1 μmol of PCP per body weight were reduced to 15% of those observed in mice not pretreated with PCP. The same pretreatment of comparable mice with PCP also reduced the average number of hepatomas per mouse at 10 months to less than 10% of that observed for 1′-hydroxysafrole in the absence of pretreatment with PCP. No effect of pretreatment with PCP was noted on hepatoma formation by diethylnitrosamine, a carcinogen which is not activated by sulfuric acid esterification (PREUSSMANN and STEWART 1984). Likewise, continuous dietary administration of PCP strongly inhibited hepatoma formation by dietary safrole or 1′-hydroxysafrole in adult female CD-1 mice. A similar dependence of DNA adduct and hepatoma formation in mouse liver upon 1′-sulfooxysafrole formation was noted

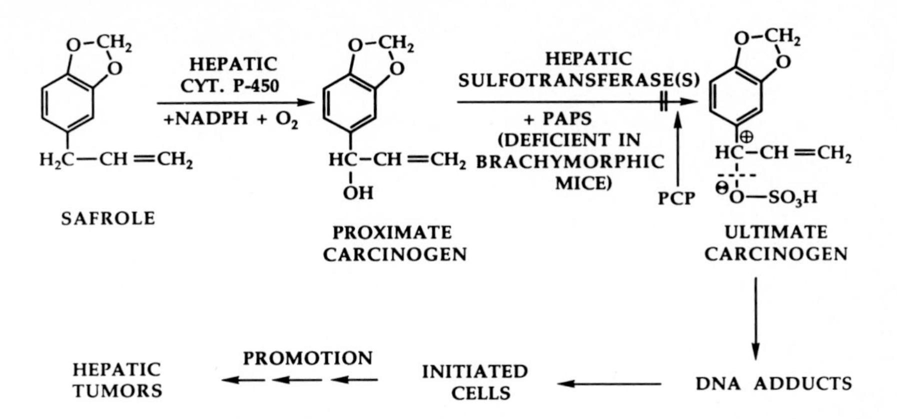

Fig. 4. The hepatic metabolism of *safrole* to the electrophilic 1′-sulfooxy-safrole, the initiation of carcinogenesis in the preweanling male $B6C3F_1$ mouse liver, and the promotion of the initiated cells to gross liver tumors in adulthood. *PCP*, pentachlorophenol; *NADPH*, reduced nicotinamide adenine dinucleotide phosphate; *PAPS*, 3′-phosphoadenosine-5′-phosphosulfate

in the PAPS-deficient brachymorphic mice. When these mice were administered 1′-hydroxysafrole, the level of DNA adducts in the livers of 12-day-old male $B6C3F_2$ brachymorphic mice was only 15% as high as in the livers of their phenotypically normal littermates given the same treatment. Similarly, the average number of hepatomas in the brachymorphic mice was no more than 10% of that found in the normal littermates. Thus, these data strongly support the conclusion that 1′-sulfooxysafrole is a critical metabolite of 1′-hydroxysafrole for the formation of DNA adducts and hepatomas in the male $B6C3F_1$ mice (Fig. 4).

2. 1′-Hydroxy-2′,3′-Dehydroestragole

Carcinogenicity tests of the synthetic acetylenic compound (1′-hydroxy-2′,3′-dehydroestragole (1′-hydroxy-DHE) showed that it was approximately ten times more active in the infant male $B6C3F_1$ mouse liver in the induction of hepatomas than the allylic compound 1′-hydroxyestragole (E.C. MILLER et al. 1983; FENNELL et al. 1985). 1′-Hydroxy-DHE formed approximately three times as much covalently bound adducts in mouse liver DNA in vivo as were obtained with 1′-hydroxyestragole (FENNELL et al. 1985). The acetic acid ester of 1′-hydroxy-DHE was electrophilic, and the nuclear magnetic resonance (NMR) spectra of the adducts formed from it in vitro showed that the triple bond remained at the 2′,3′ position. This was in contrast to the adducts from 1′-hydroxy-estragole, where two of the five DNA adducts formed in vivo contained the double bond in the original 2,3′ position, while three of the adducts had the double bond in the 1′,2′ position (an allylic shift). Only one adduct, N^2-(2′,3′-dehydroestragol-1′-yl) deoxyguanosine, was found in the hepatic DNA of mice administered 1′-hydroxy-DHE. This suggested that adducts at the 1′ position of the allylic carcinogens safrole and estragole were more active in the induction of tumors than the adducts at the 3′ position.

No cytosolic coenzyme A-dependent acetyltransferase activity for 1′-hydroxy-HDHE was detected in the livers of male B6C3F$_1$ mice. This suggested that 1′-acetoxy-DHE is not a metabolite of 1′-hydroxy-DHE. However, sulfotetransferase activity was found for this carcinogen in the cytosols of these mice, and it was strongly inhibited by PCP. Pretreatment of 12-day-old male B6C3F$_1$ mice by PCP lowered by 87% the level of the DNA adduct formed from 1′-hydroxy-DHE. Similarly, the formation of hepatomas at 10 months in comparably treated mice was reduced by 94% by the pretreatment with PCP. Thus, as noted above for the sulfuric acid ester metabolites of 1′-hydroxysafrole and 1′-hydroxyestragole, it appears that 1′-sulfooxy-DHE is a major electrophilic and carcinogenic metabolite of 1′-hydroxy-DHE (Fig. 5).

III. Polynuclear Aromatic Hydrocarbons

1. Methyl-Substituted Aromatic Hydrocarbons

Following the pioneer study of SIMS et al. (1974), extensive studies have demonstrated the importance of "bay-region" dihydrodiolepoxides as reactive ultimate electrophilic and carcinogenic metabolites of the majority of polynuclear aromatic hydrocarbons (PAHs; JERINA et al. 1986). This bay-region theory has been widely accepted as a general concept in determining the carcinogenicity of PAHs in general. However, recent studies have characterized new DNA adducts formed from enzymatic one-electron oxidations of benzo[a]pyrene and 7,12-dimethylbenz[a]anthracene (RAMAKRISHNA et al. 1992a,b; DEVANESAN et al. 1992; CAVALIERI and ROGAN 1985, 1992). Determination of the relative significances of the dihydrodiol epoxide and radical cation metabolites and their DNA adducts in carcinogenesis by the PAHs will be of great interest. For methyl-substituted PAHs, hydroxylation of *meso*-methyl groups with subsequent formation of reactive benzylic esters bearing a good leaving group such as sulfate, phosphate, or acetate has been proposed as a possible biochemical mechanism of activation, DNA binding, and carcinogenicity of these hydrocarbons (FLESHER and SYDNOR 1971, 1973). Recently, direct evidence for the metabolic formation of such electrophilic esters of PAHs has been reported (WATABE et al. 1982). These investigators have provided definitive data on the formation of a highly mutagenic sulfuric acid ester metabolite from 7-hydroxymethyl-12-methylbenz[a]anthracene (Fig. 6, part 1a), which is a major metabolite of the potent carcinogen 7,12-dimethylbenz[a]anthracene. The formation of this reactive sulfuric acid ester was catalyzed by sulfotransferase cativity in rat liver cytosol. In later studies, other hydroxymethyl PAHs have also been found to be metabolically activated to electrophilic and mutagenic sulfuric acid esters. These include

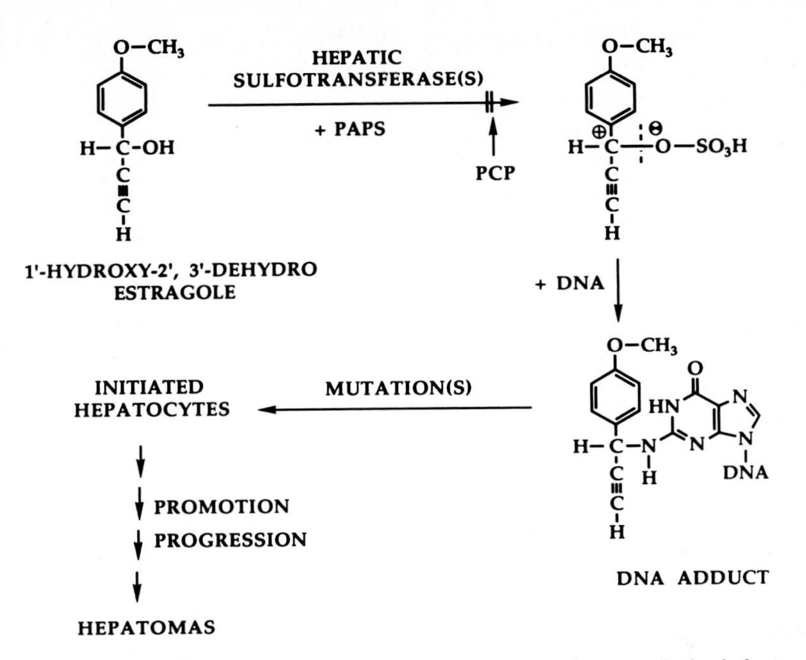

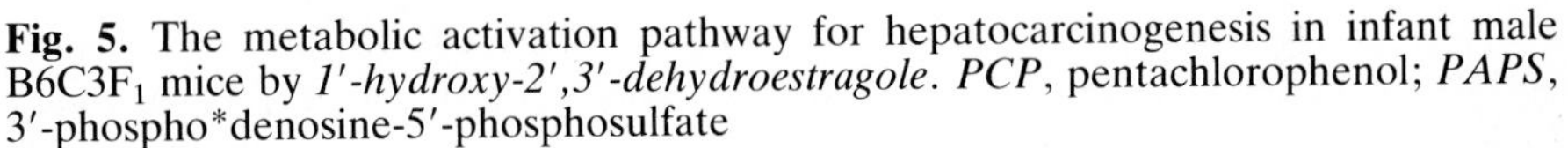
Fig. 5. The metabolic activation pathway for hepatocarcinogenesis in infant male $B6C3F_1$ mice by *1′-hydroxy-2′,3′-dehydroestragole*. *PCP*, pentachlorophenol; *PAPS*, 3′-phospho*denosine-5′-phosphosulfate

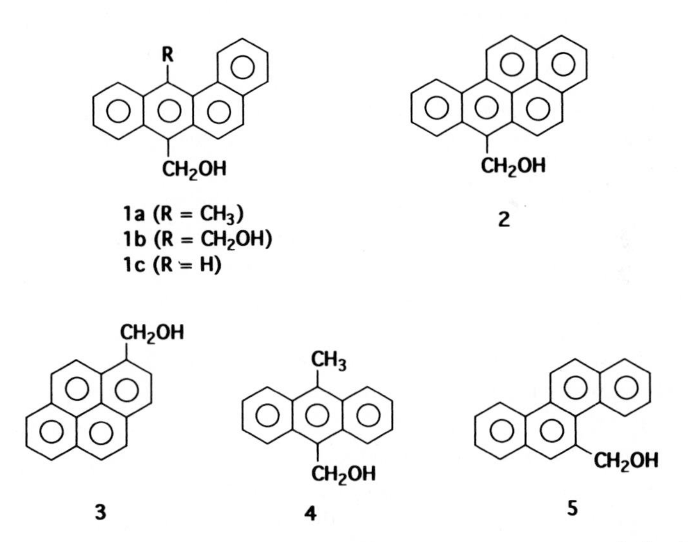

Fig. 6. Structural formulae for hydroxymethyl polynuclear aromatic hydrocarbons that are activated by hepatic sulfotransferase activities in rats and mice. *1a*, 7-Hydroxymethyl-12-methylbenz[a]anthracene; *1b*, 7,12-dihydroxymethylbenz[a]-anthracene; *1c*, 7-hydroxymethylbenz[a]-anthracene; *2*, 6-hydroxymethylbenzo[a]-pyrene; *3*, 1-hydroxy-methylpyrene; *4*, 9-hydroxymethyl-10-methylanthracene; *5*, 5-hydroxymethylchrysene

7,12-dihydroxymethylbenz[a]anthracene (Fig. 6, part 1b; WATABE et al. 1987), 7-hydroxymethylbenz[a]anthracene (Fig. 6, part 1c; WATABE et al. 1986), 5-hydroxy-methylchrysene (Fig. 6, part 5; OKUDA et al. 1989), 6-hydroxymethylbenzo[a]pyrene (Fig. 6, part 2; SURH et al. 1989), 9-hydroxymethyl-10-methylanthracene (Fig. 6, part 4; SURH et al. 1990a), and 1-hydroxymethylpyrene (Fig. 6, part 3; SURH et al. 1990a, 1991a; GLATT et al. 1990). In the presence of rodent liver cytosol and PAPS, all of these hydroxymethyl aromatic hydrocarbons induced His^+ revertants in *Salmonella typhimurium* TA98 in the Ames assay and also produced covalently bound benzylic adducts with deoxyguanosine and deoxyadenosine residues in calf thymus DNA. DHEA, a typical substrate for hydroxysteroid sulfotransferase, strongly inhibited the sulfotransferase-mediated mutagenicity and DNA binding of 7-hydroxymethyl-12-methylbenz[a]anthracene and other hydroxymethyl PAHs. Phenol sulfotransferase inhibitors PCP and DCNP were not inhibitory in this regard. Hydroxysteroid sulfotransferase purified from Sprague-Dawley rats showed high catalytic activity for hydroxymethyl PAHs as well as DHEA (OGURA et al. 1990a). Recently, cDNA encoding this enzyme has been cloned and its sequence was analyzed (OGURA et al. 1989, 1990b). Age-dependent gender differences were also observed for sulfotransferase activity toward 7-hydroxymethyl-12-methylbenz[a]anthracene (SURH et al. 1991b) and 6-hydroxymethylbenzo[a]pyrene (SURH et al. 1989); sulfotransferase activities for these hydrocarbons diminished with age much faster in male rats than in females. 7-Hydroxymethyl-12-methylbenz[a]-anthracene, 6-hydroxymethylbenzo[a]pyrene, 9-hydroxymethyl-10-methylanthracene, and 1-hydroxymethylpyrene formed the same benzylic DNA adducts in rodent livers in vivo as those obtained from these hydrocarbons by incubation with cytosol and PAPS (SURH et al. 1987, 1989, 1990a, 1991a; recently reviewed by J.A. MILLER et al. 1991). Levels of these hepatic DNA adducts were reduced by DHEA pretreatment.

The chemically synthesized sulfuric acid esters of aforementioned hydroxymethyl PAHs are extremely potent mutagens and directly interact with guanine, adenine, and cytosine bases in DNA to produce the benzylic DNA adducts in high yield (OKUDA et al. 1989; SURH et al. 1987, 1989, 1990a, 1991a; WATABE et al. 1985, 1987). These sulfooxymethyl PAHs produced much higher amounts of hepatic benzylic DNA adducts than did the corresponding parent hydroxymethyl hydrocarbons when administered i.p. to infant rats (SURH et al. 1987, 1989, 1990a, 1991a). The carcinogenicities of electrophilic sulfuric acid esters of hydroxymethyl PAHs have recently been assessed. 6-Sulfooxymethylbenzo[a]pyrene (Fig. 7) was found to be a strong hepatocarcinogen in male B6C3F1 mice and induced a much higher incidence and multiplicity of liver tumors than 6-hydroxymethylbenz-[a]pyrene and benzol[a]pyrene (SURH et al. 1990b). Repeated topical applications of this reactive sulfuric acid ester to female Swiss mice also produced high incidences of skin tumors (CAVALIERI et al. 1978). 9-Sulfooxymethyl-10-methylanthracene and 1-sulfooxymethylpyrene were relatively weak skin

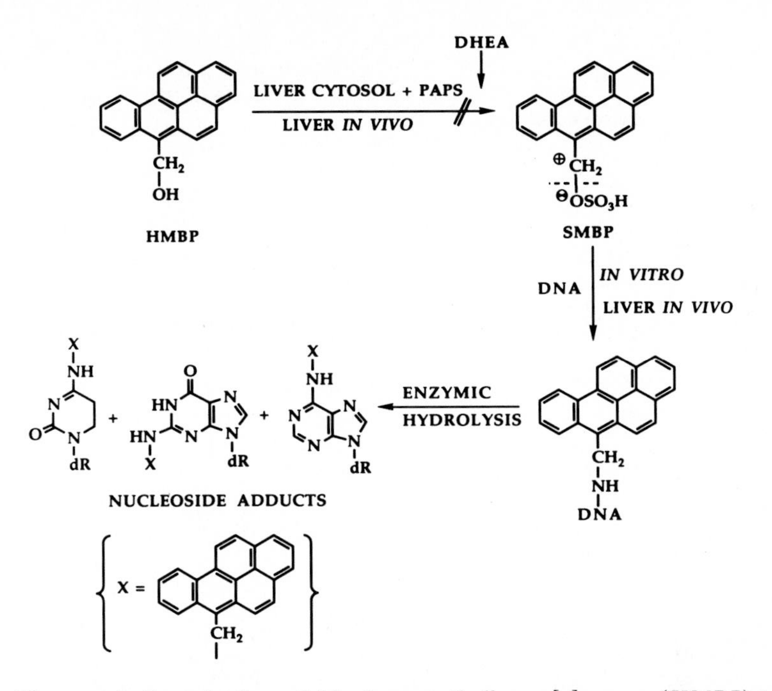

Fig. 7. The metabolic activation of 6-hydroxymethylbenzo[a]pyrene (*HMBP*) to the potent hepatocarcinogen 6-sulfooxymethylbenzo[a]pyrene (*SMBP*) in the infant male $B6C3F_1$ mouse liver. *DHEA*, dehydroepiandrosterone; *PAPS*, 3′-phosphoadenosine-5′-phosphosulfate

tumor initiators, but they were more active than the parent compounds in this regard (SURH et al. 1990a). 7-Sulfooxymethyl-12-methylbenz[a]-anthracene was not more carcinogenic than the parent hydroxymethyl hydrocarbons, as determined in various animal tumor models (SURH et al. 1991c).

2. Cyclopenta-Fused Aromatic Hydrocarbons

Cyclopenta[cd]pyrene (CPP) is a ubiquitous environmental and occupational pollutant which is produced during combustion of coal, gasoline, and diesel fuels (LEE et al. 1977; TONG and KARASEK 1984). It is also detected in carbon black soots and cigarette smoke, representing a potential health hazard. CPP is one of a unique group of PAHs, since it contains a cyclopenta-fused ring, but lacks a bay-region. 3,4-Dihydroxy-3,4-dihydrocyclopenta[cd]pyrene (3,4-DHDCPP; Fig. 8) and 4-hydroxy-3,4-dihydrocyclopenta[cd]pyrene (4-HDCPP; Fig. 8) have been identified as metabolites of CPP in rodent and human liver microsomal systems (EISENSTADT et al. 1981; SAHALI et al. 1992; KWON et al. 1992). These mono- and dihydroxy metabolites contain secondary benzylic hydroxyl group(s) in the cyclopenta ring. When 3,4-

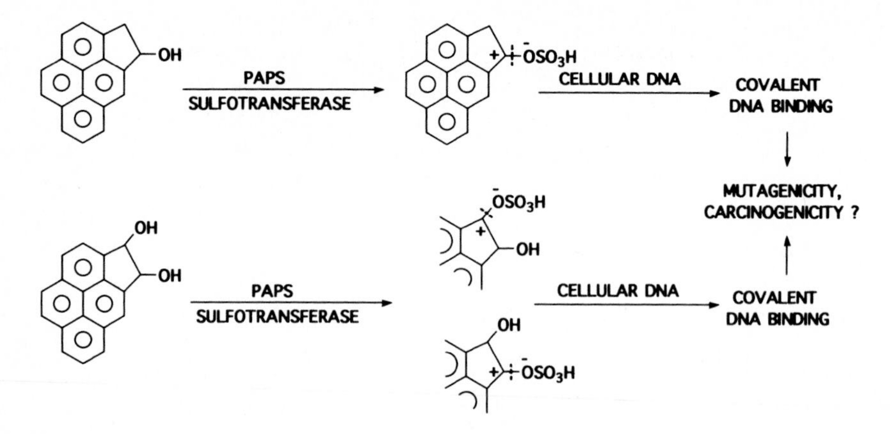

Fig. 8. Proposed pathways for metabolic activation of 4-hydroxy- and 3,4,-dihydroxy-3,4-dihydrocyclopenta[cd]pyrene to electrophilic, mutagenic, and carcinogenic sulfuric acid esters. *PAPS*, 3′-phosphoadenosine-5′-phosphosulfate

DHDCPP and 4-HDCPP were incubated with calf thymus DNA and rodent liver cytosol fortified with PAPS, significant covalent DNA binding was observed (SURH et al. 1992). The cytosol and PAPS-dependent DNA binding was inhibited by both DCNP and DHEA. Of the two isomers of 3,4-DHDCPP, the *trans*-diol produced DNA adducts to a much greater extent than did the *cis* counterpart via sulfotransferase (SURH et al. 1992). 4-HDCPP and 3,4-DHDCPP were also mutagenic toward bacteria in the presence of hepatic cytosol and PAPS. The synthetic sulfuric acid ester sodium 4-sulfooxy-3,4-dihydrocyclopenta[cd]pyrene was directly mutagenic without any activation system (SURH et al. 1992). These results suggest that other cyclopenta-fused PAHs such as 3-methylcholanthrene and benz[j]-aceanthrylene can be activated likewise through metabolic hydroxylation and subsequent sulfuric acid esterification. A novel carcinogen. 1,2,3,4-tetrahydro-7,12-dimethylbenz[a]anthracene, has very recently been postulated to be activated to an electrophilic sulfuric acid ester metabolite following hydroxylation at the benzylic C_1 atom in the saturated hexacyclic A ring (RINDERLE et al. 1992; NAIR et al. 1992).

3. Phenols, Bay-Region Dihydrodiols, Tetraols of Polynuclear Aromatic Hydrocarbons

Phenols, dihydrodiols, tetraols, and quinones are common metabolites of the majority of PAHs. These primary metabolites may undergo phase II reactions to yield more polar water-soluble conjugates. Sulfate conjugation of primary metabolites of benzo[a]pyrene has been investigated in vivo (BOROUJERDI et al. 1981) as well as in vitro with cell-free extracts (NEMOTO et al. 1978), isolated hepatocytes (ZALESKI et al. 1983), and cells in culture

(MOORE and COHEN 1978; AUTRUP 1979; TEFFERA et al. 1991). In most cases, sulfates of phenolic derivatives of benzo[a]pyrene were predominant (COHEN et al. 1977; MOORE and COHEN 1978). Sulfonation of dihydrodiol derivatives of benzo[a]pyrene is controversial. Little or no diol sulfonation was observed (NEMOTO et al. 1978; MOLLIERE et al. 1987; PIAKUNOV et al. 1987). RAO and DUFFEL (1992) have very recently reported that both (+)- and (−)-enantiomers of benzo[a]pyrene *trans*-7,8-dihydrodiol are inhibitors of rat arylsulfotransferase IV and that neither of these enantiomers is a substrate for sulfotransferase. In contrast to the above observations, *trans*-7,8-dihydro-7,8-dihydroxybenzo[a]pyrene was reported to be a major substrate for sulfotransferase in cultured human colon (AUTRUP 1979). Benzo[a]pyrene tetraols and quinones were also found to form conjugates with sulfate (NEMOTO et al. 1978). In the same study, only trace amounts of sulfate conjugates were formed from benzo[a]pyrene 7,8-dihydrodiol-9,10-epoxides I and II. Although sulfate conjugation of phenolic derivatives of BP is considered a detoxification pathway, an exceptional finding has been recently reported. Thus, benzo[a]pyrenyl-1-sulfate is directly mutagenic toward *Salmonella typhimurium* TA98 (IRWIN et al. 1992). Sulfonation of benzylic hydroxyl groups in benzo[a]pyrene dihydrodiols and tetraols may lead to the formation of reactive benzylic esters. However, neither significant DNA binding nor mutagenicity was observed with dihydrodiol and tetrol derivatives of benzo[a]pyrene in the presence of sulfotransferase activity (SURH and TANNENBAUM, unpublished observations).

IV. Nitrotoluenes

The mono- and dinitrotoluenes have been used as industrial intermediates in the manufacture of dyes and plastics, respectively. Both 2-nitrotoluene (2-NT) and 2,6-dinitrotoluene (2,6-DNT) have been reported to be genotoxic (MIRSALIS and BUTTERWORTH 1982; DOOLITTLE et al. 1983). 2,6-DNT has been shown to produce hepatocellular carcinomas when fed to male Fischer-344 rats (LEONARD et al. 1987). Previous studies demonstrated the covalent binding of 2-NT (RICKERT et al. 1984a; CHISM and RICKERT 1985) and 2,6-DNT (RICKERT et al. 1983; KEDDERIS et al. 1984) to rat hepatic macromolecules in vivo. This hepatic macromolecular binding was markedly reduced by prior administration of the sulfotransferase inhibitors PCP and DCNP, suggesting the involvement of sulfuric acid esters as ultimate electrophilic metabolites in bioactivation of 2-NT and 2,6-DNT (RICKERT et al. 1984b; KEDDERIS et al. 1984). Metabolism studies have shown that 2-NT and 2,6-DNT are oxidized by cytochrome P-450 to 2-nitrobenzyl alcohol and 2,6-dinitrobenzyl alcohol, respectively (CHISM et al. 1984; CHISM and RICKERT 1985; LONG and RICKERT 1982). These benzyl alcohols are further conjugated with glucuronic acid to form the corresponding glucuronides, which are then excreted in the bile (CHISM and RICKERT 1985; LONG and RICKERT 1982). Intestinal microflora hydrolyze each glucuronide and reduce a nitro group to yield 2-aminobenzyl alcohol and possibly 2-amino-6-nitrobenzyl alcohol, which are considered to be reabsorbed from the intestine and further metabolized in the liver to reactive species (RICKERT et al. 1984a,b). Several possible routes of bioactivation of 2-aminobenzyl alcohol and 2-amino-6-nitrobenzyl alcohol have been suggested recently (CHISM and RICKERT 1989; Fig. 9). One route is direct sulfonation of these aminobenzyl alcohols by sulfotransferase activity in the liver cytosol to *O*-sulfates which may form electrophilic carbonium ions. Another mechanism is N-hydroxylation of 2-amino- and 2-amino-6-nitrobenzyl alcohols followed by sulfotransferase-dependent formation of unstable *N,O*-sulfates. Alternatively, the above aminobenzyl alcohols may undergo N-acetylation by cytosolic *N*-acetyltransferase. Hydroxylation of the resulting *N*-acetyl arylamines and subsequent sulfuric acid esterification would yield highly reactive nitrenium ions as previously suggested for other N-substituted arylamines such as AAF and benzidine (see Sects. I.1 and I.7). The roles of electrophilic sulfuric acid esters in carcinogenesis by parent (di)nitrotoluene compounds are not known at the present time and need further investigation. Another toluene derivative, 2,4-dinitrotoluene, which is structurally related to 2,6-DNT, has been shown to be metabolized by *Escherichia coli* present in human intestine (MORI et al. 1984) and by rat cecal microflora (MORI

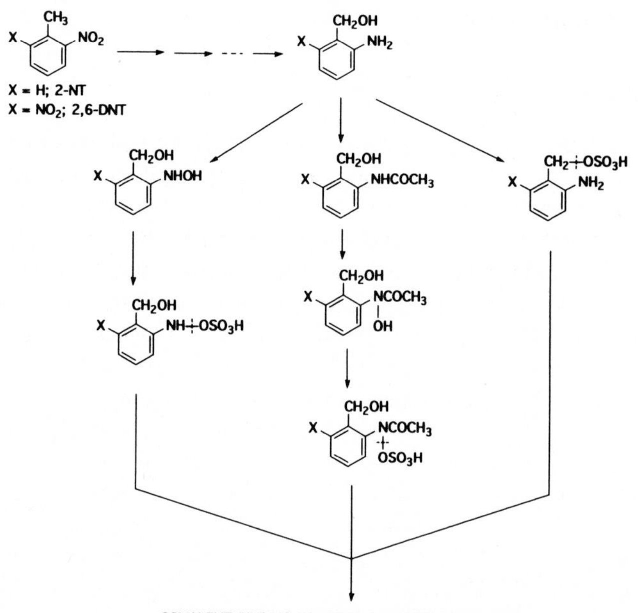

Fig. 9. Possible routes for the formation of hepatic macromolecular adducts from mono- and dinitrotoluenes following metabolic activation by various enzymes (CHISM and RICKERT 1989)

et al. 1985) to produce two aminonitrotoluenes, 2,4-diaminotoluene, 2-hydroxylamino-4-nitrotoluene, and 4-hydroxylamino-2-nitrotoluene. 2,4-Diaminotoluene also covalently bound to DNA in primary cultures of hepatocytes from male Fischer-344 rats, and this DNA binding was decreased by inhibitors of cytochrome P-450 and sulfotransferase (FURLONG et al. 1987).

V. β-Hydroxynitrosamines

MICHEJDA and his coworkers (1979) have previously postulated that β-hydroxylated nitrosamines are metabolically activated through conjugation with a good leaving group. Initial studies by these investigators demonstrated the direct mutagenicity and alkylating activity of tosyl (*p*-toluene sulfonate) esters of certain β-hydroxyalkylnitrosamines (MICHEJDA et al. 1979; KOEPKE et al. 1979). These results led to the speculation that a possible metabolic process equivalent to tosylation might be the formation of electrophilic sulfuric acid esters from the parent β-hydroxynitrosamines (MICHEJDA et al. 1979). Since then, evidence has accumulated that sulfate conjugation plays a crucial role in activation of β-hydroxylalkyl amines to electrophilic, mutagenic, and carcinogenic metabolites (reviewed by MICHEJDA et al. 1987). Thus, *N*-nitroso(2-hydroxypropyl)(2-oxopropyl)-amine, which induces pancreatic adenocarcinomas in hamsters, has been found to be efficiently sulfonated in these animals, whereas only a trace level of sulfoconjugation has been observed in rats which are resistant to the pancreotropic effect of this β-hydroxynitrosamine (KOKKINAKIS et al. 1985, 1987). Studies by German scientists (STERZEL and EISENBRAND 1986) showed that single-strand breaks in rat hepatic DNA induced by *N*-nitrosodiethanolamine were prevented by pretreatment of rats with the selective phenol sulfotransferase inhibitor DCNP. More recently, KROEGER-KOEPKE et al. (1992) have provided evidence for the involvement of sulfotransferase activity in the formation of an ultimate DNA alkylating species from *N*-nitrosomethyl(2-hydroxyethyl)-amine, which is a potent hepatocarcinogen in female Fischer-344 rats (Fig. 10). In contrast to the previous finding by STERZEL and EISENBRAND (1986),

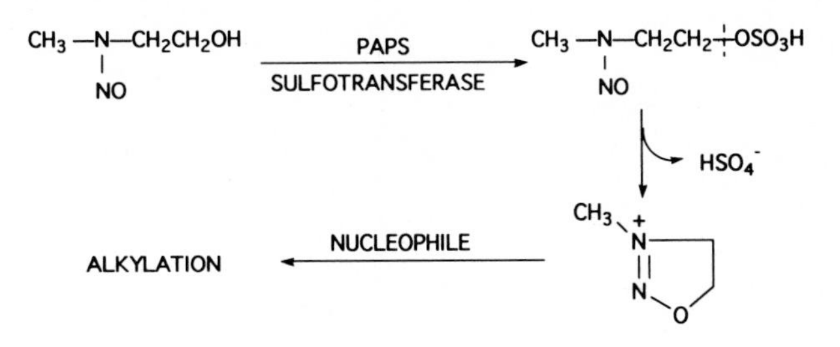

Fig. 10. A proposed scheme for the formation of an alkylating species from *N*-nitrosomethyl(2-hydroxyethyl)amine by sulfotransferase activity (adapted from KROEGER-KOEPKE et al. 1992). *PAPS*, 3′-phosphoadenosine-5′-phosphosulfate

DCNP pretreatment did not inhibit the DNA alkylation induced by this nitrosamine in rat liver in vivo, while propylene glycol had a profound inhibitory effect on the alkylation under the same experimental conditions (KROEGER-KOEPKE et al. 1992). It appears that sulfonation of *N*-nitrosomethyl(2-hydroxyethyl)amine is catalyzed by alcohol sulfotransferase or hydroxysteroid sulfotransferase, rather than by phenol sulfotransferase as previously suggested by KOKKINAKIS et al. (1987) for sulfonation of *N*-nitroso(2-hydroxypropyl)(2-oxopropyl)amine. It would be useful to examine the effect of sulfotransferase inhibitors on the induction of tumors by *β*-hydroxynitrosamines.

VI. Miscellaneous Compounds

1. 3-Hydroxypurines

Certain *N*-hydroxypurines such as 3-hydroxyxanthine and 3-hydroxyguanine are known to be potent carcinogens (SUGIURA et al. 1970; BROWN et al. 1973; LEE et al. 1979; ANDERSON et al. 1978). The oncogenicity of these 3-hydroxypurines has been shown to be correlated with the chemical reactivities of their esters. Thus, the synthetic *N*-acetoxy and tosyloxy derivatives of 3-hydroxyxanthine undergo an SN1′ reaction with several nucleophiles to yield 8-substituted xanthines (WÖLCKE et al. 1969; BIRSDSALL et al. 1971, 1972). Enzymatic conversion of 3-hydroxyxanthine to a reactive ester was proposed (STÖHRER and BROWN 1970), and sulfotransferase activity has been found to play a role in this process (ANDERSON et al. 1978; STÖHRER et al. 1972; MCDONALD et al. 1973). However, no definitive data have been

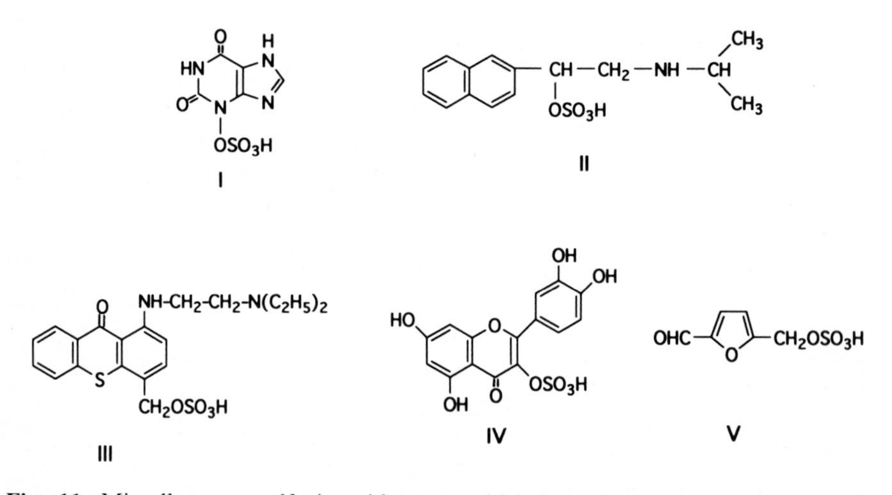

Fig. 11. Miscellaneous sulfuric acid esters which have been suggested as reactive metabolites of parent hydroxy compounds. *I*, 3-hydroxy-xanthine; *II*, prenethalol; *III*, hycanthone; *IV*, quercetin; *V*, 5-hydroxymethylfurfural

reported concerning the role of an electrophilic sulfuric acid ester (Fig. 11, part I) in carcinogenesis by 3-hydroxyxanthine as well as its formation in vivo.

2. β-Aminoalcohols

Certain β-aminoalcohols such as pronethalol (alderlin), ephedrine, and chloramphenicol have been used as drugs. In addition, there are endogenous β-aminoalcohols in animals and humans, for example, adrenaline and noradrenaline. A β-adrenergic receptor blocking agent, pronethalol, was shown to produce thymic tumors in mice (PAGET 1963; HOWE 1965). By contrast, its ether homolog propranolol without the benzyl alcohol functionality was not carcinogenic (BLACK et al. 1964). Interestingly, there was a striking increase in the incidence of thymic tumors in male mice treated with the chloro derivative of pronethalol, in which the benzylic hydroxyl group is replaced by a good leaving group, chloride ion (HOWE 1965). Based on these findings, HOWE (1965) supposed that the β-hydroxyethylamine side chain of pronethalol might be converted to an ethyleneimine to form a chemically reactive "aziridine" and that the aziridine could be an ultimate carcinogenic form of pronethalol. Results from later studies by BICKER and FISCHER (1974) have suggested that enzymatic formation of aziridines from β-aminoalcohols proceeds through unstable sulfuric acid ester metabolites (Fig. 11, part II). These aziridines might be formed from biogenic β-aminoalcohols as well as the aforementioned drugs *via* sulfotransferase activities. This aziridine synthesis might be responsible for the incidence of spontaneous tumors in animals and humans. Further investigations are needed to test this hypothesis.

3. Hycanthone

Hycanthone is an antischistosomal drug (ROSI et al. 1965, 1967). It has been reported to be a frameshift mutagen (HARTMAN et al. 1971). It is also carcinogenic in some experimental animals (HAESE and BUEDING 1976). HARTMAN and HUBERT (1975) previously proposed that metabolic esterification, particularly sulfuric acid esterification of the benzylic alcohol group of hycanthone, could account for the mutagenicity and carcinogenicity of this drug. Data to support this hypothesis have been recently provided by others (CIOLI et al. 1985; ARCHER et al. 1988). In these studies, a model ester, hycanthone *N*-methylcarbamate, was synthesized and its alkylating activity and schistosomicidal activity were determined. The synthetic *N*-methylcarbamate derivative of hycanthone alkylated 4-(*p*-nitrobenzyl)-pyridine and irreversibly inhibited nucleic synthesis in both sensitive and insensitive worms, while the parent hycanthone did not show alkylating activity and inhibited the nucleic acid synthesis in only sensitive worms (CIOLI et al. 1985). Significant covalent DNA binding was observed in HeLa cells exposed to tritium-labeled hycanthone *N*-methylcarbamate, while very little tritiated hycanthone bound to DNA under the same experimental conditions (Archer et al. 1988). These results suggest that benzylic esterification followed by alkylation of DNA applies to the mutagenicity and carcinogenicity of hycanthone as well as to its antischistosomal action. It remains unclear, however, whether sulfotransferase activity in the host or parasites converts hycanthone to an electrophilic sulfuric acid ester (Fig. 11, part III) with schistosomicidal, mutagenic, and carcinogenic activity.

4. Quercetin

Sulfate conjugates of flavonoids are widely present in many edible plants (Barron et al. 1988; Harborne 1975). Recently, sulfotransferases catalyzing the sulfonation of flavonols and other polyphenols have been partially purified from certain plant tissue extracts (Varin and Ibrahim 1989, 1991). A novel sulfotransferase from human intestinal bacteria has also been reported to catalyze the sulfoconjugation of quercetin and other related compounds (Koizumi et al. 1990). Quercetin 3-sulfate (Fig. 11, part IV) and isorhamnetin 3-sulfate contained in the aqueous extracts of dill weed and dill seeds of certain *Umbelliferae* plants were found to be mutagenic towards *Salmonella typhimurium* TA98 in the presence of S_9 fraction in an Ames-reversion assay (Fukuoka et al. 1980). Carcinogenic activities of these flavonoid sulfates have not been directly tested, although no significant carcinogenicity was observed in rats kept on a diet containing 33% dill seeds (Fukuoka et al. 1980).

5. 5-Hydroxymethylfurfural

5-Hydroxymethylfurfural (HMF) is one of the most common furfurals occurring in foodstuffs subjected to heat treatment. Thus, whenever plant or animal tissues containing hexoses are treated with heat during cooking or sterilization, HMF is formed via a sequence of reactions, collectively called "Maillard reactions" (Ulbricht et al. 1984). HMF isolated from a model browning system consisting of glucose and lysine was found to have mutagenic and DNA strand-breaking activity (Omura et al. 1983). However, the mechanism of genotoxic action of HMF is not known. In view of its structure, HMF might undergo metabolic activation at the 5-hydroxy group. One of the possible metabolic pathways responsible for HMF activation is esterification of an allylic hydroxyl group. If the resulting allylic ester possesses a good leaving group such as sulfate or phosphate, it can produce a highly reactive carbonium ion which is resonance-stabilized by distribution of charges on the furan ring. In support of this concept, the chemically synthesized sulfuric acid ester sodium 5-sulfooxymethylfurfural (Fig. 11, part V) is directly mutagenic in bacteria without metabolic activation and is tumorigenic in mouse skin (Surh et al., manuscript in preparation). Sulfotransferase activity responsible for the formation of this reactive sulfuric acid ester has been detected in the hepatic cytosols of rats and mice (Surh and Tannenbaum, unpublished observation).

C. Concluding Remarks

It is very likely that further research will reveal the occurrence of reactive sulfuric acid ester metabolites of other carcinogens belonging to the chemical classes discussed above and, possibly, to classes of carcinogens not yet studied in this respect. Of course, the electrophilic metabolites noted in this review react with cellular nucleophiles other than DNA such as RNAs, proteins, glutathione, and water. While it is possible that some of these reactions might be involved in carcinogenesis, it is more probable that most of them are conjugative detoxifications. Lastly, toxicity tests of drugs in animals pretreated with the sulfonation inhibitors PCP, DCNP, and DHEA might help to reveal unsuspected sulfonation-dependent toxicities, including mutagenicity and carcinogenicity.

Acknowledgements. Our studies in sulfonation-dependent chemical carcinogenesis were supported by grants CA-07175 and CA-22848 from the National Cancer Institute, U.S. Department of Health and Human Services.

References

Andersen RA, Enomoto M, Miller EC, Miller JA (1964) Carcinogenesis and inhibition of the Walker 256 tumor in the rat by *trans*-4-acetylaminostilbene, its N-hydroxy metabolite, and related compounds. Cancer Res 24:128–143

Anderson LM, McDonald JJ, Budinger JM, Mountain IM, Brown GB (1978) 3-Hydroxyxanthine: transplacental effects and ontogeny of related sulfate metabolism in rats and mice. J Natl Cancer Inst 61:1405–1410

Archer S, Pica-Mattoccia L, Cioli D, Seyed-Mozaffari A, Zayed A-H (1988) Preparation and antischistosomal and antitumor activity of hycanthone and some of its congeners. Evidence for the mode of action of hycanthone. J Med Chem 31:254–260

Autrup H (1979) Separation of water-soluble metabolites of benzo[a]pyrene formed by cultured human colon. Biochem Pharmacol 28:1727–1730

Barron D, Varian L, Ibrahim RK, Harborne JB, Williams CA (1988) Sulphated flavonoids – an update. Phytochemistry 27:2375–2395

Beland FA, Kadlubar FF (1990) Metabolic activation and DNA adducts of aromatic amines and nitroaromatic hydrocarbons. In: Cooper CS, Glover PL (eds) Chemical carcinogenesis and mutagenesis I. Springer, Berlin Heidelberg New York, pp 267–325

Beland FA, Tullis DL, Kadlubar FF, Straub KM, Evans FE (1980) Characterization of DNA adducts of the carcinogen *N*-methyl-4-aminoazobenzene in vitro and in vivo. Chem Biol Interact 31:1–17

Benkovic SJ, Hevey RC (1970) Studies in sulfate esters. V. The mechanism of hydrolysis of phenyl phosphosulfate, a model system for 3′-phosphoadenosine 5′-phosphosulfate. J Am Chem Soc 92:4971–4977

Bicker U, Fischer W (1974) Enzymatic aziridine synthesis from β-aminoalcohols – a new example of endogenous carcinogen formation. Nature 249:344–345

Birsdall NJM, Lee T-C, Wölcke U (1971) Purine N-oxides. XXXIX. N-Acetoxy derivatives of N-hydroxyxanthines. Tetrahedron 27:5961

Birdsall NJM, Wölcke U, Parham JC, Brown GB (1972) Purine N-oxides. XLI. The 3-acyloxypurine 8-substitution reaction: on the mechanism of the reaction. Tetrahedron 28:3–13

Black JW, Crowther AF, Shanks RG, Smith LH, Dornhurst AC (1964) A new adrenergic beta-receptor antagonist. Lancet i:1080–1081

Boberg EW, Miller EC, Miller JA, Liem A (1983) Strong evidence from studies with brachymorphic mice and pentachlorophenol that 1′-sulfooxysafrole is the major ultimate electrophilic and carcinogenic metabolite of 1′-hydroxysafrole in mouse liver. Cancer Res 43:5163–5173

Borchert P, Wislocki PG, Miller JA, Miller EC (1973a) The metabolism of the naturally occurring hepatocarcinogen safrole to 1′-hydroxysafrole and the electrophilic reactivity of 1′-acetoxysafrole. Cancer Res 33:575–589

Borchert P, Miller JA, Miller EC, Shires TK (1973b) 1′-Hydroxysafrole, a proximate carcinogenic metabolite of safrole in the rat and mouse. Cancer Res 33:590–600

Boroujerdi M, Kung H-C, Wilson AGE, Anderson MW (1981) Metabolism and DNA binding of benzo[a]pyrene in vivo in the rat. Cancer Res 41:951–957

Brown GB, Teller MN, Smullyan I, Birdsall NJM, Lee T-C, Parham JC, Stöhrer G (1973) Correlations between oncogenic and chemical properties of several derivatives of 3-hydroxyxanthine and 3-hydroxyguanine. Cancer Res 33:1113–1118

Buonarati MH, Turtletaub KW, Shen NH, Felton JS (1990) Role of sulfation and acetylation in the activation of 2-hydroxyamino-1-methyl-6-phenylimidazo [4,5-b]pyridine to intermediates which bind DNA. Mutat Res 245:185–190

Calder IC, Goss DE, Williams PJ, Funder CG, Green LR, Hann KN, Tange JD (1976) Neoplasms in the rat induced by *N*-hydroxyphenacetin, a metabolite of phenacetin. Pathology 8:1–6

Cavalieri EL, Rogan EG (1985) Role of radical cations in aromatic hydrocarbon carcinogenesis. Environ Health Perspect 64:69–84

Cavalieri EL, Rogan EG (1992) The approach to understand aromatic hydrocarbon carcinogenesis. The central role of radical cations in metabolic activation. Pharmacol Ther (in press)

Cavalieri EL, Roth RW, Grandjean C, Althoff J, Patil K, Liakus S, Marsh S (1978) Carcinogenicity and metabolic profiles of 6-substituted benzo[a]pyrene derivatives on mouse skin. Chem Biol Interact 22:53–67

Chism JP, Rickert DE (1985) Isomer- and sex-specific bioactivation of mononitrotoluenes: role of enterohepatic circulation. Drug Metab Dispos 13:651–657

Chism JP and Rickert DE (1989) In vitro activation of 2-aminobenzyl alcohol and 2-amino-6-nitrobenzyl alcohol, metabolites of 2-nitrotoluene and 2,6-dinitrotoluene. Chem Res Toxicol 2:150–156

Chism JP, Turner MJ, Rickert DE (1984) The metabolism and excretion of mononitrotoluenes by Fischer-344 rats. Drug Metab Dispos 12:596–602

Cioli D, Pica-Mattoccia L, Rosenberg S, Archer S (1985) Evidence for the mode of antischistosomal action of hycanthone. Life Sci 37:161–167

Cohen GM, Moore BP, Bridges JW (1977) Organic solvent soluble sulphate ester conjugates of monohydroxybenzo[a]pyrenes. Biochem Pharmacol 26:551–553

Cramer JW, Miller JA, Miller EC (1960) *N*-Hydroxylation: a new metabolic reaction observed in the rat with the carcinogen 2-acetylaminofluorene. J Biol Chem 235:885–888

DdBaun JR, Rowley JY, Miller EC, Miller JA (1968) Sulfotransferase activation of *N*-hydroxy-2-acetylaminofluorene in rodent livers susceptible and resistant to this carcinogen. Proc Soc Exp Biol Med 129:268–273

DeBaun JR, Miller EC, Miller JA (1970) *N*-Hydroxy-2-acetylaminofluorene sulfotransferase: its probable role in carcinogenesis and in protein-(methion-*S*-yl) binding in rat liver. Cancer Res 30:577–595

Delclos KB, Tarpley WG, Miller EC, Miller JA (1984) 4-Aminoazobenzene and *N*,*N*-dimethyl-4-aminoazobenzene as equipotent hepatic carcinogens in male C57BL/6 × C3H/He F_1 mice and characterization of *N*-(deoxyguanosin-8-yl)-4-aminoazobenzene as the major persistent hepatic DNA-bound dye in these mice. Cancer Res 44:2540–2550

Delclos KB, Miller EC, Miller JA, Liem A (1986) Sulfuric acid esters as major ultimate electrophilic and hepatocarcinogenic metabolites of 4-aminoazobenzene and its *N*-methyl derivatives in infant male C57BL/6J × C3H/HeJ F_1 ($B6C3F_1$) mice. Carcinogenesis 7:277–287

Devanesan PD, RamaKrishna NVS, Todorovic R, Rogan FG, Cavalieri EL, Jeong H, Jankowiak R, Small GJ (1992) Identification and quantitation of benzo[a]-pyrene-DNA adducts formed by rat liver microsomes in vitro. Chem Res Toxicol 5:302–309

Dooley KL, Von Tungein LS, Bucci T, Fu PP, Kadlubar FF (1992) Comparative carcinogenicity of 4-aminobiphenyl and the food pyrolysates, Glu-P-1, IQ, PhIP, and MeIQx in the neonatal $B6C3F_1$ male mouse. Cancer Lett 62:205–209

Doolittle DJ, Sherrill JM, Butterworth BE (1983) The influence of intestinal bacteria, sex of the animal, and position of the nitro group on the hepatic genotoxicity of nitrotoluene isomers in vivo. Cancer Res 43:2836–2842

Drinkwater NR, Miller EC, Miller JA, Pitot HC (1976) The hepatocarcinogenicity of estragole (1-allyl-4-methoxybenzene) and 1′-hydroxyestragole in the mouse and mutagenicity of 1′-acetoxyestragole in bacteria. J Natl Cancer Inst 57:1323–1331

Eisenstadt E, Shpizner B, Gold A (1981) Metabolism of cyclopenta[cd]pyrene at the K-region by microsomes and a reconstituted cytochrome P-450 system from rat liver. Biochem Biophys Res Commun 100:965–967

Felton JS, Knize MG (1990) Heterocyclic-amine mutagens/carcinogens in foods. In: Cooper CS, Glover PL (eds) Chemical carcinogenesis and mutagenesis I. Springer, Berlin Heidelberg New York, pp 471–502

Felton JS, Knize MG, Shen NH, Wu R, Becher G (1988) Mutagenic heterocyclic imidazoamines in cooked foods. In: King CM, Romano LJ, Schuetzle D (eds) Carcinogenic and mutagenic responses to aromatic amines and nitroarenes. Elsevier, New York, pp 73–85

Fennell TR, Miller JA, Miller EC (1984) Characterization of the biliary and urinary glutathione and *N*-acetylcysteine metabolites of the hepatic carcinogen 1′-hydroxysafrole and its 1′-oxo metabolite in rats and mice. Cancer Res 44: 3231–3240

Fennell TR, Wiseman RW, Miller JA, Miller EC (1985) Major role of hepatic sulfotransferase activity in the metabolic activation, DNA adduct formation, and carcinogenicity of 1′-hydroxy-2′,3′-dehydroestragole in infant male C57BL/6J × $C3H/HeJF_1$ mice. Cancer Res 45:5310–5320

Flesher JW, Sydnor KL (1971) Carcinogenicity of derivatives of 7,12-dimethylbenz[a]anthracene. Cancer Res 31:1951–1954

Flesher JW, Sydnor KL (1973) Possible role of 6-hydroxymethylbenzo[a]pyrene as a proximate carcinogen of benzo[a]pyrene and 6-methylbenzo[a]pyrene. Int J Cancer

Fukuoka M, Yoshihira K, Natori S, Sakamoto K, Iwahara S, Hosaka S, Hirono I (1980) Characterization of mutagenic principles and carcinogenicity test of dill weed and seeds. J Pharm Dyn 3:236–244

Furlong BB, Weaver RP, Goldstein JA (1987) Covalent binding to DNA and mutagenicity of 2,4-dinitrotoluene metabolites produced by isolated hepatocytes and 9000 g supernatant from Fischer 344 rats. Carcinogenesis 8:247–251

Glatt H, Henschler R, Phillips DH, Blake JW, Steinberg P, Seidel A, Oesch F (1990) Sulfotransferase-mediated chlorination of 1-hydroxymethylpyrene to a mutagen capable of penetrating indicator cells. Environ Health Perspect 88: 43–48

Haese WH, Bueding E (1976) Long-term hepatocellular effects of hycanthone and of two other antischistosomal drugs in mice infected with *Schistosoma mansoni*. J Pharmacol Exp Ther 197:703–713

Harborne JB (1975) Flavonoid sulphates: a new class of natural sulphur compounds in higher plants. Phytochemistry 14:1147–1155

Hartman PE, Hulbert PB (1975) Genetic activity spectra of some antischistosomal compounds, with particular emphasis on thioxanthenones and benzothiopyranoindazoles. J Toxicol Environ Health 1:243–270

Hartman PE, Levine K, Hartman Z, Berger H (1971) Hycanthone: a frameshift mutagen. Science 172:1058–1060

Howe R (1965) Carcinogenicity of alderlin (pronethalol) in mice. Nature 207:594–595

IARC (1972) IARC monographs of the evaluation of carcinogenic risk of chemicals in man, vol 1. 4-Aminobiphenyl. International Agency for Research on Cancer. World Health Organization, Lyon, pp 74–79

IARC (1987) IARC monographs of the evaluation of carcinogenic risk of chemicals in man, Supplement 7, an updating of IARC monographs, volumes 1 to 42. Phenacetin. International Agency for Research on Cancer, World Health Organization, Lyon, pp 310–312

Irving CC, Janss DH, Russell LT (1971) Lack of *N*-hydroxy-2-acetylaminofluorene sulfotransferase activity in the mammary gland and Zymbal's gland of the rat. Cancer Res 31:387–391

Irwin SE, Kwei GY, Blackburn GR, Thurman R, Kauffman FC (1992) Mutagenicity of benzo[a]pyrenyl-1-sulfate in the Ames test. Environ Mol Mutagen 19:253–258

Isaka H, Yoshi H, Otsuji A, Koike M, Nagai Y, Koura M, Sugiyasu K, Kanabayashi T (1979) Tumors of Sprague-Dawley rats induced by long-term feeding of phenacetin. Gann 70:29–36

Jerina DM, Sayer JM, Agarwal, Yagi H, Levin W, Wood AW, Conney AH, PreussSchwartz D, Baird WM, Pigott MA, Dipple A (1986) Reactivity and tumorigenicity of bay-region diol epoxides derived from polycyclic aromatic hydrocarbons. In: Kocsis JJ, Jollow DJ, Witmer CM, Nelson JO, Snyder R (eds) Biological reactive intermediates III. Plenum, New York, pp 11–30

Johansson S, Angervall L, Bengdtsson U, Wahlquist L (1974) Uroepithelial tumors of the renal pelvis associated with abuse of phenacetin-containing analgesics. Cancer 33:743–753

Kadlubar FF, Miller JA, Miller EC (1976a) Microsomal *N*-oxidation of the hepatocarcinogen *N*-methyl-4-aminoazobenzene and the reactivity of *N*-hydroxy-*N*-methylaminoazobenzene. Cancer Res 36:1196–1206

Kadlubar FF, Miller JA, Miller EC (1976b) Hepatic metabolism of *N*-hydroxy-*N*-methyl-4-aminoazobenzene to reactive sulfuric acid esters. Cancer Res 36: 2350–2359

Kato R (1986) Metabolic activation of mutagenic heterocyclic aromatic amines from protein pyrolysates. CRC Crit Rev Toxicol 16:307–348

Kato R, Yamazoe Y (1987) Metabolic activation and covalent binding to nucleic acids of carcinogenic heterocyclic amines from cooked food and amino acid pyrolysates. Gann 78:297–311

Kawazoe Y, Huang G-F (1972) Direct C-amination of guanosine with hydroxylamine-*O*-sulfonic acid. Simplest model reaction possibly involved in DNA damage leading to carcinogenesis by *N*-arylhydroxylamines. Chem Pharm Bull 20: 2073–2074

Kedderis GL, Dyoff MC, Rickert DE (1984) Hepatic macromolecular covalent binding of the hepatocarcinogen 2,6-dinitrotoluene and its 2,4-isomer in vivo: modulation by the sulfotransferase inhibitors pentachlorophenol and 2,6-dichloro-4-nitrophenol. Carcinogenesis 5:1199–1204

King CM, Phillips B (1968) Enzyme-catalyzed reactions of the carcinogen *N*-hydroxy-2-fluorenylacetamide with nucleic acid. Science 159:1351–1453

Koepke SR, Kupper R, Michejda CJ (1979) Unusually facile solvolysis of primary tosylates. A case for participation by the N-nitroso group. J Org Chem 44: 2718–2722

Koizumi M, Shimizu M, Kobashi K (1990) Enzymatic sulfation of quercetin by arylsulfotransferase from a human intestinal bacterium. Chem Pharm Bull 36:794–798

Kokkinakis DM, Hollenberg PF, Scarpelli DG (1985) Major urinary metabolites in hamsters and rats treated with *N*-nitroso(2-hydroxypropyl)(2-oxopropyl)-amine. Cancer Res 45:3586–3592

Kokkinakis DM, Scarpelli DG, Subbarao V, Hollenberg PF (1987) Species differences in the metabolism of *N*-nitroso(2-hydroxypropyl)(2-oxopropyl) amine. Carcinogenesis 8:295–303

Kriek E (1992) Fifty years of research on *N*-acetyl-2-aminofluorene, one of the most versatile compounds in experimental cancer research. Cancer Res Clin Oncol 118:481–489

Kriek E, Miller JA, Juhl U, Miller EC (1967) 8-(*N*-2-fluorenylacetamido)-guanosine, an arylamidation reaction product of guanosine and the carcinogen *N*-acetoxy-N-2-fluorenylacetamide in neutral solution. Biochemistry 6:177–182

Kroeger-Koepke MB, Koepke SR, Hernandez L, Michejda CJ (1992) Activation of a β-hydroxyalkylnitrosamine to alkylating agents: evidence for the involvement of a sulfotransferase. Cancer Res 52:3300–3305

Kwon H, Sahali Y, Skipper PL, Tannenbaum SR (1992) Metabolism of cyclopenta-[cd]pyrene by human and mouse microsomes and selected P-450 isozymes: a comparative study. Chem Res Toxicol (in press)

Lai C-C, Miller JA, Miller EC, Liem A (1985) *N*-Sulfooxy-2-aminofluorene is the major ultimate electrophilic and carcinogenic metabolite of *N*-hydroxy-2-acetylaminofluorene in the livers of infant male C57BL/6J × C3H/HeJ F_1 $(B6C3F)_1$ mice. Carcinogenesis 6:1037–1045

Lai C-C, Miller EC, Miller JA, Liem A (1987) Initiation of hepatocarcinogenesis in infant male $B6C3F_1$ mice by *N*-hydroxy-2-aminofluorene or *N*-hydroxy-2-acetylaminofluorene depends primarily on metabolism to *N*-sulfooxy-2-aminofluorene and formation of DNA-(deoxyguanosin-8-yl)-2-aminofluorene Carcinogenesis 8:471–478

Lai C-C, Miller EC, Miller JA, Liem A (1988) The essential role of microsomal deacetylase in the metabolic activation, DNA-(deoxyguanosin-8-yl)-2-aminofluorene adduct formation and initiation of liver tumors by N-hydroxy-2-acetylaminofluorene in the livers of infant male $B6C3F_1$ mice. Carcinogenesis 9:1295–1302

Lee ML, Prado GP, Howard JB, Hites RA (1977) Source identification of urban airborne polycyclic aromatic hydrocarbons by gas chromatographic mass spectrometry and high resolution mass spectrometry. Biomed Mass Spectrom 4: 182–186

Lee T-C, Teller MN, Budinger JM, Klötzer W, Brown GB (1979) Chemical reactivities and oncogenicities of a series of N-hydroxyheterocycles. Chem Biol Interact 25:369–372

Leonard TE, Graichen ME, Popp JE (1987) Dinitrotoluene isomer-specific hepatocarcinogenesis in F344 rats. J Natl Cancer Inst 79:1313–1319

Leung L (1980) Encyclopedia of common natural ingredients used in foods, drugs, and cosmetics. Wiley, New York

Long RM, Rickert DE (1982) Metabolism and excretion of 2,6-dinitro[^{14}C]toluene in vivo and in isolated perfused rat livers. Drug Metab Dispos 10:455–458

Maher VM, Miller EC, Miller JA, Szybalski W (1968) Mutations and decreases in density of transforming DNA produced by derivatives of the carcinogens 2-acetylaminofluorene and *N*-methyl-4-aminoazobenzene. Mol Pharmacol 4:411–426

McDonald JJ, Stöhrer G, Brown GB (1973) Oncogenic purine N-oxide derivatives as substrates for sulfotransferase. Cancer Res 33:3319–3323

Michejda CJ, Andrews AW, Koepke SR (1979) Derivatives of side-chain hydroxylated nitrosamines. Direct acting mutagens in *Salmonella typhimurium*. Mutat Res 67:301–308

Michejda CJ, Koepke SR, Kroeger-Koepke MB, Bosan W (1987) Recent findings on the metabolism of β-hydroxyalkylnitrosamines. In: Bartsch H, O'Neill IK, Schulte-Hermann R (eds) Relevance of N-nitroso compounds to human cancer: exposures and mechanisms. IARC, Lyon, pp 77–82

Miller EC, Sandin RB, Miller JA, Rusch HP (1956) The carcinogenicity of compounds related to 2-acetylaminofluorene. III. Aminobiphenyl and benzidine derivatives. Cancer Res 16:525–534

Miller EC, Miller JA, Hartmann HA (1961a) *N*-Hydroxy-2-acetylaminofluorene: a metabolite of 2-acetylaminofluorene with increased carcinogenic activity in the rat. Cancer Res 21:815–824

Miller EC, Lotlikar PD, Pitot HC, Fletcher TL, Miller JA (1966) *N*-Hydroxy metabolites of 2-acetylaminophenanthrene and 7-fluoro-2-acetylaminofluorene as proximate carcinogens in the rat. Cancer Res 26:2239–2247

Miller EC, Miller JA (1981) Searches for ultimate chemical carcinogens and their reactions with cellular macromolecules. Adv Cancer Res 47:2327–2345

Miller EC, Swanson AB, Phillips DH, Fletcher TL, Liem A, Miller JA (1983) Structure-activity studies of the carcinogenicities in the mouse and rat of some naturally occurring and synthetic alkenylbenzene derivatives related to safrole and estragole. Cancer Res 43:1124–1134

Miller JA, Miller EC (1953) The carcinogenic amino-azo dyes. Adv Cancer Res 1:339–396

Miller JA, Wyatt CS, Miller EC, Hartmann HA (1961b) The *N*-hydroxylation of 4-acetylaminobiphenyl by the rat and dog and the strong carcinogenicity of N-hydroxy-4-acetylaminobiphenyl in the rat. Cancer Res 21:1465–1473

Miller JA, Surh YJ, Liem A, Miller EC (1991) Electrophilic sulfuric acid ester metabolites of hydroxymethyl aromatic hydrocarbons as precursors of hepatic benzylic DNA adducts in vivo. In: Witmer CM, Snyder RR, Jollow DJ, Kalf GF, Kocsis JJ, Sipes IG (eds) Biological reactive intermediates IV. Plenum, New York (Adv Exp Med Biol 283:555–567)

Mirsalis JC, Butterworth BE (1982) Induction of unscheduled DNA synthesis in rat hepatocytes following in vivo treatment with dinitrotoluene. Carcinogenesis 3:241–245

Molliere M, Foth H, Kahl GF (1987) Comparison of benzo[a]pyrene metabolism in isolated perfused rat lung and liver. Arch Toxicol 60:270–277

Moore BP, Cohen GM (1978) Metabolism of benzo[a]pyrene and its major metabolites to ethyl acetate-soluble and water-soluble metabolites by cultured rodent trachea. Cancer Res 38:3066–3075

Mori M, Miyahara T, Hasegawa Y, Kudo Y, Kozuka H (1984) Metabolism of dinitrotoluene isomers by *Escherichia coli* isolated from human intestine. Chem Pharm Bull 32:4070–4075

Mori M, Kudo Y, Nunozawa T, Miyahara T, Kozuka H (1985) Intestinal metabolism of 2,4-dinitrotoluene in rats. Chem Pharm Bull 33:327–332

Mulder GJ, Hinson JA, Gillette JR (1978) Conversion of the *N-O*-glucuronide and *N-O*-sulfate conjugates of *N*-hydroxy-phenacetin to reactive intermediates. Biochem Pharmacol 27:1641–1649

Mulder GJ, Jakoby WB (1990) Sulfation. In: Mulder GJ (ed) Conjugation reactions in drug metabolism. Taylor and Francis, London, pp 107–161

Nair RV, Walker SE, Sharma PK, Witiak DT, DiGiovanni J (1992) Mouse skin tumor initiating activity of fluorinated derivatives of 1,2,3,4-tetrahydro-7,12-dimethylbenz[a]anthracene. Chem Res Toxicol 5:153–156

Nakanishi K, Kurata Y, Oshima M, Fukushima S, Ito N (1982) Carcinogenicity of phenacetin: long-term feeding study in B6C3F1 mice. Int J cancer 29:439–444

Nemoto N, Takayama S, Gelboin HV (1978) Sulfate conjugation of benzo[a]pyrene metabolites and derivatives. Chem Biol Interact 23:19–30

Ogura K, Kajita J, Narihata H, Watabe T, Ozawa S, Nagata K, Yamazoe Y, Kato R (1989) Cloning and sequence analysis of a rat liver cDNA encoding hydroxysteroid sulfotransferase. Biochem Biophys Res Commun 165:168–174

Ogura K, Sohtome T, Sugiyama A, Okuda H, Hiratsuka A, Watabe T (1990a) Rat liver cytosolic hydroxysteroid sulfotransferase (sulfotransferase a) catalyzing the formation of reactive sulfate esters from carcinogenic polycyclic hydroxymethylarenes. Mol Pharmacol 37:848–854

Ogura K, Kajita J, Narihata H, Watabe T, Ozawa S, Nagata K, Yamazoe Y, Kato R (1990b) cDNA cloning of the hydroxysteroid sulfotransferase STa sharing a strong homology in amino acid sequence with the sentence marker protein SMP-2 in rat livers. Biochem Biophys Res Commun 166:1494–1500

Okuda H, Nojima H, Miwa K, Watanabe N, Watabe T (1989) Selective covalent binding of the active sulfate ester of the carcinogen 5-(hydroxymethyl)chrysene to the adenine residue of calf thymus DNA. Chem Res Toxicol 2:15–22

Omura H, Jahan N, Shinohara K, Murakami H (1983) Formation of mutagens by the Maillard reaction. In: Waller GR, Feather M (eds) ACS symposium series 215. American Chemical Society, Washington DC, pp 536–563

Oswald EO, Fishbein L, Corbett BJ, Walker MP (1971) Identification of tertiary aminomethylenedioxypropiophenones as urinary metabolites of safrole in the rat and guinea pig. Biochim Biophys Acta 230:237–247

Paget GE (1963) Carcinogenic action of pronethalol. Br Med J 11:1266–1267

Phillips DH, Miller JA, Miller EC, Adams B (1981a) Structures of the DNA adducts formed in mouse liver after administration of the proximate hepatocarcinogen 1′-hydroxyestragole. Cancer Res 41:176–186

Phillips DH, Miller JA, Miller EC, Adams B (1981b) The N^2-atom of guanine and the N^6-atom of adenine residues as sites for covalent binding of metabolically activated 1′-hydroxysafrole to mouse liver DNA in vivo. Cancer Res 41:2664–2671

Piakunov I, Smolarek TA, Fischer DL, Wiley JC, Baird WM (1987) Separation by ion-pair high-performance liquid chromatography of the glucuronide, sulfate and glutathione conjugates formed from benzo[a]pyrene in cell cultures from rodents, fish and humans. Carcinogenesis 8:59–66

Poirier LA, Miller JA, Miller EC, Sato K (1967) *N*-Benzoyloxy-*N*-methyl-4-aminoazobenzene: its carcinogenic activity in the rat and its reactions with proteins and nucleic acids and their constituents in vitro. Cancer Res 27:1600–1613

Preussmann R, Stewart BW (1984) N-Nitroso compounds. In: Searle CE (ed) Chemical carcinogens, 2nd edn. American Chemical Society, Washington DC (ACS monograph 182)

RamaKrishna NVS, Devanesan PD, Rogan EG, Cavalieri EL, Jeong H, Jankowiak R, Small GJ (1992a) Mechanism of metabolic activation of the potent carcinogen 7,12-dimethylbenz[a]anthracene. Chem Res Toxicol 5:220–226

RamaKrishna NVS, Gao F, Padmavathi NS, Cavalieri EL, Rogan EG, Cerny RL, Gross ML (1992b) Model adducts of benzo[a]pyrene and nucleosides formed from its radical cation and diol epoxide. Chem Res Toxicol 5:293–302

Rao SI, Duffel MW (1992) Inhibition of rat hepatic aryl sulphotransferase IV by dihydrodiol derivatives of benzo[a]pyrene and naphthalene. Xenobiotica 22: 247–255

Rickert DE, Schnell SR, Long RM (1983) Hepatic macromolecular covalent binding and intestinal disposition of ^{14}C-dinitrotoluenes. J Toxicol Environ Health 11:555–567

Rickert DE, Long RM, Dyroff MC, Kedderis GL (1984a) Hepatic macromolecular covalent binding of mononitrotoluenes in Fischer-344 rats. Chem Biol Interact 52:131–139

Rickert DE, Butterworth BE, Popp JA (1984b) Dinitrotoluene: acute toxicity, oncogenicity, and metabolism. CRC Crit Rev Toxicol 13:217–234

Rinderle SJ, Black SD, Sharma PK, Witiak DT (1992) Comparative metabolism in vitro of a novel carcinogenic polycyclic aromatic hydrocarbon, 1,2,3,4-tetrahydro-7,12-dimethylbenz[a]anthracene, and its two regioisomeric B-ring fluoro analogues. Cancer Res 52:3035–3042

Robbins PW, Lipmann F (1957) Isolation and identification of active sulfate. J Biol Chem 229:837–851

Rosi D, Peruzzotti EW, Dennis DA, Berberian H, Freele H, Archer S (1965) A new active metabolite of "Miracil D". Nature 208:1005–1006

Rosi D, Peruzzotti EW, Dennis EW, Berberian H, Freele H, Tullar BF, Archer S (1967) Hycanthone, a new active metabolite of lucanthone. J Med Chem 10: 867–876

Sahali Y, Kwon H, Skipper PL, Tannenbaum SR (1992) Microsomal metabolism of cyclopenta[cd]pyrene: identification of new metabolites, absolute configuration and mechanisms. Chem Res Toxicol 5:157–162

Sato K, Poirier LA, Miller JA, Miller EC (1966) Studies on the *N*-hydroxylation and carcinogenicity of 4-aminoazobenzene and related compounds. Cancer Res 26:1678–1687

Scribner JD, Naimy NK (1975) Adducts between the carcinogen 2-acetamidophenanthrene and adenine and guanine of DNA. Cancer Res 35:1416–1421

Sims P, Grover PL, Swaisland A, Pal K, Hewer A (1974) Metabolic activation of benzo[a]pyrene proceeds by a diol-epoxide. Nature 252:326–328

Smith BA, Gutmann HR, Springfield JR (1985) Interaction of nucleophiles with the enzymatically-activated carcinogen, *N*-hydroxy-2-acetylaminofluorene, and with the model ester, *N*-acetoxy-2-acetylaminofluorene. Carcinogenesis 6:271–277

Smith BA, Springfield JR, Gutmann HR (1986) Interaction of the synthetic ultimate carcinogens, N-sulfonoxy- and N-acetoxy-2-acetylaminofluorene, and of enzymatically activated N-hydroxy-2-acetylaminofluorene with nucleophiles. Carcinogenesis 7:405–411

Sterzel W, Eisenbrand G (1986) N-Nitrosodiethanolamine is activated in the rat to an ultimate genotoxic metabolite by sulfotransferase. J Cancer Res Clin Oncol 111:20–24

Stöhrer G, Brown GB (1970) Oncogenic purine derivatives: evidence for a possible proximate oncogen. Science 167:1622–1624

Stöhrer G, Corbin G, Brown GB (1972) Enzymatic activation of the oncogen 3-hydroxyxanthine. Cancer Res 32:637–642

Sugimura T (1986) Past, present, and future of mutagens in cooked foods. Environ Health Perspect 67:5–10

Sugiura K, Teller MN, Parham JC, Brown GB (1970) A comparison of the oncogenicities of 3-hydroxyxanthine, guanine 3-N-oxide, and some related compounds. Cancer Res 30:184–188

Surh Y-J, Lai C-C, Miller JA, Miller EC (1987) Hepatic DNA and RNA adduct formation from the carcinogen 7-hydroxymethyl-12-methylbenz[a]anthracene and its electrophilic sulfuric acid ester metabolite in preweanling rats and mice. Biochem Biophys Res Commun 144:576–582

Surh Y-J, Liem A, Miller EC, Miller JA (1989) Metabolic activation of the carcinogen 6-hydroxymethylbenzo[a]pyrene: formation of an electrophilic sulfuric acid ester and benzylic DNA adducts in rat liver in vivo and in reactions in vitro. Carcinogenesis 10:1519–1528

Surh Y-J, Blomquist JC, Liem A, Miller JA (1990a) Metabolic activation of 9-hydroxymethyl-10-methylanthracene and 1-hydroxymethylpyrene to electrphilic, mutagenic, and tumorigenic sulfuric acid esters by rat hepatic sulfotransferase activity. Carcinogenesis 11:1451–1460

Surh Y-J, Liem A, Miller EC, Miller JA (1990b) The strong hepatocarcinogenicity of the electrophilic and mutagenic metabolite 6-sulfooxymethylbenzo[a]pyrene and its formation of benzylic DNA adducts in the livers of infant male $B6C3F_1$ mice. Biochem Biophys Res Commun 172:85–91

Surh Y-J, Blomquist JC, Miller JA (1991a) Activation of 1-hydroxymethylpyrene to an electrophilic and mutagenic metabolite by rat hepatic sulfotransferase activity. In: Witmer CM, Snyder RR, Jollow DJ, Kalf GF, Kocsis JJ, Sipes IG (eds) Biological reactive intermediates IV. Plenum, New York (Adv Exp Med Biol 283:383–391)

Surh Y-J, Liem A, Miller EC, Miller JA (1991b) Age- and sex-related differences in activation of the carcinogen 7-hydroxymethyl-12-methylbenz[a]anthracene to an electrophilic sulfuric acid ester metabolite in rats. Biochem Pharmacol 41:213–221

Surh Y-J, Liem A, Miller EC, Miller JA (1991c) 7-Sulfooxymethyl-12-methylbenz[a]-anthracene is an electrophilic mutagen, but does not appear to play a role in carcinogenesis by 7,12-dimethylbenz[a]anthracene or 7-hydroxymethyl-12-methylbenz[a]anthracene. Carcinogenesis 12:339–347

Surh Y-J, Kwon H, Tannenbaum SR (1992) Sulfotransferase-mediated activation of 4-hydroxy- and 3,4-dihydroxycyclopenta[cd]pyrene, major metabolites of cyclopenta[cd]pyrene. Cancer Res (submitted)

Swanson AB, Miller EC, Miller JA (1981) The side-chain epoxidation and hydroxylation of the hepatocarcinogens safrole and estragole and some related compounds by rat and mouse liver microsomes. Biochim Biophys Acta 673:504–516

Teffera Y, Baird WM, Smith DL (1991) Determination of benzo[a]pyrene sulfate conjugates from benzo[a]pyrene-treated cells by continuous-flow fast atom bombardment mass spectrometry. Anal Chem 63:453–456

Tong HY, Karasek FW (1984) Quantitation of polycyclic aromatic hydrocarbons in diesel exhaust particular matter by high-performance liquid chromatography fractionation and high resolution gas chromatography. Anal Chem 56:2129–2134

Ulbricht RJ, Northup SJ, Thomas JA (1984) A review of 5-hydroxymethylfurfural (HMF) in parenteral solutions. Fund Appl Toxicol 4:843–853

Varian L, Ibrahim RK (1989) Partial purification and characterization of three flavonol-specific sulfotransferases from *Flaveria chloraefolia*. Plant Physiol 90: 977–981

Varian L, Ibrahim RK (1991) Partial purification and some properties of flavonol 7-sulfotransferase from *Flaveria bidentis*. Plant Physiol 95:1254–1258

Watabe T, Ishizuka T, Isobe M, Ozawa N (1982) 7-Hydroxymethylsulfate ester as an active metabolite of 7,12-dimethylbenz[a]anthracene. Science 215:403–405

Watabe T, Fujieda T, Hiratsuka A, Ishizuka T, Hakamata Y, Ogura K (1985) The carcinogen, 7-hydroxymethyl-12-methylbenz[a]anthracene, is activated and covalently binds to DNA via a sulphate ester. Biochem Pharmacol 34:3002–3005

Watabe T, Hakamata Y, Hiratsuka A, Ogura K (1986) A 7-hydroxymethyl sulphate ester as an active metabolite of the carcinogen, 7-hydroxymethylbenz[a]anthracene. Carcinogenesis 7:207–214

Watabe T, Hiratsuka A, Ogura K (1987) Sulfotransferase-mediated covalent binding of the carcinogen 7,12-dihydroxymethylbenz[a]anthracene to calf thymus DNA and its inhibition by glutathione transferase. Carcinogenesis 8:445–453

Williams RT (1959) Detoxication mechanisms, 2nd edn. Chapman Hall, London

Wiseman RW, Fennell TR, Miller JA, Miller EC (1985) Further characterization of the DNA adducts formed by electrophilic esters of the hepatocarcinogens 1′-hydroxysafrole and 1′-hydroxyestragole in vitro and in mouse liver in vivo, including new adducts at C-8 and N-7 of guanine residues. Cancer Res 45: 3096–3105

Wislocki PG, Borchert P, Miller JA, Miller EC (1976) The metabolic activation of the carcinogen 1′-hydroxysafrole in vivo and in vitro and the electrophilic activities of possible ultimate carcinogens. Cancer Res 36:1686–1695

Wislocki PG, Miller EC, Miller JA, McCoy EC, Rosenkranz HS (1977) Carcinogenic and mutagenic activities of safrole, 1′-hydroxysafrole, and some known and possible metabolites. Cancer Res 37:1883–1891

Wölcke U, Birdsall NJM, Brown GB (1969) The preparation of 8-substituted xanthines and guanines by a nucleophilic displacement of a 3-substituent. Tetrahedron Lett 10:785–788

Zaleski J, Bansal SK, Gessner T (1983) Formation of glucuronide, sulphate and glutathion conjugates of benzo[a]pyrene in hepatocytes isolated from inbred strains of mice. Carcinogenesis 4:1359–1366

CHAPTER 16

Glutathione Conjugate-Mediated Toxicities

T.J. MONKS and S.S. LAU

A. Introduction

Glutathione (γ-glutamylcysteinylglycine; GSH) is the predominant intracellular nonprotein sulfhydryl present in the cytosol of animal and plant cells. GSH plays an integral role in a large number of biologically important reactions (SIES and KETTERER 1988; TANIGUCHI et al. 1989; VINA 1990). The numerous reactions that GSH participates in can be divided into those involving the γ-glutamyl moiety of the tripeptide and those of the sulfhydryl moiety. Those reactions involving the latter function can be further divided into either oxidation–reduction reactions or nucleophilic reactions. In its reduced form, GSH is a strong nucleophile and can react with electrophiles via a direct Sn2 reaction to form a thioether. These reactions may also be catalyzed by one or more of the cytosolic, microsomal, or mitochondrial GSH *S*-transferase isoenzymes. Most compounds that are conjugated with GSH are ultimately excreted in urine as the corresponding mercapturic acid, which are S-conjugates of *N*-acetylcysteine. Conjugation with GSH has usually been considered a detoxication reaction. The increased water solubility and the active secretion of organic acids by renal tubules greatly facilitates mercapturic acid excretion. However, the principal detoxication function of GSH conjugation, namely, the inactivation of a reactive electrophile by the initial attack of the GSH thiolate anion (REED and MEREDITH 1985), does not necessitate mercapturate formation. Conjugation with GSH has now been implicated in the bioactivation of a variety of chemicals to mutagenic, carcinogenic, and cytotoxic metabolites. This chapter will describe the most recent advances in our knowledge of the mechanism(s) by which xenobiotic conjugations with GSH can result in toxicity.

B. Glutathione-Dependent Activation of Halogenated Alkanes and Alkenes

I. Glutathione-Dependent Mutagenicity

GSH-dependent metabolic activation of 1,2-dichloroethane was demonstrated in the Ames test (BREM et al. 1974; RANNUG et al. 1978). 1,2-

Dicholoroethane was mutagenic only if a post-mitochondrial liver fraction was used, the addition of a pure microsomal fraction being inactive. Thus, metabolic activation was dependent upon enzymes other than those of the microsomal mixed-function oxidases and was subsequently demonstrated to be dependent upon the presence of both GSH and GSH *S*-transferases (Rannug et al. 1978; Rannug and Beije 1979). Moreover, the GSH *S*-transferase-mediated activation of dihaloethanes resulted in the preferential alkylation of DNA and RNA (Guengerich et al. 1980; Sundheimer et al. 1982) rather than of protein. The mechanism of this novel form of metabolic activation appeared to be via the initial enzyme-catalyzed displacement of a chlorine atom by GSH. This reaction gives the *S*-(2-chloroethyl)-GSH conjugate, which subsequently gives rise to the sulfur mustard, or half-mustard. Rearrangement to an electrophilic episulfonium (thiiranium) ion occurs via internal displacement (β-elimination) of the second chlorine atom by the sulfur atom (Fig. 1). The episulfonium ion then interacts with nucleophilic sites on tissue macromolecules. The alkylation of DNA by this mechanism may be responsible for both the mutagenic (Rannug et al. 1978) and carcinogenic (Olson et al. 1973) effects of 1,2-dichloroethane. The carcinogenic and mutagenic potential of such β-halogen thioethers has been recognized for a number of years (Auberbach and Robson 1946).

Insight into the mechanism of the GSH-mediated activation of dihaloalkanes to mutagenic metabolites was obtained from the elegant studies by Van Bladeren et al. (1979, 1980, 1981). Experiments with a series of *S*-(2-haloethyl)-cysteine analogs demonstrated that the GSH-dependent mutagenicity of vicinal dihalogen compounds was also dependent on both the nature and stereochemistry of the substituent. The more heavily substituted the vicinal dihalogen compound, the lower was its mutagenic activity. Introducing a small amount of steric hindrance into the molecule, such as a

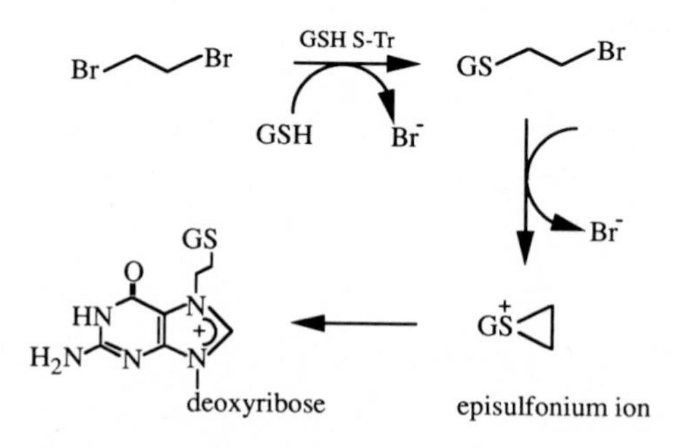

Fig. 1. Glutathione (*GSH*) *S*-transferase (*GSH S*-Tr) catalyzed dehalogenation of dihaloalkanes. The GSH catalyzed addition/elimination of bromine (*Br*) leads to the formation of an *episulfonium ion* that reacts with DNA to form a variety of adducts. The major adduct, *S*-[2-(N^7-guanyl)ethyl]-GSH is illustrated

methyl group, almost completely abolished the mutagenic activity of the conjugate, and the insertion of one or two methylene groups lowered the ratio of DNA binding to GSH conjugation by 100-fold (INSKEEP and GUENGERICH 1984). Thus, although 1,3-dibromopropane and 1,4-dibromobutane are more readily conjugated with GSH than 1,2-dibromoethane, they are less likely to form an equivalent sulfur half-mustard because of the increased chain-length between the two bromine atoms (SMIT et al. 1979). In contrast, the better the leaving group ability of the halogen substituent, the higher the mutagenic effect (VAN BLADEREN et al. 1981). For example, 1,2-dibromoethane undergoes GSH-dependent activation to both mutagenic and carcinogenic metabolites and is far more mutagenic, on a per-dose basis, than 1,2-dichloroethane, even though the *S*-(2-chloroethyl) conjugate is highly mutagenic. Moreover, the specific activity of rat liver GSH *S*-transferases toward 1,2-dichloroethane was much lower than toward 1,2-dibromoethane. Introduction of a second chlorine molecule, as in *S*-(2,3-dichloropropyl)-*N*-acetyl-L-cysteine, increases mutagenic activity, possibily via cross-link formation mediated by the generation of two consecutive episulfonium ions (VAN BLADEREN et al. 1987). However, 1,2-dibromo-3-chloropropane and *tris*-(2,3-dibromopropyl)-phosphate bind less effectively to DNA in vivo than 1,2-dibromoethane (INSKEEP and GUENGERICH 1984). These observations are consistent with those of VAN BLADEREN et al. (1981), who demonstrated that alkyl substitution of vicinal dihalides decreased both the GSH *S*-transferase-catalyzed conjugation of these compounds and their in vitro mutagenicity. Thus, this type of GSH-mediated DNA binding might be expected to be a major process only with vicinal dihalogen compounds.

Although *S*-(2-bromoethyl)GSH is very unstable, it is stable enough to diffuse out of isolated hepatocytes and react with exogenously added DNA (OZAWA and GUENGERICH 1983), even though the estimated half-life of the conjugate is less then 10 s (INSKEEP et al. 1986). The sulfur half-mustard of *S*-(2-chloroethyl)GSH is more stable than the bromo analog and has been isolated in relatively pure form (SCHASTEEN and REED 1983; REED and FOUREMAN 1986). Moreover, the formation of *S*-[2-(N^7-guanyl)-ethyl]GSH occurs in incubation mixtures containing deoxyguanosine and *S*-(2-chloroethyl)GSH; *S*-[2-(N^7-guanyl)ethyl]-L-cysteine was also formed in incubation mixtures containing deoxyguanosine and *S*-(2-chloroethyl)-L-cysteine (FOUREMAN and REED 1987). The latter adduct was detectable at lower concentrations of alkylating agent than was the corresponding GSH adduct, which suggests that *S*-(2-chloroethyl)-L-cysteine is a more potent alkylating agent than *S*-(2-chloroethyl)-GSH.

The major (>95%) DNA adduct formed both in vivo and in isolated hepatocytes from the coincubation of 1,2-dibromoethane and GSH was also identified as *S*-[2-(N^7-guanyl)ethyl]GSH (Fig. 1; OZAWA and GUENGERICH 1983; INSKEEP et al. 1986), and structural (COSY NMR) and kinetic evidence supported the involvement of an episulfonium intermediate in the reaction (PETERSON et al. 1988). A minor (approximately 2%) adduct, *S*-[2-

(N'^1-adenyl)ethyl]GSH, is also formed (KIM and GUENGERICH 1990). S-[2-(N^3-Deoxycytidyl)ethyl]GSH, S-[2-(O^6-deoxyguanosyl)ethyl]GSH, and S-(2-[N^2-deoxyguanosyl]ethyl)GSH have also been identified (<0.2%) as adducts formed in calf thymus DNA treated with 1,2-dibromoethane and GSH (CMARIK et al. 1992). Since the mutagencity of several small alkylating agents appears to lie in their ability to form O^6-guanyl and/or O^4-thymidyl adducts, the carcinogenic and/or toxicologic significance of the N^7-guanyl adducts is unclear. Although several alkylating agents that form only N^7-guanyl adducts appear to be weak mutagens, several lines of evidence suggest that the major S-[2-(N^7-guanyl)ethyl]GSH adduct plays a major role in 1,2-dibromoethane carcinogencity. Thus, S-[2-(N^7-guanyl)ethyl]GSH is mutagenic in bacteria (CMARIK et al. 1992), and structural changes to the GSH moiety have significant effects on the mutagenicity of the adducts (KIM and GUENGERICH 1990).

CMARIK et al. (1992) subsequently investigated the type, site, and frequency of mutagens in a portion of the *lacZ* gene resulting from the in vitro modification of bacteriophage M13mp18DNA with S-(2-chloroethyl)GSH. Using the repair-deficient *Salmonella typhimurium* TA 100 as the test strain, sequence analysis of the resulting mutants demonstrated that the spectrum of mutations consisted primarily of base substitutions, of which G:C to A:T transitions accounted for 70% of the total mutations. Results from the sequence selectivity assay demonstrated that adduct formation occurred at all guanines within the *lacZ* sequence. Consistent with other N^7-guanyl-alkylating agents, adjacent guanines, particularly those within a run of three or more, represented sites of the highest levels of S-[2-(N^7-guanyl)ethyl] GSH adduct formation. Although the data indicated that S-[2-(N^7-guanyl) ethyl]GSH was a mutagenic lesion, not all such adducts were processed to yield mutations. By preparing several oligonucleotides containing the S-[2-(N^7-guanyl)ethyl]GSH lesion, OIDA et al. (1991) were able to show that the pairing of guanine to cytosine was considerably weakened by its N^7-alkylation. However, no evidence for a more favorable interaction with another base was observed. Several reasons for the inability of the N^7-guanyl adduct to form a preferential base pair with thymine in this model, which must occur within the cell in order for the adduct to drive a mutation, have been presented (OIDA et al. 1991).

Studies on the hydrolysis and alkylating activities of S-(2-haloethyl)-L-cysteines demonstrated an increase in hydrolysis rate at alkaline pH. It was suggested that the amine moiety was responsible for this observation, and the formation of 3-(thiomorpholine)-carboxylic acid was proposed as an alternative pathway to the generally accepted hydrolysis mechanism for S-(2-haloethyl)-L-cysteine analogs (SCHASTEEN and REED 1983). In addition, during studies on the interactions of S-(2-haloethyl)-mercapturic acid analogs with plasmid DNA (VADI et al. 1985), it was noted that S-(2-chloroethyl) GSH did not affect supercoiled plasmid DNA. This finding was in marked contrast to the data obtained with S-(2-chloroethyl)-L-cysteine, whereas the

N-acetylated analog was also prevented from interacting with DNA. Blocking the cysteine amine moeity, as in the GSH and mercapturic acid conjugates, decreased the enhanced hydrolysis of *S*-(2-chloroethyl)-L-cysteine under alkaline conditions and thereby prevented the formation of 3-(thiomorpholine)-carboxylic acid (SCHASTEEN and REED 1983). This inhibitory effect is probably responsible for the observed differences in reaction with plasmid DNA exhibited by the different analogs.

1,2-Dibromo-3-chloropropane causes renal necrosis and testicular atrophy in laboratory animals and infertility in humans exposed to the chemical during manufacture. Three DNA adducts of 1,2-dibromo-3-chloropropane have been isolated and characterized as *S*-[*bis*-(N^7-guanylmethyl)methyl]GSH and the two diastereoisomers of *S*-[1-(hydroxymethyl)-2-(N^7-guanyl)ethyl)GSH (HUMPHREYS et al. 1991). Formation of these adducts probably occurs via formation of two consecutive episulfonium ion intermediates with subsequent attack at the unsubstituted methyl carbon. Although these adducts are structurally similar to the major adduct derived from 1,2-dibromoethane, the GSH conjugate of 1,2-dibromo-3-chloropropane was not mutagenic in bacterial assays, but was cytotoxic. Moreover, only low levels of the N^7-guanyl adducts were found in the livers of rats treated with 1,2-dibromo-3-chloropropane, the reason for which is unclear. The cytotoxicity of the GSH conjugate has been attributed to its ability to behave as a cross-linking agent, as evidenced by the formation of the *bis*-guanyl adduct, which appears to be formed more readily between adjacent intrastrand guanines (HUMPHREYS et al. 1990).

II. Cysteine Conjugate *β*-Lyase-Dependent Mutagenicity

Hexachloro-1,3-butadiene (HCBD) is nephrocarcinogenic when chronically administered to rats. Both the GSH (VAMVAKAS et al. 1988a) and cysteine conjugate (DEKANT et al. 1986) of HCBD have been reported to be bacterial mutagens. The mutagenicity of the cysteine conjugate was reduced in the presence of aminooxyacetic acid, an inhibitor of cysteine conjugate *β*-lyase(s). Thus, the mutagenicity of chloroalkenyl cysteine *S*-conjugates is dependent upon *β*-lyase (DEKANT et al. 1986; VAMVAKAS et al. 1988a,b,c, 1989), and such conjugates induced unscheduled DNA synthesis, albeit at a relatively slow rate, in mammalian cell cultures (VAMVAKAS et al. 1988b). Only S-conjugates that are metabolized to thioketenes (see below) appear to be mutagenic. Interestingly, the binding of radiolabeled HCBD was higher to mitochondrial DNA than to nuclear DNA (SCHRENK and DEKANT 1989).

III. Glutathione-Dependent Nephrotoxicity

To understand why the kidney is especially susceptible to the toxicity of mercapturic acid pathway metabolites, an appreciation of the biochemical and physiological functions of the kidney is required. Kidneys possess relatively high activities of the enzymes involved in mercapturic acid biosynthesis, i.e., γ-glutamyl transpeptidase (γ-GT), cysteinylglycine dipeptidase (s), and *N*-acetyltransferases (GOLDSTEIN 1993). The first step in the metabolism of GSH conjugates involves either hydrolysis or transamination by γ-GT and transfer of the γ-glutamyl group to an appropriate acceptor (MEISTER and TATE 1980). γ-GT is an ubiquitous membrane-bound enzyme (TATE 1980), the active site of which is oriented on the outer surface of the cell (HORIUCHI et al. 1978). Kidneys possess the highest level of γ-GT activity, followed by the pancreas, which in the rat has 20% of the level of the kidney (GOLDBAG et al. 1960). Most other tissues have less than 1% of the activity found in the kidney, although it is important to note that γ-GT activity is usually localized to one cell type within an organ and to one area of the membrane, where it may be highly concentrated. The product of the γ-GT-catalyzed reaction is the S-substituted cysteinylglycine dipeptide which, in turn, is subject to hydrolytic cleavage of the glycine residue. Several membrane-bound peptidases may catalyze this reaction (TATE 1980). The detoxication function of mercapturic acid biosynthesis is completed by the transfer of an acetyl group from acetyl coenzyme A to the S-substituted cysteine conjugate, catalyzed by cysteine-thioether *N*-acetyltransferase (DUFFEL and JAKOBY 1982), which is also located in renal proximal tubular cells (HUGHEY et al. 1978). However, whereas γ-GT and dipeptidases are located in the brush border membrane, *N*-acetyltransferase is associated with the heavy microsomal fraction.

In contrast to the detoxication function of the mercapturic acid pathway, the elucidation of the "thiomethyl shunt" pathway (JAKOBY and STEVENS 1984; JAKOBY et al. 1985) provided a biochemical basis upon which to rationalize possible mechanism(s) of GSH S-conjugate-mediated nephrotoxicity. Cysteine conjugate β-lyase(s) catalyze the formation of reactive thiol fragments (see below) from cysteine conjugates of several halogenated alkanes and alkenes via a β-elimination mechanism (TATEISHI et al. 1978; STEVENS and JAKOBY 1983). The enzyme therefore competes with the pathway leading to mercapturic acid formation and plays a major role in the nephrotoxicity of a variety of GSH–cysteine conjugates (see below). Both liver and kidney (BHATTACHARYA and SCHULTZE 1967; STEVENS and JAKOBY 1983) possess β-lyase activity, although the enzymes from these two tissues are not identical (STEVENS and JAKOBY 1983). Liver β-lyase copurifies and possesses characteristics identical to those of kynureninase (STEVENS 1985), whereas both mitochondrial and cytosolic β-lyase activity from rat kidney cortex copurify with glutamine transaminase K (STEVENS et al. 1986). Several gastrointestinal bacteria also possess β-lyase activity (STEVENS and JONES 1989; STEVENS and BAKKE 1990).

The metabolism of haloalkenal and haloalkanal cysteine conjugates by β-lyase(s) has been suggested to be the key step in their bioactivation. β-Lyase is dependent upon pyridoxal phosphate for activity and exhibits activity toward a number of aliphatic and aromatic thioethers of cysteine, including

S-(1,2-dichlorovinyl)-L-cysteine (DCVC; Stevens and Jakoby 1983). Renal β-lyase(s) are localized in both the cytosolic and mitochondrial compartments (Dohn and Anders 1982; Stevens 1985; Lash et al. 1986a). The latter activity is important, because mitochondria appear to be the cellular target of DCVC toxicity (see below), and mitochondrial β-lyase activity was more susceptible to inhibition by aminooxyacetic acid than the cytosolic enzyme. Further fractionation showed that mitochondrial β-lyase activity was localized in the outer mitochondrial membrane (Lash et al. 1986a), although other workers have suggested β-lyase activity to be preferentially localized to the inner mitochondrial membrane (Robbins and Stevens 1986). In addition, a second pathway for the formation of thiol-containing metabolites from cysteine conjugates which involves an initial deamination reaction followed by cleavage of the resultant thiopyruvic acid conjugate has been described (Tomisawa et al. 1986). This activity appears distinct from that catalyzed by β-lyase, at least in liver cytosol. However, the contribution of this pathway to the renal formation of thiol compounds from cysteine conjugates remains to be established. Thus, because of the relatively low activity of renal P-450, the high activity of GSH-related enzymes, and the rapid turnover of GSH, it is likely that GSH-dependent metabolic activation within the kidney has greater toxicological significance than that mediated by the cytochrome(s) P-450.

The ability of the kidney to concentrate tubular fluid also predisposes this organ to toxicity. For example, many organic compounds are secreted into the tubular lumen by organic acid or base transport mechanisms, thereby passing through or accumulating within proximal tubular cells and exposing these cells to relatively high concentrations. Kidneys also remove a large proportion of plasma GSH (Hahn et al. 1978; Griffith and Meister 1979; McIntyre and Curthoys 1980) and as much as 70% of plasma GSH clearance is renal (Haberle et al. 1979). One mechanism for the delivery of GSH and GSH S-conjugates to the kidneys is glomerular filtration. However, although 80% of plasma GSH is removed by the kidney (Haberle et al. 1979), only 25% is removed by the glomeruli. The fraction that enters the tubular lumen is hydrolyzed by γ-GT and cysteinylglycine dipeptidase (see above). A significant amount of circulating GSH is also removed by a nonfiltration mechanism which involves transport into renal cells across the basal–lateral membrane (Rankin and Curthoys 1982; Lash and Jones 1983, 1984). Lash and Jones (1984) characterized an electrogenic, Na^+-coupled, and probenecid-sensitive transport system for the uptake of intact GSH into renal basal–lateral membrane vesicles. A similar mechanism for the delivery of GSH S-conjugates to the kidneys, in addition to glomerular filtration, may also be operating. For example, GSH and GSH S-conjugates undergo a similar pattern of interorgan metabolism (Stevens and Jones 1989), and the same enzymes are responsible for the conversion of both GSH and GSH S-conjugates to cysteine and cysteine S-conjugates, respectively (Jones et al. 1979). In addition, the Na^+-coupled, probenecid-sensitive, basal–lateral-membrane GSH transport system exhibits a broad substrate specificity for γ-glutamyl compounds (LASH and JONES 1984). However, since γ-GT is also found in the basal–lateral membrance of kidney epithelia (SPATER et al. 1982), the relative contribution of Na^+-coupled and γ-GT-mediated GSH transport to total renal plasma GSH clearance is debatable. In vivo evidence suggests that the ability of the kidney to utilize GSH is due to GSH breakdown mediated by γ-GT both in the tubule and basal–laterally (ANDERSON et al. 1980; ABBOT et al. 1984). In either case, it appears that basal–laterally mediated uptake accounts for the ability of the kidney to extract a significant portion of the GSH passing through the renal circulation.

The transport of GSH by renal brush border membrane vesicles, in which γ-GT was inhibited with AT-125 (L(α5*S*)-2-amino-α-chloro-4,5-dihydro-isoxazoleacetic acid), has also been demonstrated (DASS and WELBOURNE 1982). This GSH transport system was dependent upon the membrane potential and involved the transfer of negative charge. Thus, GSH, which is secreted into the tubular lumen by a specific translocase in the luminal membranes or filtered by the glomerulus, may subsequently be degraded by γ-GT and peptidase activities. The resulting free amino acids can then be reabsorbed into tubule cells by the Na^+-dependent transport system in renal cortical brush border membranes. The presence of similar export systems for GSH S-conjugates formed intracellularly has also been demonstrated in erythrocyte membranes (KONDO et al. 1982) and hepatic canalicular plasma membranes (INNOUE et al. 1984). Thus, because of its physiological function and biochemical profile, the kidney is particularly susceptible to the toxicity of GSH–cysteine conjugates.

1. The Role of Renal Transport

GSH conjugation and subsequent metabolism to the cysteine conjugate mediates the nephrotoxicity caused by several halogenated alkanes and alkenes. For example, DCVC, the cysteine conjugate of trichloroethylene (TCE), is a potent nephrotoxicant that produces renal failure characterized by severe proximal tubular necrosis (TERRACINI and PARKER 1965). The transport of *S*-(1,2-dichlorovinyl)GSH (DCVG) was investigated in renal basal–lateral membrane vesicles and isolated kidney cells (LASH and JONES 1985). Vesicular uptake was demonstrated to be Na^+ dependent and was inhibited by GSH, oxidized GSH (GSSG), and γ-glutamyl glutamate, but not by DCVC. This latter observation suggested that the Na^+-dependent DCVG uptake system exhibits specificity for the γ-glutamyl moiety. Conversely, DCVG inhibited the Na^+-dependent uptake of GSH into basal–lateral membrane vesicles, providing evidence that uptake of GSH S-conjugates and GSH was mediated by a common Na^+-dependent mechanism. This Na^+-dependent uptake system was inhibited by probenecid. Probenecid is a selective, competitive inhibitor of organic anion transport (MUDGE 1980) without effect on either energy metabolism or transport carrier synthesis. Probenecid also has no effect on the transport of other substances, such as organic cations or sugars that are also actively accumulated by the kidney.

Adminstration of probenecid (0.175 mmol/kg) also protected against DCVC-mediated nephrotoxicity in vivo, as evidenced by decreased elevations in urinary glucose excretion rates (ELFARRA et al. 1986). The mechanism and polarity of DCVC transport was subsequently investigated in rat kidney cortex membrane vesicles (SCHAEFFER and STEVENS 1982). It was shown that Na^+-dependent transport on the luminal side was responsible for the uptake of cysteine conjugates across the apical membrane. No Na^+-stimulated transport was found on the basal–lateral side, and uptake of DCVC in brush border membrane vesicles was inhibited by a variety of neutral amino acids and cysteine conjugates, but not by polar amino acids. The amino acid transport system L-specific substrate, 2-amino-2-norborane carboxylic acid, was not inhibitory. SCHAEFFER and STEVENS (1982) proposed that the driving force for the apical transport of cysteine conjugates may be the coupling of luminal transport to the Na^+ gradient. DCVC transport was also investigated in the LLC-PK_1 kidney epithelial cell line (SCHAEFFER and STEVENS 1987). In contrast to data obtained using rat kidney cortex membrane vesicles, the accumulation of DCVC into these cells involved the participation of two Na^+-independent transport systems, both of which were inhibited by the L-amino acid transport system. Although several factors might be responsible for the observed differences, it is clear that renal transport plays a key role in GSH–cysteine conjugate-mediated nephrotoxicity. This is exemplified by the fact that stimulation of DCVC uptake into LLC-PK_1 cells resulted in enhanced toxicity.

As noted above, 1,2-dichloroethane undergoes GSH-dependent bioactivation to mutagenic metabolites. 1,2-Dichloroethane also causes both kidney and liver damage. *S*-(2-Chloroethyl)-cysteine, a metabolite of 1,2-dichloroethane, also produces acute proximal tubular necrosis and elevations in blood urea nitrogen (BUN) and urinary glucose concentrations (ELFARRA et al. 1985). Protection against *S*-(2-chloroethyl)-cysteine-mediated renal necrosis was afforded by prior adminstration of probenecid (ELFARRA et al. 1985). In contrast, it was suggested that the GSH conjugate of 1,2-dichloroethane, *S*-(2-chloroethyl)GSH, rather than the cysteine conjugate, was responsible for the renal toxicity of 1,2-dichloroethane (KRAMER et al. 1987). Administration of *S*-(2-chloroethyl)-GSH (220 μmol/kg i.v.) to rats produced renal lesions that were similar to those produced by the cysteine analog. To determine whether metabolism of *S*-(2-chloroethyl)GSH to its corresponding cysteine conjugate was responsible for the toxicity, animals were pretreated with AT-125, an inhibitor of several glutamine-utilizing enzymes (WEBER 1983) including γ-GT (ALLEN et al. 1980; REED et al. 1980). AT-125 has been used to probe the role of γ-GT in the nephrotoxicity of a number of GSH conjugates. However, AT-125 pretreatment did not protect animals against the *S*-(2-chloroethyl)-GSH-induced renal

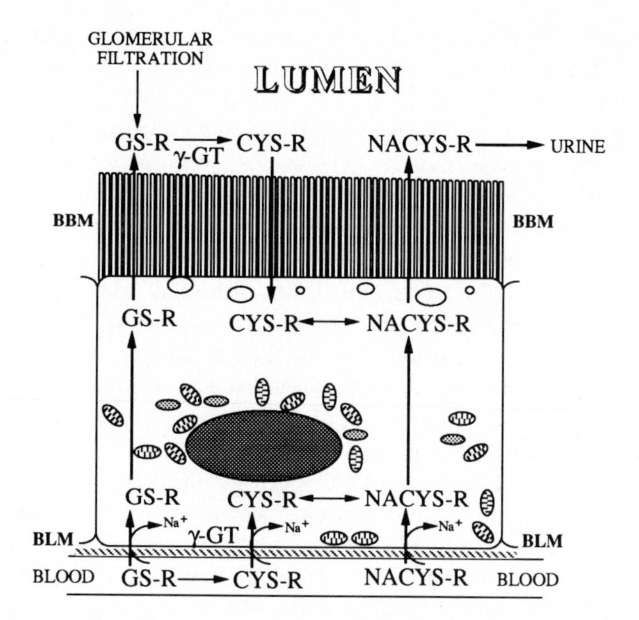

Fig. 2. Renal transport of mercapturic acid pathway metabolites. Glutathione conjugates (*GS-R*) that are filtered at the glomerulus are metabolized by γ-glutamyl transpeptidase (*γ-GT*) and dipeptidases at the brush border membrane (*BBM*) to the corresponding cysteine conjugates (*CYS-R*), which are transported into proximal tubular cells by an amino acid carrier system. GS-R that is not filtered at the glomerulus can either be transported into cells intact, via a sodium-dependant, probenecid-sensitive transport system, or metabolized by γ-GT at the basalateral membrane (*BLM*) followed by uptake of the CYS-R conjugate via a sodium-coupled transport system. Mercapturates (*NACYS-R*) are transported into proximal tubular cells from blood via the organic anion transporter present on the BLM

lesion, rather it potentiated the toxicity (Kramer et al. 1987). It is becoming increasingly apparent that multiple transport processes exist for the proximal tubular accumulation of GSH conjugates (Fig. 2; Monks and Lau 1987).

HCBD causes kidney toxicity in both rats and rabbits (Kociba et al. 1977; Lock and Ishmael 1979). Although renal organic ion transport was inhibited in slices from rats treated with HCBD in vivo (Nash et al. 1984), little effect was observed when renal slices were exposed directly to HCBD; in other words, HCBD was not a direct-acting nephrotoxicant (Berndt and Mehendale 1979). Moreover, HCBD-induced nephrotoxicity could be prevented by cannulation of the bile duct (Nash et al. 1984), indicating a role for hepatic metabolism and biliary excretion in HCBD nephrotoxicity. Administration of HCBD to rats also caused a depletion of liver, but not kidney, nonprotein sulfhydryl groups (Kluwe et al. 1985; Lock and Ishmael 1981), suggesting that conjugation of HCBD with GSH in the liver and subsequent transport of the conjugate to the kidney may play a role in toxicity. The formation of the GSH conjugate was catalyzed by the microsomal GSH *S*-transferases, which were more active than the soluble enzymes at catalyzing the addition–elimination reaction of HCBD with GSH, resulting in the formation of the vinyl-GSH adduct *S*-(1,2,3,4,4-pentachloro-1,3-butadienyl) GSH (PCBG; WOLF et al. 1984). PCBG was subsequently identified as both an in vitro and in vivo metabolite of HCBD (WOLF et al. 1984; NASH et al. 1984) and was suggested to be responsible for HCBD-mediated nephrotoxicity, via metabolism to the corresponding cysteine conjugate and β-lyase-catalyzed conversion to the ultimate nephrotoxic metabolite (WOLF et al. 1984). In support of this sequence of events, PCBG, *S*-(1,2,3,4,4-pentachloro-1,3-butadienyl)-cysteine (PCBC), and *S*-(1,2,3,4,4-pentachloro-1,3-butadienyl)-*N*-acetylcysteine (PCBNAC) were all shown to cause a similar toxicity. Moreover, PCBC was a substrate for β-lyase (GREEN and ODUM 1985). Adminstration of either PCBC or PCBNAC to rats or mice resulted in acute renal necrosis of the pars recta segment of the proximal tubule (LOCK and ISHMAEL 1985), that portion of the nephron associated with organic anion secretion (ROCH-RAMEL and WEINER 1980). Administration of probenecid (500 μmol/kg) to rats reduced the renal cortex to plasma ratio of PCBNAC, reduced the renal cortical concentration of PCBNAC, and reduced renal cortical covalent binding (LOCK and ISHMAEL 1985). Moreover, probenecid also protected rats against the nephrotoxicity of PCBNAC, PCBC, and PCBG, as assessed by decreases in BUN and by histological examination of kidney slices (LOCK and ISHMAEL 1985). These data supported the hypothesis that the renal cortical accumulation and selective proximal tubular toxicity of HCBD and its sulfur conjugates were related to a carrier-mediated transport system.

2. The Role of Renal Bioactivation

Nephrotoxic GSH–cysteine conjugates are converted to electrophilic metabolites that readily alkylate tissue components. Recent investigations on the chemical nature of these intermediates and of the consequences of their interaction with cellular constituents have provided considerable insight into the mechanism of toxicity of these conjugates. The elegant studies recently reported by DEKANT and colleagues have provided insight into the chemical nature of the reactive intermediates generated by the β-lyase-catalyzed metabolism of haloalkenal cysteine conjugates. Whereas chloroalkenes were metabolized exclusively to chlorovinyl S-conjugates (DEKANT et al. 1989), fluoroalkenes predominantly formed alkyl S-conjugates (ANDERS et al. 1988). Thus the β-lyase-catalyzed metabolism of *S*-(1,2,2-trichlorovinyl)-L-cysteine yields 1,2,2-trichlorovinylthiol, which may rearrange to either thionoacyl chloride or a thioketene (see Fig. 3 in DEKANT et al. 1993). Recent evidence suggests that 2-chlorovinylthiols yield thioketenes as the exclusive products. Similarly, a thioketene is the most likely acylating intermediate formed during the β-lyase-catalyzed metabolism of PCBC. The β-lyase catalyzed metabolism of *S*-(2-chloro-1,1,2-trifluoroethyl)-L-cysteine (CTFC) yields 2-

chloro-1,1,2-trifluoroethane thiol as the initial metabolite (Dekant et al. 1987). Subsequent loss of hydrogen fluoride produces the corresponding thionoacetyl fluoride (see Fig. 4 in Dekant et al. 1993), the putative thionoacyl reactive metabolite that covalently binds to tissue macromolecules. Indeed, Harris et al. (1992) provided indirect evidence for the generation of thioacyl fluorides in vivo by demonstrating the presence of N^{ε}-(chlorofluoroacetyl)-L-lysine in renal protein from *S*-(1-chloro-1,2,2-trifluoroacetyl)-L-cysteine treated rats.

Hayden et al. (1991a) investigated the potential selectivity of S-(1,1,2,2-tetra-fluoroethyl)-L-cysteine (TFEC) protein adduct formation immunohistochemically, utilizing antibodies raised against adducts which were formed by the interaction of halothane metabolites with protein and which cross-reacted with the TFEC adducts. The anti-trifluoroacetyl antibody raised against the halothane adducts apparently displays a high specificity for halogen-substituted epsilon amides of lysine. Hayden et al. (1991b) subsequently demonstrated the formation of difluorothionoacetyl adducts with nucleophiles within bovine serum albumin (BSA) and provided convincing evidence that a major portion of the stable adducts are formed with lysine residues, by isolating and characterizing an N^2-acetyl-N^{ε}-(difluorothionoacetyl)lysine adduct. Two intriguing and insightful observations led to the proposal that the reaction of difluorothionoacetyl fluoride with protein occurs first at tyrosine or histidine residues followed by transfer of the difluorothionoacetyl group to lysine, which then forms a stable thioamide adduct. Thus, although lysyl residues on BSA were particularly reactive toward β-lyase-catalyzed metabolites of TFEC, *N*-acetyllysine was a poor inhibitor of TFEC binding to BSA; in addition, the binding of TFEC metabolites to BSA was facilitated by the presence of either N^{α}-acetylhistidine or *N*-acetyltyrosine. The nucleophilic catalysis of stable lysyl adduct formation by histidine and tyrosine was supported by experiments which demonstrated that a variety of primary amines all inhibited TFEC binding to BSA, whereas a variety of nucleophilic catalysts, such as aromatic amines and phenols, all facilitated TFEC binding.

These studies demonstrated that the difluorothionoamide protein adducts formed in vitro also arise as a consequence of TFEC metabolism in vivo. Sodium dodecyl sulfate polyacrylamide gel electrophoresis (SDS-PAGE) immunoblot analysis of kidney homogenate from TFEC-treated rats revealed the presence of three major immunoreactive proteins with molecular masses of 87, 79, and 61 kDa that were principally localized to the mitochondrial fraction (Hayden et al. 1991b). Thus, despite the presence of both cytosolic and mitochondrial forms of β-lyase, lysyl-directed adducts of TFEC were predominantly localized within mitochondria. Immunoreactivity occured within 6 h of TFEC treatment and persisted for 2–3 days, after which immunoreactive protein could no longer be detected. Immunohistochemical staining of kidney slices revealed that although immunoreactive protein could be detected in cells that appeared to be morphologically healthy, death occurred only in those cells that contained the TFEC protein adducts (HAYDEN et al. 1991b). Although the nature of the immunoreactive proteins is not known, cysteine conjugates have been shown to inhibit a number of enzymes, including pyruvate and 2-oxoglutarate dehydrogenases (STONARD and PARKER 1971), succinate/cytochrome c, isocitrate dehydrogenase (LASH and ANDERS 1987), and lipoyl dehydrogenase (LOCK and SCHNELLMAN 1990). These enzyme complexes are comprised of subunits with molecular masses in the range of the identified immunoreactive proteins; however, the potential interaction of TFEC metabolites with cysteine residues within the same and additional proteins precludes a definitive assignment of the immunoreactive proteins. For example, TFEC metabolites are reactive toward thiol nucleophiles such as GSH and *N*-acetylcysteine (HAYDEN et al. 1991a). However, the anticipated difluorodithioester adducts could not be isolated, and blocking the single cysteinyl sulfhydryl group in BSA had no effect on the binding of TFEC metabolites. Thus, the apparently unstable nature of difluorodithioester protein adducts precludes an informed discussion on the potential role of these adducts in TFEC-mediated nephrotoxicity (HAYDEN et al. 1991a). STONARD (1973) reported that reactive metabolites of DCVC inhibited hepatic GSH reductase and mitochondrial lipoyl dehydrogenase. Subsequently, LOCK and SCHNELLMAN (1990) demonstrated that PCBNAC, TFEC, and DCVC were noncompetitive inhibitors of both renal cytosolic GSH reductase and of mitochondrial lipoyl dehydrogenase. Since both these enzymes possess essential sulfhydryl group(s) within their active sites, it seems likely that the reactive metabolites generated by β-lyase target these groups to cause enzyme inhibition. Interestingly, the reactive metabolites of PCBC, TFEC, and DCVC appear to exhibit a certain degree of selectivity in terms of their ability to inhibit these sulfhydryl-dependent enzymes. For example, the reactive thiol generated from the metabolism of PCBC inhibited GSH reductase activity more effectively than it inhibited lipoyl dehydrogenase. Conversely, TFEC and DCVC were relatively poor inhibitors of GSH reductase, but effective inhibitors of lipoyl dehydrogenase (LOCK and SCHNELLMAN 1990).

In addition to forming covalent adducts with both DNA and protein, CTFC and TFEC also form phospholipid adducts in isolated kidney mitochondria (HAYDEN et al. 1992). Lipids extracted from both [^{35}S]CTFC- and [^{35}S]TFEC-exposed mitochondria contained almost 42% of the mitochondria-associated [^{35}S]-radiolabel. The major adducts of both cysteine conjugates were thioamides of phosphotidylethanolamine, which presumably form via nucleophilic attack of the polar amine head group on the reactive thionoacyl halide arising from the β-lyase-catalyzed cleavage of the conjugate (HAYDEN et al. 1992). Thionoacyl halides have been shown to react with a variety of nucleophilic amines (DEKANT et al. 1987; COMMANDEUR et al. 1989; HAYDEN et al. 1991a,b). PCBC and DCVC also gave rise to lipid-derived adducts, although structural elucidation of these adducts was not possible.

3. Mechanisms of Toxicity

Although it is well established that many chemicals require metabolism to reactive intermediates which can bind to cellular macromolecules, the events that occur subsequent to bioactivation, and which ultimately lead to cell death, are less clearly understood. Thus, although DCVC is metabolized by β-lyase to a reactive intermediate that covalently binds to tissue macromolecules and although the extent of such binding correlates with the extent of cell death, the challenge is to link these two events. Results from a number of laboratories studying a variety of chemicals suggest that a cascade of interrelated events are triggered following bioactivation and that several of these events can be inhibited in the absence of any effects on the interaction of the reactive intermediate with tissue macromolecules. Such findings have led some investigators to claim that not only can covalent binding be dissociated from cell death, but that covalent binding per se is unrelated to cytotoxicity. A more likely scenario suggests that covalent binding is necessary, but insufficient for cell death to occur, and several groups have attempted to elucidate events that link covalent binding to cell death. CHEN et al. (1992) showed that DCVC induced the expression of the growth arrest and DNA damage-inducible gene *gadd153* and suggested that the covalent binding of DCVC metabolites to cellular macromolecules served as the signal for gene induction. The inhibition of DCVC metabolism and covalent binding prevented *gadd153* induction. Events subsequently triggered by *gadd153* and their relationship to cytotoxicity remain to be determined.

Studies with rat kidney slices and isolated mitochondria demonstrated that both mitochondrial respiration and 2-oxoacid dehydrogenases were inhibited by DCVC (PARKER 1965; STONARD and PARKER 1971). These data suggested that mitochondria may be the cellular target of DCVC-mediated toxicity and were consistent with the finding that β-lyase activity is present in rat kidney mitochondria (see above). DCVC and CTFC, both of which require metabolism by β-lyase for their expression of toxicity, were potent inhibitors of state 3 respiration in isolated mitochondria. Furthermore, the addition of aminooxyacetic acid (AOA), an inhibitor of pyridoxal phosphate-requiring enzymes, protected against this toxicity. However, neither *S*-(1,2-dichlorovinyl)-DL-α-methyl cysteine nor the α-methyl analog of CTFC were toxic to mitochondria. The α-methyl cysteine analogs, which lack a proton on the α-carbon, cannot be metabolized by the pyridoxal phosphate-dependent β-lyase. The effects of these cysteine conjugates were further investigated in rat kidney mitoplasts (inner mitochondrial plasma membrane fractions). Since renal mitochondrial β-lyase appears to be localized in the outer mitochondrial membrane, mitoplasts should be devoid of β-lyase activity. Consistent with these findings, neither DCVC nor CTFC had any effect on state 3 respiration in mitoplasts.

A potential role for lipid peroxidation in DCVC-mediated nephrotoxicity was suggested by SCHMID et al. (1983). Treatment of mice with DCVC caused a dose-dependent elevation in renal cortical malondialdehyde (MDA) concentrations and increased the exhalation of ethane. In addition, DCVC also increased MDA formation in renal cortical slices (BEUTER et al. 1989) and in isolated renal cortical mitochondria (LASH and ANDERS 1987), but not when incubated with isolated rat renal epithelial cells (LASH and ANDERS 1986). Moreover, DCVC had no effect on GSH concentrations and only weakly inhibited GSH synthesis. Since no effects on GSSG concentrations or lipid peroxidation were observed, oxidative stress was ruled out as a possible mechanism of DCVC toxicity (LASH et al. 1986b). However, in contrast to the effects of DCVC on intact isolated kidney cells, DCVC did cause GSH oxidation and lipid peroxidation in isolated renal mitochondria. The relevance of these findings to DCVC toxicity in vivo is unclear, but, as noted by LASH and ANDERS (1987), the effects of a localized mitochondrial oxidative stress induced by DCVC may be limited in intact cells by the presence of extramitochondrial protective processes. The initial effects of DCVC on renal mitochondria appear to involve the inhibition of energy metabolism (succinate-linked state 3 respiration) and GSH oxidation. CHEN et al. (1990) subsequently showed that several antioxidants, especially *N,N'*-diphenyl-*p*-phenylene-diamine (DPPD) inhibited DCVC-induced lipid peroxidation and cytotoxicity in several in vitro renal epithelial cell models. DPPD did not prevent depletion of nonprotein thiols. The protective effects of DPPD occurred in the absence of any effects on the covalent binding of DCVC. These authors concluded that DCVC (and CTFC and TFEC) was toxic to renal epithelial cells via a combination of covalent binding, depletion of nonprotein thiols, and lipid peroxidation.

GROVES et al. (1991a) extended these findings by investigating the role of lipid peroxidation in DCVC-, PCBC-, TFEC-, and CTFC-mediated toxicity in isolated suspensions of rabbit renal proximal tubules. The results from these studies suggested that iron-dependent lipid peroxidation may contribute to PCBC-, DCVC-, and CTFC-mediated cytotoxicity. However, the finding that cytotoxicity occurred even when the iron was chelated and lipid peroxidation inhibited indicated that nonperoxidative events probably play a major role in the cytotoxicity of these conjugates. Indeed, TFEC-mediated cytotoxicity to isolated rabbit renal proximal tubules was independent of lipid peroxidation (GROVES et al. 1991a).

A potential role for Ca^{2+}-deregulation in cysteine conjugate-mediated cytotoxicity was suggested by JONES et al. (1986), who showed that treatment of isolated renal epithelial cells with $100\,\mu M$ PCBG resulted in blebbing of the plasma membrane, which was associated with the loss of mitochondrial Ca^{2+} and a concomitant elevation of cytosolic Ca^{2+}. Cellular respiration was also inhibited, with a marked depletion of cellular adenosine triphosphate (ATP) concentrations, suggesting that mitochondria were also a subcellular target of PCBG metabolites. The subcellular toxicity of PCBC was subsequently investigated in isolated rabbit renal proximal tubules (SCHNELLMAN et al. 1987). PCBC severely inhibited mitochondrial function, uncoupled oxidative phosphorylation, and caused an initial increase in mitochondrial respiration. Subsequent alterations in mitochondrial respiration were a consequence of severe mitochondrial damage, characterized by the inhibition of state 3 respiration, inhibition of cytochrome C/cytochrome oxidase, and electron transport. PCBC also caused a dose-dependent loss in mitochondrial Ca^{2+} retention, which was associated with a sudden collapse of the mitochondrial membrane potential in isolated rat renal cortical mitochondria (Wallin et al. 1987). Lash et al. (1986a) also reported that the inhibition of cellular respiration in isolated rat kidney cells caused by DCVC was associated with the release of mitochondrial Ca^{2+}. DCVC had no effect on microsomal Ca^{2+} sequestration, but did inhibit mitochondrial Ca^{2+} sequestration. DCVC also inhibited cellular respiration (see above) and decreased mitochondrial Ca^{2+} sequestration and cellular ATP concentrations (Lash and Anders 1987). Vamvakas et al. (1990) subsequently investigated the relationship between perturbations in intracellular Ca^{2+} homeostasis and DCVC toxicity in LLC-PK_1 cells. Exposure of growth-arrested (serum-depleted and hydroxyurea-treated) cells to $100\,\mu M$ DCVC resulted in an approximately fivefold increase in average $[Ca^{2+}]$ within 24 h. At this time, it appeared that the mitochondria contained lower $[Ca^{2+}]$ than other cellular compartments, although the loss of Ca^{2+} was not associated with a concomitant collapse of the mitochondrial membrane potential. However, the maintenance of the mitochondrial membrane potential allows continued Ca^{2+} cycling, as the effluxed Ca^{2+} is subject to reuptake via the mitochondrial Ca^{2+} uniporter. The continued efflux of Ca^{2+} eventually results in a depletion of mitochondrial energy stores (reduced pyridine nucleotides) and in a complete collapse of the mitochondrial membrane potential. Indeed, by 72–96 h, Vamvakas et al. (1990) observed the complete absence of rho-123 staining in DCVC-treated LLC-PK_1 cells.

4. The Role and Regulation of β-Lyase

The activity of cysteine conjugate β-lyase can be regulated at the chemical (Stevens 1985; Stevens and Jones 1989), biochemical (Stevens et al. 1986; Stevens and Jones 1989), and physiological level (Stevens and Jones 1989), and the fraction of any given cysteine conjugate that undergoes β-lyase-mediated bioactivation will therefore depend upon a combination of factors. The cysteine conjugate may be excreted unchanged from the body or it can be converted to the corresponding mercapturic acid by *N*-acetyltransferase (Duffel and Jakoby 1982). The mercapturate may then be excreted or the cysteine conjugate regenerated by the action of a deacetylase enzyme (Suzuki and Tateishi 1981). Thus, the intracellular concentration of a cysteine conjugate will depend upon the relative activity of these two enzymes and the relative rate of export from the cell of both the mercapturate and cysteine conjugate. Indeed, Commandeur et al. (1989) reported that a high in vivo N-deacetylation to N-acetylation ratio for *S*-(1,1,2,2-terafluoroethyl)-*N*-acetyl-L-cysteine and TFEC may result in a rapid depletion of acetyl CoA. As the availability of this cofactor becomes rate limiting, accumulation of the cysteine conjugate may cause a greater fraction of the conjugate to be converted to reactive metabolites by the action of β-lyase. Alternatively, another pathway for the formation of thiol-containing metabolites from cysteine conjugates has been described (TOMISAWA et al. 1986), involving an initial deamination reaction followed by cleavage of the resulting thiopyruvate conjugate. This activity appears distinct from that catalyzed by β-lyase, at least in liver cytosol. The role of this enzyme in the bioactivation of cysteine conjugates in the kidney remains to be determined. Finally, the thiol may be inactivated by thiol *S*-methyltransferase (BREMER and GREENBERG 1961; BORCHARDT and CHENG 1978; WEISIGER and JAKOBY 1979) to form an inactive thiomethyl compound. Thus, the factors regulating the formation of a potentially reactive thiol from a cysteine conjugate are complex, and prediction of the potential toxicity of any given GSH or cysteine conjugate will be difficult to determine.

Although the balance of the evidence supports the hypothesis that β-lyase plays a major role in haloalkenal- and haloalkanal-mediated nephrotoxicity, there remain a few inconsistencies with this scenario. For example, based on immunohistochemical studies, JONES et al. (1988) were unable to demonstrate a correlation between the renal tubular distribution of β-lyase and the site-selective injury caused by DCVC. This finding suggested that factors other than β-lyase, such as the tubular distribution of renal transporters, also contribute to the segment specificity of toxic cysteine conjugates. In contrast, MCFARLANE et al. (1989) demonstrated a correlation between the immunohistochemical localization of β-lyase and HCBD nephrotoxicity. When HAYDEN and STEVENS (1990) investigated the metabolism and covalent binding of a series of nephrotoxic cysteine conjugates in isolated rat kidney mitochondria, they demonstrated that both DCVC and PCBC inhibited state 3 respiration, but only PCBC uncoupled oxidative phosphorylation. Moreover, although AOA prevented both DCVC- and PCBC-mediated inhibition of state 3 respiration, the uncoupling effects of PCBC were insensitive to the effects of AOA. GROVES et al. (1991b) also showed that whereas AOA decreased the effects of PCBC on rabbit renal proximal tubule respiration and cellular ATP concentrations, it did not prevent cytotoxicity. In addition, cell death occurred despite the ability of AOA to inhibit the covalent binding of PCBC to tubular protein by almost 90% (GROVES et al. 1991b). AOA also blocked the covalent binding of [^{35}S]PCBC to mitochondrial macromolecules by 93%, but was ineffective at preventing PCBC-mediated decreases in mitochondrial function (HAYDEN and STEVENS 1990).

Recently, SAUSEN and ELFARRA (1990) reported the presence of a reduced nicotinamide adenosine dinucleotide phosphate (NADPH)-dependent cysteine conjugate *S*-oxidase activity in both renal and hepatic microsomal preparations. The *S*-oxidase activity was characterized utilizing *S*-benzyl-L-cysteine as the substrate, and sulfoxidation of this substrate was inhibited by

DCVC, suggesting that DCVC may also be a substrate for the microsomal flavin-containing monooxygenase (FMO). In contrast, PARK et al. (1992) were unable to demonstrate S-oxidation of *S*-benzyl-cysteine in rat kidney microsomes, although purified hog liver FMO catalyzed the S-oxygenation of *cis*- and *trans*-1,3-dichloropropene. Differences in the sensitivity of the assays for *S*-oxidase activity may account for this discrepancy (SAUSEN et al. 1993). Subsequently, SAUSEN et al. (1993) reported the characterization and purification of a flavin-dependent *S*-benzyl-L-cysteine oxidase activity from rat liver and kidney microsomes. Immunological characterization of the purified rat kidney *S*-oxidase and determination of the N-terminal amino acid sequence suggest that this enzyme exhibits properties similar to that of the known FMO 1A1 isozymes.

SAUSEN and ELFARRA (1991) also investigated the reactivity of *S*-(1,2-dichlorovinyl)-L-cysteine sulfoxide and demonstrated the formation of *S*-[1-chloro-2-(*S*-glutathionyl)vinyl]-L-cysteine sulfoxide in the presence of GSH. In addition, when the sulfoxide of DCVC was administered to rats, both hepatic and renal nonprotein sulfhydryls were significantly reduced and the sulfoxide was a more potent nephrotoxicant than DCVC itself. Moreover, methimazole, a competitive inhibitor of the FMOs, reduced DCVC nephrotoxicity when administered 30 min prior to DCVC (SAUSEN et al. 1992). PARK et al. (1992) were also able to inhibit *S*-(*cis*-3-chloro-2-propenyl)-*N*-acetyl-L-cysteine and *S*-(*cis*-3-chloro-2-propenyl)-L-cysteine toxicity to isolated rat renal epithelial cells by inclusion of methimazole, leading these authors also to infer a role for FMO in cytotoxicity. Methimazole also prevented cephaloridine-mediated oxidation of nonprotein thiols, suggesting that its antioxidant properties may also be involved in its cytoprotective effects (SAUSEN et al. 1992). Interestingly, AOA (0.5 m*M*) did not inhibit *S*-(*cis*-3-chloro-2-propenyl)-L-*N*-acetylcysteine (0.1 m*M*) cytotoxicity in $LLCPK_1$ cells (PARK et al. 1992), suggesting that this mercapturate is bioactivated by a β-lyase-independent pathway.

C. Glutathione- and Quinone-Mediated Toxicities

The reactivity of quinones resides in their ability to undergo "redox cycling" and to create an oxidative stress (SMITH et al. 1985) and/or to react directly with cellular nucleophiles such as protein and nonprotein sulfhydryls (JOCELYN 1972; FINLEY 1974). GSH is the major nonprotein sulfhydryl present in cells (REED and MEREDITH 1985). The addition of a thiol to the double bond of a quinone represents nucleophilic addition to an α,β-unsaturated carbonyl. Although there are several studies on the addition of sulfur nucleophiles to quinones, there is little information available on the biological consequences of these reactions. Recent evidence indicates that a variety of quinone-thioethers possess biological (re)activity (MONKS and LAU 1992).

I. Biological (Re)activity of Quinone-Thioethers

One of the earliest examples of quinones retaining biological activity following the addition of thiols was published by FRIEDMANN et al. (1948), who showed that the GSH conjugate of menadione retained the antimitotic properties of the unsubstituted quinone in cultures of chick fibroblasts. In contrast, addition of GSH to 1,4-naphthoquinone effectively eliminated the activity of this quinone. NICKERSON et al. (1963) subsequently showed little difference between the reduction potentials of menadione and its GSH conjugate, and a similar lack of effect was reported for the one-electron reduction potentials (WILSON et al. 1986). In contrast, BUFFINTON et al. (1989) found that the addition of GSH and *N*-acetylcysteine to menadione resulted in a lowering of the redox potential. The addition of cysteine to 3,4-dihydroxyphenylalanine (dopa) also lowered the oxidation potential of dopa by about 45–50 mV (HANSSON et al. 1980; ITO et al. 1980). Thus, cystein-*S*-yl-dopa is easier to oxidize than dopa itself. Metabolism of 2-bromo-3-(glutathion-*S*-yl)hydroquinone through the mercapturic acid pathway also has significant effects on the ease of oxidation of the intermediates (MONKS and LAU 1990; LAU and MONKS 1991). Thus, the activity of γ-GT appeared to facilitate oxidation of the quinol moiety. Oxidation of 2-bromohydroquinone (2-BrHQ) is therefore exquisitely regulated by its passage through the mercapturic acid pathway. The potential toxicological significance of this relationship has been discussed (MONKS and LAU 1990).

Both the GSH and *N*-acetylcysteine conjugates of menadione retain the ability to redox cycle, with the concomitant formation of reactive oxygen species (WEFERS and SIES 1983; BROWN et al. 1991). In this respect, the conjugation of menadione with GSH cannot be considered a true detoxication reaction, although excretion of the quinone is facilitated by conjugation with GSH, as the conjugate is actively excreted from liver cells (SIES 1988; SIES et al. 1989). The formation of reactive oxygen species from menadione and its GSH conjugate was enhanced in the presence of dicumarol, an inhibitor of NAD(P)H quinone: oxidoreductase (DT-diaphorase), suggesting that both compounds were substrates for two-electron reduction by this enzyme (WEFERS and SIES 1983). This was later confirmed when several quinone–GSH conjugates, including 2-methyl-3-(glutathion-*S*-yl)-1,4-naphthoquinone, were shown to be effective substrates for DT-diaphorase (BUFFINTON et al. 1989).

II. Enzyme Inhibition by Quinone-Thioethers

The rather unique bifunctional nature of quinone-thioethers apparently contributes to their ability to interact with several enzymes that have either quinones as their usual substrates and/or GSH as a cofactor. For example "NADP-linked" 15-hydroxyprostaglandin dehydrogenases (WESTBROOK et al. 1977) which catalyze oxidoreduction at the 9 and 15 positions of various prostaglandins (HASSID and LEVINE 1977; LIN and JARABAK 1978) exhibit carbonyl reductase activity toward a variety of other substrates. Thus, several quinones (JARABAK et al. 1983), including menadione and toluquinone (CHUNG et al. 1987a), are reduced by these enzymes far more effectively than the prostaglandins. The placental NADP-linked 15-hydroxyprostaglandin dehydrogenase also contains a GSH-binding site located close to the active site of the enzyme (CHUNG et al. 1987b). In fact, the km of the GSH conjugates of menadione and toluquinone for NADP-linked 15-hydroxyprostaglandin dehydrogenase were two- and tenfold lower, respectively, than the quinones (CHUNG et al. 1987a). Both of the quinone-thioethers were also mixed-type inhibitors of prostaglandin B_1 oxidation with IC_{50} values in the n*M* range. JARABAK (1991) has shown that the placental carbonyl reductase also catalyzes redox cycling of 2-methyl-3-(glutathion-*S*-yl)-1,4-naphthoquinone and 4-(glutathion-*S*-yl)-1,2-naphthoquinone and noted that "it is unlikely that polycyclic aromatic hydrocarbon quinones or their GSH adducts are inert products of detoxication in tissues that contain the carbonyl reductase or another enzyme with similar substrate specificity."

The GSH *S*-transferases utilize GSH for the enzymatic detoxication of a large number of electrophiles, as reviewed in Chap. 3 of this volume. Several forms of GSH *S*-transferase have been found to be overexpressed in a variety of tumor cells that have either inherent or acquired resistance to cytotoxic chemotherapeutic agents (HAYES et al. 1990). Thus, the GSH *S*-transferases play an important role in the development of the so-called drug-resistant phenotype. Several quinones are known to inhibit the GSH *S*-transferases (MOTOYAMA et al. 1978; DIERICKX 1983). GSH conjugates of several halogenated quinones have been synthesized as potentially specific irreversible inhibitors of the GSH *S*-transferases (VOS et al. 1989; VAN OMMEN et al. 1988, 1989, 1991). The quinone-thioethers exhibited reactivity toward sulfhydryl groups and affinity for the GSH-binding site of the enzyme. Thus, the GSH conjugates inactivated GSH *S*-transferase more rapidily than the corresponding quinones; 2,6-dichloro-3-(glutathion-*S*-yl)-1,4-benzoquinone caused a 41-fold increase in the rate of enzyme inhibition when compared to the parent quinone. Quinone-thioethers might provide a basis for the development of drugs designed to augment the efficacy of those chemotherapeutic agents, primarily alkylating agents, that are substrates for GSH *S*-transferases within tumor-resistant cells. The potential for quinone-thioethers to interact with other enzymes that possess either a GSH-binding site and/or cysteine residues critical for enzyme function clearly exists, and the toxicological consequences of these interactions deserve attention.

III. Free Radical Formation by Quinone-Thioethers

At least seven GSH conjugates have been isolated from the peroxidase-catalyzed oxidation of *p*-phenetidine, several of which exist in both oxidized and reduced forms and are readily interconverted by redox processes (Ross et al. 1985). Interestingly, the peroxidase-mediated covalent binding of *p*-phenetidine to protein was inhibited by the addition of GSH (ANDERSSON et al. 1983), whereas binding to DNA was enhanced by GSH (ANDERSSON et al. 1984). Subsequently, a diglutathionyl adduct of *N*-(4-ethoxy-phenyl)-*p*-benzoquinoneimine was shown to bind to calf thymus DNA (LARSSON et al. 1988). Although neither the mechanism of this binding nor the nature of the adduct have been elucidated. POTTER et al. (1986) demonstrated that the GSH conjugate of acetaminophen was readily oxidized to a free radical intermediate. The cytotoxicity of 2,6-dimethoxyquinone to lens epithelial cells in culture was also related to reactive oxygen generation and the formation of a stable free radical (WOLFF and SPECTOR 1987). The latter was dependent upon the conjugation of 2,6-dimethoxyquinone with GSH. The electron spin resonance (ESR) spectrum of the radical was consistent with the one-electron oxidation of 2,6-dimethoxy-3,5-(di-glutathion-*S*-yl) hydroquinone. Since oxidant-mediated alterations to lens constituents may play an important role in the pathogenesis of human cataracts (AUGUSTEYN 1981; SPECTOR 1984), the redox activity of 2,6-dimethoxy-3,5-(di-glutathion-*S*-yl)hydroquinone was considered to be consistent with this hypothesis (WOLFF and SPECTOR 1987). The cataractogenicity of naphthalene has been attributed to 1,2-naphthoquinone (REES and PIRIE 1967; WELLS et al. 1989) and possibly to its cysteine and GSH conjugates, which were very effective at catalyzing the oxidation of ascorbic acid (REES and PIRIE 1967). Ascorbate levels decrease precipitously during cataract formation. ESR studies also support the formation of GSH-conjugated semiquinone free radicals from 2-methyl-3-(glutathion-*S*-yl)-1,4-naphthoquinone, 3-(glutathion-*S*-yl)-1,4-naphthoquinone, 2,3-(di-glutathion-*S*-yl)-1,4-naphthoquinone, and 2-*S*-glutathion-*S*-yl)-1,4-benzoquinone (TAKAHASHI et al. 1987; RAO et al. 1988).

IV. Quinone-Thioether-Catalyzed Methemoglobinemia

Methemoglobinemia is a common event following in vivo exposure to aminophenols (KIESE 1974). Elegant studies by EYER and KIESE (1976) demonstrated that when GSH concentrations within red blood cells were high, the binding of oxidized 4-(*N*-dimethyl)aminophenol (DMAP) to hemoglobin was decreased, with the concomitant formation of 4-*N*-dimethyl-*p*-amino-2,3,6-(tri-glutathion-*S*-yl)phenol. In contrast, when GSH concentrations were low, the principal product was 4-dimethyl-*p*-amino-2, 6-(di-glutathion-*S*-yl)phenol (*bis*-[G*S*yl]-DMAP), which also catalyzed the formation of ferrihemoglobin. However, substantial differences occurred in the kinetics of ferrihemoglobin formation from DMAP and *bis*-(G*S*yl)-DMAP. Thus, superoxide anion radicals, produced in the reaction between *bis*-(G*S*yl)-DMAP and hemoglobin, or in the autooxidation of *bis*-(G*S*yl)-DMAP, increased the rate of ferrihemoglobin formation by *bis*-(G*S*yl)-DMAP, a portion of which could be attributed to hydrogen peroxide produced via dismutation of superoxide anion. In contrast, superoxide anion and hydrogen peroxide could not be detected in the reaction of DMAP with hemoglobin. In addition, the autoxidation of *bis*-(G*S*yl)-DMAP was more rapid than its oxidation by oxyhemoglobin, whereas DMAP oxidation by oxyhemoglobin was greater than its rate of autoxidation. DMAP has also been shown to be nephrotoxic in rats and cytotoxic to isolated rat kidney tubules (Kiese et al. 1975; Szinicz and Weger 1980). Whether quinone-thioethers are involved in this toxicity is not known.

V. Quinone-Thioethers and Nephrotoxicity

Conjugation of some quinones with GSH, however, does result in the formation of potent, and selective, nephrotoxicants (Monks et al. 1985, 1988a; Lau et al. 1988a, 1990; Mertens et al. 1991). Thus, the nephrotoxicity of bromobenzene in rats is probably mediated via its metabolism to 2-bromo-(di-glutathion-*S*-yl)hydroquinone (Monks et al. 1985, 1988a). As little as 10 μmol/kg of 2-bromo-(di-glutathion-*S*-yl)hydroquinone is sufficient to cause glucosuria, enzymuria, and renal proximal tubular cell necrosis. GSH conjugates of 1,4-benzoquinone are also nephrotoxic. In particular, 2,3,5-(tri-glutathion-*S*-yl)hydroquinone (10–20 μmol/kg) caused severe renal proximal tubular necrosis when administered to male Sprague-Dawley rats (Lau et al. 1988a). Hydroquinone has been reported to be nephrocarcinogenic in male rats, as shown by marked increases in tubular cell adenomas of the kidneys (Kari 1989; Shibata et al. 1991). Based upon the known nephrotoxicity of several GSH conjugates of hydroquinone, in particular, 2,3,5-(tri-glutathion-*S*-yl)hydroquinone, such adducts may contribute to hydroquinone-mediated nephrocarcinogenicity. 2,3,5-(triglutathion-*S*-yl)hydroquinone has been reported as an in vivo metabolite of hydroquinone in the rat (Hill et al. 1993).

The tissue selectivity of 2-bromo-(di-glutathion-*S*-yl)hydroquinone and 2,3,5-(tri-glutathion-*S*-yl)hydroquinone appears to be a consequence of their targeting to renal proximal tubule cells by brush border γ-GT. Thus, inhibition of γ-GT by pretreatment of animals with AT-125 protected them against both 2-bromo-(di-glutathion-*S*-yl)hydroquinone-mediated (Fig. 3; Monks et al. 1988a) and 2,3,5-(tri-glutathion-*S*-yl)hydroquinone-mediated (Lau et al. 1988a) nephrotoxicity. The uptake of 2-bromo-(di-glutathion-*S*-yl)hydroquinone by freshly isolated kidney slices was also inhibited by AT-125 (Lau et al. 1988b). Probenecid, which inhibited the toxicity of PCBNAC, DCVC, and *S*-(2-chloroethyl)GSH (see above), did not protect against either 2-bromo-(di-glutathion-*S*-yl)hydroquinone-mediated (Fig. 3) or 2,3,5-(tri-GSH-*S*-yl)hydroquinone-mediated nephrotoxicity (Monks et al. 1988a; Lau et al. 1988a).

The nephrotoxicity of GSH and cysteine-conjugated halogenated alkanes and alkenes is dependent upon their metabolism by cysteine conjugate β-lyase (see above). However, β-lyase does not appear to play a major role in

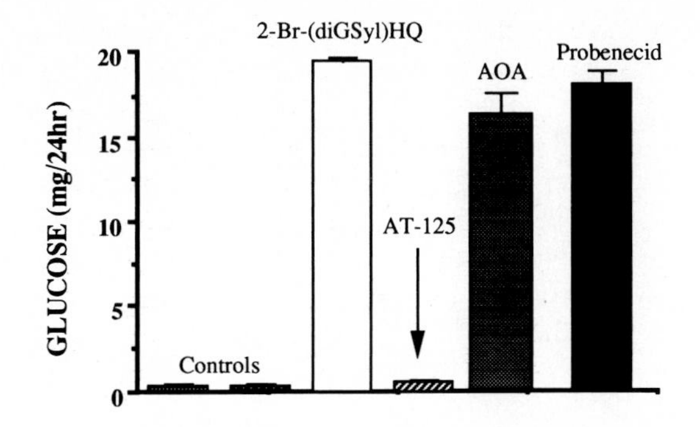

Fig. 3. 2-Bromo-(diglutathion-*S*-yl)hydroquinone (*2-Br-(diGSyl)HQ*)-mediated nephrotoxicity is prevented by inhibition of γ-glutamyl transpeptidase, but not by inhibition of either cysteine conjugate β-lyase or of the organic anion transporter. 2-Br-(diGSyl)HQ-mediated nephrotoxicity (□) was monitored by the urinary excretion of *glucose*. *AT-125* (L(α5*S*)-2-amino-α-chloro-4,5-dihydroisoxazoleacetic acid; (▨) was used to inhibit γ-glutamyl transpeptidase, aminooxyacetic acid (*AOA*); (▩) to inhibit cysteine conjugate β-lyase, and *probenecid* (■) to inhibit the organic anion transporter

either 2-Br-(di-glutathion-*S*-yl)hydroquinone-mediated (Fig. 3) or 2,3,5-(tri-glutathion-*S*-yl)hydroquinone-mediated nephrotoxicity. For example, pretreatment of rats with AOA did not protect animals from 2-Br-(di-glutathion-*S*-yl)hydroquinone-mediated nephrotoxicity (Monks et al. 1988a), and the nephrotoxicity of 6-bromo-2,5-dihydroxy-thiophenol, a putative β-lyase-catalyzed metabolite of 2-bromo-3-(glutathion-*S*-yl)hydroquinone, was dependent upon the quinone, rather than the thiol, function (Monks et al. 1988b). Studies on the relative toxicity of 2-Br-(di-cystein-*S*-yl)hydroquinone and 2-Br-(di-*N*-acetylcystein-*S*-yl)-hydroquinone provided further evidence against a major role for β-lyase. Both 2-Br-(di-cystein-*S*-yl)hydroquinone and 2-Br-(di-*N*-acetylcystein-*S*-yl)hydroquinone caused renal proximal tubular necrosis in male rats. However, whereas the toxicity of the cysteine conjugate was not inhibited by pretreatment of animals with either AOA or probenecid, which was consistent with findings obtained with 2-Br-(di-glutathion-*S*-yl)hydroquinone, inhibition of β-lyase and the organic anion transporter did protect against the toxicity of the mercapturate (Monks et al. 1991). The data were consistent with earlier studies which indicated that metabolism of 2-Br-(di-glutathion-*S*-yl)hydroquinone to the mercapturate was a minor metabolic pathway. Mercapturic acid formation from quinone–GSH conjugates may also be limited by the ability of either the cysteinylglycine and/or cysteine conjugate to undergo an oxidative cyclization reaction that results in formation of a 1,4-benzothiazine (Fig. 4). This reaction can therefore channel the products of the γ-GT-catalyzed metabolism of quinone–GSH conjugates away from the classic mercapturic acid pathway (Monks et al. 1990).

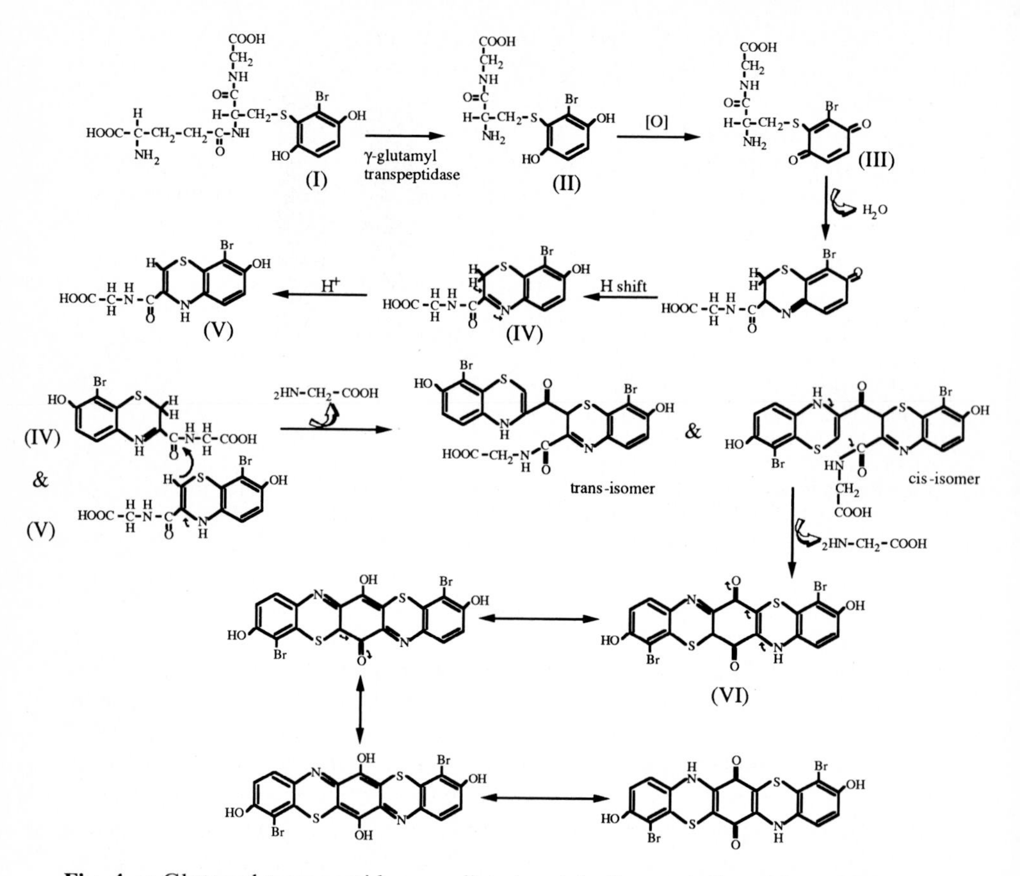

Fig. 4. γ-Glutamyl transpeptidase-mediated metabolism and disposition of 2-bromo-3-(glutathion-*S*-yl)hydroquinone (from MONKS and LAU 1992, with permission). 2-Bromo-3-(glutathion-*S*-yl)hydroquinone (*I*) is metabolized by γ-glutamyl transpeptidase to the corresponding dipeptide, 2-bromo-3-(cystein-*S*-ylglycine)hydroquinone (*II*). The dipeptide is readily oxidized to 2-bromo-3-(cystein-*S*-ylglycine)-1,4-benzoquinone (*III*). The quinone carbonyl condenses with the free cysteinyl amino group to yield a cyclic quinoneimine intermediate (*IV*) that rearranges via a hydride shift to give the corresponding 1,4-benzothiazine (*V*). Elimination of glycine and coupling of the carbon atoms *ortho* to the nitrogen atom in one benzothiazine (*V*) and *ortho* to the sulfur atom in the second benzothiazine (*VI*) results in formation of the dimeric 2,3-*bis*-(1,4-benzothiazine) (*VIII*). The dimer can readily tautomerize to one of several forms which can undergo further coupling to melanin-like polymers

Experiments with [^{14}C]-labeled GSH conjugates of 2-BrHQ demonstrated that the majority of the reactive metabolites generated from these conjugates are a consequence of oxidation to the corresponding quinone (MONKS et al. 1988a). Thus, ascorbic acid significantly decreased the in vitro covalent binding of the conjugates. To examine this question in more detail, the GSH conjugates of 2,5-dichloro-1,4-benzoquinone and tetrachloro-1,4-

benzoquinone were synthesized (MERTENS et al. 1991). These conjugates have certain similarities to the 2-BrHQ and HQ conjugates, the major difference being that they reside in the quinone form. However, when administered by intravenous injection to rats, 2,5-dichloro-3-(glutathion-*S*-yl)hydroquinone and 2,5,6-trichloro-3-(glutathion-*S*-yl)hydroquinone, were more potent nephrotoxicants than 2,5-dichloro-3-(glutathion-*S*-yl)-1,4-benzoquinone and 2,5,6-trichloro-3-(glutathion-*S*-yl)-1,4-benzoquinone (MERTENS et al. 1991). The quinone-thioethers probably react extensively with extra-renal nucleophiles, including plasma proteins, decreasing the effective dose delivered to the kidney. Interestingly, the nephrotoxicity of both 2,5-dichloro-3-(glutathion-*S*-yl)hydroquinone and 2,5,6-trichloro-3-(glutathion-*S*-yl)hydroquinone was potentiated by inhibition of γ-GT with AT-125 (MERTENS et al. 1991).

4-Aminophenol causes acute renal proximal tubular necrosis following administration to rats (GREEN et al. 1969; NEWTON et al. 1982). GARTLAND et al. (1989) demonstrated that either depletion of hepatic GSH by pretreatment of animals with buthionine sulfoximine, or cannulation of the bile duct to decrease the delivery of hepatic metabolites to the kidney, afforded protection against 4-aminophenol nephrotoxicity, suggesting a role for GSH conjugation in 4-aminophenol nephrotoxicity. Indeed, oxidation of 4-aminophenol to the quinoneimine and reaction with GSH gave rise to several isomeric, multisubstituted conjugates (ECKERT et al. 1990). Subsequently, FOWLER et al. (1991) demonstrated that 4-amino-3-(glutathion-*S*-yl)-phenol reproduced 4-aminophenol nephrotoxicity in male Fischer 344 rats at doses three- to fourfold lower than that of 4-aminophenol. KLOS et al. (1992) subsequently identified 4-amino-2-(glutathion-*S*-yl)phenol, 4-amino-3-(glutathion-*S*-yl)-phenol, 4-amino-2,5-(di-glutathion-*S*-yl)phenol, and 4-amino-2,3,5 (or 6)-(tri-glutathion-*S*-yl)-phenol in the bile of Wistar rats following administration of 4-aminophenol (100 mg/kg; i.p.). The latter three conjugates were all capable of causing cytotoxicity when incubated with rat kidney cortical cells, and the toxicity was prevented by inhibition of γ-GT.

2-Methyl-3-(*N*-acetylcystein-*S*-yl)-1,4-naphthoquinone, but not 2-methyl-3-(glutathion-*S*-yl)-1,4-naphthoquinone, produced renal proximal tubular necrosis when administered to male Sprague-Dawley rats (LAU et al. 1990). Consistent with these observations, only the mercapturate, and not the GSH conjugate of menadione was cytotoxic when incubated with isolated rat kidney cortical epithelial cells (BROWN et al. 1991). The differences between the mercapturate and GSH conjugate of menadione are most likely related to the ability of the latter to undergo γ-GT-catalyzed oxidative cyclization and 1,4-benzothiazine formation (BROWN et al. 1991). This reaction eliminates the reactive quinone function from the molecule and prevents redox cycling of the thioether. In contrast, the presence of the *N*-acetyl group in the mercapturate effectively prevents the cysteinyl amino group from condensing with the quinone carbonyl group. Consequently, 2-methyl-3-(*N*-acetylcystein-*S*-yl)-1,4-naphthoquinone retains the ability to redox cycle with the concomitant formation of reactive oxygen species (BROWN et al. 1991). The GSH conjugate of menadione (600 μM) has been shown to cause toxicity in the isolated perfused rat kidney (REDEGELD et al. 1989).

3-*Tert*-butyl-4-hydroxyanisole increases the formation of preneoplastic and neoplastic foci in rat kidney (TSUDA et al. 1984), and thioether metabolites have been reported in rat urine (TAJIMA et al. 1991). 2-*Tert*-butylhydroquinone, a metabolite of 3-*tert*-butyl-4-hydroxyanisole, is oxidized in rat liver microsomes and in the presence of GSH forms 2-*tert*-butyl-5-(glutathion-*S*-yl)hydroquinone and 2-*tert*-butyl-6-(glutathion-*S*-yl)hydroquinone (TAJIMA et al. 1991). Whether the GSH conjugates are involved in the carcinogenic effects of 3-*tert*-butyl-4-hydroxyanisole remains to be determined.

VI. Quinone-Thioethers and Neurotoxicity

Defects in catecholamine metabolism have also been implicated in several neurological disorders. For example, a defect in the metabolism of the neurotransmitter 5-hydroxytryptamine (serotonin: 5-HT) has been implicated in various neurodegenerative, neuropsychiatric, and behavioral disorders (WOOLEY and SHAW 1954). Thus, 5-HT may be converted to several polyhydroxylated metabolites (MCISSAC and PAGE 1959; ERICKSEN et al. 1960), including 5,6- and 5,7-dihydroxytryptamine, both of which have been shown to be potent neurotoxicants (BAUMGARTEN et al. 1971, 1972a,b). Serotonergic abnormalities have been reported extensively in dementia of the Alzheimer type (PERRY et al. 1983; BOWEN et al. 1983; PALMER et al. 1987), and the cerebrospinal fluid (CSF) of Alzheimer patients apparently contains a product with properties consistent with an oxidized form of 5-HT (BOWEN et al. 1983) suggested to be tryptamine-4,5-dione (MATSON et al. 1984). Tryptamine-4,5-dione caused the release of 5-HT from serotonergic neurons (CHEN et al. 1989) similar to that caused by 5,6-dihydroxytryptamine, a known neurotoxicant (WOLF and BOBIK 1988). Thus, tryptamine-4,5-dione might also exhibit neurodegenerative properties and possibly play a role in the etiology of Alzheimer's disease. However, GSH is present in relatively high concentrations (2 mM) throughout the brain (SLIVKA et al. 1987) and it has been suggested that the release of 5-HT mediated by tryptamine-4,5-dione may be a consequence of its interaction with GSH or protein sulfhydryls (CHEN et al. 1989). At physiological pH, tryptamine-4,5-dione reacts rapidly with GSH to form 7-*S*-(glutathionyl)-tryptamine-4,5-dione (WONG and DRYHURST 1990). Moreover, a putative GSH conjugate of tryptamine-4,5-dione has been identified from an acid-soluble extract of rat brain homogenate (CHEN et al. 1989), and it has been suggested that 7-*S*-(glutathionyl)-tryptamine-4,5-dione may in fact be the species responsible for the neurodegenerative effects of tryptamine-4,5-dione (WONG and DRYHURST 1990), although this remains to be determined.

Several oxidases catalyze the oxidation of 5,6-dihydroxytryptamine to its corresponding *ortho*-quinone (SINGH and DRYHURST 1991). In the presence of GSH, the *ortho*-quinone forms 4-(glutathion-*S*-yl)-5,6-dihydroxytryptamine, which can undergo further oxidation and GSH conjugation to 4,7-(di-glutathion-*S*-yl)-5,6-dihydroxytryptamine and 4,4′-(di-glutathion-*S*-yl)-2,7′-*bis*-(5,6-dihydroxytryptamine). Further reaction between 4-(glutathion-*S*-yl)-tryptamine-5,6-dione and 4,7-(di-glutathion-*S*-yl)-5, 6-dihydroxytryptamine gives 4,7,4′-(tri-glutathion-*S*-yl)-2,7′-*bis*(5,6-dihydroxytryptamine). The susceptibility of the initial conjugate to further oxidation and the reactivity of the quinone–GSH conjugates toward sulfhydryl groups suggests that these metabolites may exhibit neurotoxic properties.

The amphetamine analogs, 3,4-(methylenedioxy)amphetamine and 3, 4-(methylenedioxy)-methamphetamine are serotonergic neurotoxins that undergo enzymatic demethylenation to 3,4-dihydroxyamphetamine (α-methyldopamine) and 3,4-dihydroxymethamphetamine (*N*-methyl-α-methyldopamine; Fig. 5; FUKUTO et al. 1991; LIN et al. 1992). In NG 108-15 cells (a murine blastoma–glioma hybrid cell line), α-methyldopamine was metabolized via oxidation to the corresponding *ortho*-quinone followed by conjugation with GSH (Fig. 5; PATEL et al. 1991). Rat liver microsomes also metabolized 3,4-(methylenedioxy)methamphetamine to the corresponding

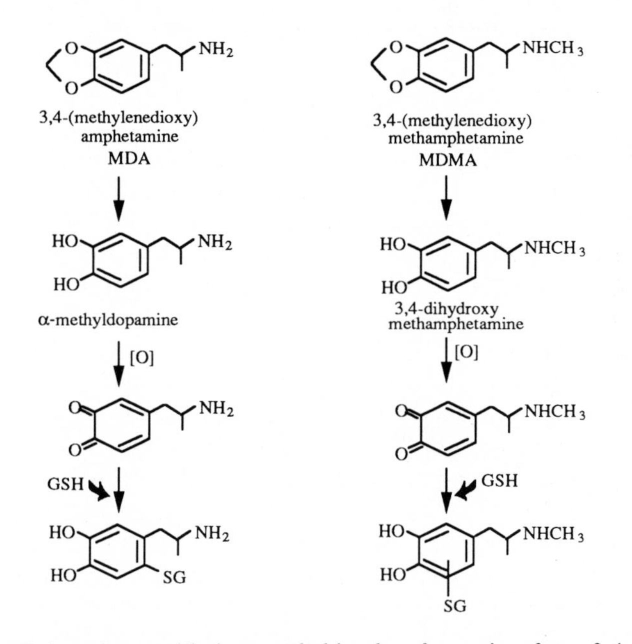

Fig. 5. Demethylenation, oxidation, and thioether formation from 3,4-(methylenedioxy)-amphetamine (*MDA*) and *3,4-(methylenedioxy)methamphetamine (MDMA)* (from MONKS and LAU 1992, with permission)

catechol, followed by *ortho*-quinone formation and GSH conjugation (Fig. 5; HIRAMATSU et al. 1990). The potential role, if any, of the quinone-thioether metabolites of these amphetamine analogs in neurotoxicity has yet to be established.

VII. Quinone-Thioethers and Alcoholism?

COLLINS (1982) suggested that a variety of tetrahydroisoquinoline alkaloids, which are elevated in the brains of chronic alcoholics, may undergo oxidation to neurotoxic metabolites and play a role in the various physical and behavioral changes that accompany chronic alcoholism (COHEN and COLLINS 1970). For example, salsolinol (1,2,3,4-tetrahydro-1-methyl-6,7-isoquinoline

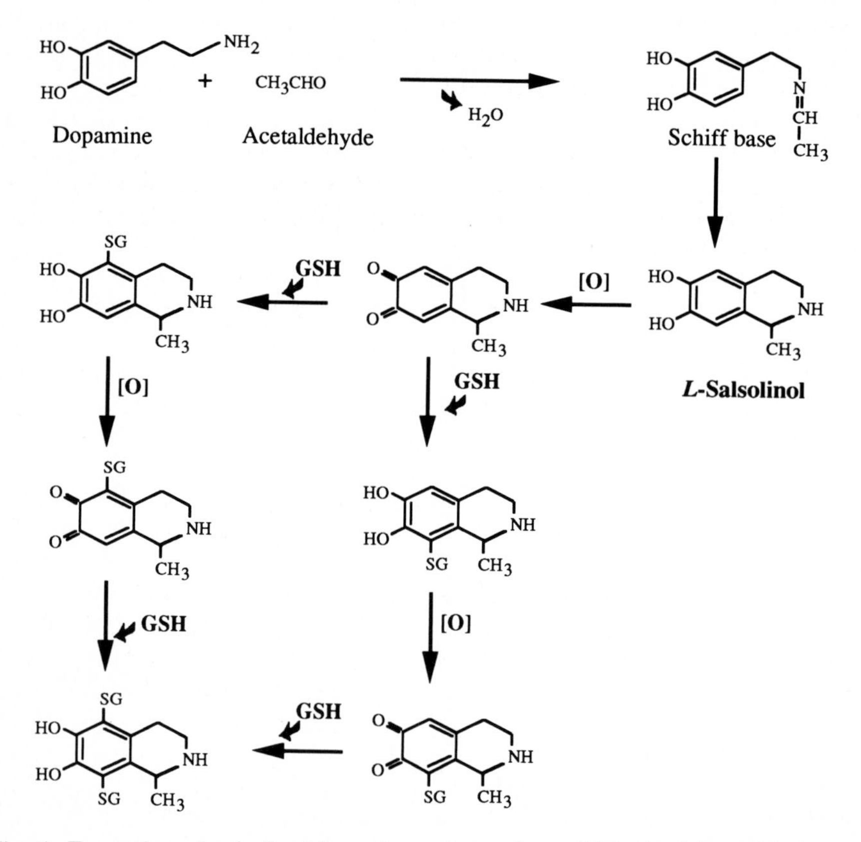

Fig. 6. Formation of *salsolinol* from *dopamine* and *acetaldehyde*, followed by oxidation and thioether formation. Condensation of dopamine with acetaldehyde gives rise to a *Shiff base*, which rearranges to the tetrahydroisoquinoline alkaloid, salsolinol. Salsolinol may undergo both enzymatic and non-enzymatic oxidation to the ortho-quinone, followed by glutathione (*GSH*) conjugation. The initial thioether may also undergo oxidation, with subsequent formation of the *bis*-substituted conjugate

diol) is formed via condensation of dopamine with acetaldehyde (Fig. 6; WHALEY and GOVINDACHARI 1951), a metabolite of ethanol, and concentrations of salsolinol are elevated in discrete regions of the brain in rats which chronically consume ethanol (SJOQUIST et al. 1982; MYERS et al. 1984; MATSUBARA et al. 1987). FA and DRYHURST (1991a,b) subsequently studied the electrochemical and enzymatic oxidation of salsolinol and showed that it was readily oxidized to a variety of products following initial oxidation to the *ortho*-quinone. In the presence of GSH, the *ortho*-quinone underwent nucleophilic attack to yield the 5-S- and 8-S-conjugates, both of which were further oxidized to the 5,8-*bis*-glutathionyl conjugate (FA and DRYHURST 1991a; Fig. 6).

It has also been suggested that chronic consumption of alcohol results in increased concentrations of acetaldehyde, inhibition of aldehyde dehydrogenase, and accumulation of 3,4-dihydroxyphenylacetaldehyde, a dopamine metabolite, which then condenses with dopamine to form tetrahydropapaveroline (Fig. 7; DAVIS and WALSH 1970), an alkaloid that demonstrates addictive properties in rats (MYERS and MELCHIOR 1977). Tetrahydropapaveroline was readily oxidized by a variety of oxidases and peroxidases to a diquinone intermediate, which, in the presence of GSH gave 1,2,3,4-tetrahydro-1-[(6-*S*-glutathionyl-3,4-dihydroxyphenyl)-methyl]-6,7-isoquinolinediol (Fig. 7; ZHANG and DRYHURST 1991). The conjugate was also further oxidized, followed by addition of a second molecule of GSH to 1,2,3,4-tetrahydro-[6-*S*-glutathionyl-3,4-dihydroxyphenyl)-methyl-]8-*S*-glutathionyl-6,7-isoquinoline-diol (ZHANG and DRYHURST 1991; Fig. 7). Thus, oxidation of tetrahydropapaveroline within the brain could cause toxicity either indirectly, via depletion of GSH concentrations, or directly, via the concomitant formation of potentially neurotoxic quinone-thioethers.

VIII. γ-Glutamyl Transpeptidase and Quinone-Thioether-Mediated Toxicities

The potential for quinone-thioethers to cause toxicity to cells other than those of the renal proximal tubules and expressing high γ-GT activity has been discussed (MONKS and LAU 1989, 1992). γ-GT is also present in embryonic yolk sac, and enzyme activity increases with gestational age, suggesting that the developing yolk sac might be at risk from maternal exposure to quinone-thioethers. Indeed, ANDREWS et al. (1993) reported that in vitro exposure of embryos having intact visceral yolk sacs to 2-Br-6-(glutathion-*S*-yl)hydroquinone (120 μM) caused significant decreases in yolk sac diameter, crown to rump length, head length, total protein, developmental score, and somite number and a significant increase in the percent of abnormal embryos. Embryos exposed to 2-Br-(diglutathion-*S*-yl)hydroquinone (80 μM) had significantly lower developmental scores, and at 120 μM, embryos also exhibited significantly lower yolk sac diameters with a

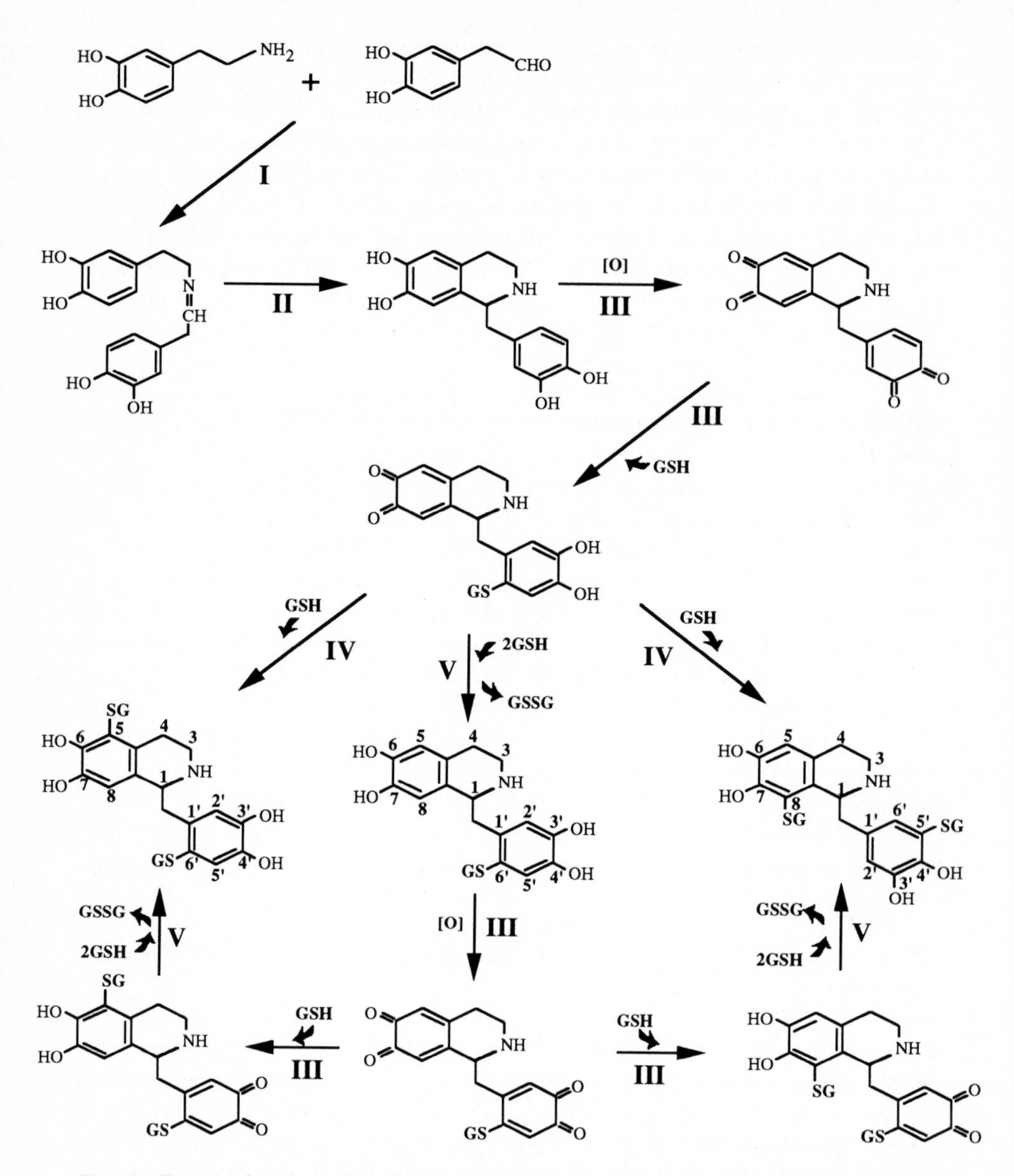

Fig. 7. Tetrahydropaveroline formation from dopamine and its deaminated metabolite, 3,4-dihydroxyphenylacetaldehyde, followed by oxidation and thioether formation. Tetrahydropaveroline is probably formed via condensation of dopamine with 3,4-dihydroxy-phenylacetaldehyde (I & II) the monoamine oxidase-catalyzed metabolite of dopamine. It has been suggested that high levels of acetaldehyde, resulting from chronic alcohol consumption, inhibit aldehyde dehydrogenase, causing the accumulation of 3,4-dihydroxyphenylacetaldehyde (Davis and Walsh 1970), which then condenses with dopamine. Tetrahydropaveroline is readily oxidized (III) and in the presence of glutathione (*GSH*) forms a variety of mono- and *bis*-substituted thioethers (IV & V) *GSSG*, glutathione disulfide

higher percentage of abnormalities. Studies on the potential in vivo developmental toxicity of 2-Br-(diglutathion-*S*-yl)hydroquinone were complicated by maternal toxicity (ANDREWS et al. 1993). The ability of γ-GT to predispose certain cells to the adverse effects of quinone-thioethers might have some potential chemotherapeutic applications. For example, γ-GT is widely used as a marker of preneoplastic lesions in the liver during chemical carcinogenesis (PERAINO et al. 1983), and abnormally high levels of γ-GT were also observed in tumors of a variety of tissues, including hepatocellular carcinomas (FIALA et al. 1976; WILLIAMS et al. 1980), malignant squamous carcinomas of the skin (DEYOUNG et al. 1978), squamous cell carcinomas of the buccal pouch epithelium (SOLT 1981), adenocarcinomas of the lungs (DEMPO et al. 1981), and some mammary tumors (JAKEN and MASON 1978). Suffice it here to note that such toxicity can be modulated by a variety of factors, including the relative activities of cysteine conjugate *N*-acetyltransferase and the corresponding *N*-deacetylase, the relative activities of one- and two-electron reductases, and the availability of various antioxidants, such as ascorbic acid, GSH, and NAD[P]H. The combination of all these factors will determine both species and tissue susceptibility of γ-GT-containing cells to the toxicity of quinone-thioethers. However, it is clear that quinone-thioethers possess a variety of biological and toxicological activity (MONKS and LAU 1992). The ubiquitous nature of quinones and the high concentrations of GSH within cells virtually guarantees that humans will be exposed to the potential adverse effects of the resulting quinone-thioethers. Knowledge of the disposition of quinone-thioethers will, therefore, be an important prerequiste to understanding their mechanism of action and studies on the occurrence and biological and toxicological activity of quinone-thioethers will be an important area for future research.

D. Reversible Glutathione Conjugations and Their Toxicological Significance

Recently, a new class of toxic GSH conjugates has been described in which the parent compound is in equilibrium with its GSH conjugate. These reactions are of particular toxicological significance because they provide a means by which a reactive molecule may initially be detoxified via conjugation with GSH, only for release of the reactive moiety to occur distal to its site of formation. A succinct and insightful review of these reactions has been published (BAILLIE and SLATIER 1991).

GSH may also play a role in the delivery of some heavy metals to the kidney. For example, both methylmercury and inorganic mercury are carried in blood to the kidney as complexes with GSH (NAGANUMA et al. 1988; TANAKA et al. 1990). Renal methylmercury concentrations were reduced, and urinary methylmercury excretion increased in animals treated with AT-125, implicating a role for γ-GT in renal methylmercury accumulation (NAGANUMA et al. 1988). In addition, renal methylmercury uptake can occur through the basolateral membrane, via the inorganic anion transport system (TANAKA et al. 1992). In contrast, cadmium is believed to be delivered to the kidney as a complex with metallothionein (FOULKES 1978), although renal uptake of cadmium can be demonstrated in the presence of cysteine and GSH (FELLEY-BOSCO and DIEZI 1987; FOULKES and BLANCK 1990). The relative importance of the metallothionein and GSH delivery systems in heavy metal-mediated nephrotoxicity requires clarification.

I. Isothiocyanates

Isothiocyanates are naturally occurring compounds (FENWICK et al. 1982) which are of toxicological interest, since amyl isothiocyanate has been shown to be a bladder carcinogen in rats (DUNNICK et al. 1982), whereas benzyl isothiocyanate exhibits anticarcinogenic activity (WATTENBURG 1981). These compounds are extensively metabolized via conjugation with GSH, since most of the urinary metabolites are derived from the mercapturate pathway (BRUSEWITZ et al. 1977; MENNICKE et al. 1983). Isothiocyanates are relatively unstable and react readily with a variety of nucleophiles. The reaction with thiols is reversible (DROBNICA et al. 1977), the dithiocarbamate being in equilibrium with the parent compound. For example, the mercapturate derived from benzyl isothiocyanate is unstable, and in urine containing this metabolite, free isothiocyanate is released (BRUSEWITZ et al. 1977). The thiol conjugates of amyl and benzyl isothiocyanate were subsequently demonstrated to exhibit toxicity almost identical to that of the parent compounds. Thiol conjugates of amyl isothiocyanate were just as toxic as amyl isothiocyanate, whereas benzyl isothiocyanate was more toxic than its thiol conjugates (BRUGGEMAN et al. 1986). In a clonogenic assay, the benzyl derivatives were slightly more toxic than the amyl derivaties, and in both instances the cysteine conjugates were more potent than the GSH conjugates, the mercapturates exhibiting the least toxicity (BRUGGEMAN et al. 1986). Since the position of the dithiocarbamate–isothiocyanate equilibrium is influenced by pH and concentration of the reactants, it is possible that the isothiocyanates become conjugated with GSH at one site and subsequently, when conditions of pH and GSH concentrations are favorable, become released at a second site. Thus, amyl isothiocyanate exerts its carcinogenic activity in the bladder of the rat (DUNNICK et al. 1982), where the pH of urine is usually basic, favoring release of free isothiocyanate from its mercapturic acid pathway metabolites, which are readily excreted in urine.

The mechanism of both allyl and benzyl isothiocyanate cytotoxicity probably involves the thiocarbamoylation of nucleophilic sites in cellular membranes and other macromolecules (TEMMINK et al. 1986). Morphological studies demonstrated that the thiol conjugates exhibited similar effects to those produced by the free isothiocyanates, consistent with the role of reversible conjugation. The isothiocyanates caused an initial blebbing and swelling of the dictyosomal cisternae in suspensions of RL-4 hepatocytes (TEMMINK et al. 1986). Higher concentrations caused swelling of the endoplasmic reticulum. These alterations suggested that the primary targets of isothiocyanates and their thiol conjugates were the plasma membrane and intracellular membrane systems. Such changes were indicative of alterations in cellular monovalent cation and water homeostasis. In contrast, mitochondria were not affected until the cells reached the necrotic phase of cell injury.

II. α,β-Unsaturated Aldehydes (Acrolein)

TEMMINK et al. (1986) suggested that a similar role for GSH could occur with other chemicals, such as α,β-unsaturated carbonyls, where a reversible Michael addition can be proposed. Although such reactions are theoretically reversible, most such adducts are quite stable. However, thiol adducts of several α,β-unsaturated aldehydes are cytotoxic. For example, the crotonaldehyde cysteine and *trans*-4-hydroxypentenal-cysteine adducts are carcinostatic, probably via release of the active aldehyde (TILLIAN et al. 1976, 1978; CONROY et al. 1977). *S*-(3-Oxopropyl)GSH, the GSH conjugate of acrolein, is nephrotoxic when administered to male Sprague-Dawley rats (HORVATH et al. 1992). Whether the nephrotoxicity is due to release of acrolein is not known, but this appears likely in view of the recently proposed bioactivation mechanism for *S*-(3-oxopropyl)-*N*-acetyl-L-cysteine (HASHMI et al. 1992). Thus, although base-catalyzed release of acrolein could not be demonstrated from *S*-(3-oxopropyl)-*N*-acetyl-L-cysteine, the corresponding *S*-oxide readily eliminated acrolein. Both the mercapturate and the *S*-oxide were cytotoxic to LLC PK_1 cells and in isolated renal proximal tubular cells. However, only the toxicity of the mercapturate was inhibited by the inclusion of methimazole, an inhibitor of FMOs. Thus, the toxicity of *S*-(3-oxopropyl)-*N*-acetyl-L-cysteine appears to involve FMO-mediated sulfoxidation followed by β-elimination of the cytotoxic acrolein (HASHMI et al. 1992). Acrolein has also been implicated in the bladder toxicity associated with cyclophosphamide chemotherapy (STILLWELL and BENSON 1988). Subsequently, acrolein in urine following cyclophosphamide administration appeared to be present in a "bound" form (FRAISER and KEHRER 1992). FRAISER et al. (1993) then provided evidence that the bladder toxicity may involve *S*-oxidation of *S*-(3-oxopropyl)-*N*-acetyl-L-cysteine (Fig. 8). Thus, the *S*-oxide released significant amounts of acrolein in vitro, and instillation of the *S*-oxide into the bladder resulted in a hemorrhagic cystitis similar to that seen after either cyclophosphamide or acrolein administration.

III. Isocyanates

More recently, attention has focused on the role of GSH in the toxicological activity of isocyanates, particularly since the catastrophic release of methyl

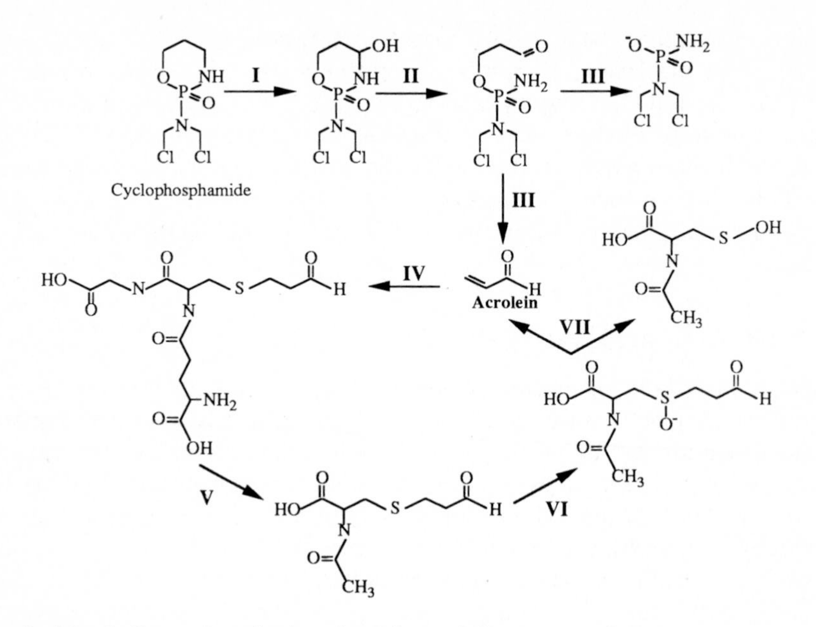

Fig. 8. Metabolism of *cyclophosphamide* to *S*-(3-oxopropyl)-*N*-acetyl-L-cysteine-*S*-oxide, a putative bladder toxic and nephrotoxic metabolite. Cyclophosphamide is metabolized by either cytochrome(s) P-450 and/or prostaglandin H synthase to 4-hydroxycyclophosphamide (*I*), which may (*II*) tautomerize to aldophosphamide, an unstable product that (*III*) rearranges to phosphoramide mustard and *acrolein*. Acrolein, an α-β-unsaturated aldehyde, subsequently (*IV*) reacts with glutathione (GSH) to form *S*-(3-oxopropyl)GSH, which is then metabolized (*V*) to the corresponding mercapturic acid, *S*-(3-oxopropyl)-*N*-acetyl-L-cysteine. Sulfoxidation (*VI*) of the mercapturate by renal flavin-containing monooxygenase(s) gives the *S*-oxide, which can then undergo a base-catalyzed rearrangement that releases acrolein and *N*-acetyl-L-cysteine sulfenate

isocyanate at Bhopal caused the death of several thousand residents and many of the survivors have experienced a variety of other adverse reactions. It is with respect to these latter toxicities that a potential role for GSH as a transporter of methyl isothiocyanate has been proposed. Evidence in support of this proposal has been provided by a number of elegant studies by BAILLIE and coworkers. For example, administration of methyl isocyanate to rats results in the biliary and urinary exeretion of *S*-(*N*-methylcarbamyl) GSH and *S*-(*N*-methylcarbamyl)-*N*-acetylcysteine, respectively (PEARSON et al. 1990; SLATTER et al. 1991) Both these carbamyl thioesters and the corresponding cysteine conjugate were capable of carbamylating a variety of sulfhydryl acceptors (PEARSON et al. 1990, 1991; BAILLIE and SLATTER 1991). Moreover, the carbamylating properties of the carbamyl thioesters was probably mediated by the release of free ethyl isocyanate (PEARSON et al. 1991). *S*-(*N*-Methylcarbamyl)GSH has also been shown to be toxic to mouse embryos in culture (GUEST et al. 1992). The conjugate caused decreased growth and development in explanted embryos, but was not lethal over the concentration range 0.1–0.2 m*M*. Spinal kinks and somite pair distortion, in the region of the forelimb, were found in about 40% of the embryos. *S*-(*N*-Methylcarbamyl)GSH also decreased DNA content and thymidine incorporation by both the embryos and the yolk sac. Thus, the embryotoxic and dysmorphogenic effects of the conjugate may play a role in the systemic toxicity of methyl isocyanate (Guest et al. 1992).

Methyl isocyanate might also play a role in *N*-methylformamide-mediated hepatotoxicity (Kestell et al. 1987). Since *S*-(*N*-methylcarbamyl) GSH is a biliary metabolite of *N*-methylformamide in the rat (Threadgill et al. 1987), and since such carbamate thioesters kill isolated hepatocytes (Han et al. 1990), it is possible that the GSH adduct plays a role in *N*-methylformamide liver injury. The rate at which the conjugate is exported from the hepatocytes into bile in vivo, the intracellular GSH concentration, and the rate of release of methyl isocyanate will all determine whether the conjugate participates in *N*-methylformamide liver injury. *S*-(2-Chloroethylcarbamyl)GSH, the thioester formed from the decomposition of the antitumor agent carmustine (BCNU), is a potent mutagen, causing single-strand breaks in DNA (Stahl et al. 1988, 1992).

E. Pharmacologically Active Glutathione Conjugates

I. Leukotrienes

Several endogenous compounds have been shown to require conjugation with GSH and/or cysteine for the expression of their pharmacological activity. For example, each of the leukotrienes which constitute the slow-reacting substance of anaphylaxis (SRS-A), namely, 5-(*S*)-hydroxy-6(*R*)-*S*-glutathionyl-7,9-*trans*-11,14-*cis*-eicosatetraenoic acid (leukotriene C, LTC) and the 6-*S*-cysteinylglycyl (LTD) and 6-*S*-cysteinyl (LTE) analogs exhibit significant biological potency as nonvascular smooth muscle spasmogens for guinea pig pulmonary parenchymal strips and guinea pig ileum (Drazen et al. 1980; Lewis et al. 1980). It is interesting that the conjugation of an endogenous, lipophilic fatty acid with GSH results in the formation of such biologically active compounds. By inference, the conjugation of lipophilic xenobiotics with GSH might also result in the formation of novel compounds possessing significant pharmacological properties. With the exception of the organic nitrates discussed below, the potential pharmacological activity of GSH and cysteine conjugates synthesised during xenobiotic metabolism has not been investigated.

II. Nitric Oxide and Endothelium-Derived Relaxing Factor

The possibility that xenobiotics exhibit activity via an interaction with specific endogenous receptors is worthy of consideration. For example, organic nitrates require metabolism in order to express their vasodilatory activity, and the thionitrites *S*-nitroso-GSH and/or the cysteine analog have been suggested to be the proximal activators of guanyl cyclase, resulting in the relaxation of vascular smooth muscle (Ignarro et al. 1981; Yeates et al. 1985) and inhibition of platelet aggregation (Mellion et al. 1983). There has been a veritable explosion of information published on the role of nitric oxide as a mediator of vascular tone and as a retrograde messenger in the central nervous system, and there is widespread acceptance of the assertion that endothelium-derived relaxing factor (EDRF) is nitric oxide. However, there are several reports that challenge this position. As early as 1987, Long et al. discriminated, on a chromatographic basis, between EDRF and NO in smooth muscle, and Rosenblum (1992) has summarized the available evidence indicating that at least in the cerebral cerebellum NO is not EDRF. If NO is not EDRF, then what constitutes EDRF? The most popular alternative is that either NO is produced from a precursor, most likely a *S*-nitroso derivative, or that a nitrosothiol itself is EDRF, a view supported by the observation that nitrosothiols are potent vasodilators (Meyers et al. 1990; Rubanyi et al. 1991). In addition, *S*-nitrosothiols have been suggested as the active intermediates involved in vascular smooth muscle relaxation mediated by a variety of nitroso vasodilators (Ignarro et al. 1981). Clancy and Abramson (1992a) have described some of the functional properties of *S*-nitroso GSH. Thus, *S*-nitroso-GSH was capable of inhibiting platelet aggregation, promoting adenine diphosphate ribosylation of a cytosolic 32-kDa protein in neutrophils, and increasing cyclic guanosine monophosphate synthesis in cultured lymphocytes. NO and/or *S*-nitrosothiol derivatives also inhibit the formation of superoxide anion, adhesion (of neutrophils) to vascular endothelium, and leukotriene B_4 synthesis in activated neutrophils (Ney et al. 1990; Kubes et al. 1991; Clancy and Abramson 1992b).

The catechol estrogens are also known to form various thiol adducts, the properties of which have yet to be determined. The cysteine conjugates of dopa play an integral role in the biosynthesis of the sulfur-containing pheomelanins (Prota 1988), and polymerization of both free and S-substituted catecholamines results in the deposition of neuromelanin (Prota 1988), a phenomenon associated with the aging process.

F. Summary

From the preceeding discussion it should be clear that GSH conjugation no longer represents a mechanism for the detoxication of xenobiotics and/or their metabolites. Although the vast majority of conjugations with GSH do facilitate the efficient excretion of xenobiotics from the body, many examples now exist where this process results in enhanced biological (re)activity. The number of examples in which GSH conjugation plays an important role in the generation of biologically reactive intermediates is expanding rapidly. In addition, GSH-dependent toxicity is being manifest in many diverse ways. Thus, GSH and/or the corresponding cysteine conjugates are (i) mutagenic and (ii) probably carcinogenic, (iii) nephrotoxic, (iv) embryotoxic, (v) cataractogenic, (vi) catalyze methemoglobinemia, (vii) inhibit a variety of enzymes, (viii) may be neurotoxic, and (ix) may be involved in the delivery of a variety of toxic agents to target tissue. The generation of a biologically reactive intermediate is usually the initial and necessary step that eventually results in cell death, tissue necrosis and/or tumor formation. The myriad ways in which reactive intermediates interact with cellular constituents and trigger events that lead to cell death or cell transformation, are only now becoming unravelled. Changes in intracellular energy and ion homeostasis are inevitably interlinked, and the consequences of such alterations probably converge in creating a stress that most cells cannot survive. It is therefore the linking of metabolism to toxicity that is necessary for understanding the mechanism(s) of GSH conjugate mediated toxicities. Several laboratories are making great advances in this area, and we should look forward to the many exciting years that lie ahead.

References

Abbot WA, Bridges RJ, Meister A (1984) Extracellular metabolism of glutathione accounts for its disappearance from the basolateral circulation of the kidney. J Biol Chem 259:15393–15400

Allen L, Meck RA, Yunis A (1980) The inhibition of γ-glutamyl transpeptidase from human pancreatic carcinoma cells by (αS,$5S$)-α-amino-3-chloro-4,5-dihydro-5-isoxazoleacetic acid (AT-125; NSC-163501). Res Commun Chem Pathol Pharmacol 27:175–182

Anders MW, Lash LH, Dekant W, Elfarra AA, Dohn DR (1988) Biosynthesis and biotransformation of glutathione S-conjugates to toxic metabolites. CRC Crit Rev Toxicol 18:311–341

Anderson ME, Bridges RJ, Meister A (1980) Direct evidence for inter-organ transport of glutathione and that the non-filtration renal mechanism for glutathione utilization involves γ-glutamyl transpeptidase. Biochem Biophys Res Commun 96:848–853

Andersson B, Larsson R, Rahimtula A, Moldeus P (1983) Hydroperoxide-dependent activation of *p*-phenetidine catalyzed by prostaglandin synthase and other peroxidases. Biochem Pharmacol 32:1045–1050

Andersson BR, Larsson A, Rahimtula A, Moldeus P (1984) Prostaglandin synthase and horseradish peroxidase catalysed DNA binding of *p*-phenetidine. Carcinogenesis 5:161–165

Andrews JE, Rogers JM, Ebron-McCoy M, Logsdon TR, Monks TJ, Lau SS (1993) Developmental toxicology of bromohydroquinone and bromohydroquinone-glutathione conjugates in vivo and in whole embryo culture. Toxicol Appl Pharmacol 120:1–7

Auberbach C, Robson JM (1946) Chemical production of mutations. Nature 157:302

Augusteyn RC (1981) Protein modification of cataract: possible oxidative mechanisms. In: Duncan G (ed) Mechanisms of cataract formation in the human lens. Academic, London, pp 71–115

Baille TA, Slatter JG (1991) Glutathione: a vehicle for the transport of chemically reactive metabolites in vivo. Acc Chem Res 24:264–270

Baumgarten HG, Bjorklund A, Lachenmayer L, Nobin A, Stenevi U (1971) Long-lasting selective depletion of brain serotonin by 5,6-dihydroxytryptamine. Acta Physiol Scand 373:1–15

Baumgarten HG, Evetts KD, Holman RB, Iverson LL, Vogt M, Wilson G (1972a) Effects of 5,6-dihydroxytryptamine on monoaminergic neurones in the central nervous system of the rat. J Neurochem 19:1587–1597

Baumgarten HG, Goethert M, Holstein AF, Schlossberger G (1972b) Chemical sympathectomy induced by 5,6-dihydroxytryptamine. Z Zellforsch 128:115–134

Berndt WO, Mehendale HM (1979) Effects of hexachlorobutadiene (HCBD) on renal function and renal organic ion transport in the rat. Toxicology 14:55–65

Beuter W, Cojocel C, Muller W, Donaubauer HH, Mayer D (1989) Peroxidative damage and nephrotoxicity of dichlorovinylcysteine in mice. J Appl Toxicol 9:181–186

Bhattacharya RK, Schultze MO (1967) Enzymes from bovine and turkey kidneys which cleave *S*-(1,2-dichlorovinyl)-L-cysteine. Comp Biochem Physiol 22: 723–735

Borchardt RT, Cheng CF (1978) Purification and characterization of rat liver microsomal thiol methyltransferase. Biochim Biophys Acta 522:340–353

Bowen DM, Allen SJ, Benton JS, Goodhardt MJ, Haan MJ, Palmer AM, Sims NR, Smith CCT, Spillane JA, Esiri MM, Neary D, Snowden JS, Wilcock GK, Davison AN (1983) Biochemical assessment of serotonergic and cholinergic dysfunction and cerebral atrophy in Alzheimer's disease. J Neurochem 41: 266–272

Brem H, Stein AB, Rosenkranz HS (1974) The mutagenicity and DNA-modifying effects of haloalkanes. Cancer Res 34:2576–2579

Bremer J, Greenberg DM (1961) Enzymic methylation of foreign sulphydryl compounds. Biochim Biophys Acta 46:217–224

Brown PC, Dulik DM, Jones TW (1991) The toxicity of menadione (2-methyl-1, 4-naphthoquinone) and two thioether conjugates studied with isolated renal epithelial cells. Arch Biochem Biophys 285:187–196

Bruggeman JM, Temmink JMH, van Bladeren PJ (1986) Glutathione- and cysteine-mediated cytotoxicity of allyl and benzyl isothiocyanate. Toxicol Appl Pharmacol 83:349–359

Brusewitz G, Cameron BD, Chasseaud LF, Görler K, Hawkins DR, Kock H, Mennicke WH (1977) The metabolism of benzyl isothiocyanate and its cysteine conjugate. Biochem J 162:99–107

Buffinton GD, Ollinger K, Brunmark A, Cadenas E (1989) DT-diaphorase-catalysed reduction of 1,4-naphthoquinone derivatives and glutathionyl-quinone conjugates. Biochem J 257:561–571

Chen J-C, Crino PB, Schnepper PW, To AS, Volicer L (1989) Increased serotonin efflux by a partially oxidized serotonin: tryptamine-4,5-dione. J Pharmacol Exp Ther 250:141–148

Chen Q, Jones TW, Brown PC, Stevens JL (1990) The mechanism of cysteine conjugate cytotoxicity in renal epithelial cells. J Biol Chem 265:21603–21611

Chen Q, Yu K, Holbrook NJ, Stevens JL (1992) Activation of the growth arrest and DNA damage-inducible gene *gadd* 153 by nephrotoxic cysteine conjugates and dithiothreitol. J Biol Chem 267:8207–8212

Chung H, Harvey RG, Armstrong RN, Jarabak J (1987a) Polycyclic aromatic hydrocarbon quinones and glutathione thioethers as substrates and inhibitors of the human placental NADP-linked 15-hydroxyprostaglandin dehydrogenase. J Biol Chem 262:12448–12451

Chung H, Fried J, Williams-Ashman E, Jarabak J (1987b) Glutathione mixed disulfide inhibitors of the human placental NADP-linked 15-hydroxyprostaglandin dehydrogenase. Prostaglandins 33:383–390

Clancy RM, Abramson SB (1992a) Clin Res 40:248A, 262A

Clancy RM, Abramson SB (1992b) Novel synthesis of *S*-nitrosoglutathione and degradation by human neutrophils. Anal Biochem 204:365–371

Cmarik JL, Humphreys WG, Bruner KL, Lloyd RS, Tibbetts C, Guengrich FP (1992) Mutation spectrum and sequence alkylation selectivity resulting from modification of bacteriophage M13mp18DNA with *S*-(2-chloroethyl)glutathione. J Biol Chem 267:6672–6679

Cohen G, Collins MA (1970) Alkaloids from catecholamines in adrenal tissue: possible role in addiction. Science 167:1749–1751

Collins MA (1982) A possible neurochemical mechanism for brain and nerve damage associated with chronic alcoholism. Trends Pharmacol Sci 3:373–375

Commandeur JNM, De Kanter FJJ, Vermeulen NPE (1989) Bioactivation of the cysteine-*S*-conjugate and mercapturic acid of tetrafluoroethylene to acylating reactive intermediates in the rat: dependence of activation and deactivation activities on acetyl coenzyme A availability. Mol Pharmacol 36:654–663

Conroy PJ, Nodes JT, Slater TF, While GW (1977) The inhibitor effects of a 4-hydroxypentenal: cysteine adduct against sarcoma 180 cells in mice. Eur J Cancer 13:55–63

Dass PD, Welbourne TC (1982) Effects of AT-125 on renal γ-glutamyl-transferase activity. FEBS Lett 144:21–24

Davis VE, Walsh MJ (1970) Alcohol, amines and alkaloids: a possible biochemical basis for alcohol addiction. Science 167:1005–1007

Dekant W, Vamvakas S, Berthold K, Schmidt S, Wild D, Henschler D (1986) Bacterial β-lyase mediated cleavage and mutagenicity of cysteine conjugates derived from the nephrocarcinogenic alkenes trichloroethylene, tetrachloroethylene and hexachlorobutadiene. Chem Biol Interact 60:31–45

Dekant W, Lash LH, Anders MW (1987) Bioactivation mechanism of the cytotoxic and nephrotoxic *S*-conjugate *S*-(2-chloro-1,1,2-trifluoroethyl)-L-cysteine. Proc Natl Acad Sci USA 84:7443–7447

Dekant W, Vamvakas S, Anders MW (1989) Bioactivation of nephrotoxic haloalkenes by glutathione conjugation: formation of toxic and mutagenic intermediates by cysteine conjugate β-lyase. Drug Metab Rev 20:43–83

Dekant W, Anders MW, Monks TJ (1993) Bioactivation of halogenated xenobiotics by *S*-conjugate formation. In: Anders MW, Dekant W, Henschler D, Oberleithner H, Silbernagl S (eds) Renal disposition and nephrotoxicity of xenobiotics. Academic, New York, pp 187–215

Dempo K, Elliot KA, Demond W, Fishman WH (1981) Demonstration of gamma glutamyl transpeptidase, alkaline phosphatase, CEA and HGG in human lung cancer. Oncodev Biol Med 2:21–37

DeYoung LM, Richards WL, Bonzelet W, Tsai LL, Boutwell RK (1978) Localization and significance of γ-glutamyl transpeptidase in normal and neoplastic mouse skin. Cancer Res 38:3697–3701

Dierickx PJ (1983) Interaction of benzo- and naphthoquinones with soluble glutathione *S*-transferases from rat liver. Pharmacol Res Commun 15:581–591

Dohn DR, Anders MW (1982) The enzymatic reaction of chlorotrifluoroethylene with glutathione. Biochem Biophys Res Commun 109:1339–1345

Drazen JM, Austen KF, Lewis RA, Clark DA, Goto G, Marfat A, Corey EJ (1980) Comparative airway and vascular activities of leukotrienes C-1 and D in vivo and in vitro. Proc Natl Acad Sci USA 77:4354–4358

Drobnica L, Kristian P, Augustin J (1977) The chemistry of the isothiocyanate group. In: Patai S (ed) The chemistry of cyanates and their thio-derivatives. Wiley, Chichester, pp 1003–1221

Duffel MW, Jakoby WB (1982) Cysteine *S*-conjugate *N*-acetyltransferase from rat kidney microsomes. Mol Pharmacol 21:444–448

Dunnick JK, Prejean JD, Haseman J, Thompson RB, Giles HD, McConnell EE (1982) Carcinogenesis bioassay of allyl isothiocyanate. Fund Appl Toxicol 2:114–120

Eckert K-G, Eyer P, Sonnenbichler J, Zetl I (1990) Activation and detoxication of aminophenols. II. Synthesis and structural elucidation of various thiol addition products of 1,4-benzoquinoneimine and *N*-acetyl-1,4-benzoquinoneimine. Xenobiotica 20:333–350

Elfarra AA, Baggs RB, Anders MW (1985) Structure nephrotoxicity relationships of *S*-(2-chloroethyl)-*DL*-cysteine and analogs. Role for an episulfonium ion. J Pharmacol Exp Ther 233:512–516

Elfarra AA, Jakobson I, Anders MW (1986) Mechanism of *S*-(1,2 dichlorovinyl) glutathione-induced nephrotoxicity. Biochem Pharmacol 35:283–288

Ericksen N, Martin GM, Benditt EP (1960) Oxidation of the indole nucleus of 5-hydroxytryptamine and the formation of pigments: isolation and partial characterization of a dimer of 5-hydroxytryptamine. J Biol Chem 235:1662–1667

Eyer P, Kiese M (1976) Biotransformation of 4-dimethylaminophenol: reaction with glutathione, and some properties of the reaction products. Chem Biol Int 14:165–178

Fa Z, Dryhurst G (1991a) Interactions of salsolinol with oxidative enzymes. Biochem Pharmacol 42:2209–2397

Fa A, Dryhurst G (1991b) Oxidation chemistry of the endogenous central nervous system alkaloid salsolinol. I. Electrochemical studies. Bioorg Chem 19:384–397

Felley-Bosco E, Diezi J (1987) Fate of cadmium in rat renal tubules: a microinjection study. Toxicol Appl Pharmacol 91:204–211

Fenwick GR, Heany RK, Mullin WJ (1982) Glucosinulates and their breakdown products in food and food plants. CRC Crit Rev Food Sci Nutr 181:123–201

Fiala S, Mohindru A, Kettering WG, Fiala AE, Morris HP (1976) Glutathione and gamma glutamyl transpeptidase in rat liver during chemical carcinogenesis. J Natl Cancer Inst 57:591–598

Finley KT (1974) The addition and substitution chemistry of quinones. In: Patai S (ed) The chemistry of the quinonoid compounds, part 2. Wiley, New York, pp 877–1144

Foulkes EC (1978) Renal tubular transport of cadmium metallothionein. Toxicol Appl Pharmacol 45:505–512

Foulkes EC, Blanck S (1990) Acute cadmium uptake by rabbit kidneys: mechanism and effect. Toxicol Appl Pharmacol 102:464–473

Foureman GL, Reed DJ (1987) Formation of *S*[2-(N^7-guanyl)ethyl] adducts by the postulated *S*(2-chloroethyl)cysteinyl and *S*(2-chloroethyl)glutathionyl conjugates of 1,2-dichloroethane. Biochemistry 26:2028–2033

Fowler LM, Moore RD, Foster JR, Lock EA (1991) Nephrotoxicity of 4-aminophenol glutathione conjugate. Hum Exp Toxicol 10:451–459

Fraiser L, Kehrer JP (1992) Murine strain differences in metabolism and bladder toxicity of cyclophosphamide. Toxicology 75:257–273

Fraiser L, Skarovsky C, Kehrer JP (1993) Bioactivation of a glutathione-acrolein conjugate to bladder toxic species. Toxicologist 13:226

Friedmann E, Marrian DH, Simon-Ruess I (1948) Sulfhydryl addition compounds of some quinones and related substances and their action on the growth of normal cells. Br J Pharmacol 3:335–340

Fukuto JM, Kumagai Y, Cho AK (1991) Determination of the mechanism of demethylenation of (methylenedioxy)phenyl compounds by cytochrome P450 using deuterium isotope effects. J Med Chem 34:2871–2876

Gartland KPR, Bonner FW, Timbrell JA, Nicholson JK (1989) Biochemical characterization of 4-aminophenol-induced nephrotoxic lesions in the F344 rat. Arch Toxicol 63:97–106

Goldbag JA, Friedman OM, Pineda EP, Smith EE, Chatterji RR, Stein EH, Rutenberg AM (1960) The colorimetric determination of γ-glutamyl transpeptidase with a synthetic substrate. Arch Biochem Biophys 91:61–70

Goldstein RS (1993) Biochemical heterogeneity and site-specific tubular injury. In: Hook JR, Goldstein RS (eds) Tocicology of the kidney, 2nd edn. Raven, New York, pp 201–247

Green CR, Ham KN, Tange JD (1969) Kidney lesions induced in rats by 4-aminophenol. Br Med J 1:162–164

Green T, Odum J (1985) Stucture/activity studies of the nephrotoxic and mutagenic action of cysteine conjugates of chloro- and fluoroalkenes. Chem Biol Interact 54:15–31

Griffith OW, Meister A (1979) Glutathione. Interorgan translocation, turnover and metabolism. Proc Natl Acad Sci USA 76:5606–5610

Groves CE, Lock EA, Schnellmann RG (1991a) Role of lipid peroxidation in renal proximal tubule cell death induced by haloalkene cysteine conjugates. Toxicol Appl Pharmacol 107:54–62

Groves CE, Schnellman RG, Sokol PP, Steffens TG, Lock EA (1991b) Pentachlorobutadienyl-L-cysteine (PCBC) toxicity: the importance of mitochondrial dysfunction. J Biochem Toxicol 6:253–260

Guengerich FP, Crawford WM, Domoradzki JY, MacDonald TL, Watanabe PG (1980) In vitro activation of 1,2-dichloroethane by microsomal and cytosolic enzymes. Toxicol Appl Pharmacol 55:303–317

Guest I, Baillie TA, Varma DR (1992) Toxicity of the methyl isocyanate metabolite *S*-(*N*-methylcarbamoyl) GSH on mouse embryos in culture. Teratology 46: 6167

Haberle D, Wahllander A, Sies H (1979) Assessment of the kidney function in maintenance of plasma glutathione concentration and redox state in anaesthetized rats. FEBS Lett 108:335–340

Hahn R, Wendel A, Flohe L (1978) The fate of extracellular glutathione in the rat. Biochim Biophys Acta 539:324–337

Han H, Pearson PG, Baillie TA, Dayal R, Tsang LH, Gescher A (1990) Chemical synthesis and cytotoxic properties of *N*-alkylcarbamic acid thioesters, metabolites of hepatotoxic formamides. Chem Res Toxicol 3:118–124

Hansson C, Rorsman H, Rosengren E (1980) 5-*S*-Cysteinyldopa as a substrate for tyrosinase. Acta Derm (Stockh) 60:399–402

Hashmi M, Vamvakas S, Anders MW (1992) Bioactivation mechanisms of *S*(3-oxopropyl)-*N*-acetyl-L-cysteine, the mercapturic acid of acrolein. Chem Res Toxicol 5:360–365

Hassid A, Levine L (1977) Multiple molecular forms of prostaglandin 15-hydroxydehydrogenase and 9-ketoreductase in chicken kidney. Prostaglandins 13:503–516

Harris JW, Dekant W, Anders MW (1992) In vivo detection and characterization of protein adducts resulting from bioactivation of haloethene cysteine *S*-conjugates by ^{19}FNMR: chlorotrifluoroethene and tetrafluoroethene. Chem Res Toxicol 5:34–41

Hayden PJ, Stevens JL (1990) Cysteine conjugate toxicity, metabolism, and binding to macromolecules in isolated rat kidney mitochondria. Mol Pharmacol 37: 468–476

Hayden PJ, Ichimura T, McCann DJ, Pohl LR, Stevens JL (1991a) Detection of cysteine conjugate metabolite adduct formation with specific mitochondrial proteins using antibodies raised against halothane metabolite adducts. J Biol Chem 266:18415–18418

Hayden PJ, Yang Y, Ward AJI, Dulik DM, McCann DJ, Stevens JL (1991b) Formation of difluorothionacetyl-protein adducts by *S*-(1,1,2,2-tetrafluoroethyl)-L-cysteine metabolites: nucleophilic catalysis of stable lysyl adduct formation by histidine and tyrosine, Biochemistry 30:5935–5943

Hayden PJ, Welsh CJ, Yang Y, Schaefer WH, Ward AJI, Stevens JL (1992) Formation of mitochondrial phospholipid adducts by nephrotoxic cysteine conjugate metabolites. Chem Res Toxicol 5:231–237

Hayes JD, Pickett CB, Mantle TJ (1990) Glutathione *S*-transferases and drug resistance. Taylor and Francis, London

Hill BA, Kleiner HE, Ryan EA, Dulik DM, Monks TJ, Lau SS (1993) Identification of multi-*S*-substituted conjugates of hydroquinone by HPLC-coulometric electrode array analysis and mass spectroscopy. Chem Res Toxicol 6:459–469

Hiramatsu M, Kumagai Y, Unger SE, Cho AK (1990) Metabolism of methylenedioxymethamphetamine: formation of dihydroxymethamphetamine and a quinone identified as its glutathione adduct. J Pharmacol Exp Ther 254:512–527
Horiuchi S, Inoue M, Morino Y (1978) γ-Glutamyl transpeptidase. Sidedness of its active site on renal brush-border membrane. Eur J Biochem 87:429–437
Horvath JJ, Witmer CM, Witz G (1992) Nephrotoxicity of the 1:1 acrolein-glutathione adduct in the rat. Toxicol Appl Pharmacol 117:200–207
Hughey R, Rankin B, Elce J, Curthoys N (1978) Specificity of a particulate rat renal peptidase and its localization along with other enzymes of mercapturic acid synthesis. Arch Biochem Biophys 186:211–217
Humphreys WG, Kim K-H, Cmarik JL, Shimada T, Guengerich FP (1990) Comparison of the DNA-alkylating properties and mutagenic responses of a series of *S*-(2-haloethyl)-substituted cysteine and glutathione derivatives. Biochemistry 29:10342–10350
Humphreys WG, Kim DH, Guengerich FP (1991) Isolation and characterization of *N*-[7]-guanyl adducts derived from 1,2-dibromo-3-chloropropane. Chem Res Toxicol 4:445–453
Ignarro LJ, Lippton H, Edwards JC, Baricos WH, Hyman AL, Kadowitz PJ, Gruetter CA (1981) Mechanism of vascular smooth muscle relaxation by organic nitrates, nitroprusside and nitric oxide: evidence for the involvement of *S*-nitrosothiols as active intermediates. J Pharmacol Exp Ther 218:739–749
Innoue M, Okajima K, Morino Y (1984) Hepato-renal cooperation in biotransformation, membrane transport and elimination of cysteine-*S*-conjugates of xenobiotics. J Biochem 95:247–254
Inskeep PB, Guengerich FP (1984) Glutathione-mediated binding of dibromoalkanes to DNA: specificity of rat glutathione-*S*-transferases and dibromoalkane structure. Carcinogenesis 5:805–808
Inskeep PB, Koga N, Cmarik JL, Guengerich FP (1986) Covalent binding of 1,2-dihaloalkanes to DNA and stability of the major DNA adduct *S*-[2-(*N*-[7]-guanyl) ethyl]glutathione. Cancer Res 46:2839–2844
Ito S, Novellino E, Chioccara F, Misuraca G, Prota G (1980) Co-polymerization of dopa and cysteinyldopa in melanogenesis in vitro. Experientia 36:822–823
Jaken S, Mason M (1978) Differences in the isoelectric focussing patterns of γ-glutamyl transpeptidase from normal and cancerous rat mammary tissue. Proc Natl Acad Sci USA 75:1750–1753
Jakoby WB, Stevens J (1984) Cysteine conjugate β-lyase and the thiomethyl shunt. Biochem Soc Trans 12:33–35
Jakoby WB, Stevens J, Duffel MW, Weisiger RA (1985) The terminal enzymes of mercapturate formation and the thiomethyl shunt. Rev Biochem Toxicol 6:97–115
Jarabak J (1991) Polycyclic aromatic hydrocarbon quinone-mediated oxidation reduction cycling catalyzed by a human placental NADPH-linked carbonyl reductase. Arch Biochem Biophys 291:334–338
Jarabak J, Luncsford A, Berkantz D (1983) Substrate specificity of three prostaglandin dehydrogenases. Prostaglandins 26:849–904
Jocelyn PC (1972) Biochemistry of the SH Group. Academic, London
Jones DP, Moldeus P, Stead J, Ormstad K, Jornvall H, Orrenius S (1979) Metabolism of glutathione and glutathione conjugates by isolated kidney cells. J Biol Chem 254:2787–2792
Jones TW, Chen Q, Schaeffer VH, Stevens JL (1988) Immunocytochemical localization of glutamine transaminase K, a cysteine conjugate β-lyase, and the relationship to the segment specificity of cysteine conjugate nephrotoxicity. Mol Pharmacol 34:621–627
Jones TW, Wallin A, Thor H, Gerdes RG, Ormstad K, Orrenius S (1986) The mechanism of pentachlorobutadienyl-glutathione nephrotoxicity studied with isolated rat renal epithelial cells. Arch Biochem Biophys 251:504–513

Kari FW (1989) Toxicology and carcinogenesis studies of hydroquinoine in F344/N rats and B6C3F1 mice (Gavage Studies), National Toxicology Program Technical Report 366. US Department of Health and Human Services, PHS, NIH

Kestell P, Threadgill MD, Gescher A, Gledhill AP, Shaw AJ, Farmer PB (1987) An investigation of the relationship between the hepatotoxicity and the metabolism of *N*-alkylformamides. J Pharmacol Exp Ther 240:265–270

Kiese M (1974) Methemoglobinemia: a comprehensive treatise. CRC Press, Boca Raton

Kiese M, Szinicz L, Thiel N, Weger N (1975) Ferrihemoglobin and kidney lesions in rats produced by 4-aminophenol or 4-dimethylaminophenol. Arch Toxicol 34:337–340

Kim D-H, Guengerich FP (1990) Formation of the adduct *S*-[2-(N^7-guanyl)ethyl] glutathione from ethylene dibromide: effects of modulation of glutathione and glutathione *S*-transferase levels and lack of a role for sulfation. Carcinogenesis 11:419–424

Klos C, Koob M, Kramer C, Dekant W (1992) *p*-Aminophenol nephrotoxicity: biosynthesis of toxic glutathione conjugates. Toxicol Appl Pharmacol 115:98–106

Kluwe WM, McNish R, Smithson K, Hook JB (1985) Depletion by 1,2-dibromoethane, 1,2-dibromo-3-chloropropane, *tris*-(2,3-dibromopropyl)phosphate and hexachloro-1,3-butadiene of reduced non-protein sulfhydryl groups in target and non-target organs. Biochem Pharmacol 30:2265–2271

Kociba RJ, Schwetz BA, Keyes DG, Jersey GC, Ballard JJ, Dittenber DA, Quast JF, Wade CE, Humiston CG (1977) Chronic toxicity and reproduction studies of hexachlorobutadiene in rats. Environ Health Perspect 21:49–53

Kondo T, Murao M, Taniguchi N (1982) Glutathione *S*-conjugate transport using inside-out vesicles from human erythrocytes. Eur J Biochem 125:551–554

Kramer RA, Foureman G, Greene KE, Reed DJ (1987) Nephrotoxicity of *S*-(2-chloroethyl)glutathione in the Fischer rat: evidence for γ-glutamyl transpeptidase-independent uptake by the kidney. J Pharmacol Exp Ther 242:741–748

Kubes P, Suzuke M, Granger DN (1991) Nitric oxide: an endogenous modulator of leukocyte adhesion. Proc Natl Acad Sci USA 88:4651–4655

Larsson R, Boutin J, Moldeus P (1988) Peroxidase-catalysed metabolic activation of xenobiotics. In: Gorrod JW, Oelschlager H, Caldwell J (eds) Metabolism of xenobiotics. Taylor and Francis, New York, pp 43–50

Lash LH, Anders MW (1986) Cytotoxicity of *S*-(1,2-dichlorovinyl)glutathione and *S*-(1,2-dichlorovinyl)-L-cysteine in isolated rat kidney cells. J Biol Chem 261:13076–13081

Lash LH, Anders MW (1987) Mechanism of *S*-(1,2-dichlorovinyl)-L-cysteine and *S*-(1,2-dichlorovinyl)-L-homocysteine-induced renal mitochondrial toxicity. Mol Pharmacol 32:549–556

Lash LH, Jones DP (1983) Transport of glutathione by renal basal-lateral membrane vesicles. Biochem Biophys Res Commun 112:55–60

Lash LH, Jones DP (1984) Renal glutathione transport. Characteristics of the sodium-dependent system in the basal-lateral membrane. J Biol Chem 259: 14508–14514

Lash LH, Jones DP (1985) Uptake of the glutathione conjugate *S*-(1,2-dichlorovinyl) glutathione by renal basal-lateral membrane vesicles and isolated kidney cells. Mol Pharmacol 28:278–282

Lash LH, Elfarra AA, Anders MW (1986a) Renal cysteine conjugate β-lyase: bioactivation of nephrotoxic cysteine *S*-conjugates in mitochondrial outer membrane. J Biol Chem 261:5930–5935

Lash LH, Elfarra AA, Anders MW (1986b) *S*-(1,2-dichlorovinyl)-L-homocysteine-induced cytotoxicity in isolated rat kidney cells. Arch Biochem Biophys 251: 432–439

Lau SS, Hill BA, Highet RJ, Monks TJ (1988a) Sequential oxidation and glutathione addition to 1,4-benzoquinone: correlation of toxicity with increased glutathione substitution. Mol Pharmacol 34:829–836
Lau SS, McMenamin MG, Monks TJ (1988b) Differential uptake of isomericbromo-hydroquinone conjugates into kidney slices. Biochem Biophy Res Commun 152:233–230
Lau SS, Jones TW, Highet RJ, Hill BA, Monks TJ (1990) Differences in the localization and extent of the renal proximal tubular necrosis caused by mercapturic acid and glutathione conjugates of menadione and 1,4-naphthoquinone. Toxicol Appl Pharmacol 104:334–350
Lau SS, Monks TJ (1991) Glutathione conjugation as a mechanism of targeting latent quinones to the kidney. In: Witmer CM, Snyder RR, Jollow DJ, Kalf GF, Kocsis JJ, Sipes IG (eds) Biological reactive intermediates IV. Molecular and cellular effects and human Impact. Plenum, New York, pp 457–464
Lewis RA, Drazen JM, Austen KF, Clark DA, Corey EJ (1980) Identification of the C(6)-*S*-conjugate of leukotriene A with cysteine as a naturally occuring slow reacting substance of anaphylaxis. Importance of the II-*cis*-geometry for biological activity. Biochem Biophys Res Commun 96:271d–277d
Lin LY, Kumagai Y, Cho AK (1992) Enzymatic and chemical demethylenation of (methylenedioxy)amphetamine and (methylenedioxy)methamphetamine by rat brain microsomes. Chem Res Toxicol 5:401–406
Lin Y-M, Jarabak J (1978) Isolation of two proteins with 9-keto-prostaglandin reductase and NADP-linded 15-hydroxyprostaglandin dehydrogenase activities and studies on their inhibition. Biochem Biophys Res Commun 81:1227–1234
Lock EA, Ishmael J (1979) The acute toxic effects of hexachloro-1,3-butadeine on the rat kidney. Arch Toxicol 43:47–57
Lock EA, Ishmael J (1981) Hepatic and renal non-protein sulfhdryl concentrations following toxic doses of hexachloro-1,3-butadiene in the rat: the effect of Aroclor 1254, phenobarbitone or SKF 525A treatment. Toxicol Appl Pharmacol 57:79–87
Lock EA, Ishmael J (1985) Effect of the organic acid transport inhibitor probenecid on renal cortical uptake and proximal tubular toxicity of hexachloro-1,3-butadiene and its conjugates. Toxicol Appl Pharmacol 81:32–42
Lock EA, Schnellmann RG (1990) The effect of haloalkene cysteine conjugates on rat renal glutathione reductase and lipoyl dehydrogenase activities. Toxicol Appl Pharmacol 104:180–190
Matson WR, Langlais P, Volicer L, Gamache PH, Bird E, Mark KA (1984) *n*-Electrode three-dimensional chromatography with electrochemical detection for determination of neurotransmitters. Clin Chem 30:1477–1488
Matsubara K, Fukishima S, Fukui Y (1987) A systematic regional study of brain salsolinol levels during and immediately following chronic ethanol injection in rats. Brain Res 413:336–343
McFarlane M, Foster JR, Gibson GG, King LJ, Lock EA (1989) Cysteine conjugate β-lyase of rat kidney cytosol: characterization, immunocytochemical localization and correlation with hexachlorobutadiene nephrotoxicity. Toxicol Appl Pharmacol 98:185–197
McIntyre TM, Curthoys NP (1980) The interorgan metabolism of glutathione. Int J Biochem 12:545–551
McIsaac WM, Page, IH (1959) The metabolism of serotonin (5-hydroxytryptamine). J Biol Chem 234:858–864
Meister A, Tate SS (1980) Glutathione and related γ-glutamyl compounds. Biosynthesis and utilization. Annu Rev Biochem 45:559–604
Mellion BT, Ignarro LJ, Myers CB, Ohlstein EH, Ballot BA, Hyman AL, Kadowitz PJ (1983) Inhibition of human platelet aggregation by *S*-nitrothiols. Heme-dependent activation of soluble guanylate cyclase and stimulation of cyclic GMP accumulation. Mol Pharmacol 23:653–664
Mennicke WH, Görler K, Krumbiegel G (1983) Metabolism of some naturally occurring isothiocyanates in the rat. Xenobiotica 13:203–207

Mertens JJWM, Temmink JHM, van Bladeren PJ, Jones TW, Lo H-H, Lau SS, Monks TJ (1991) Inhibition of γ-glutamyl transferase potentiates the nephrotoxicity of glutathione conjugated chlorohydroquinones. Toxicol Appl Pharmacol 110:45–60

Meyers PR, Minor RLJ, Guerra R Jr, Bates JN, Harrison DG (1990) Vasorelaxant properties of the endothelium-derived relaxing factors more closely resemble *S*-nitroso-cysteine than nitric oxide. Nature 345:161–163

Monks TJ, Lau SS, Highet RJ, Gillette JR (1985) Glutathione conjugates of 2-bromohydroquinone are nephrotoxic. Drug Metab Dispos 13:553–559

Monks TJ, Lau SS (1987) Commentary: renal transport processes and glutathione conjugate-mediated nephrotoxicity. Drug Metab Dispos 15:437

Monks TJ, Highet RJ, Lau SS (1988a) 2-Bromo-(diglutathion-*S*-yl)hydroquinone nephrotoxicity: physiological, biochemical and electrochemical determinants. Mol Pharmacol 34:492–500

Monks TJ, Highet RJ, Chu PS, Lau SS (1988b) Synthesis and nephrotoxicity of 6-bromo-2,5-dihydroxythiophenol. Mol Pharmacol 34:15–22

Monks TJ, Lau SS (1989) Sulfur conjugate-mediated toxicities. Rev Biochem Toxicol 10:41–90

Monks TJ, Highet RJ, Lau SS (1990) Oxidative cyclization, 1,4-benzothiazine formation and dimerization of 2-bromo-3-(glutathion-*S*-yl)hydroquinone. Mol Pharmacol 38:121–127

Monks TJ, Lau SS (1990) Glutathione, γ-glutamyl transpeptidase and the mercapturic acid pathway as modulators of 2-bromohydroquinone oxidation. Toxicol Appl Pharmacol 103:557–563

Monks TJ, Jones TW, Hill BA, Lau SS (1991) Nephrotoxicity of 2-bromo-(cystein-*S*-yl)hydroquinone and 2-bromo-(*N*-acetylcystein-*S*-yl)hydroquinone thioethers. Toxicol Appl Pharmacol 111:279–298

Monks TJ, Lau SS (1992) Toxicology of quinone-thioethers. CRC Crit Rev Toxicol 22:243–270

Motoyama N, Kulkarni AP, Hodgson E, Dauterman WC (1978) Endogenous inhibitors of glutathione *S*-transferases in house flies. Pesticide Biochem Physiol 9:255–262

Mudge GH (1980) Inhibitors of tubular transport of organic compounds. In: Gilman AG, Goodman LS, Gilman (eds) The pharmacologic basic of therapeutics, vol 6. MacMillan, New York, pp 929–934

Myers RD, Melchior CL (1977) Alcohol drinking: abnormal intake caused by tetrahydropapaveroline in brain. Science 196:554–556

Myers WD, Mackenzie L, Ng KT, Singer G, Smythe GA, Duncan MW (1984) Salsolinol and dopamine in rat medial basal hypothalamus after chronic ethanol exposure. Life Sci 36:309–314

Naganuma A, Oda-Urano N, Tanaka T, Imura N (1988) Possible role of hepatic glutathione in transport of methylmercury into mouse kidney. Biochem Pharmacol 37:291–296

Nash JA, King LJ, Lock EA, Green T (1984) The metabolism and disposition of hexachloro-1,3-butadiene in the rat and its relevance to nephrotoxicity. Toxicol Appl Pharmacol 73:124–137

Newton JF, Kuo C-H, Gemborys MW, Mudge GH, Hook JB (1982) Nephrotoxicity of 4-aminophenol, a metabolite of acetaminophen in the F344 rat. Toxicol Appl Pharmacol 65:336–344

Ney P, Schroder H, Schror K (1990) Nitrovasodilator-induced inhibition of LTB4 release from human PMN may be mediated by cyclic GMP. Eicosanoids 3:243–245

Nickerson WJ, Falcone G, Strausse G (1963) Studies on quinone-thioethers. I. Mechanism of formation and properties of thiodone. Biochemistry 2:537–543

Oida T, Humphreys WG, Guengerich FP (1991) Preparation and characterization of oligonucleotides containing *S*-[2-(N^7-guanyl)ethyl] glutathione. Biochemistry 30:10513–10522

Olson WA, Habermann RT, Weisburger EK, Ward JM, Weisburger JH (1973) Induction of stomach cancer in rats and mice by halogenated aliphatic fumigants. J Natl Cancer Inst 51:1993–1995

Ozawa N, Guengerich FP (1983) Evidence for formation of an *S*-[2-(*N*-guanyl)ethyl] glutathione adduct in glutathione-mediated binding of the carcinogen 1,2-dibromoethane to DNA. Proc Natl Acad Sci 80:5266–5270

Palmer AM, Francis PT, Benton JS, Sims NR, Mann DMA, Neary D, Snowdon JS, Bowen DM (1987) Presynaptic serotonergic dysfunction in patients with Alzheimer's disease. J Neurochem 48:8–15

Park SB, Osterloh JD, Vamvakas S, Hashmi M, Anders MW, Cashman JR (1992) Flavin-containing monooxygenase-dependent stereoselective *S*-oxygenation and cytotoxicity of cysteine *S*-conjugates and mercapturates. Chem Res Toxicol 5:193–201

Parker VH (1965) A biochemical study of the toxicity of *S*-dichlorovinyl-L-cysteine. Food Cosmet Toxicol 3:75–84

Patel N, Kumagai Y, Unger SE, Fukuto JM, Cho AK (1991) Transformation of dopamine and α-methyldopamine by NE 108–15 cells: formation of thiol adducts. Chem Res Toxicol 4:421–126

Pearson PG, Slatter JG, Rashed MR, Han D-H, Grillo MP, Baillie TA (1990) *S*-(*N*-methylcarbamoyl)glutathione: a reactive *S*-linked metabolite of methyl isocyanate. Biochem Biophys Res Commun 166:245–250

Pearson PG, Slatter JG, Rashed MS, Han D-H, Baillie TA (1991) Carbamoylation of peptides and proteins in vitro by *S*-(*N*-methylcarbamoyl) glutathione and *S*-(*N*-methyl-carbamoyl) cysteine, two electrophilic *S*-linked conjugates of methyl isocyanate. Chem Res Toxicol 4:436–444

Peraino C, Richards WL, Stevens FJ (1983) Multi-stage-hepatocarcinogenesis. In: Slaga TJ (ed) Mechanisms of tumor promotion, vol I. Tumor promotion in internal organs. CRC Press, Florida, pp 1–53

Perry EK, Marshal EF, Blessed G (1983) Decreased imipramine binding in the brains of patients with depressive illness. Br J Psychiatry 142:188–192

Peterson LA, Harris TM, Guengerich FP (1988) Evidence for an episulfonium ion intermediate in the formation of *S*-[2(N^7-guanyl)ethyl]glutathione in DNA. J Am Chem Soc 110:3284–3291

Potter DW, Miller DW, Hinson JA (1986) Horseradish peroxidase-catalysed oxidation of acetaminophen to intermediates that form polymers or conjugate with glutathione. Mol Pharmacol 29:155–162

Prota G (1988) Progress in the chemistry of melanins and related metabolites. Med Res Rev 87:525–556

Rankin BB, Curthoys NP (1982) Evidence for the renal paratubular transport of glutathione. FEBS Lett 108:193–196

Rannug U, Beije B (1979) The mutagenic effect of 1,2-dichloroethane on *Salmonella typhimurium*. II. Activation by the isolated perfused rat liver. Chem Biol Interact 24:265–285

Rannug U, Sundvall A, Ramel C (1978) The mutagenic effect of 1,2-dichloroethane on *Salmonella typhimurium*. I. Activation through conjugation with glutathione in vitro. Chem Biol Interact 20:1–16

Rao DNR, Takahashi N, Mason RP (1988) Characterization of a glutathione conjugate of the 1,4-benzosemiquinone-free radical formed in rat hepatocytes. J Biol Chem 263:1798–17986

Redegeld FAM, Hofman GA, van der Loo PGF, Koster AS, Noordhoek J (1989) Nephrotoxicity of the GSH conjugate of menadione (2-methyl-1,4-naphthoquinone) in the isolated perfused rat kidney. Role of metabolism by γ-glutamyl transpeptidase and probenecid-sensitive transport. J Pharmacol Exp Ther 256:665–669

Reed DJ, Ellis WW, Meck RA (1980) The inhibition of γ-glutamyl transpeptidase and glutathione metabolism of isolated rat kidney cells by L-(αS,$5S$)-α-amino-3-chloro-4,5-dihydro-5-isoxazoleacetic acid (AT-125;NSC-163501). Biochem Biophys Res Commun 94:1273–1277

Reed DJ, Foureman GL (1986) A comparison of the alkylating capabilities of the cysteinyl and glutathionyl conjugates of 1,2-dichloroethane. In: Snyder R, Nelson JO, Witmer CM, Jollow DJ, Kocsis JJ (eds) Biological reactive intermediates III. Mechanisms of action in animal models and human disease. Plenum, New York, pp 469–475

Reed DJ, Meredith MJ (1985) Cellular defense mechanisms against reactive metabolites. In: Anders MW (ed) Bioactivation of foreign compounds. Academic, New York, pp 71–108

Rees JR, Pirie A (1967) Possible reactions of 1,2-naphthoquinone in the eye. Biochem J 102:853–863

Robbins JD, Stevens JL (1986) Purification and characterization of a cysteine conjugate β-lyase activity from rat kidney mitochondria and its dependence on an α-keto acid for activity. Pharmacologist 28:196

Roch-Ramel F, Weiner IM (1980) Renal urate excretion. Factors determining the action of drugs. Kidney Int 18:665–676

Rosenblum WI (1992) Endothelium-derived relaxing factor in brain blood vessels is not nitric oxide. Stroke 23:1527–1532

Ross D, Larsson R, Norbeck K, Ryhage R, Moldeus P (1985) Characterization and mechanism of formation of reactive products formed during peroxidase-catalysed oxidation of p-phenetidine. Mol Pharmacol 27:277–288

Rubanyi GM, John WD, Bates FN, Harrison D (1991) Evidence that a *S*-nitrosothiol, but not nitric oxide, may be identical with endothelium derived relaxing factor. J Cardiovasc Pharmacol 17 [Suppl 3]:S41–S45

Sausen PJ, Elfarra AA (1990) Cysteine conjugate *S*-oxidase. Characterization of a novel enzymatic activity in rat hepatic and renal microsomes. J Biol Chem 265:6139–6145

Sausen PJ, Elfarra AA (1991) Reactivity of cysteine *S*-conjugate sulfoxides: formation of *S*-[1-chloro-2-(*S*-glutathionyl)vinyl]-L-cysteine sulfoxide by the reaction of *S*-(1,2-dichlorovinyl)-L-cysteine sulfoxide with glutathione. Chem Res Toxicol 4:655–660

Sausen PJ, Elfarra AA, Cooley AJ (1992) Methimazole protection of rats against chemically induced kidney damage in vivo. J Pharmacol Exp Ther 260:393–401

Sausen PJ, Duescher RJ, Elfarra AA (1993) Further characterization and purification of the flavin-dependent *S*-benzyl-L-cysteine *S*-oxidase activities of rat liver and kidney microsomes. Mol Pharmacol 43:388–396

Schaeffer VH, Stevens JL (1982) Mechanism of transport for toxic cysteine conjugates in rat kidney cortex membrane vesicles. Mol Pharmacol 32:293–298

Schaeffer VL, Stevens JL (1987) The transport of *S*-cysteine conjugates in LLC-PK1 cells and its role in toxicity. Mol Pharmacol 31:506–512

Schasteen CS, Reed DJ (1983) The hydrolysis and alkylation activities of *S*-(2-haloethyl)-L-cysteine analogs. Evidence for extended half-life. Toxicol Appl Pharmacol 70:423–432

Schmid A, Beuter W, Mayring L (1983) Untersuchungen zum wirkungsmechanismus von *S*-(dichlorvinyl)-L-cystein. Zentralbl Veterinarmed [A] 30:511–520

Schnellman RG, Lock EA, Mandel LJ (1987) A mechanism of *S*-(1,2,3,4,4-pentachloro-1,3-butadienyl)-L-cysteine toxicity to rabbit renal proximal tubules. Toxicol Appl Pharmacol 90:513–521

Schrenk D, Dekant W (1989) Covalent binding of hexachlorobutadiene metabolites to renal and hepatic mitochondrial DNA. Carcinogenesis 10:1139–1141

Shibata M-A, Hirose M, Tanaka H, Asakawa E, Shirai T, Ito N (1991) Induction of renal cell tumors in rats and mice, and enhancement of hepatocellular tumor development in mice after long-term hydroquinone treatment. Jpn J Cancer Res 82:1211–1219

Sies H (1988) Intracellular effects of glutathione conjugates and their transport from the cell. In: Sies H, Ketterer B (eds) Glutathione conjugation mechanisms and biological significance. Academic, New York, pp 175–192

Sies H, Ketterer (1988) Glutathione conjugation: mechanisms and biological significance. Academic, San Diego

Sies H, Akerboom T, Ishikawa T (1989) Glutathione conjugates: Transport from the cell and intracellular effects. In: Taniguchi N, Higashi T, Sakamoto Y, Meister A (eds) Glutathione centennial. Molecular perspectives and clinical implications. Academic, New York, pp 357–367

Singh S, Dryhurst G (1991) Reactions of the serotonergic neurotoxin 5,6-dihydroxytryptamine with glutathione. J Org Chem 56:1767–1773

Sjoquist B, Liljequist S, Engel J (1982) Increased salsolinol levels in rat striatum and limbic forebrain following chronic ethanol treatment. J Neurochem 39:259–262

Slatter JG, Rashed MS, Pearson PG, Han D-H, Bailie TA (1991) Biotransformation of methyl isocyanate in the rat. Evidence for glutathione conjugation as a major pathway of metabolism and implications for isocyanate-mediated toxicities. Chem Res Toxicol 4:157–161

Slivka A, Spina MB, Cohen G (1987) Reduced and oxidized glutathione in human and monkey brain. Neurosci Lett 74:112–118

Smit WA, Zefirov NS, Bodrikov IV, Krimer MZ (1979) Episulfonium ions: myth and reality. Acc Chem Res 12:282–288

Smith MT, Evans CG, Thor H, Orrenius S (1985) Quinone-induced oxidative injury to cells and tissues. In: Sies H (ed) Oxidative stress. Academic, London, pp 91–113

Solt DB (1981) Localization of gamma glutamyl transpeptidase in hamster buccal pouch epithelium treated with 7,12-dimethylbenz[a]anthracene. J Natl Cancer Inst 67:193–197

Spater HW, Poruchynsky MS, Quintana N, Innoue M, Novikoff AB (1982) Immunocytochemical localization of γ-glutamyltransferase in rat kidney with protein A-horseradish peroxidase. Proc Natl Acad Sci USA 79:3547–3550

Spector A (1984) Towards a solution of senile cataracts. Invest Opthamol Vis Sci 25:130–146

Stahl W, Denkel E, Eisenbrand G (1988) Influence of glutathione on the mutagenicity of 2-chloroethylnitrosoureas. Mutagenic potential of glutathione derivatives formed from 2-chloroethylnitrosoureas and glutathione. Mutat Res 206:459–465

Stahl W, Lenhardt S, Przybylski M, Eisenbrand G (1992) Mechanism of glutathione-mediated DNA damage by the antineoplastic agent 1,3-bis(2-chloroethyl)-*N*-nitrosourea. Chem Res Toxicol 5:106–109

Stevens J, Hayden P, Taylor G (1986) The role of glutathione conjugate metabolism and cysteine conjugate β-lyase in the mechanism of *S*-cysteine conjugate toxicity in LLC-PK1 cell. J Biol Chem 261:3325–3332

Stevens J, Jakoby WB (1983) Cysteine conjugate β-lyase. Mol Pharmacol 23:761–765

Stevens JL (1985) Isolation and characterization of a rat liver enzyme with both cysteine conjugate β-lyase and kynureninase activity. J Biol Chem 260:7954–7950

Stevens JL, Jones DP (1989) The mercapturic acid pathway: biosynthesis, intermediary metabolism and physiological disposition. In: Dolphin D, Poulson D, Avramovic O (eds) Coenzymes and cofactors, vol 3: glutathione: chemical, biochemical and medical aspects. Wiley, New York, pp 45–85

Stevens JL, Bakke J (1990) *S*-Methylation. In: Mulder GJ (ed) Conjugation reactions in drug metabolism. Taylor and Francis, London, pp 233–250

Stillwell TJ, Benson RC (1988) Cyclophosphamide-induced hemorrhagic cystisis. Cancer 61:451–457

Stonard MD (1973) Further studies on the site and mechanism of action of *S*-(1,2-dichlorovinyl)-L-cysteine and *S*-(1,2-dichlorovinyl)-3-mercaptopropionic acid in rat liver. Biochem Pharmacol 22:1329–1335

Stonard MD, Parker VH (1971) 2-Oxo acid dehydrogenases of rat liver mitochondria as the site of action of *S*-(1,2-dichlorovinyl)-L-cysteine and *S*-(1,2-dichlorovinyl)-3-mercaptopropionic acid. Biochem Pharmacol 20:2417–2427

Sundheimer DW, White RD, Brendel K, Sipes JG (1982) The bioactivation of 1,2-dibromoethane in rat hepatocytes: covalent binding to nucleic acids. Carcinogenesis 3:1129–1133

Suzuki S, Tateishi M (1981) Purification and characterization of a rat liver enzyme catalysing *N*-deacetylation of mercapturic acid conjugates. Drug Metab Dispos 9:573–577

Szinicz LL, Weger N (1980) Effects of 4-dimethylaminophenol in rat kidneys, isolated kidney tubules and hepatocytes. Xenobiotica 10:611–620

Tajima K, Hashizaki M, Yamamoto K, Mizutani T (1991) Identification and structure characterization of *S*-containing metabolites of 3-*tert*-butyl-4-hydroxyanisole in rat urine and liver microsomes. Drug Metab Dispos 19:1028–1033

Takahashi N, Schreiber J, Fischer V, Mason R (1987) Formation of glutathione-conjugated semiquinones by the reaction of quinones with glutathione; an ESR study. Arch Biochem Biophys 252:41–48

Tanaka T, Naganuma A, Imura N (1992) Routes for renal transport of methylmercury in mice. Eur J Pharmacol 228:9–14

Tanaka TA, Naganuma A, Imura N (1990) Role of γ-glutamyltranspeptidase in renal uptake and toxicity of inorganic mercury in mice. Toxicology 60:187–198

Taniguchi N, Higashi T, Sakamoto Y, Meister A (eds) (1989) Glutathione centennial: molecular perspectives and clinical implications. Academic, San Diego

Tate SS (1980) Enzymes of mercapturic acid formation. In: Jakoby WB (ed) Enzymatic basis of detoxification, vol 2. Academic, Orlando, pp 95–120

Tateishi M, Suzuki S, Shimizu H (1978) Cysteine conjugate β-lyase in rat liver. A novel enzyme catalyzing formation of thiol-containing metabolites of drugs. J Biol Chem 253:8854–8859

Temmink JHM, Bruggeman IM, van Bladeren PJ (1986) Cytomorphological changes in liver cells exposed to allyl and benzyl isothiocyanate and their cysteine and glutathione conjugates. Arch Toxicol 59:103–110

Terracini B, Parker VH (1965) A pathological study of *S*-dichlorovinyl-L-cysteine. Food Cosmet Toxicol 3:67–74

Threadgill MD, Axworthy DB, Baillie TA, Farmer PB, Farrow KC, Gescher A, Kestell P, Pearson PG, Shaw AJ (1987) Metabolism of *N*-methylformamide in mice: primary kinetic deuterium isotope effect and identification of *S*-(*N*-methylcarbamoyl)glutathione as a metabolite. J Pharmacol Exp Ther 242: 312–319

Tillian H, Schauenstein E, Ertyl A, Esterbauer H (1976) Therapeutic effects of cysteine adducts of α,β-unsaturated aldehydes on Ehrlich ascites tumor of mice I. Eur J Cancer 12:989–993

Tillian H, Schauenstein E, Ertyl A, Esterbauer H (1978) Therapeutic effects of cysteine adducts of α,β-unsaturated aldehydes on Ehrlich ascites tumor of mice II. Eur J Cancer 14:533–536

Tomisawa H, Fukazawa H, Ichihara S, Tateishi M (1986) A novel pathway for formation of thiol-containing metabolites from cysteine conjugates. Biochem Pharmacol 35:2270–2272

Tsuda H, Fukushima S, Imaida K, Sakata T, Ito N (1984) Modification of carcinogenesis by antioxidants and other compounds. Acta Pharmacol Toxicol 55: 125–143

Vadi HV, Schasteen CS, Reed DJ (1985) Interaction of *S*-(2-haloethyl)-mercapturic acid analogs with plasmid DNA. Toxicol Appl Pharmacol 80:386–396

Vamvakas S, Elfarra AA, Dekant W, Henschler D, Anders MW (1988a) Mutagenicity of amino acid and glutathione *S*-conjugates in the Ames test. Mutat Res 206:83–90

Vamvakas S, Berthold K, Dekant W, Henschler D (1988b) Bacterial cysteine conjugate β-lyase and the metabolism of cysteine *S*-conjugates: structural requirements for the cleavage of *S*-conjugates and the formation of reactive intermediates. Chem Biol Int 65:59–71

Vamvakas S, Kordowich FJ, Dekant W, Neudecker T, Henschler D (1988c) Mutagenicity of hexachloro-1,3-butadiene and its *S*-conjugates in the Ames test – role of activation by the mercapturic acid pathway in its nephrocarcinogenicity. Carcinogensis 9:907–910

Vamvakas S, Herkenhoff M, Dekant W, Henschler D (1989) Mutagenicity of tetrachloroethylene in the Ames-test – metabolic activation by conjugation with glutathione. J Biochem Toxico 4:21–27
Vamvakas S, Sharma VK, Sheu S-S, Anders MW (1990) Perturbations of intracellular calcium distribution in kidney cells by nephrotoxic haloalkenyl cysteine *S*-conjugates. Mol Pharmacol 38:455–461
van Bladeren PJ, Van der Gen A, Breimer DD, Mohn GR (1979) Stereoselective activation of vicinal dihalogen compounds to mutagens by glutathione conjugation. Biochem Pharmacol 28:2521–2524
van Bladeren PJ, Breimer DD, Rotteveel-Smijs GMT, de Jong RAW, Buijs W, van der Gen A, Mohn GR (1980) The role of glutathione conjugation in the mutagenicity of 1,2-dibromoethane. Biochem Pharmacol 29:2975–2982
van Bladeren PJ, Breimer DD, Rotteveel-Smijs GMT, De Knijff P, Mohn GR, van Meeteren-Walchi B, Buijs W, van der Gen A (1981) The relation between the structure of vicinal dihalogen compounds and their mutagenic activation via conjugation to glutathione. Carcinogenesis 2:499–505
van Bladeren PJ, Bruggeman IM, Jongen WMF, Scheffer AG, Temmink JHM (1987) The role of conjugating enzymes in toxic metabolite formation. In: Benford DJ, Bridges JW, Gibson GG (eds) Drug metabolism. From molecule to man. Taylor and Francis, London, pp 151–171
van Ommen B, Den Besten C, Ruttern ACM, Ploemen JHTM, Voo RME, Muller M, van Bladeren PJ (1988) Active site-directed irreversible inhibition of glutathione *S*-transferases by the glutathione conjugate of tetrachloro-1,4-benzoquinone. J Biol Chem 263:12939–12942
van Ommen B, Ploemen JHTM, Ruven HJ, Vos RME, Boggards JJP, van Berkel WJH, van Bladeren PJ (1989) Studies on the active site of rat glutathione *S*-transferase isoenzyme 4-4. Chemical modification by tetrachloro-1,4-benzoquinone and its glutathione conjugate. Eur J Biochem 181:423–429
van Ommen B, Ploemen JP, Bogaards JJP, Monks TJ, Lau SS, van Bladeren PJ (1991) Irreversible inhibition of rat glutathione *S*-transferase 1-1 by quinones and their glutathione conjugates: structure-activity relationship and mechanism. Biochem J 276:661–666
Vina J (ed) (1990) Glutathione: metabolism and physiological functions. CRC Press, Boca Raton
Vos RME, van Ommen B, Hoekstein MSJ, de Goede JHM, van Bladeren PJ (1989) Irreversible inhibition of rat hepatic glutathione *S*-transferase isoenzymes by a series of structurally related quinones. Chem Biol Int 71:381–392
Wallin A, Jones TW, Vercesi AE, Cotgreave I, Ormstad K, Orrenius S (1987) Toxicity of *S*-pentachlorobutadienyl-L-cysteine studied with isolated rat renal cortrical mitochondria. Arch Biochem Biophys 258:365–372
Wattenberg LW (1981) Inhibition of carcinogen-induced neoplasia by sodium cyanate, tertbutyl isocyanate and benzyl isothiacyanate administered subsequent to carcinogen exposure. Cancer Res 41:2991–2994
Weber G (1983) Biochemical strategy of cancer cells and the design of chemotherapy. Cancer Res 43:3466–3492
Wefers H, Sies H (1983) Hepatic low-level chemiluminesence during redox cycling of menadione and the menadione-glutathione conjugate: relation to glutathione and NAD(P)H: quinone reductase (DT-diaphorase) activity. Arch Biochem Biophys 224:568–578
Weisiger RA, Jakoby WB (1979) Thiol *S*-methyltransferase from rat liver. Arch Biochem Biophys 196:631–637
Wells PG, Wilson B, Lubek BM (1989) In vivo murine studies on the biochemical mechanism of naphthalene cataractogenesis. Toxicol Appl Pharmacol 99: 466–473
Westbrook C, Lin Y-M, Jarabak J (1977) NADP-linked 15-hydroxyprostaglandin dehydrogenase from human placenta: partial purification and characterization of

the enzyme and identification of an inhibitor in placental tissue. Biochem Biophys Res Commun 76:943–946
Whaley MW, Govindachari TR (1951) The Pictet-Spengler synthesis of tetrahydroisoquinolines and related compounds. In: Rogers A (ed) Organic reactions VI. Wiley, New York, pp 151–190
Williams G, Ohmori T, Katayama S, Rice J (1980) Alteration by phenobarbital of membrane-associated enzymes including gamma glutamyl transpeptidase. Carcinogenesis 1:813–818
Wilson I, Wardman P, Lin T, Sartorelli AC (1986) One-electron reduction of 2- and 6-methyl-1,4-naphthoquinone bioreductive alkylating agents. J Med Chem 29:1381–1384
Wolf CR, Berry PN, Nash JA, Green T, Lock EA (1984) Role of microsomal and cytosolic glutathione *S*-transferases in the conjugation of hexachloro-1,3-butadiene in the rat and its possible relevance to nephrotoxicity. J Pharmacol Exp Ther 228:202–208
Wolf WA, Bobik A (1988) Effects of 5,6-dihydroxytryptamine on the release, synthesis and storage of serotonin: studies using rat brain synaptosomes. J Neurochem 50:536–542
Wolff SP, Spector A (1987) Pro-oxidant activation of occular reductants. 2 Lens epithelial cell cytotoxicity of a dietary quinone is associated with a stable free radical formed with glutathione in vitro. Exp Eye Res 45:791–801
Wong K-S, Dryhurst G (1990) Tryptamine-4,5-dione: properties and reaction with glutathione. Bioorg Chem 18:253–264
Wooley DW, Shaw E (1954) A biochemical and phamacological suggestion about certain mental disorders. Proc Natl Acad Sci USA 40:228–231
Yeates RA, Laufen H, Leitold M (1985) The reaction between organic nitrates and sulfhydryl compounds. A possible model system for the activation of organic nitrates. Mol Pharmacol 28:555–559
Zhang F, Dryhurst G (1991) Electrochemical and enzyme-mediated oxidation of tetrahydropapaveroline. J Org Chem 56:7113–7121

CHAPTER 17

Challenges and Directions for Future Research

F.C. Kauffman

A. Introduction

It is clear from material reviewed in the preceding chapters that application of the tools of molecular biology to enzyme reactions catalyzing conjugating and deconjugating enzymes has greatly advanced understanding of the expression and regulation of these important drug-metabolizing systems in a variety of tissues. In addition to better understanding the biology of transferases involved in conjugation of biotic and xenobiotic metabolites, it is clear that various hydrolases such as β-glucuronidase, aryl-sulfatase, amidases, and carboxylesterases have critical functions in the net formation and biological activity of many drug and toxic chemical conjugates. Molecular biological approaches being used to define the genetic regulation and tissue distribution of hydrolases involved in processing chemical conjugates are reviewed in several chapters of this volume, since their role in regulating net conjugate production in intact cells is beginning to be recognized.

Material reviewed in the preceding chapters of this book also emphasizes that many products of phase II conjugation reactions possess biological activity of their own. Promising new areas of drug discovery and development will flow from future studies directed at understanding the mechanism of biologically active chemical conjugates. The purpose of this chapter is to identify some of the challenging questions that have arisen from recent studies of conjugation–deconjugation reactions reviewed in this volume and to provide suggestions for future research.

B. Search for Factors Regulating Polymorphic Expression of Phase II Conjugating and Deconjugating Enzymes

Enormous progress has been made over the last 5 years in knowledge concerning the molecular structure of transferases and hydrolases involved in phase II conjugation reactions. It is now clear that, as with the cytochrome P450 supergene family, many of the enzymes involved in phase II reactions are also members of supergene families. Developing appropriate nomenclatures based on evolutionary divergence schemes remains a challenge for workers in the field, although considerable progress has been made for major classes of these enzymes such as the uridine diphosphate (UDP)-glucuronosyl gene superfamily (BURCHELL et al. 1991) and sulfotransferases (WEINSHILBOUM 1988). Knowledge concerning the regulation of expression of various transferases and hydrolases has grown at a rapid rate. A summary of some immediate questions being given attention is presented below.

I. Genetic Factors

Full-length genes of many transferases involved with phase II conjugation reactions have now been cloned, including UDP-glucuronosyltransferase (UDPGT; BURCHELL et al. 1991), sulfotransferase (WEINSHILBOUM 1988; OTTERNESS et al. 1992), glutathione *S*-transferases (PICKETT et al. 1984; TELAKOWSKI-HOPKINS et al. 1985), *N*-acetyltransferase (BLUM et al. 1990), thiopurine (HONCHEL et al. 1993), catechol, and phenylethanolamine transferases (GROSSMAN et al. 1992a). Similarly, many genes for hydrolases such as carboxylesterase (OVNIC et al. 1991) and β-glucuronidase (WAWRZYNIAK et al. 1989) have been cloned and expressed. This work has contributed greatly to better understanding the structure and regulation of these enzymes. A challenge for future investigations is to identify natural and xenobiotic substrates for many of the individual isoenzymes identified by molecular cloning. For example, eight different rat UDPGTs and ten human UDPGTs have been identified to date (BURCHELL et al. 1991). It has been suggested that the UDPGT multigene family, in fact, may be similar in size to the cytochrome P450 family, which has more than 30 members (GONZALEZ 1992). Many of the UDPGT isoforms in rat are known to glucuronidate at least one endogenous acceptor; however, despite extensive studies, endogenous acceptors for the planar UDPGT have not been found. On the other hand, isoforms that glucuronidate many drugs have not been identified either by purification or by cDNA cloning (reviewed in Chap. 1 of this volume). Identifying substrates for various isoforms remains a challenge for sulfotransferases, where substrate specificities for only half of the reported cDNAs have been determined.

The role of alternative splicing of a common precursor RNA to explain the generation of different isoforms of gene complexes, although possible, has not received much attention. Based on recent findings (OWENS and RITTER 1992) it has been suggested that transcription of UDPGTs is under the control of its own promoter. Additional studies are also needed to determine whether expression of separate isoforms of transferases are regulated individually, as demonstrated recently for angiotensin-converting enzymes (KUMAR et al. 1991).

Research directed at determining molecular events involved in the expression of various transferases and hydrolases in different tissues during development or exposure to xenobiotic-inducing agents is needed. Factors regulating ontogenic expression of most enzymes involved in conjugation–

deconjugation reactions are poorly understood. In this regard, it is important to note that corticosteroids (DUTTON 1980) and thyroid hormones (LABRUNE et al. 1991) have been implicated in the expression of phenol UDPGTs during development. In view of recent studies made in understanding the regulation of the steroid supergene family, studies designed to identify *cis* and *trans* elements that regulate gene expression for UDPGTs as well as other phase II conjugating enzymes are needed. Such information is necessary for understanding mechanisms involved in the induction, tissue distribution, and ontogeny of these proteins.

A powerful tool being applied to analyzing relationships between molecular structure and function is site-directed mutagenesis. As more cDNAs for transferases and hydrolases are expressed in prokaryotic cell systems, increased opportunities for studies employing site-directed mutagenesis will be realized. A recent application of site-directed mutagenesis demonstrated that mutations in His-159 produced a change in the activity of glutathione transferase (R.N. WANG et al. 1992). The availability of large amounts of enzyme protein made possible by molecular cloning and expression procedures should also foster crystallographic structural analyses of enzyme–substrate complexes. An example of this approach was demonstrated recently for the mu-class of glutathione *S*-transferase (REINEMER et al. 1992; LIU et al. 1992).

Chromosome mapping procedures have been applied to establish the genetic basis of human polymorphism with respect to conjugation–deconjugation reactions (MOGHRABI et al. 1992; MONAGHAN et al. 1992; OWENS and RITTER 1992). For example, human N-acetylation polymorphism associated with slow and fast acetylation of a variety of drug substrates typified by isoniazid and sulfamethazine is related to variants in the NAT2 locus (BLUM et al. 1990; VATSIS and WEBER 1991). Slow acetylation is apparently related to reduced amounts of the cytosolic enzyme *N*-acetyl-transferase without alteration of the kinetic properties of the enzyme. Mechanisms suggested for the reduced enzyme include impaired translational efficiency of mutant NAT2 mRNA or enhanced degradation of mutant protein (BLUM et al. 1990; DEGUCHI 1992). Unraveling the molecular basis for impaired expression of the NAT2 product will likely serve as a useful approach to deciphering other human genetic polymorphisms.

Interindividual variation in the methylation of endogenous and xenobiotic compounds has been implicated in the pharmacological activity and toxicity of thiopurines and catecholamines (WEINSHILBOUM 1989; LENNARD et al. 1987). In a recent series of studies, Weinshilbaum and his colleagues (GROSSMAN et al. 1992b) measured methyltransferase activities in human erythrocytes and showed that variations in enzyme activities correlated with therapeutic effects and toxicities of different drugs. The molecular basis for the inherited variations in methyltransferases is currently an area of active research.

II. Environmental Factors

It is clear that many enzymes involved in conjugation–deconjugation reactions are induced by enhanced transcription of genes regulating their expression (PICKETT et al. 1984). Molecular mechanisms underlying induction of these enzymes by environmental factors is a very active area of current research. An exciting example of work in this area is illustrated by studies on the regulation of expression of rat liver glutathione *S*-transferases by xenobiotics and antioxidants, reviewed extensively in Chap. 3 of this volume. Initial work on the regulation of the GST *Ya* subunit gene showed that at least two *cis*-acting sequences between nucleotides 1651 and 663 of the flanking region were necessary for maximal basal and inducible expression of the reporter gene, *CAT* (TELAKOWSKI-HOPKINS et al. 1985). Subsequent use of deletion constructs spanning the entire 1717 bp of the flanking region, transfection in HepG2 cells, and measurement of *CAT* activity in the presence or absence of several inducers indicated five distinct regulatory elements in the rat *Ya* subunit gene (RUSHMORE et al. 1991). One of the *cis*-acting regulatory elements in the flanking region was identified by its ability to mediate induction of the *Ya* subunit gene by *β*-naphthoflavone and 3-methylcholan-threne. Extensive analyses of the rat gene suggest that this regulatory element, designated the antioxidant responsive element (ARE), is similar to the Ah receptor-independent mechanism accounting for the induction of several phase II conjugating enzymes by phenolic antioxidants reported by TALALAY et al. (1988). A similar electrophilically responsive element having significant sequence homology to ARE has been noted in the flanking region of a mouse GST *Ya* subunit gene (FRILING et al. 1992). These recent experiments raise the intriguing possibility that a pro-oxidative environment within cells may activate transcription through ARE. Induction of enzymes that protect cells from endogenous or exogenous compounds that form reactive O_2 species would follow from this activation. In accord with this hypothesis, genes for at least one other enzyme associated with protection of cells against oxidative stress, reduced nicotinamine adenosine dinucleotide (phosphate) (NAD(P)H)-quinone reductase, contain a functional ARE sequence (FAVREAU and PICKETT 1991; JAISWAL 1991). Further studies to test the idea that electrophilic signals activate ARE and subsequently lead to the protection of a variety of cells from oxidative stress is an important direction for future research.

C. Net Conjugate Production by Intact Cells

Material reviewed in several earlier chapters of this volume emphasizes the variety of factors, in addition to activities of phase II conjugating and deconjugating emzymes, that regulate the production of conjugates in intact cells. These factors include availability of cofactors, futile cycling between transferases and hydrolases, and transport of metabolites and cofactors across biological membranes. Selected highlights of research in this area and potential directions for future studies are discussed briefly here.

I. Interaction Between Transferases and Hydrolases

Studies concerning futile cycling of metabolites via specific transferases and associated hydrolases have been carried out for only a limited number of substrates such as hydroxycoumarin (KAUFFMAN et al. 1991), bilirubin (DWIVEDI et al. 1987), and *p*-nitrophenol (BELINSKY et al. 1984). Although these studies demonstrate the potential for futile cycling of phase I and phase II metabolites in intact hepatocytes, further work is needed to test the generality of this phenomenon with other compounds and other cell types. Studies carried out to date (KAUFFMAN et al. 1991; EL MOUELHI and KAUFFMAN 1986) suggest that the kinetic properties and subcellular location of sulfotransferase(s) and arylsulfatase(s) may be particularly favorable for futile cycling of sulfate conjugates (EL MOUELHI and KAUFFMAN 1986). This possibility should be tested using drugs and hormones that are primarily converted to sulfate conjugates by the liver such as estrogen (TSENG et al. 1983), catecholamines (GAUDIN et al. 1985), and thyroxin (KUNG et al. 1988).

A key determinant of futile cycling of sulfate and glucuronide conjugates may involve the localization of arylsulfatase (KAUFFMAN et al. 1991) and β-glucuronidase (SOKOLOVE et al. 1984) in membranes of the endoplasmic reticulum (ER). A challenge in this area is to determine whether alterations in arylsulfatase or β-glucuronidase targeted for the ER change net glucuronide and sulfate production.

Considerable progress has been made in understanding mechanisms targeting enzymes for the ER. One of the best examples of targeting of an enzyme to the ER concerns the interaction between β-glucuronidase and its membrane-anchoring protein egasyn (MEDDA and SWANK 1985). Based on immunochemical and sequencing studies (SWANK et al. 1986), egasyn is a microsomal carboxylesterase. Organophosphates, which are well-known inhibitors of various esterases, cause a rapid and profound release of liver ER enzyme into plasma (WILLIAMS 1969). The mechanism(s) underlying the specific and massive release of β-glucuronidase are not known, and clarification of this interesting phenomenon is needed.

II. Cofactor Supply

Generation of cofactors such as UDP-glucuronic acid (UDPGA), phosphoadenosine phosphosulfate (PAPS), and *S*-adenosylmethionine (SAM) via energy-dependent reactions is an important determinant of rates of phase II conjugation reactions in intact cells (reviewed in Chap. 8 of this volume). In general, intracellular levels of activated substrates required for conjugation are in the range of K_m values for related transferases. For example, the K_m values of UDPGA for glucuronosyltransferase are in the range of 0.1–0.4 mM (BOCK et al. 1973), which are similar to concentrations of UDPGA in liver (GREENBAUM et al. 1971). Thus, metabolic events that alter intracellular concentrations of UDPGA would be expected to change rates of net conjugate production by intact cells. Indeed, several laboratories (REINKE et al. 1981) have shown that such is the case for a variety of substrates. A challenge facing investigators in the field is to determine the extent to which various metabolic burdens such as compromised nutritional status or exposure to toxic agents alters conjugation of metabolites of commonly used therapeutic agents.

Although there is considerable information on relationships between cofactor supply and rates of sulfation and glucuronidation, little information exists concerning the role of cofactor supply in determining rates of methylation, acetylation, and amino acid conjugation of drugs and their metabolites, and there is a need for research in this area. For example, it would be important to determine whether high rates of lipogenesis limit acetylation of drugs such as sulfamethoxazole, which are acetylated at high rates (HELLERSTEIN et al. 1991), by competing for limited intracellular pools of acetyl-coenzyme A (CoA). Steady state concentrations of acetyl-CoA are estimated to range from 20 to 50 nmol/gm liver (GREENBAUM et al. 1971).

Further research concerning alterations in normal hepatic function caused by interactions between various pathways generating cofactors and drugs metabolized at high rates is needed. For example, highly reactive intermediates may deplete intracellular reduced glutathione nonenzymatically and promote oxidative stress. Drugs or toxic agents undergoing high rates of acetylation may impair lipogenesis by competing for limited pools of acetyl-CoA as mentioned above.

III. Transport of Conjugated Metabolites

Vectorial anion transport of drug conjugates into plasma and bile is an important determinant of their net formation by intact hepatoctyes. Recent development of techniques for the preparation of highly purified basolateral and canalicular membrane vesicles has led to great progress in characterizing molecular features of transport systems for drug conjugates (MEIER 1988; SZTUL et al. 1987; VORE and HOFFMAN 1992). Evidence is accumulating that many drug conjugates are transported from plasma into hepatocytes by a multispecific Na^+–taurocholate cotransport system (ZIMMERLI et al. 1989). A cDNA encoding a functional glycosylated protein for the Na^+–taurocholate cotransport system has been expressed in *Xenopus* oocytes (HAGENBUCH et al. 1991). It would be important to determine whether the broad range of drug conjugates (e.g., estradiol-3-sulfate) implicated as substrates for this transport system are true substrates for the Na^+–taurocholate cotransporter, as suggested by Vore in Chap. 11 of this volume. It will also be important to determine whether this system functions as a bidirectional transporter for drug conjugates.

Further characterizing of adenosine triphosphate (ATP)-dependent systems involved in the transport of drugs and drug conjugates across canalicular membranes of hepatocytes into bile has been accomplished. Antibodies for various *P*-glycoproteins related to the multidrug-resistant glucoprotein (MDR) have been produced in mice (BUSCHMAN et al. 1992). One of these antibodies, Mdr2, was present in high amounts in canalicular, but not in sinusoidal, membrane vesicles from mouse liver. The function of this protein is not known, and additional research is needed to determine its potential role in transporting xenobiotics and endogenous metabolites such as bilirubin mono- and diglucuronides. Phase I clinical trials employing inhibitors of *P*-glycoprotein to inhibit MDR-mediated efflux of chemotherapeutic agents are beginning. One of these agents, cyclosporine, caused hyperbilirubinemia (YAHANDA et al. 1989), consistent with the idea that MDR is involved in the transport of conjugated bilirubin in the bile.

Further characterization of mechanisms associated with the transport of drug conjugates across basolateral and canalicular membranes in hepatocytes from various species is needed in view of the critical roles that have been established for these systems in biotic and xenobiotic metabolism and toxicity.

D. Mechanisms of Biologically Active Conjugates

Ample evidence, reviewed in the chapters above, documents the biological activity of many phase II conjugates. Although the activity of a number of compounds has been known for some years, knowledge concerning their precise mechanisms of action is sparse. In general, conjugates described in this volume either act directly or serve as carrier molecules of biological activity. Compounds acting directly are exemplified by compounds that behave as electrophiles, e.g., certain sulfonates and acyl-linked glucuronides, or agents interacting with receptor molecules, e.g., minoxidil sulfate. A brief overview of some major questions concerning biologically active conjugates is given below.

I. Chemically Active Toxic Conjugates

1. Sulfonates

Sulfuric acid esters that are unstable in water were among the first active conjugates studied in a systematic fashion. Acetyl-aminofluorene-*N*-sulfate is one of the most studied chemical carcinogens (BAMFORTH et al. 1992). Although it is known that heterolytic cleavage of such compounds generates sulfate ion and highly reactive electrophiles that combine covalently with nucleophilic groups in cellular macromolecules to form adducts, the exact relationship of such adducts to mutagenic and carcinogenic processes is not clear. An unstable sulfuric acid ester has only been isolated once from tissues (Watabe et al. 1986). Much of the evidence implicating sulfonates in carcinogenesis has been obtained primarily by indirect means, such as using various inhibitors of sulfotransferases (Michejda et al. 1987; Kroeger-Koepke et al. 1992). Although it is probably correct to assume that mutagenesis and carcinogenesis arise from DNA adducts of various sulfonates, these compounds interact with other cellular constituents including RNAs, proteins, and glutathione and the possibility that some of these reactions are involved in carcinogenesis needs to be more critically evaluated.

2. Acyl Glucuronides

Another class of compounds that readily undergo spontaneous chemical reactions is 1-*O*-acyl glucuronides. The potential physiological actions of this class of compounds involving transacylation reactions was pointed out more than 10 years ago (Olson et al. 1992). Virtually all xenobiotic and endogenous organic acids have the capacity to form 1-*O*-acyl glucuronides, i.e., glycosidic bonds are incorporated into ester linkages, that may undergo spontaneous nucleophilic displacement (Bradow et al. 1989). Many acyl glucuronides bind covalently to serum albumin (van Breemen and Fenselau 1984), casein (Smith et al. 1990), and polylysine (Manafo et al. 1990). Such studies argue strongly that formation of covalent bonds between 1-*O*-acyl glucuronides and biopolymers occur in vivo. Since many drugs including hypolipidic agents (van Breemen and Fenselau 1984), diuretics (Olson et al. 1992), anticonvulsants, and nonsteroidal anti-inflammatory agents (Volland et al. 1991; Watt and Dickinson 1990) can be metabolized to 1-*O*-acyl glucuronides, it is important that the occurrence of transacylation from these compounds be further studied in vivo and the role of such reactions in toxicity, drug allergy, and carcinogenicity be evaluated.

3. Glutathione Conjugates

Considerable information concerning the activation of a variety of xenobiotics and their metabolites by conjugation with reduced glutathione (GSH) has been obtained over the last decade. Some of the more widely studied for which mechanistic data are beginning to emerge include haloalkanes (Vamvakas et al. 1990; Dekant et al. 1993), menadione (Brown et al. 1991), bromobenzene, and bromohydroquinones (Andrews et al. 1993). Application of techniques in molecular biology have led to insights for the mechanisms of growth arrest by nephrotoxic cysteine conjugates and dithiothreitol (Chen et al. 1992). This approach has also defined the mutation caused by a mutagenic glutathione conjugate (Cmarik et al. 1992), and it is anticipated that similar studies will shed light on the actions of glutathione conjugates at the gene level. Recent work has also shown that the actions of biologically active glutathione conjugates display considerable heterogeneity with respect to tissue injury (GOLDSTEIN 1993). The basis of the actions of GSH conjugates has been studied most extensively in the kidney, and there is a need to consider the biochemical action on other tissues. Information recently acquired indicates significant actions of bromohydroquinone–GSH conjugates on the developing organism (ANDREWS et al. 1993). Studying the ontogenetic actions of other GSH conjugates represents one of many areas of study required for this important group of biologically active conjugates.

II. Pharmacologically Active Conjugates

1. Direct Acting Conjugates

In contrast to progress that has been made in understanding the toxic mechanism of chemically reactive conjugates, the actions of pharmacologically active conjugates such as morphine-6-glucuronide (MULDER 1992) and minoxidil sulfate (MEISHERI et al. 1993) are only beginning to be understood. A major challenge facing investigators in this area is to determine the nature of receptors for such conjugates. Morphine-6-glucuronide binds $\mu 1$ and $\mu 2$ opiate receptors with affinities similar to morphine in mouse brain (MULDER 1992). Further studies determining whether the addition of hydrophilic groups to low molecular weight ligands improves their interaction at peptide receptor sites, as suggested earlier (MULDER 1992), are clearly needed.

2. Carrier Conjugates

Innovative techniques employing the use of antibody-linked hydrolases to target conjugates formed by phase II enzymes in vivo or synthesized chemically ex vivo have recently been used to deliver drugs to specific target tissues (HELLSTROM and SENTER 1992; S.-M. WANG et al. 1992). Further work in this area should enhance methods to deliver drugs to specific sites in the body and limit their toxicity. Linking drug substrates to endogenous compounds such as bile acids handled by tissue-specific transport systems (KRAMER et al. 1992) also promises to be a fruitful area of research in the near future. Although there is evidence that conjugates of carcinogen metabolites, e.g., glucuronide conjugates of aromatic amines (BELAND and KADLUBAR 1990; WANG et al. 1987) and benzo(a)pyrene phenols (IRWIN et al. 1992), serve as carriers of toxicity to certain target tissues, additional research to test the importance of this phenomenon is needed. Finally, the discovery that carcinogenicity of certain compounds is related to the distribution of acetyltransferases in the intestines of rapid and slow acetylator rabbits (ILETT et al. 1991) suggests the availability of carcinogenic products of various conjugates may be influenced by pharmacogenetic mechanisms.

E. Conclusion

Material presented in this volume would be considerably shorter were it not for the tremendous advances that have been made in characterizing enzymes involved in conjugation–deconjugation reactions of xenobiotics and endogenous metabolites of phase I reactions through molecular cloning techniques. It is now clear that multiple gene families have evolved for most, if not all, of the enzymes involved in conjugation–deconjugation reactions in mammalian tissues. Understanding the broad substrate specificity and regulation of enzymes involved in these reactions has been advanced greatly by the clearer perspective, gained largely through the application of molecular biological techniques to this field.

It is also clear that phase II conjugations participate in the activation of drugs and toxic chemicals to a much greater extent than traditionally believed. Although conjugation via phase II reactions function primarily to detoxify metabolites and facilitate their excretion, examples of the formation of biologically active conjugates that are toxic or pharmacologically active continues to increase. Thus, a major conclusion emphasized throughout this volume is that phase II conjugation reactions, as phase I monooxygenase reactions, both activate as well as deactivate biologically important molecules.

References

Andrews JE, Robers JM, Ebron-McCoy M, Logsdon RT, Monks TJ, Lau SS (1993) Developmental toxicology of bromohydroquinone and bromohydroquinone-glutathione conjugates in vivo and in whole embryo culture. Toxicol Appl Pharmacol (in press)

Bamforth KJ, Dalgliesh K, Coughtrie MWH (1992) Inhibition of human liver steroid sulfotransferase activities by drugs: a novel mechanism of drug toxicity? Eur J Pharmacol 228:15–21

Beland FA, Kadlubar FF (1990) Chemical carcinogenesis and mutagenesis I. Springer, Berlin Heidelberg New York, pp 267–325

Belinsky SA, Kauffman FC, Sokolove PM, Tsukuda T, Thurman RG (1984) Calcium-mediated inhibition of glucuronide production by epinephrine in the perfused rat liver. J Biol Chem 259(12):7705–7711

Blum M, Grant DM, McBride W, Heim M, Meyer UA (1990) Human arylamine N-acetyltransferase genes: isolation, chromosomal localization, and functional expression. DNA Cell Biol 9:193–203

Bock KW, Frohling W, Remmer H, Rexer B (1973) Effects of phenobarbital and 3-methylcholanthrene on substrate specificity of rat liver microsomal UDP-glucuronyltransferase. Biochim Biophys Acta 327:46–56

Bradow G, Kan L, Fenslau C (1989) Studies of intramolecular rearrangements of acyl-linked glucuronides using salicylic acid, flufenamic acid, and [S]- and [R]- benoxaprofen and confirmation of isomerization in acyl-linked delta-9-11-carboxytetrahydro-cannabinol glucuronide. Chem Res Toxicol 2:316–324

Brown PC, Dulik DW, Jones TW (1991) The toxicity of menadione (2-methyl-1, 4-naphthoquinone) and two thioethers conjugates studied with isolated renal epithelial cells. Arch Biochem Biophys 285:187–196

Bunton CA (1949) Oxidation of alpha-diketones and alpha-ketoacids by hydrogen peroxide. Nature 163:444

Burchell B, Nebert DW, Nelson DR, Bock KW, Iyanagi T, Jansen PLM, Lancet D et al. (1991) The UDP-glucuronosyltransferase gene superfamily: suggested nomenclature based on evolutionary divergence. DNA Cell Biol 10:487–494

Buschman E, Arceci RJ, Croop JM, Che M, Arias IM, Housman DE, Gros P (1992) *mdr2* encodes P-glucoprotein expressed in the bile canalicular membrane as determined by isoform-specific antibodies. J Biol Chem 267:18093–18099

Chen Q, Yu K, Holbrook NJ, Stevens JL (1992) Activation of the growth arrest and DNA damage-inducible gene *gadd* 153 by nephrotoxic cyteine conjugates and dithiothreitol. J Biol Chem 267:8207–8212

Cmarik JL, Humphreys WG, Bruner KL, Lloyd RS, Tibbetts C, Guengrich FP (1992) Mutation spectrum and sequence alkylation selectivity resulting from modification of bacteriophage M13mp18DNA with *S*-(2-chloroethyl) glutathione. J Biol Chem 267:6672–6679

Deguchi T (1992) Sequence and expression of alleles of polymorphic arylamine N-acetyltransferase of human liver. J Biol Chem 267:18140–18147

Dekant W, Anders MW, Monks TJ (1993) Bioactivation of halogenated xenobiotics by *S*-conjugate formation. In: Anders MW, Dekant W, Henschler D, Oberleithner H, Silbernagl S (eds) Renal disposition and nephrotoxicity of xenobiotics. Academic, New York, pp 187–215

Dutton GJ (1980) Glucuronidation of drugs and other compounds. CRC, Boca Raton

Dwivedi C, Downie A, Webb T (1987) Net glucuronidation in different rat strains: importance of microsomal β-glucuronidase. FASEBJ 1:303–307

El Mouelhi M, Kauffman FC (1986) Sublobular distribution of transferases and hydrolases associated with glucuronide, sulfate and glutathione conjugation in human liver. Hepatology 6:450–456

Favreau LV, Pickett CB (1991) Transcriptional regulation of the rat NAD(P)H: quinone reductase gene. Identification of regulatory elements controlling basal level expression and inducible expression by planar aromatic compounds and phenolic antioxidants. J Biol Chem 266:4556–4561

Friling RS, Bergelson S, Daniel V (1992) Two adjacent AP-1-like binding sites from the electrophilic responsive element of the murine glutathione S-transferase Ya subunit gene. Proc Natl Acad Sci USA 89:668–672

Garcia JH, Kamijyo Y (1974) Cerebral infarction – evolution of histopathological changes after occlusion of a middle cerebral artery in primates. J Neuropathol Exp Neurol 33:408–421

Gaudin C, Ruget G, Selz F, Cuche JL (1985) Free and conjugated catecholamines in digestive tissues of rats. Life Sci 37:1469–1474

Goldstein RS (1993) Biochemical heterogeneity and site-specific tubular injury. In: Hook JR, Goldstein RS (eds) Toxicology of the kidney. Raven, New York, pp 201–247

Gonzalez FJ (1992) Molecular genetics of the P-450 superfamily. In: Kalow W (ed) Pharmacogenetics of drug metabolism. Pergamon, New York, pp 413–452

Greenbaum AL, Gumaa KA, McLean P (1971) The distribution of hepatic metabolites and the control of the pathways of carbohydrate metabolism in animals of different dietary and hormonal status. Arch Biochem Biophys 143:617–663

Grossman MH, Emanuel BS, Budarf ML (1992a) Chromosomal mapping of the human catechol-*O*-methyltransferase gene to 22q11.1 to q11.2. Genomics 12: 822–825

Grossman MH, Szumlanski C, Littrell JB, Weinstein R, Weinshilboum RM (1992b) Electrophoretic analysis of low and high activity forms of catechol-*O*-methyltransferase in human erythrocytes. Life Sci 50:473–480

Hagenbuch B, Stieger B, Foguet M, Lubbert H, Meier PJ (1991) Functional expression cloning and characterization of the hepatocyte Na^+/bile acid cotransport system. Proc Natl Acad Sci USA 88:10629–10633

Hellerstein MK, Wu K, Kaempfer S, Kletke C, Shackleton CHL (1991) Sampling the lipogenic hepatic acetyl-CoA pool in vivo in the rat: comparison of xenobiotic

probe to values predicted from isotopomeric distribution in circulating lipids and measurement of lipogenesis and acetyl-CoA dilution. J Biol Chem 266:10912–10919
Hellstrom KE, Senter PD (1992) Activation of prodrugs by targeted enzymes. Eur J Cancer 27:1342–1343
Honchel R, Aksoy IA, Szumlanski C, Wood TC, Otterness DM, Wieban ED, Weinshilboum RM (1993) Human thiopurine methyltransferase: molecular cloning and expression of T84 colon carcinoma cell cDNA. Mol Pharmacol (in press)
Ilett KF, Reeves PT, Minchin RF, Kinnear BF, Watson HF, Kadlubar FF (1991) Distribution of acetyltransferase activities in the intestines of rapid and slow acetylator rabbits. Carcinogenesis 12:1465–1469
Irwin SE, Kwei GY, Blackburn GR, Thurman R, Kauffman FC (1992) Mutagenicity of benzo(a)pyrenyl-1-sulfate in the Ames test. Environ Mol Mutagen 19:235–243
Jaiswal AK (1991) Human NAD(P)H:quinone oxidoreductase (NQ01) gene structure and induction by dioxin. Biochemistry 30:10647–10653
Kauffman FC, Whittaker M, Anundi I, Thurman RG (1991) Futile cycling of a sulfate conjugate by isolated hepatocytes. Mol Pharmacol 39:414–420
Kramer W, Wess G, Schubert G, Bickel M, Girbig F, Gutjar U, Kowalewski S et al. (1992) Liver-specific drug targeting by coupling to bile acids. J Biol Chem 267:18598–18604
Kroeger-Koepke MB, Koepke SR, Hernandez L, Michejda CJ, (1992) Activation of a β-hydroxyalkylnitrosamine to alkylating agents: evidence for the involvement of a sulfotransferase. Cancer Res 52:3300–3305
Kumar RS, Thekkumkara TJ, Sen GC (1991) The mRNAs encoding the two angiotensin-converting isozymes are transcribed from the same gene by a tissue specific choice of alternative transcription initiation sites. J Biol Chem 266:3854–3862
Kung MP, Spaulding SW, Roth JA (1988) Desulfation of 3,5,3′-triiodothronine sulfate by microsomes from human and rat tissues. Endocrinology 122:1195–1200
Labrune P, Myara A, Huguet P, Foliot A, Vial M, Trivin F, Odievre M (1991) Bilirubin UDP-glucuronosyltransferase hepatic activity in jaundice associated with congenital hypothyroidism. J Pediatr Gastroenterol Nutr 14:79–82
Lennard L, van Loon JA, Lilleyman JS, Weinshilboum RM (1987) Thiopurine pharmacogenetics in leukemia: correlation of erthrocyte thiopurine methyltransferase activity and 6-thioguanine nucleotide concentrations. Clin Pharmacol 41:18–25
Liu S, Zhang P, Ji X, Johnson WW, Gilliland GL, Armstrong RN (1992) Contribution of tyrosine 6 to the catalytic mechanism of isozyme 3-3 of glutathione S-transferase. J Biol Chem 267:4296–4299
Manafo A, McDonagh AF, Smith PC, Benet LZ (1990) Irreversible binding of tolmetin glucuronic acid esters to albumin in vitro. Pharm Res 7:21–27
Medda S, Swank RT (1985) Egasyn, a protein which determines the subcellular distribution of β-glucuronidase, has esterase activity. J Biol Chem 260:15802–15808
Meier PJ (1988) Transport polarity of hepatocytes. Sem Liver Dis 8:293–307
Meisheri KD, Garland M, Johnson A, Puddinoton L (1993) Enzymatic and non-enzymatic sulfation mechanisms in the biological actions of minoxidil. Biochem Pharmacol 20 (in press)
Michejda CJ, Koepke SR, Kroeger-Koepke MB, Bosan W (1987) Recent findings on the metabolism of β-hydroxyalkylnitrosamines. In: Bartsch H, O'Neill IK, Schulte-Hermann R (eds) Relevance of *N*-nitroso compounds to human cancer: exposure and mechanisms. IARC, Lyon, pp 77–82
Moghrabi N, Sutherland L, Wooster R, Povey S, Boxer M, Burchell B (1992) Chromosome assignment of human phenol and bilirubin UDP-glucuronosyltransferase genes (UGT1A-Subfamily). Ann Hum Genet 56:83–93

Monaghan G, Povey S, Burchell B, Boxer M (1992) Localization of a bile acid UDP-glucuronosyltransferase gene (UGT2B) to chromosome 4 using the polymerase chain reaction. Genomics 13:908–909
Mulder GJ (1992) Pharmacological effects of drug conjugates: is morphine 6-glucuronide an exception? Trends Pharmacol Sci 13:302–304
Olson JA, Moon RC, Anders MW, Fenselau C, Shane B (1992) Enhancement of biological activity by conjugation reactions. J Nutr 122:615–624
Otterness DM, Weiben ED, Wood TC, Watson RWG, Madden BJ, McCormick DJ, Weinshilboum RM (1992) Human liver dehydroepiandrosterone sulfotransferase: molecular cloning and expression of cDNA. Mol Pharmacol 41:865–872
Ovnic M, Swank RT, Fletcher C, Zhen L, Novak EK, Baumann H, Heintz N et al. (1991) Characterization and functional expression of a cDNA encoding egasyn (esterase-22): the endoplasmic reticulum targeting protein of β-glucuronidase. Genomics 11:956–967
Owens IS, Ritter JK (1992) The novel bilirubin/phenol UDP-glucuronosyltransferase UGT1 gene locus: implications for multiple non-hemolytic familiar hyperbilirubinemia phenotypes. Pharmacogenetics 2:93–108
Pickett CB, Telakowski-Hopkins CA, Ding GJ-F, Argenbright L, Lu AYH (1984) Rat liver glutathione S-transferases. Complete nucleotide sequence of a glutathione S-transferase mRNA and the regulation of the Ya, Yb, and Yc MRNAs by 3-methylcholanthrene and phenobarbital. J Biol Chem 259:5182–5188
Reinemer P, Dirr HW, Ladenstein R, Huber R, Lo Bello M, Federici G, Parker W (1992) Three-dimensional structure of class Pi glutathione S-transferase from human placenta in complex with S-hexylglutathione at 2.8A resolution. J Mol Biol 227:214–226
Reinke LA, Belinsky SA, Evans RK, Kauffman FC, Thurman RG (1981) Conjugation of p-nitrophenol in the perfused rat liver: the effect of substrate concentration and carbohydrate reserves. J Pharmacol Exp Ther 217:863–870
Rushmore TH, Morton MR, Pickett CB (1991) The antioxidant responsive element. Activation by oxidative stress and identification of the DNA consensus sequence required for functional activity. J Biol Chem 266:11632–11639
Smith PC, Benet LZ, McDonagh AF (1990) Covalent binding of zomepirac glucuronide to proteins: evidence for a Schiff base mechanism. Drug Metab Dispos 18:639–644
Sokolove PM, Wilcox MA, Thurman RG, Kauffman FC (1984) Stimulation of hepatic microsomal β-glucuronidase by calcium. Biochem Biophys Res Commun 121:987–993
Swank RT, Pfister K, Miller D, Chapman V (1986) The egasyn gene affects the processing of oligosaccharides of lysosomal β-glucuronidase in liver. Biochem J 240:445–454
Sztul ES, Biemesderfer D, Caplan MJ, Kashgarian M, Boyer JL (1987) Localization of Na^+-, K^+-ATPase alpha-subunit to the sinusoidal and lateral but not canalicular membranes of rat hepatocytes. J Cell Biol 104:1239–1248
Talalay P, DeLong MJ, Prochaska HJ (1988) Identification of a common chemical signal regulating the induction of enzymes that protect against chemical carcinogenesis. Proc Natl Acad Sci USA 85:8261–8265
Telakowski-Hopkins CA, Rodkey JA, Bennett CD, Lu AYH, Pickett CB (1985) Rat liver glutathione S-transferases. Construction of a cDNA clone complementary to a Yc mRNA and prediction of the complete amino acid sequence of a Yc subunit. J Biol Chem 260:5820–5825
Tseng L, Mazella J, Lee LY, Stone ML (1983) Estrogen sulfatase and estrogen sulfotransferase in human primary mammary carcinoma. J Steroid Biochem 19:1413–1417
Vamvakas S, Sharma VK, Sheu S-S, Anders MW (1990) Perturbations of intracellular calcium distribution in kidney cells by nephrotoxic haloalkenyl cysteine S-conjugates. Mol Pharmacol 38:455–461
Van Breemen RB, Fenselau C (1984) Acylation of albumin by 1-*O*-acyl glucuronides. Drug Metab Dispos 13:318–320

Vatsis KP, Weber WW (1991) Genetic variation in human N-acetyltransferase at the *NAT1* and *NAT2* loci. Am J Hum Genet 49:112
Volland C, Sun H, Dammeyer J, Benet LZ (1991) Stereoselective degradation of the fenoprofen acyl glucuronide enantiomers and irreversible binding to plasma protein. Drug Metab Dispos 19:1080–1086
Vore M, Hoffman T (1992) ATP-dependent transport of estradiol-17β-(β-D-glucuronide) in canalicular plasma membranes (Abstr). Hepatology 16:146A
Wang CY, Zukowski K, Lee MS, Imaida K (1987) Production of urothelial tumors in the heterotopic bladder of rats by instillation of N-glucuronosyl or N-acetyl derivates of N-hydroxy-2-aminofluorene. Cancer Res 47:3406–3409
Wang RN, Newton DJ, Huskey S-E, McKeever BM, Pickett CB, Lu AYH (1992) Site-directed mutagenesis of glutathione S-transferase YaYa – important roles of tyrosine-9 and aspartic acid-101 in catalysis. J Biol Chem 267:19866–19871
Wang S-M, Chern J-W, Yeh M-Y, Ng JC, Tung E, Roffler SR (1992) Specific activation of glucuronide prodrugs by antibody-targeted enzyme conjugates for cancer therapy. Cancer Res 52:4484–4491
Watabe T, Hakamata Y, Hiratsuka A, Ogura K (1986) A 7-hydroxymethyl sulphate ester as an active metabolite of the carcinogen, 7-hydroxymethylbenz-[a] anthracene. Carcinogenesis 7:207–214
Watt JA, Dickinson RG (1990) Reactivity of diflunisal acyl glucuronide in human and rat plasma a albumin solutions. Biochem Pharmacol 39:1067–1075
Wawrzyniak CJ, Gallagher PM, D'Amore MA, Carter JE, Rinchik EM, Ganschow RE (1989) DNA determinants of structural and regulatory variation within the murine β-glucuronidase gene complex. Mol Cell Biol 9:4074–4078
Weinshilboum R (1988) Phenol sulfotransferase inheritance. Cell Mol Neurobiol 8:27–34
Weinshilboum R (1989) Methyltransferase pharmacogenetics. Pharmacol Ther 43: 77–90
Williams CH (1969) β-Glucuronidase activity in serum and liver of rats administered pesticides and hepatotoxic agents. Toxicol Appl Pharmacol 14:283–292
Yahanda AM, Adler KM, Fisher GA, Brophy NA, Halsey J, Hardy RI, Gosland MP et al. (1989) Phase I trial of etoposide with cyclosporine as a modulator of multidrug resistance. J Clin Oncology 10:1624–1634
Zimmerli B, Valantinas J, Meier PJ (1989) Multispecificity of Na^+-dependent taurocholate uptake in basolateral (sinusoidal) rat liver plasma membrane vesicles. J Pharmacol Exp Ther 250:301–308

Subject Index

Springer-Verlag and the Environment

We at Springer-Verlag firmly believe that an international science publisher has a special obligation to the environment, and our corporate policies consistently reflect this conviction.

We also expect our business partners – paper mills, printers, packaging manufacturers, etc. – to commit themselves to using environmentally friendly materials and production processes.

The paper in this book is made from low- or no-chlorine pulp and is acid free, in conformance with international standards for paper permanency.

Printing: Saladruck, Berlin
Binding: Buchbinderei Lüderitz & Bauer, Berlin